Progress in China Epidemiology

Dong-Qing Ye
Editor

Progress in China Epidemiology

Volume 1

PMPH PEOPLE'S MEDICAL PUBLISHING HOUSE
Springer

Editor
Dong-Qing Ye
Epidemiology and Biostatistics
Anhui Medical University
Hefei, China

ISBN 978-981-19-2198-8 ISBN 978-981-19-2199-5 (eBook)
https://doi.org/10.1007/978-981-19-2199-5

Jointly published with People's Medical Publishing House, PR of China

This Springer imprint is published by the registered company Springer Nature Singapore Pte Ltd.
The registered company address is: 152 Beach Road, #21-01/04 Gateway East, Singapore 189721, Singapore

Preface

It is well-known that China's modern history was an era that is full of suffering and precariousness. So, it is not surprised that the development of epidemiology in China has experienced many challenges and epidemics. In the history of epidemiology in China, there is a landmark event worth mentioning, that is, the famous epidemiologist Liande Wu directed the eradication of the Northeast plague in 1910. Fortunately, the People's Republic of China was established in 1949. The development of epidemiology in China has thus ushered in a new era. For instance, smallpox has been successfully eliminated, and great success has been achieved in the prevention and control of infectious diseases such as schistosomiasis, malaria, and plague. After that, the Chinese economy continuously grew due to the Economic Reform and open up policy, non-communicable disease prevention and control thus has received more focus. As a consequence, chronic non-communicable disease control has also made tremendous progress. Today, the average life expectancy in China has reached 76.5 years, more than twice that of 70 years ago (35 years).

Truth comes from practice. Chinese epidemiologists and CDC workers have accumulated much experience in disease prevention and control from countless epidemiological practices. Naturally, China's epidemiological research and disease prevention and control work has made world-renowned achievements in last decades.

Therefore, at the beginning of 2020, the heads of Springer Nature and PMPH and I had the idea of planning and publishing a book that can fully reflect the progress of epidemiology in China. To this end, I invited Chinese professors, academicians, well-known experts, and scholars engaged in epidemiology research to compile this book jointly. We aim to share Chinese valuable experience and achievement in disease control in recent decades with the world. Moreover, we hope this book can facilitate the development of epidemiology and promote human health around the world.

Given the excessive content, we have to publish this book in volumes. Currently, this edition is the first volume of this series, but more fantastic research fruits will be shared with readers in the future. This book covers three major parts. Part 1 is about infectious diseases. We focus on dengue fever, and tuberculosis, which have very successful prevention and control experience in China. In Part 2, we selected chronic non-communicable diseases such as injury, lung cancer, and pharmacoepidemiology as the main content. Part 3 is about the epidemiological method, which includes a detailed introduction to the improvement of methods in the prediction model of diseases.

We are very proud that all authors of this book have excellent writing ability and vast academic influence. I believe this book will bring a feast of Chinese epidemiological experiences sharing to the world.

The publication of *Progress in China Epidemiology* is one of my dreams that I have strived for years. In writing this book, we invited well-known experts in the field of epidemiology to carry out multiple and mutual reviews to ensure professional and academic value. Special thanks to my old friend, also the main reviewer of the book, Professor Liming Li from the School of Public Health, Peking University, for giving his constructive comments on the topic and content of this book. Thanks to Dr. Xinyu Fang, the secretary of this book, for her hard work. Besides, I would like to thank the Inflammation and Immune-mediated Diseases Laboratory of Anhui Province, Anhui University of Science and Technology, and my alma mater, Anhui Medical University, for providing me with lots of support. Also, many thanks to all authors of this book and Mr. Bin Hu. I'm here sincerely thank you all for your hard work and unreserved trust!

Hefei, China Dongqing Ye

Contents

1 The Infectious Diseases Associated with Behavior and Ecological Changes

Jianguo Xu

Abstract

In recent years, there have been significant changes in the causes and manifestations of infectious diseases, which are closely related to the changes of social behavior, personal behavior, development models, lifestyles, the environment, and ecology. Some of them were associated with large-scale breeding of economic animals, such as SARS, human infection with *Streptococcus suis*, avian influenza A (H5N1) and (H7N9). Some were associated with personal dietary preferences. For instance, most cases of infection with *Vibrio cholerae* O139 in China were related to turtles. Some were associated with the large-scale trade of sheep and other bacteria-carrying food animals, such as brucellosis. Some were associated with the global sales and transportation of vegetables, such as Shiga toxin-producing *Escherichia coli* O104:H4. Some were related to the distribution and scale of modern drug production, such as the outbreak of fungal meningitis caused by the transmission of *Exserohilum monoceras* through drugs in the USA in 2012. Some were related to increased densities of vectors (such as ticks) carrying pathogens, such as *Anaplasma phagocytophilum* infection. And many were related to wildlife, such as SARS. These behavior and ecological infectious diseases are associated with the model of social and economic development.

Keywords

Infectious disease · Behavior and ecology-induced infectious diseases · Behavior · Ecology · Prevention and control

1.1 Introduction

The emergence of Severe Acute Respiratory Syndrome (SARS) in China in 2003 triggered a high attention to emerging infectious diseases. In the spring of 2013, the emergence of Avian influenza A (H7N9) infection in human in China aroused reflection on the factors that contribute to the occurrence of emerging infectious diseases [1]. The re-emergence of Ebola virus disease in 2015 and the imported infection cases with Zika and yellow fever viruses in 2016 brought awareness of the global and long-term transmission of infectious diseases.

During the two decades from 1983 to 2002, about 10 emerging infectious diseases were

J. Xu (✉)
State Key Laboratory of Infectious Disease Prevention and Control, National Institute for Communicable Disease Control and Prevention, Chinese Center for Disease Control and Prevention, Beijing, China

Institute of Public Health, Nankai University, Tianjin, China
e-mail: xujianguo@icdc.cn

D.-Q. Ye (ed.), *Progress in China Epidemiology*, https://doi.org/10.1007/978-981-19-2199-5_1

identified in China, including Lyme disease, *Legionella* pneumonia, *Yersinia enterocolitica* infection, *Escherichia coli* O157:H7 infection, rotavirus infection in adults, hemorrhagic fever with renal syndrome, hepatitis C, *Campylobacter jejuni* infection, HIV infection (or AIDS), and *Vibrio cholerae* O139. From 2003 to 2021, approximately 20 emerging and re-emerging infectious diseases were identified in China, including SARS, avian influenza A (H5N1) infection in human, avian influenza A (H7N9) infection in human, H1N1 influenza, human granulocytic anaplasmosis, *Streptococcus suis* serotype 7 infection in human, Group C Neisseria meningitidis [2], Middle East respiratory syndrome (MERS), hand-foot-and-mouth disease, dengue, Zika virus infection, yellow fever, Huaiyangshan hemorrhagic fever caused by a novel tick-borne Bunyavirus [3], the Wenzhou virus infection [4], Jingmen virus infection [5, 6], infection of *Anaplasma capra* [7], plague [8], and COVID-19 caused by the novel coronavirus [9–11]. In the same period, China has also responded to the threat of imported infectious diseases such as yellow fever, Zika virus infection, MERS, malaria, Rift Valley fever, and dengue [12, 13].

The above are only emerging and re-emerging infectious diseases widely reported in the media. Chinese scientists have also reported many new bacteria, viruses, parasites, and so on, especially emerging infectious diseases, in professional journals. But they have not attracted widespread attention from the media, the public, or even the academic community. For example, the team of Yongzhen Zhang discovered 143 novel viruses in specimens of arthropods (such as mosquitoes, flies, cockroaches, ticks, and spiders) and rodents (such as rats) collected in Hubei Province, Zhejiang Province, Xinjiang Uygur Autonomous Region, and other regions [14, 15]. The team of Wuchun Cao found that the dominant tick species in China carried over 30 microorganisms, more than 20 of which are pathogenic to humans [16]. They also found that *Rickettsia tarasevichiae*, *Borrelia valaisiana*, *Rickettsia sibirica* subspecies *sibirica* BJ-90, and *Anaplasma capra* have caused human infections [17, 18]. Cases of *Rickettsia raoultii*, *Babesia venatoru*, and *Anaplasma ovis* have been identified in China [19]. Our laboratory isolated *Helicobacter himalayanus* and *Escherichia marmotae* from *Marmota himalayana* [20, 21]. We also isolated a variety of bacteria pathogenic to humans from feces of *Marmota himalayana*, including enteropathogenic, entero-aggregative, Shiga-toxin-producing, and uropathogenic *E. coli*.

It can be easily seen that the frequency of emerging and re-emerging infectious diseases in China is increasing; the size of the affected population is expanding; and the range of pathogens is widening. Each year, China has to deal with one or more emerging and re-emerging infectious diseases, with a variety of new pathogens discovered.

While people's living conditions, hygiene, and food quality continue to improve with the social and economic development, the infectious diseases are not gradually reduced or even eliminated as people expected, but are increasing. This is because the infectious diseases are not just a biological issue as we thought, but also a sociological one. The infection diseases were somehow induced or expanded by the dramatic changes in production model and scale, in the lifestyles, environment, and ecology [22, 23]. The COVID-19 pandemic is the best example.

1.2 Examples of Behavior and Ecology-Induced Infectious Diseases

A review of the history clearly reveals the close relation between infectious diseases and social behavior, individual behavior, production model, lifestyles, environment, and ecology. While much attention has been paid to pathogens, the behavioral and ecological aspects are largely ignored. A review of the major infectious diseases that have occurred in China will provide distinctive insights [22].

1.2.1 Plague

Plague is a Class A notifiable infectious disease in China caused by *Yersinia pestis*, with rodents as important animal reservoirs. More than ten million people died of plague in the history of China. The only literature recorded the outbreak of plague in Harbin in 1910 with about 60,000 deaths, the major event in the modern history of infectious diseases in China. The approaches, strategies, techniques, and methods in China's response to emerging and re-emerging infectious diseases were basically established from Dr. Wu Lien-teh's response to the plague in Harbin in 1910. While it had been widely believed that the plague in Harbin in 1910 was a "natural disaster," it was actually a "human disaster," a major epidemic caused by improper behavior, when the history was re-visited.

When Dr. Wu Lien-teh arrived in Harbin in 1910, he found that "all of the first infected people were migrants from inside Shanhaiguan Pass who were hunting marmots in the grasslands around Manzhouli." In the early twentieth century, marmot hunters were active in North Manchuria and Siberia. In 1910, the price of a marmot skin soared more than six times compared with 1907. Driven by the huge profits, many Chinese and Russian businessmen recruited Chinese laborers to hunt marmots. The number of marmot skins exported from Manzhouli increased from 700,000 in 1907 to 2.5 million in 1910, and the demand from the international market stimulated the boom of marmot hunting. At that time, continuous natural disasters in Shandong and Zhili provinces drove a large number of refugees to Northeast China for a living. At one time, there were more than 10,000 marmot hunters on the Manzhouli grasslands, many of whom had no hunting experience. In tracing the source of the epidemic, *Shengjing Times* described it as follows: The jobless from Shandong and Zhili provinces hunted in the mountains of Manzhouli one after another, causing a mess of the valley littered with blood and flesh everywhere. Experienced hunters could recognize the weak and probably infected marmots and would not bring them back. Stimulated by the high profits, many wandering laborers from Shandong province hunted without choice and would cook the meat of the marmots when they were hungry. The hunters spent the night in humble inns. Where dozens of people often crowded on a big heatable brick bed. In winter days, the doors and windows of the inns were closed to keep warm. The closed, warm, humid environment is very suitable for the spread of *Yersinia pestis*: no one in the inn would be spared once someone was infected. The plague spread wildly along the Chinese Eastern Railroad, where Harbin was hit the hardest. At that time, the plague was believed to spread via rats. However, no *Yersinia pestis* were found in the captured rats, which meant there was no evidence that the plague was carried by rats. Dr. Wu Lien-teh confirmed that the plague in Harbin in 1910 was caused by marmots. Apparently, the commercial acquisition and hunting of marmots was the direct cause and driving force of the plague [23].

Since the foundation of New China, China has made great achievements in plague prevention and control, and the annual number of cases reduced from about 10,000 in 1949 to less than five cases per year in recent years, and even no case reported in most of the time. Careful analysis reveals that in the past 50 years, the plague cases were mainly found in the natural focus of *Marmota himalayana* plague in Qinghai-Tibet Plateau. For a long time, Qinghai province has been a province with the most plague cases in China. The plague in Qinghai is basically caused by human's direct contact with marmots, and hunting marmots is the first cause of the disease. If people did not contact marmots actively, there is basically no chance of contracting the plague [24]. Therefore, for the plague in Qinghai province, measures can be taken to prevent human exposure to marmots and other animals, if pathogen in wild animal was detected [25]. So the prevention and control of the plague starts with controlling the human exposure to rather than relying on vaccines or other measures [26].

1.2.2 Acquired Immune Deficiency Syndrome (AIDS) in China

The pathogen of AIDS is HIV (human immunodeficiency virus), which mainly detected in the blood, semen, vaginal secretions, and breast milk of infected persons. It can be transmitted through sexual contact (including heterosexual sex, homosexual sex between men, and bisexual sex), blood and blood products (including needle sharing in intravenous drug use, transfusion of contaminated blood or blood products and unclean interventional medical operations), and mother-to-child transmission (including prenatal and peripartum transmission and postpartum breastfeeding). The main transmission modes of HIV vary in different countries and regions. In developing countries, HIV is mainly transmitted via heterosexual sex; in developed countries, it is mainly transmitted via homosexual sex; and in middle income countries, especially in Asia, it is mainly transmitted by drug abuse and sex contact.

In the history of AIDS in China, drug abuse was the main transmission mode in the early stage, and illegal blood collection and supply in the middle stage caused much transmission and infection. Recently, sexual transmission has become the most dominant route of transmission, with the most rapid rise in the population of homosexual behavior between men. Sexual transmission is the main mode of HIV transmission from high-risk groups to the general population. In recent years, the increasing percentage of farmers, workers, students, and officials among the newly discovered AIDS patients and HIV-infected patients every year indicates that the AIDS epidemic in China has entered the stage of spreading from a limited number of specific high-risk groups to a huge number of members of general public. Therefore, the transmission of HIV is closely related to behavior, and the prevention and control of HIV should start with behavior, especially in the context of setbacks in vaccine development [27–29].

1.2.3 Severe Acute Respiratory Syndrome (SARS)

Caused by SARS-CoV, SARS appeared in Guangdong province in the winter of 2002 and spread rapidly to several countries around the world. In May 2003, Yi Guan's research team isolated the SARS-CoV like viruses from masked palm civets sold in a wildlife market in Shenzhen, Guangdong Province, and focus was gradually placed on the wildlife to identify the origin of SARS-CoV. In December 2003 and January 2004, four more mild cases of SARS were identified in Guangzhou Province. The S gene sequence of SARS-CoV detected from the patients' clinical specimens was consistent with the sequence of SARS-CoV detected from masked palm civets in the wildlife market. All masked palm civets in the Xinyuan Market in Guangzhou in January 2004 were tested positive for SARS-CoV; while masked palm civets raised in captivity in 14 other provinces and cities were tested negative for SARS-CoV. All four patients reported in 2004 had dined at a restaurant that provided masked palm civets. The whole genome sequence of SARS-CoV detected from the restaurant's masked palm civets was highly homologous to the virus isolated from the patients [30].

Before the Government of Guangdong Province took action to completely cull masked palm civets and other wild animals from the markets and restaurants, we collected throat and anal swab specimens from masked palm civets, racoon dogs, and poultry in the market for real-time fluorescence PCR and nested PCR to detect SARS-CoV. Those positive for both P and N genes were marked as positive specimens. Of the 91 randomly collected masked palm civets' specimens from the market, 84 were positive for both throat and anal swabs (the others were positive for a single specimen); 12 of the 15 racoon dogs were positive for both throat and anal swabs; and 22 of the 24 environmental specimens from the market (including smear specimens from animal cages and walls) were positive. So, where did the SARS-CoV carried by the masked palm civets in the Xinyuan Market come from? According to the investigation of the source of the masked palm civets sold in the Xinyuan Market, since January 2004, more than 1400 civets collected from more than 20 farms in 14 provinces of China were found to be negative for SARS-CoV detection. These results showed that the SARS-CoV like virus carried by masked palm civets in the Guangzhou Xinyuan Market was not introduced by masked palm civets from farms in other provinces, but probably by some other wild animals. Animals such as masked palm civets and racoon dogs are very sensitive to SARS-CoV, which can play the role of reproduction, amplification, and transmission of SARS-CoV. Xinyuan Market was like an "incubator" of SARS-CoV, where the new entry of healthy animals such as masked palm civets could be quickly infected. Therefore, masked palm civets raised in other provinces and cities did not carry the SARS-CoV. However, the wildlife market in Guangzhou was highly contaminated, and masked palm civets were infected with SARS-CoV immediately after arriving at the market [31]. These masked palm civets, carrying SARS-CoV, were sold to restaurants and then infected people dining there and the restaurant employees, triggering the outbreak of SARS [31–33].

The dietary civets in winter had been popular in Guangdong region for hundred years, since people believed in a myth that it is good for health. The high demand for civets dramatically increased along with the booming economy in the region, which induced the large-scale civet farming industry. Therefore, when large number of civets gathered in animal market of Guangzhou city, it provided ideal incubator for SARS virus and resulted into the large epidemic. We believe that the SARS epidemic was associated with the large-scale civet industry. This animal has been consumed for hundred years in the region, and no associated disease has been noticed.

1.2.4 *Escherichia coli* O157:H7 Infection

In 1999, an outbreak of *E. coli* O157:H7 infection occurred in Jiangsu and Anhui provinces. 194 patients were admitted to hospital with early symptoms of diarrheal disease, oliguria, and anuria, and 177 died of sudden kidney failure and other organ failure; it is estimated that over 20,000 people were infected. As the cause of the disease was unknown, there was no specific control measures could be taken, some social and economic order was disrupted. Unlike the common mode of transmission through food, vegetables, or beverages, extensively reported in other countries, the outbreak of *E. coli* O157:H7 infection in Jiangsu and Anhui provinces confirmed a new transmission model. About 10–20% domestic economic animals, such as chickens, cattle, pigs, and sheep raised in local rural households, were found carrying the pathogenic bacteria. Those pathogen-carrying economic animals contaminated the environment through fecal excretion, resulting into a widespread epidemic. It is an outbreak of *E. coli* O157:H7 infection with the largest epidemic size, the largest number of deaths, the longest duration, and the most complex transmission in the world to date. It was found that the strain isolated from Jiangsu and Anhui provinces was different from that isolated from Japan and the USA, which belonged to a unique clone (ST96). Its ability to produce Shiga toxin was significantly enhanced, and a 37 KB plasmid possibly derived from *Salmonella* was obtained. In particular, the strain from the outbreak in Jiangsu and Anhui provinces appeared only in 1999, and has not been isolated from patients or livestock or poultry since then. Combined with the above findings, we believe that the outbreak of *E. coli* O157:H7 infection in Jiangsu and Anhui provinces was caused by the large-scale promotion of Boer goats in 1997–1998. The local government hoped to improve the economy by introducing superior varieties. Unexpected, the Boer goats imported from foreign countries carried the pathogen. The economy promotion activities actually promoted a major disaster of infectious disease [34–38].

1.2.5 Human Infection of *Streptococcus suis*

S. suis is a major pathogen of zoonotic diseases. In the past, human cases of severe streptococcal infections were successively reported only in Europe and the USA. Mild cases show general symptoms of bacterial infection such as fever, chills, headache, and decreased appetite, while severe cases present sepsis and bacterial meningitis, and more severe cases can suffer toxic shock and death. Most of the scientists studying this were veterinary microbiologists in the world. The medical microbiologists were rarely engaged in the study of *S. suis*. *S. suis* is mainly transmitted through skin dam, and people involved in the slaughter of pigs, selling pork, and housewives (who handle raw pork) are the main infected population.

However, in 2005, the world's largest outbreak of human infection with *S. suis* occurred in Sichuan province, China. Among the 215 patients, 61 showed streptococcal toxic shock like syndrome, and 38 died. The rapid onset of the disease and high mortality were significantly different from the previously reported clinical features [39]. Our study revealed that the pathogen causing the human infection with *S. suis* in China was a mutational *S. suis* Sequence Type 7, which mutated from *S. suis* Sequence Type 1 with enhanced virulence. We proposed to classify *S. suis* into moderately pathogenic, highly pathogenic, and epidemic types based on data from clinical manifestations, animal experiments, and genomic analysis. The moderately pathogenic *S. suis* is mainly ST25, etc., mainly distributed in North America. While it can cause infection in pigs, few cases of human infection and no death of human infection have been reported. The highly pathogenic *S. suis* consists mainly of ST1, distributed mainly in Europe and Asia. It can cause infection in pigs, and a large number of human infections and deaths have been reported, which caused no large-scale outbreak of human infections, but mainly meningitis and occasionally reported septicemia. The only representative of the epidemic type of *S. suis* is ST7, which can cause streptococcal toxic shock and death. Accordingly, a two-stage pathogenic mechanism hypothesis of *S. suis* infection was proposed. The first stage is the onset of streptococcal toxic shock like syndrome, starting from 4 h after *S. suis* Sequence Type 7 enters the bloodstream; the second stage is the onset of meningitis. About 4 h after entering the bloodstream, *S. suis* Sequence Type 7 can stimulate the production of a cytokine storm in the organism that can trigger shock and death about 9–48 h after the onset of the disease. Therefore, the early treatment of human infection with *S. suis* should focus on the prevention and control of shock and not only on antimicrobial therapy [40–42].

The most important fact is that so far, *S. suis* Sequence Type 7 has only been found in China, which may be related to our feeding model. Our study suggests that the large-scale sales of piglets carrying pathogenic bacteria to farming households was the cause of the outbreak: it was the unhealthy commercial activities that brought pathogens to thousands of farming households. Almost all infected people had a history of contact with pigs or diseased pigs and pork. It can be seen that unhealthy feeding model, slaughter of sick pigs, and sales and disposal of sick pork are the direct cause of the outbreak. It seems that the modern mode of swine production without concern of the possible pathogen was responsible for the outbreak [43].

1.3 Behavioral and Ecological Factors that Can Cause Emerging and Re-Emerging Infectious Diseases

There are many behavioral, ecological, and other factors that can trigger an outbreak of infectious diseases. The following is a list of only a few that we currently recognize.

1.3.1 Large-Scale Farming of Economic Animals Without Concern of Infectious Diseases

Large-scale farming of economic animals (pigs, cattle, sheep, and so on) is a sign of social progress. However, it could lead to a disaster if no due attention is paid to the pathogen. The intensity of the impact depends on the size of the breeding. Many of the emerging and re-emerging infectious diseases in China are closely related to large-scale farming of economic animals: SARS is related to the large-scale farming of masked palm civets [1, 31, 40, 44–46]. Driven by the consumer demand, masked palm civets were raised in more than 10 provinces and cities in China at one time, and the largest and most concentrated masked palm civets market was formed in Guangzhou. As a result, Guangdong province became the epicenter of SARS outbreak.

1.3.2 Large-Scale Supply of Piglets and Lambs Carrying Pathogens

In the investigation of the outbreak of human infection with *S. suis* in 2005, the 84 strains of *S. suis* isolated from the patients in China had the same chromosomal PFGE (Pulse Field Gel Electrophoresis) banding pattern, and the strains isolated from all sick free-ranging pigs of the families of patients had the same PFGE banding pattern as those from the patients, suggesting the same source of infection. In other words, the breeding farms that provided free-range piglets to the farmers might be the source of infection. Only the strain isolated from a patient in Guizhou province showed a different banding pattern [40].

1.3.3 Changes in Dietary Habits

With economic and social development, people's dietary habits have changed. More and more people prefer to have salads (raw vegetables), raw seafood, and half-cooked or 70%-cooked meat, and the consumption of seafood is on the rise. Such changes have brought about changes in the types of diarrheal diseases. The isolation rate of diarrheal disease pathogens has changed in most cities in China. In Shenzhen, Shanghai and Hangzhou, *Vibrio parahaemolyticus* has overtaken *Shigella* to become the pathogen with the highest isolation rate [47].

1.3.4 Trade Activities

The epidemic situation of brucellosis was very severe in the early stage of the new China. After decades of efforts, the number of annual reported new cases dropped to 219 in 1992, bringing the incidence rate down to 0.02 in a hundred thousand, reaching the international level. In recent years, due to the increasing scale of cattle and sheep farming, the number of sick sheep and cattle is increasing, leading to a spike in the number and incidence of cases, with 40,994 new cases reported in 2012 and an incidence rate of 3.04 in a hundred thousand (194 times and 159 times of those of 1992, respectively). The increase of farming scale and areas leads to expansion of the infected area to almost every province where sheep and cattle are farmed (including Hainan), through the trade of animals carried germs [48–50].

1.3.5 Large-Scale Production, Transportation, and Distribution of Food Products

A certain food, vegetable, or other semi-manufactured food produced by a company can be supplied to consumers in a city, country, or several countries in modern time. Once contaminated, it can expose the consumers of a city, country, or several countries to a pathogen almost at the same time, leading to large-scale infections. For example, the *E. coli* O104:H4 infection occurred in Europe in 2011 through contaminated sprouts, involving 16 countries and leading to 4075 cases and 50 deaths [13, 51, 52]. In China, soft-shelled turtle cultured in a certain place became a source of *V. cholerae* O139 infection in several provinces [53].

1.3.6 Modern Pharmaceutical Production Methods that Expand the Impact of Incidental Contamination

Contamination of intravenous or intramuscular injection drugs or biologicals by non-pathogenic microorganisms can cause major public health events. In the USA in 2012, steroids and other drugs produced by New England Compounding

Center (NECC) were contaminated with *Exserohilum rostratum*, which is widely available in the environment. About 13,000 people were injected with the drugs, and more than 700 people developed fungal meningitis and nearly 50 died [54, 55]. In 1997, *Nocardia asteroides* caused hip infections in more than 100 people by contaminating the distilled water used to dissolve penicillin for injection in a hospital in Deyang, Sichuan province.

1.3.7 Unsafe Sexual Behavior

Sexually transmitted diseases are spreading in China. Through more than a decade of efforts since the foundation of the New China in 1949, it was announced in 1964 that sexually transmitted diseases had been largely eliminated in the mainland of China. Sexually transmitted diseases resurfaced in the 1980s. In recent years, there has been a rapid rise of sexually transmitted diseases (mainly gonorrhea, syphilis, AIDS, and so on) [56, 57].

1.3.8 Unprotected Exposure to Vectors Carrying Pathogens Such as Ticks

In recent years, the rural living conditions have changed considerably, and there are more trees and higher densities of vectors such as ticks. New infectious diseases have emerged, such as the *Anaplasma phagocytophilum* found in Anhui province in 2006 and the Huaiyangshan fever caused by New Bunyavirus found in Henan and Hubei provinces in 2009 [10, 58–60]. The research of Wuchun Cao's team found that the dominant tick species in China carry more than 30 kinds of microorganisms, more than 20 of which are pathogenic to humans. It is noteworthy that they were the first team internationally to have found *Rickettsia tarasevichiae*, *Borrelia valaisiana*, *Rickettsia sibirica* subspecies *sibirica* BJ-90, and *Anaplasma capra* which are capable of infecting humans and causing disease. Human cases of infection with *R. raoultii*, *Babesia venatoru*, and *Anaplasma ovis* were found in China, which were the first known cases of human infection outside Europe [16–19, 61]. These findings have greatly enriched the understanding of tick-borne human pathogens and have important public health implications, urging us to pay great attention to vectors.

1.3.9 Unprotected Exposure to Wildlife

SARS-CoV and Ebola virus are associated with bats [62, 63], and Avian influenza A (H5N1) is associated with migratory birds. It has recently been found that the distribution of Huaiyangshan virus correlates with the range of migratory birds. Therefore, Huaiyangshan virus is likely to be transmitted by tick and migratory birds [58]. Due to the lack of awareness of animal-borne diseases and lack of necessary protection, examples abound of Lyme disease and Human granulocytic anaplasmosis due to travel as well as Bartonella infections resulting from contact with pets. It has been reported in the literature that Ebola hemorrhagic fever was initially contracted by contact with orangutans that died of some disease [62–64].

1.3.10 The Large-Scale Development of Transportation Means and Methods

International communication or travel will undoubtedly bring new problems. These problems were not obvious in the past as Chinese residents rarely went abroad. With the rapid economic development, the development of overseas markets and the increase in foreign tourism, the risk of introduction of infectious diseases from abroad naturally increases. In 2016, Chinese residents traveling abroad were infected with Zika virus and yellow fever virus and brought them into China, causing public health problems [65, 66]. The introduction of infectious diseases from abroad will become the norm along with the economic development [67, 68].

1.4 Prevention and Control of Behavior and Ecology-Induced Infectious Diseases

It is generally accepted that infectious diseases are mainly prevented by vaccines, treated by drugs, so that they get controlled or eliminated. However, some infectious diseases cannot be prevented or controlled by vaccines. We have drastically reduced the number of incidences and deaths from some infectious diseases, such as plague, cholera, bacterial dysentery, and so on, where it is not vaccines that play a major role. These infectious diseases are basically related to behavioral and ecological aspects. Therefore, prevention and control of behavior and ecology-induced infectious diseases depends mainly on behavioral change and ecological improvement. Infectious diseases related to individual behavior are mainly prevented and controlled by changing individual behavior; those related to social behavior need to be prevented and controlled by changing social behavior through the power of government, which is the most economical, fast, safe, and effective way.

1.4.1 Prevention and Control of Infectious Diseases by Controlling Social Behavior

1.4.1.1 Successful Prevention of Re-Emergence of SARS by Prohibition of Large-Scale Masked Palm Civets Trade

In 2003, Yi Guan's team found that masked palm civets were the main animal hosts of SARS-COV. In the spring of 2004, SARS cases reappeared in Guangdong province. In January 2004, SARS-COV was detected in all masked palm civets from the Xinyuan Market in Guangzhou; however, none of the masked palm civets from 14 provinces and cities supplied to Xinyuan Market were detected with SARS-COV [31]. Our explanation is that the Xinyuan Market in Guangzhou was severely contaminated with SARS-COV, and masked palm civets from other provinces and cities were infected immediately after entering the market. The masked palm civets carried the SARS-COV into restaurants, and customers who dined at the restaurants providing masked palm civets were infected. Subsequently, through some unknown mutation mechanism, a regional or wider epidemic was triggered [31].

In order to effectively prevent the re-emergence of SARS, Nanshan Zhong, Academician of Chinese Academy of Engineering, and Professor Yi Guan proposed a ban on masked palm civet trade. The People's Government of Guangdong Province adopted this proposal and banned masked palm civet trade throughout the province. Despite some controversies, SARS has not re-emerged in Guangdong Province since then. Therefore, the ban on the large-scale trade of masked palm civets prevented the re-emergence of SARS [22].

The effective prevention of SARS was a victory for scientists and politicians. The politicians adopted the scientists' proposal of a ban on the trade in masked palm civets, put it into practice, changed the social behavior, prevented the re-emergence of SARS, and made a great contribution to China. This could not be achieved by relying on vaccines and drugs.

1.4.1.2 Effective Control of the Scale of the Outbreaks of H5N1 and H7N9 Avian Influenza in Humans by Closure of Live Poultry Markets

In the early stage of H5N1 avian influenza outbreak, most avian influenza patients had a contact history with sick or dead poultry before the onset of the disease, or lived in a place where there was an animal avian influenza epidemic. In contrast, the patient, who had the onset of the disease in Guangzhou in February 2006, lived in the center of Guangzhou, where there was no animal avian influenza epidemic, and he had no contact history with sick or dead poultry. So, how did he get infected? Where is the source of infection?

The investigation of Guangzhou Center for Disease Control and Prevention revealed that the patient had visited nine food markets with live poultry from January 23 to February 22, 2006 to study the feasibility of starting a condiment business. All nine markets were located in downtown Guangzhou, with an area between 200 and 2500 square meters, good sanitary conditions, and standardized management. Unlike food markets in the north of China, each market had about 2–10 stalls selling live poultry, mainly live chickens and a small number of ducks, geese, pigeons, and quails, which were slaughtered on site. The number of live poultry sold daily ranged from 100 to 1000 [69].

One of the 79 specimens of animal cage swabs from the nine food markets tested positive for HPAI H5N1, from which the virus was isolated. And 1 of the 112 serum samples from the market personnel engaged in poultry trading in the nine food markets tested positive for neutralizing antibody against H5N1. The study concluded that it was possible that some birds entering the food markets carried the avian influenza virus but did not show obvious symptoms and infected customers with a very low probability. It was recommended that the sales of live poultry by retail and on-site slaughter in food markets, farmers markets, and other locations be temporarily prohibited in provinces, cities, and autonomous regions where there were outbreaks and dissemination of avian influenza among animals and human cases of avian influenza [69].

After the occurrence of H7N9 avian influenza infection in human in 2013, we immediately pointed out that farmers markets with live poultry might be the main places where the infection occurred. The Jiangsu Provincial Center for Disease Control and Prevention soon detected nucleic acid of H7N9 avian influenza virus from environmental samples from the farmers markets with live poultry. Epidemiological investigations revealed that poultry carrying the virus were the source of infection and that farmers markets with live poultry were the main sites of human infection with the H7N9 avian influenza [70].

Theoretically, the incubation period of H7N9 avian influenza is 7 days. If effective measures are taken, no new cases will occur in principle after 7 days of the measures. Shanghai Municipal Government took decisive measures and took the lead in closing the farmers markets on April 6. Of the 27 patients reported subsequently, 22 had onset before April 6. No new infections occurred after April 13. The epidemic in Shanghai was basically under effective control. Hangzhou Municipal People's Government closed the farmers markets on April 15. Of the 23 cases reported after April 15, 18 had onset before April 15. No new infections occurred after April 22. The onset of all new infection cases occurred within no more than 7 days from the day the farmers markets in Shanghai and Hangzhou were closed. In other words, no new cases occurred after 7 days since the closure of the farmers markets. Therefore, the closure of farmers markets with live poultry during epidemic in endemic areas is an effective measure to prevent human infection with H7N9 avian influenza in highly populated cities [70]. Studies reveal that closing farmers markets with live poultry can reduce the risk of infection among urban residents by 97–99%. The study concluded that closing farmers markets was the most effective and efficient measure to control the outbreak of H7N9 avian influenza infection in human in spring 2013. In the short term, it was recommended that measures be taken promptly to close farmers markets with live poultry in areas with cases of H7N9 avian influenza infection in human or outbreaks among birds. In the long term, study should be conducted on the feasibility of regular closure, regular disinfection, centralized slaughter of live poultry, and sales of chilled or frozen poultry in farmers markets [39].

Three things are needed to control the outbreak of H7N9 avian influenza infection in human: (1) to reduce the number of cases; (2) to reduce the fatality rate; and (3) to prevent the spread of the epidemic. Closure of the farmers markets during the epidemics in endemic areas effectively reduced the number of cases. Research, development, and use of new drugs, equipment, technologies, and strategies were effective in reducing the fatality rate. However, the epidemic areas expanded as no strict measures were taken in 2013 to prohibit or restrict the spread of live poultry carrying the virus through the trade [71, 72], which provided conditions for the development of the epidemic in 2014.

Since October 2013, human infection with H7N9 avian influenza emerged successively in the year 2014. As of March 17, 2014, 384 cases were reported. Compared with the epidemic in 2013, the onset of the disease was earlier (the first case in 2013 was not confirmed and announced until March 30), and cases were found in more provinces, mainly concentrated in Jiangsu, Zhejiang, Guangdong, and other places. The epidemic was on the rise, triggering high attention from the society, media, government, and professionals. At that time, almost everyone believed that the epidemic in 2014 was coming with such intensity that the scale might be much larger than that in 2013. What's more, the unprecedented density and intensity of population movement with the approach of the Spring Festival would have an immeasurable impact on the development of the epidemic. Officials of relevant state departments in China gave several important instructions, and administrative departments, research institutions, and disease prevention and control departments had hot discussions [32].

Consumption of live poultry is deep-rooted in China, which is not only a habit but also a culture. Closing farmers markets with live poultry will cause certain economic losses and social risks. Although the role of closing farmers markets with live poultry in controlling epidemics is highly recognized by infectious disease prevention and control departments, people from different departments have different points of view, given the impact on the poultry industry and the related social and economic risks.

On January 26, 2014, National Health Commission of the PRC held a video conference. The principal leader asked the local Health Commissions where the epidemic occurred to recommend to the local governments closure of the farmers market. The prompt decision took effect. After the Spring Festival, the number of human infections with H7N9 avian influenza did not peak as expected. According to data of the epidemic in 2013, the number of cases rose rapidly in March and peaked in April. Without the action, the trend in 2014 would be like that in 2013. After measures were taken to close the farmers markets with live poultry in the affected provinces, the number of cases declined rapidly and there was no peak in March or April. Therefore, the closure of the farmers markets effectively prevented the large-scale human infection with H7N9 avian influenza in 2014, and nothing else could have achieved this goal. The decisive action of the National Health Commission of the PRC was the main and decisive factor in preventing a large-scale epidemic. Thus, the prevention and control of human infection with H7N9 avian influenza in 2014 is a model for response to unexpected major new infectious diseases by health administrations, which is worthy of further study and discussion [32].

For social behavior to prevent further infectious diseases outbreak, we must remember the following.

1. Development of healthy and safe large-scale poultry and livestock farming modes to prevent large-scale human infections with avian influenza and *S. suis*.
2. High attention to microbial contamination of food, especially the microbiological issues in large-scale food production and supply chain to prevent outbreaks of food-borne infectious diseases.
3. Strict prohibition on contact between humans and marmots for possible quick control and even elimination of the threat from plague.
4. Strengthened customs quarantine to prevent the import of infectious diseases abroad.
5. Strict management of travel-related vaccination to prevent infection with pathogens overseas.

1.4.2 Individual Behavior

For induvial behavior to prevent infection by pathogen, we must be aware the following.

1. Education on safe sex as the most important measure for prevention and control of sexually transmitted diseases such as AIDS.
2. Knowledge on pet care to help prevent infectious diseases such as cat scratch fever.

3. Knowledge on wildlife carrying pathogens to help prevent animal-borne infectious diseases.
4. Knowledge on vectors to help prevent infectious diseases transmitted by ticks and other vectors.
5. Strict implementation of vaccination recommendations before going abroad to prevent infectious diseases overseas.

References

1. Gao R, Cao B, Hu Y, Feng Z, Wang D, Hu W, et al. Human infection with a novel avian-origin influenza a (H7N9) virus. N Engl J Med. 2013;368(20):1888–97.
2. Shao Z, Li W, Ren J, et al. Identification of a new Neisseria meningitidis serogroup C clone from Anhui province, China. Lancet. 2006;367(9508):419–23.
3. Zhang YZ, He YW, Dai YA, et al. Hemorrhagic fever caused by a novel Bunyavirus in China: pathogenesis and correlates of fatal outcome. Clin Infect Dis. 2012;54(4):527–33.
4. Li K, Lin XD, Wang W, et al. Isolation and characterization of a novel arenavirus harbored by rodents and shrews in Zhejiang province. China Virol. 2015;476:37–42.
5. Wang ZD, Wang B, Wei F, et al. A new segmented virus associated with human febrile illness in China. N Engl J Med. 2019;380(22):2116–25.
6. Qin XC, Shi M, Tian JH, et al. A tick-borne segmented RNA virus contains genome segments derived from unsegmented viral ancestors. Proc Natl Acad Sci USA. 2014;111(18):6744–9.
7. Li H, Zheng YC, Ma L, et al. Human infection with a novel tick-borne Anaplasma species in China: a surveillance study. Lancet Infect Dis. 2015;15(6):663–70.
8. Zhou H, Guo S. Two cases of imported pneumonic plague in Beijing, China. Medicine (Baltimore). 2020;99(44):e22932.
9. Zhu N, Zhang D, Wang W, et al. A novel coronavirus from patients with pneumonia in China, 2019. N Engl J Med. 2020;382(8):727–33.
10. Zhang L, Liu Y, Ni D, Li Q, Yu Y, Yu XJ, et al. Nosocomial transmission of human granulocytic anaplasmosis in China. JAMA. 2008;300(19):2263–70.
11. Shao Z, Li W, Ren J, Liang X, Xu L, Diao B, et al. Identification of a new Neisseria meningitidis serogroup C clone from Anhui province. China Lancet. 2006;367(9508):419–23.
12. Liu Q, Xu W, Lu S, et al. Landscape of emerging and re-emerging infectious diseases in China: impact of ecology, climate, and behavior. Front Med. 2018;12(1):3–22.
13. Rohde H, Qin J, Cui Y, Li D, Loman NJ, Hentschke M, et al. Open-source genomic analysis of Shiga-toxin-producing E. coli O104:H4. N Engl J Med. 2011;365(8):718–24.
14. Shi M, Lin XD, Vasilakis N, Tian JH, Li CX, Chen LJ, et al. Divergent viruses discovered in arthropods and vertebrates revise the evolutionary history of the Flaviviridae and related viruses. J Virol. 2015;90(2):659–69.
15. Li CX, Shi M, Tian JH, Lin XD, Kang YJ, Chen LJ, et al. Unprecedented genomic diversity of RNA viruses in arthropods reveals the ancestry of negative-sense RNA viruses. elife. 2015;4:e05378.
16. Fang LQ, Liu K, Li XL, Liang S, Yang Y, Yao HW, et al. Emerging tick-borne infections in mainland China: an increasing public health threat. Lancet Infect Dis. 2015;15(12):1467–79.
17. Jia N, Zheng YC, Jiang JF, Ma L, Cao WC. Human infection with Candidatus rickettsia tarasevichiae. N Engl J Med. 2013;369(12):1178–80.
18. Jia N, Jiang JF, Huo QB, Jiang BG, Cao WC. Rickettsia sibirica subspecies sibirica BJ-90 as a cause of human disease. N Engl J Med. 2013;369(12):1176–8.
19. Jiang JF, Zheng YC, Jiang RR, Li H, Huo QB, Jiang BG, et al. Epidemiological, clinical, and laboratory characteristics of 48 cases of "Babesia venatorum" infection in China: a descriptive study. Lancet Infect Dis. 2015;15(2):196–203.
20. Liu S, Jin D, Lan R, Wang Y, Meng Q, Dai H, et al. Escherichia marmotae sp. nov., isolated from faeces of Marmota himalayana. Int J Syst Evol Microbiol. 2015;65(7):2130–4.
21. Hu S, Jin D, Lu S, Liu S, Zhang J, Wang Y, et al. Helicobacter himalayensis sp. nov. isolated from gastric mucosa of Marmota himalayana. Int J Syst Evol Microbiol. 2015;65(Pt 6):1719–25.
22. Xu JG. Behavioral and ecological infectious diseases: from SARS to H7N9 avian influenza outbreak in China. Zhonghua Liu Xing Bing Xue Za Zhi. 2013;34(5):417–8.
23. Flohr C. The plague fighter: Wu Lien-teh and the beginning of the Chinese public health system. Ann Sci. 1996;53(4):361–80.
24. Lu L, Ren Z, Yue Y, Yu X, Lu S, Li G, et al. Niche modeling predictions of the potential distribution of Marmota himalayana, the host animal of plague in Yushu County of Qinghai. BMC Public Health. 2016;16(1):183.
25. Yu D. Prevention of plague in China in last 50 years. Zhonghua Liu Xing Bing Xue Za Zhi. 2000;21(4):300–3.
26. Shen EL. Human plague during 1979-1988 in China and strategy of its control. Zhonghua Liu Xing Bing Xue Za Zhi. 1990;11(3):156–9.
27. Wang N, Wu G, Lu R, Feng L, Xiao Y, McFarland W, et al. Investigating HIV infection and HIV incidence among Chinese men who have sex with men with recent sexual debut, Chongqing, China, 2011. AIDS Behav. 2016;20(12):2976–82.
28. Xu W, Zheng L, Liu Y, Zheng Y. Sexual sensation seeking, sexual compulsivity, and high-risk sexual

behaviours among gay/bisexual men in Southwest China. AIDS Care. 2016;28:1138–44.
29. Zhang B, Li X, Hu T. Survey on the high risk behaviors related to acquired immunologic deficiency syndrome and sexually transmitted diseases among men who have sex with men in mainland China. Zhonghua Liu Xing Bing Xue Za Zhi. 2001;22(5):337–40.
30. Wang M, Yan M, Xu H, et al. SARS-CoV infection in a restaurant from palm civet. Emerg Infect Dis. 2005;11(12):1860–5.
31. Kan B, Wang M, Jing H, Xu H, Jiang X, Yan M, et al. Molecular evolution analysis and geographic investigation of severe acute respiratory syndrome coronavirus-like virus in palm civets at an animal market and on farms. J Virol. 2005;79(18):11892–900.
32. Xu J. Prevention and control of the social behavior associated infectious by changing social behavior. Zhonghua Liu Xing Bing Xue Za Zhi. 2014;35(5):475–6.
33. Wang M, Yan M, Xu H, Liang W, Kan B, Zheng B, et al. SARS-CoV infection in a restaurant from palm civet. Emerg Infect Dis. 2005;11(12):1860–5.
34. Xiong Y, Wang P, Lan R, Ye C, Wang H, Ren J, et al. A novel Escherichia coli O157:H7 clone causing a major hemolytic uremic syndrome outbreak in China. PLoS One. 2012;7(4):e36144.
35. Pang B, Jing H, Zheng H, Sun H, Zhao A, Xu J. Molecular typing of Shiga-toxin producing Escherichia coli O157:H7 isolated in China with pulsed field gel electrophoresis. Zhonghua Liu Xing Bing Xue Za Zhi. 2002;23(2):123–6.
36. Li H, Jing H, Pang B, Zhao G, Yang J, Xu J. Study on diarrhea disease caused by enterohemorrhagic Escherichia coli O157:H7 in Xuzhou city, Jiangsu province in 2000. Zhonghua Liu Xing Bing Xue Za Zhi. 2002;23(2):119–22.
37. Xu J, Cheng B, Feng L, Jing H, Yang J, Zhao G, et al. Serological investigations on patients with hemolytic uremic syndromes due to enterohemorrhagic Escherichia coli O157:H7 infection. Zhonghua Liu Xing Bing Xue Za Zhi. 2002;23(2):114–8.
38. Xu JG, Cheng BK, Jing HQ. Escherichia Coli O157 H7 and Shiga-like-toxin- producing Escherichia Coli in China. World J Gastroenterol. 1999;5(3):191–4.
39. Yu H, Wu JT, Cowling BJ, Liao Q, Fang VJ, Zhou S, et al. Effect of closure of live poultry markets on poultry-to-person transmission of avian influenza a H7N9 virus: an ecological study. Lancet. 2014;383(9916):541–8.
40. Ye C, Zhu X, Jing H, Du H, Segura M, Zheng H, et al. Streptococcus suis sequence type 7 outbreak, Sichuan. China Emerg Infect Dis. 2006;12(8):1203–8.
41. Ye C, Bai X, Zhang J, Jing H, Zheng H, Du H, et al. Spread of Streptococcus suis sequence type 7. China. Emerg Infect Dis. 2008;14(5):787–91.
42. Ye C, Zheng H, Zhang J, Jing H, Wang L, Xiong Y, et al. Clinical, experimental, and genomic differences between intermediately pathogenic, highly pathogenic, and epidemic Streptococcus suis. J Infect Dis. 2009;199(1):97–107.
43. Gottschalk M, Segura M, Xu J. Streptococcus suis infections in humans: the Chinese experience and the situation in North America. Anim Health Res Rev. 2007;8(1):29–45.
44. Yu H, Shu Y, Hu S, Zhang H, Gao Z, Chen H, et al. The first confirmed human case of avian influenza a (H5N1) in mainland China. Lancet. 2006;367(9504):84.
45. Yu Z, Song Y, Zhou H, Xu X, Hu Q, Wu H, et al. Avian influenza (H5N1) virus in waterfowl and chickens, Central China. Emerg Infect Dis. 2007;13(5):772–5.
46. Guan Y, Zheng BJ, He YQ, Liu XL, Zhuang ZX, Cheung CL, et al. Isolation and characterization of viruses related to the SARS coronavirus from animals in southern China. Science. 2003;302(5643):276–8.
47. Ma C, Wu S, Yang P, Li H, Tang S, Wang Q. Behavioural factors associated with diarrhea among adults over 18 years of age in Beijing. China BMC Public Health. 2014;14:451.
48. Wang W, Liao Q, Wu X, Hou S, Wang Y, Wu J, et al. Potential risk of blood transfusion-transmitted brucellosis in an endemic area of China. Transfusion. 2015;55(3):586–92.
49. Chen JD, Ke CW, Deng X, Jiang S, Liang W, Ke BX, et al. Brucellosis in Guangdong Province, People's Republic of China, 2005–2010. Emerg Infect Dis. 2013;19(5):817–8.
50. Hou Q, Sun X, Zhang J, Liu Y, Wang Y, Jin Z. Modeling the transmission dynamics of sheep brucellosis in Inner Mongolia autonomous region. China Math Biosci. 2013;242(1):51–8.
51. Buchholz U, Bernard H, Werber D, Bohmer MM, Remschmidt C, Wilking H, et al. German outbreak of Escherichia coli O104:H4 associated with sprouts. N Engl J Med. 2011;365(19):1763–70.
52. Bielaszewska M, Mellmann A, Zhang W, Kock R, Fruth A, Bauwens A, et al. Characterisation of the Escherichia coli strain associated with an outbreak of haemolytic uraemic syndrome in Germany, 2011: a microbiological study. Lancet Infect Dis. 2011;11(9):671–6.
53. Tang XF, Liu LG, Ma HL, Zhu BP, Hao CX, Wu XY, et al. Outbreak of cholera associated with consumption of soft-shelled turtles, Sichuan province, China, 2009. Zhonghua Liu Xing Bing Xue Za Zhi. 2010;31(9):1050–2.
54. Smith RM, Schaefer MK, Kainer MA, Wise M, Finks J, Duwve J, et al. Fungal infections associated with contaminated methylprednisolone injections. N Engl J Med. 2013;369(17):1598–609.
55. Kainer MA, Reagan DR, Nguyen DB, Wiese AD, Wise ME, Ward J, et al. Fungal infections associated with contaminated methylprednisolone in Tennessee. N Engl J Med. 2012;367(23):2194–203.
56. Ma Q, Zeng S, Xia S, Pan X, Wang D, Zhu H, et al. Risky sexual networks and concentrated HIV epidemics among men who have sex with men in Wenzhou, China: a respondent-driven sampling study. BMC Public Health. 2015;15:1246.

57. Huang S, Tang W, Zhu Z, Lu H, Tan X, Zhang B, et al. Higher prevalence of sexual transmitted diseases and correlates of genital warts among heterosexual males attending sexually transmitted infection clinics (MSCs) in Jiangmen, China: implication for the up-taking of STD related service. PLoS One. 2015;10(3):e0121814.
58. Zhang YZ, Xu J. The emergence and cross species transmission of newly discovered tick-borne Bunyavirus in China. Curr Opin Virol. 2016;4(16):126–31.
59. Zhang YZ, Zhou DJ, Qin XC, Tian JH, Xiong Y, Wang JB, et al. The ecology, genetic diversity, and phylogeny of Huaiyangshan virus in China. J Virol. 2012;86(5):2864–8.
60. Zhang YZ, Zhou DJ, Xiong Y, Chen XP, He YW, Sun Q, et al. Hemorrhagic fever caused by a novel tick-borne Bunyavirus in Huaiyangshan, China. Zhonghua Liu Xing Bing Xue Za Zhi. 2011;32(3):209–20.
61. Li H, Zheng YC, Ma L, Jia N, Jiang BG, Jiang RR, et al. Human infection with a novel tick-borne Anaplasma species in China: a surveillance study. Lancet Infect Dis. 2015;15(6):663–70.
62. Heymann DL, Chen L, Takemi K, Fidler DP, Tappero JW, Thomas MJ, et al. Global health security: the wider lessons from the West African Ebola virus disease epidemic. Lancet. 2015;385(9980):1884–901.
63. Faye O, Boelle PY, Heleze E, Faye O, Loucoubar C, Magassouba N, et al. Chains of transmission and control of Ebola virus disease in Conakry, Guinea, in 2014: an observational study. Lancet Infect Dis. 2015;15(3):320–6.
64. Johnson BK, Gitau LG, Gichogo A, Tukei PM, Else JG, Suleman MA, et al. Marburg and Ebola virus antibodies in Kenyan primates. Lancet. 1981;1(8235):1420–1.
65. Deng YQ, Zhao H, Li XF, Zhang NN, Liu ZY, Jiang T, et al. Isolation, identification and genomic characterization of the Asian lineage Zika virus imported to China. Sci China Life Sci. 2016;59(4):428–30.
66. Chen J, Lu H. Yellow fever in China is still an imported disease. Biosci Trends. 2016;10(2):158–62.
67. Ma T, Heywood A, MacIntyre CR. Chinese travellers visiting friends and relatives—a review of infectious risks. Travel Med Infect Dis. 2015;13(4):285–94.
68. Shi L, Fu S, Wang L, Li X, Gu D, Liu C, et al. Surveillance of mosquito-borne infectious diseases in febrile travelers entering China via Shenzhen ports, China, 2013. Travel Med Infect Dis. 2016;14(2):123–30.
69. Wang M, Di B, Zhou DH, Zheng BJ, Jing H, Lin YP, et al. Food markets with live birds as source of avian influenza. Emerg Infect Dis. 2006 November;12(11):1773–5.
70. Xu J, Lu S, Wang H, Chen C. Reducing exposure to avian influenza H7N9. Lancet. 2013;381(9880):1815–6.
71. Lu S, Chen C, Yu W, Wang H, Du P, Kan B, et al. Investigating geographical spread of the human infection with avian influenza a (H7N9)virus by online knowledge analysis of the live bird trade with a distributed focused crawler. Zhonghua Liu Xing Bing Xue Za Zhi. 2014;35(3):228–30.
72. Chen C, Lu S, Du P, Wang H, Yu W, Song H, et al. Silent geographical spread of the H7N9 virus by online knowledge analysis of the live bird trade with a distributed focused crawler. Emerg Microbes Infect. 2013;2(12):e89.

Check for updates

2 Progress in Epidemiology of Emerging Tick-Borne Infections in China

Li-Qun Fang, Wan-Jun Chen, and Wu-Chun Cao

Abstract

A total of 33 emerging tick-borne agents have been reported in the Chinese mainland from 1980 to 2015, including eight species of spotted fever group rickettsiae, seven species in the family Anaplasmataceae, six genospecies in the complex *Borrelia burgdorferi* sensu lato, 11 species of *Babesia,* and the severe fever with thrombocytopenia syndrome virus. Among them 15 emerging tick-borne agents have been identified to cause human disease, and their clinical characteristics were described and their geographic distributions mapped. The pathogenicity in humans of the other 18 tick-borne agents detected in ticks or animals is yet to be determined. Various factors have contributed to the emergence of emerging tick-borne diseases in China; for example, advances in and application of modern molecular techniques might facilitate the identification of emerging tick-borne agents and improve lab diagnosis of human cases. We anticipate that more emerging tick-borne agents will continue to be identified in ticks and animals and additional emerging tick-borne diseases will be discovered in humans.

Keywords

Tick · Emerging tick-borne infection · Geographic distribution · Influencing factors · China

2.1 Introduction

Ticks were the first arthropods recognized to be vectors that can transmit pathogens to humans, which are vectors of infectious diseases second only to mosquitoes in the world [1]. Tick-borne pathogens are usually maintained in natural cycles involving animal hosts and tick vectors, and humans are occasional hosts for tick vectors, playing no role in maintaining tick-borne pathogens in nature [2]. The risk areas of human tick-borne diseases are mainly determined by the geographic distributions of tick vectors, and which are usually shaped by their feverous biotopes or environments. Tick-borne pathogens have been emerging worldwide and becoming significant threats to humans in the past four decades [1, 3].

Although China has made tremendous progress in the prevention and control of infectious diseases, it is facing the great challenge of emerging infectious diseases [4]. While outbreaks of

L.-Q. Fang · W.-C. Cao (✉)
State Key Laboratory of Pathogen and Biosecurity, Beijing Institute of Microbiology and Epidemiology, Beijing, People's Republic of China
e-mail: caowc@bmi.ac.cn

W.-J. Chen
Zhejiang Provincial Center for Disease Control and Prevention, Hangzhou, People's Republic of China

D.-Q. Ye (ed.), *Progress in China Epidemiology*, https://doi.org/10.1007/978-981-19-2199-5_2

severe acute respiratory syndrome, H5N1 and H7N9 avian influenza virus infections, and coronavirus disease 2019 have attracted great attention, emerging tick-borne diseases are generally neglected by clinicians and primary healthcare providers. Although increasing reports of tick-borne infections have been seen in China, no comprehensive review has been reported. In this chapter, we summarize the type and distribution of emerging tick-borne infections in ticks, animal hosts, and humans, describe clinical characteristics of human tick-borne infections, and discuss possible influencing factors contributing to their emergence.

2.2 Emergence of Emerging Tick-Borne Agents in the Mainland of China

A total of 33 emerging tick-associated agents have been identified in the mainland of China from 1982 to 2015, including eight species of spotted fever group rickettsiae (SFGR) [5–11]; three species of *Ehrlichia* [12–14], three species of *Anaplasma* [15–17] and a *Candidatus* Neoehrlichia mikurensis [18] in the family Anaplasmataceae; six genospecies in the complex *Borrelia (B.) burgdorferi* sensu lato [19–23]; 11 species of *Babesia* [24–33]; and a virus causing severe fever with thrombocytopenia syndrome [34]. The majority of them (19/33) were initially detected in tick vectors, followed by six in livestock and pet animal (sheep, goat, buffalo, and dog), six in people, and two in wild animals (Chinese white-bellied rat and Chinese hare). The year and location of each tick-borne agent first identified are summarized in Table 2.1 [4].

Fifteen (45.5%) newly recognized tick-associated agents have been reported to cause human infection, including four species of SFGR [11, 35–37], an *Ehrlichia* [38], two *Anaplasma* [17, 38], and *Candidatus* Neoehrlichia mikurensis [18] in the family Anaplasmataceae, three genospecies of *B. burgdorferi* sensu lato [19, 21, 39], three species of *Babesia* [33, 40, 41], and SFTSV (Table 2.2) [34]. Six tick-borne pathogens, including *Candidatus* Rickettsia (*R.*) tarasevichiae, *Candidatus* Neoehrlichia mikurensis, *Borrelia (B.) garinii*, *B. afzelii*, "*Babesia (Ba.) venatorum*," and SFTSV, were first identified in febrile patients, and then identified in ticks (see Table 2.1) [4]. The other nine pathogens, including *R. heilongjiangensis*, *R. sibirica* sp. BJ-90, *R. raoultii*, *Ehrlichia (E.) chaffeensis*, *Anaplasma (A.) phagocytophilum*, "*A. capra*," *B. valaisiana*-related, *Ba. microti*, and *Ba. divergens* were first detected from ticks or animals and then were shown to infect humans. Among them, severe fever with thrombocytopenia syndrome virus (SFTSV) was first identified in the mainland of China [34], and subsequently reported in South Korea, Japan, and Vietnam [42, 43]. A tick-borne pathogen similar to SFTSV has also been reported in the USA [44]. Human infections with the four pathogens including *R. sibirica* sp. BJ-90, *Candidatus* R. tarasevichiae, "*A. capra*," and *B. valaisiana*-related have been exclusively diagnosed in China [11, 17, 36, 39]. Human infections with *Candidatus* Neoehrlichia mikurensis, "*Ba. venatorum*," and *R. raoultii* were first reported in Europe, and were then identified to infect humans in the mainland of China [18, 33, 37]. Five tick-borne pathogens, including *R. monacensis*, *R. slovaca*, *R. sibirica* sp. *mongolotimonae*, *B. valaisiana*, and *B. burgdorferi* sensu stricto, have been found in ticks and/or reservoir hosts, but not yet been reported to cause human infections in China [45–49]. In addition, 13 agents including *Candidatus* R. hebeiii, *Ehrlichia canis*, *Ehrlichia* sp. Tibet, *A. platys*, *B. sinica*, and eight *Ba.* species such as *Ba. ovis*, *Ba. ovata*, *Ba. orientalis*, *Ba. major*, *Ba. motasi*, *Ba. caballi*, *Ba.* sp. Kashi, and *Ba.* sp. Xinjiang, have been identified in ticks or/and animals, but their pathogenicity to humans remains to be determined.

Table 2.1 The first identified origin and locations of emerging tick-borne infections in the mainland of China from 1982 to 2015 [4]

Species	First identified origin[a]	First identified province (year)[b]	References (subsequent investigations)
Spotted fever group rickettsiae			
R. heilongjiangensis	*D. silvarum*	Heilongjiang (1982)	5 [6, 8, 35, 50–59]
R. sibirica sp. BJ-90	*D. sinicus*	Beijing (1990)	7 [36]
R. sibirica sp. *mongolotimonae*	*Hy. asiaticum kozlovi*	Inner Mongolia (1991)	7
R. monacensis	*I. persulcatus*	Henan, Anhui, and Hubei provinces (2006)	8 [58, 60]
R. Raoultii	*D. silvarum*	Xinjiang (2011)	9 [37, 61, 62]
R. slovaca	*D. silvarum*	Xinjiang (2011)	9 [62, 63]
Candidatus R. hebeiii	*H. longicornis*	Hebei (2011)	10 [64]
Candidatus R. tarasevichiae	Human (*I. persulcatus*)	Heilongjiang (2012)	11
Agents in the family Anaplasmataceae			
E. Chaffeensis	*Amblyomma testudinarium*	Yunan (1996)	12 [32, 38, 50, 65–73]
E. canis	*Rhipicephalus sanguineus* sensu stricto	Guangdong (1997)	13 [16, 68, 74]
E. Sp. Tibet	*Rhipicephalus microplus*	Tibet (2000)	14
A. Phagocytophilum	*I. persulcatus*	Heilongjiang (1997)	15 [38, 50, 63, 65, 66, 73, 75–86]
A. platys	Dog	Guangdong (1998)	16 [74]
"*A. capra*"[c]	Goat	Heilongjiang (2014)	17
Candidatus Neoehrlichia mikurensis	Human (*I. persulcatus*)	Heilongjiang (2010)	18 [87, 88]
Borrelia burgdorferi sensu lato			
B. Garinii	Human (*I. persulcatus*)	Heilongjiang (1986)	19 [21, 23, 39, 50, 65, 89–101]
B. Valaisiana	*I. granulatus (Apodemus (Ap.) agrarius)*	Zhejiang (1997)	20 [96, 102]
B. sinica	*Niviventer confucianus*	Chongqing (1997)	20
B. afzelii	Human	Heilongjiang (2000)	21 [39, 50, 89, 91, 93–95, 100]
B. Valaisiana-related	*I. Granulates, H. longicornis* (*Ap. agrarius*)	Guizhou (2006)	22 [39, 93, 96, 98]
B. Burgdorferi sensu stricto	*Caprolagus sinensis*	Hunan (2010)	23 [102]
Babesia			
Ba. Ovis	Sheep	Sichuan (1982)	24 [103]
Ba. Major	*H. longicornis* (cattle)	Henan (1988)	25 [104]
Ba. Ovata	Cattle	Henan (1990)	26 [105]
Ba. Orientalis	Buffalo	Hubei (1997)	27 [106, 107]
Ba. Motasi	Sheep	Gansu (1997)	28 [108, 109]
Ba. Caballi	*D. silvarum, D. nuttalli*	Gansu (1998)	29 [110–112]
Ba. Sp. Kashi	*Hy. anatolicum*	Xinjiang (2005)	30 [113]
Ba. Sp. Xinjiang	*R. sanguineus* sensu stricto, *Hy. anatolicum*	Xinjiang (2007)	31 [113]
Ba. Microti	*I. persulcatus, H. concinna*	Heilongjiang (2007)	32 [41, 50, 69, 114–116]
Ba. Divergens	*I. persulcatus, H. concinna, H. japonica* (*Ap. agrarius*)	Heilongjiang (2007)	32 [40, 50]
"*Ba. Venatorum*"[c]	Human	Xinjiang (2012)	33 [117]

(continued)

Table 2.1 (continued)

Species	First identified origin[a]	First identified province (year)[b]	References (subsequent investigations)
SFTSV[d]	Human	Henan (2009)	34 [118–126]

[a]To indicate the first-identified origin (human, domestic animal, rodent, and tick) of each emerging tick-associated agent. The agent identified simultaneously in other hosts or ticks is shown in parentheses

[b]Provinces also include autonomous regions and metropolis

[c]"*A. capra*" and "*Ba. venatorum*" have not been formally described in taxonomic papers and thus their names are in quotation marks

[d]SFTSV: severe fever with thrombocytopenia syndrome virus

Table 2.2 Human emerging tick-borne diseases reported in the mainland of China [4]

Emerging tick-borne disease	Pathogen	No. of patients	Diagnostic methods[a] (references)
Rickettsiosis	*R. heilongjiangensis*	34	A&B [35], B&C [57], A&C [59]
Rickettsiosis	*R. sibirica* sp. BJ-90	1	A&B [36]
Rickettsiosis	*R. Raoultii*	2	A&B [37]
Rickettsiosis	*Candidatus* R. tarasevichiae	5	B [11]
Rickettsiosis	Uncharacterized *rickettsia*	37	C [127–129], B [130], A&C [131], E [132]
Human monocytic ehrlichiosis	*E. chaffeensis*	12	B [38, 66]
Human granulocytic anaplasmosis	*A. phagocytophilum*	104	B [38, 66, 85, 86], A&B&C [84], A&B [75], E [82]
Human infection with "*A. capra*"	"*A. capra*"	28	A&B&C [17]
Human infection with *Candidatus* Neoehrlichia mikurensis	*Candidatus* Neoehrlichia mikurensis	7	B [18]
Lyme disease	*B. garinii*	30	B [21, 23, 39, 100, 101]
Lyme disease	*B. afzelii*	8	B [21, 23, 39, 100], C [133]
Lyme disease	*B. Valaisiana*-related	1	B [39]
Lyme disease	Uncharacterized *B. burgdorferi* sensu lato	2691	A [134–138], E [139]
Babesiosis	*Ba. divergens*	2	B [40]
Babesiosis	*Ba. Microti*	11	B&D [41, 116]
Babesiosis	"*Ba. Venatorum*"	49	A&B&C [33], B&C&D [117]
Babesiosis	Uncharacterized *Babesia*	3	D [140, 141]
SFTS[b]	SFTSV[c]	2543	A&B&C [34, 125], A or B or C [121, 126], A or B [122], B&C [123], B [124]

[a]Diagnostic methods: (A) a fourfold increase in the titer of specific antibodies in blood sera collected from the acute and convalescent stages of illness, or a seroconversion of specific antibodies, (B) molecular detection and sequence determination, (C) isolation of pathogens from clinical samples, (D) light or electronic micrograph identification for thin blood smear, and (E) methods were not provided

[b]SFTS severe fever with thrombocytopenia syndrome

[c]SFTSV severe fever with thrombocytopenia syndrome virus

2.3 Emerging SFGR Infections

A total of eight novel species of SFGR have been reported in the mainland of China from 1982 to 2015 (see Table 2.1) [5–11], which are mainly distributed in northern China (north of 36° north latitude).

Tick and Animal Infections

The eight novel species and uncharacterized species of SFGR have been reported to be associated with 16 tick species (Fig. 2.1) [4]. *R. heilongjiangensis* can infect a variety of tick species, three rodent species, and goats (Fig. 2.2) [4]. In Heilongjiang province of northeastern China, *R. heilongjiangensis* was detected in nine tick species and two rodent species [50–52], and was detected in *Haemaphysalis* spp. ticks from Jilin province and in *Haemaphysalis (H.) verticalis*, *Dermacentor (D.) niveus*, *Hyalomma (Hy.) asiaticum kozlovi*, *Rhipicephalus pumilio*, and *D. nuttalli* ticks, among Inner Mongolia [52, 53]. In Qinghai province of northwestern China, *R. heilongjiangensis* has been detected in *D. silvarum* ticks [54]. *R. heilongjiangensis* has been detected in *H. longicornis* ticks, goats, and Chestnut white bellied rats from Guangdong, Yunnan, and Hainan provinces of southern China, respectively [55–57]. It was also identified in *H. longicornis* from Zhejiang province and in *H. flava* ticks from Henan, Anhui, and Hubei provinces of central and eastern China [8, 58]. *R. sibirica* sp. BJ-90 was identified in *D. sinicus* from Beijing suburb [7]. *R. raoultii* was found in *D. silvarum* and *D. marginatus* in western China [9, 61], and in *H. verticalis*, *D. silvarum*,

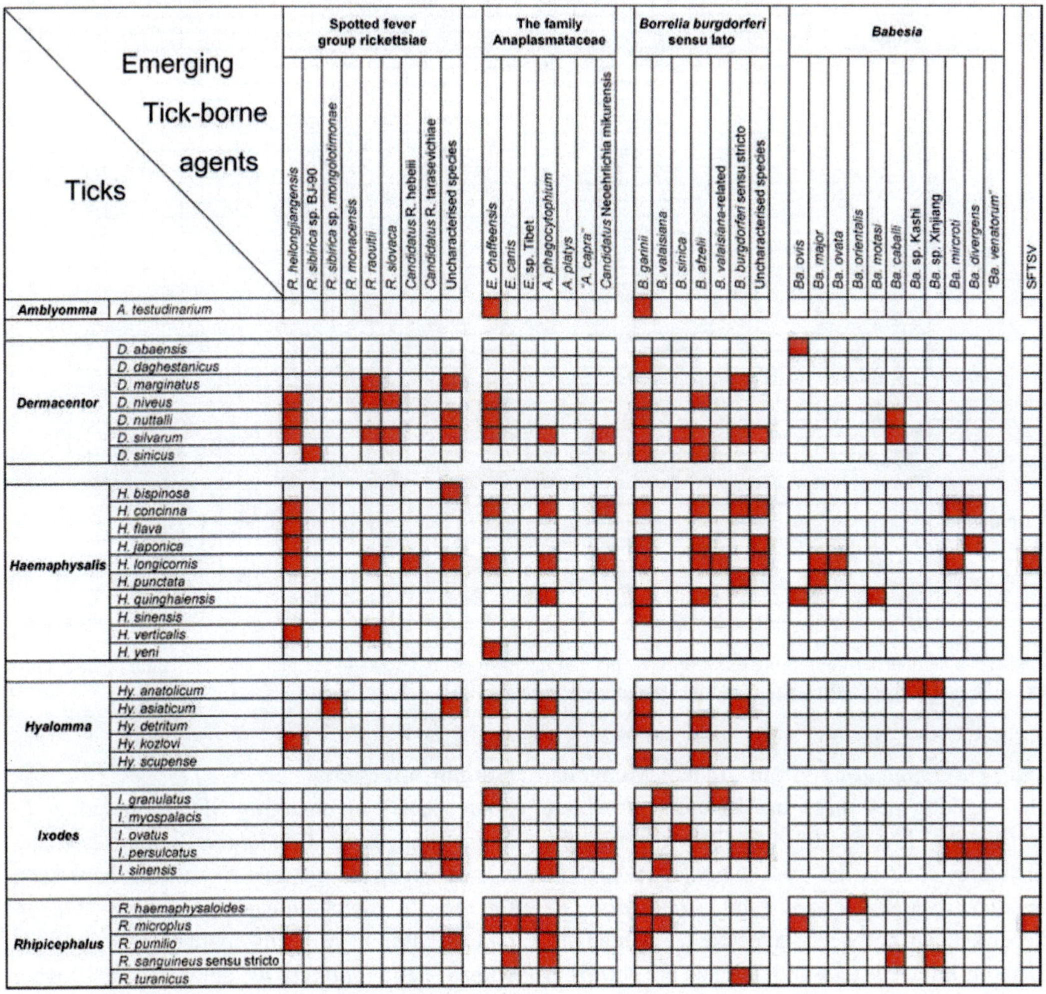

Fig. 2.1 The matrix of emerging tick-associated agents and tick species in the mainland of China. SFTSV indicates the severe fever with thrombocytopenia syndrome virus [4]

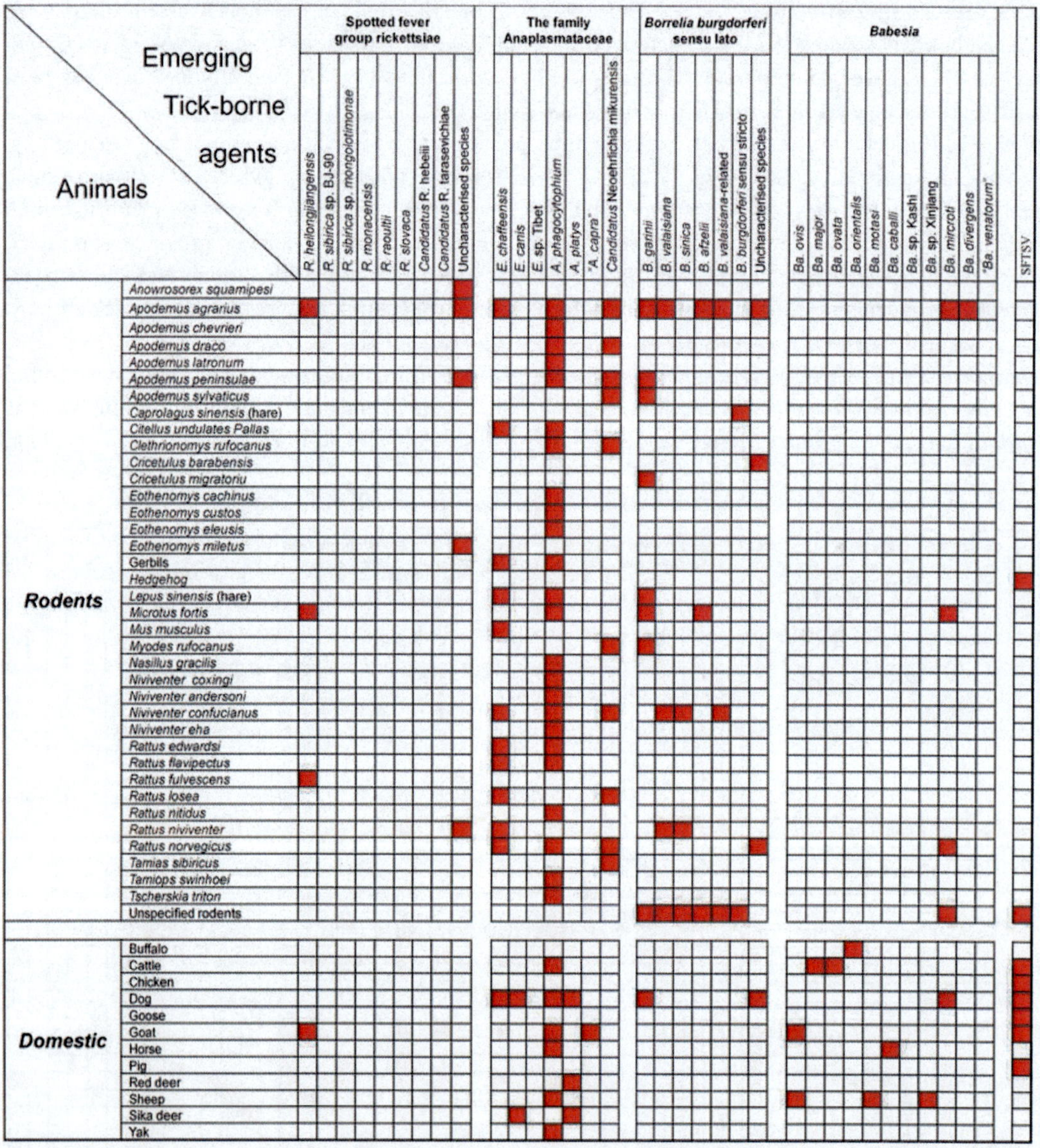

Fig. 2.2 The matrix of emerging tick-borne agents and involved animal hosts in the mainland of China. SFTSV indicates the severe fever with thrombocytopenia syndrome virus [4]

and *H. longicornis* from Inner Mongolia, Heilongjiang province, and Liaoning province, respectively [37, 53, 62, 63]. The four species, including *R. sibirica* sp. *mongolotimonae*, *R. monacensis*, *R. slovaca*, and *Candidatus* R. hebeiii, have not been detected from humans. Data on infected ticks and animals are shown in Figs. 2.1 and 2.2 [4, 7–10, 60, 64, 65, 127, 142–147].

Human Infections

Four species of emerging SFGR, including *R. heilongjiangensis*, *Candidatus* R. tarasevichiae, *R. sibirica* sp. BJ-90, and *R. raoultii*, have been reported to infect humans (see Table 2.2). 34 human cases have been reported to be infected with *R. heilongjiangensis*; among them 19 were reported in forested areas of northeastern China in the 1990s [35, 59]. The other 15 cases were diagnosed in Hainan province in 2008 [57]. Our study of the active surveillance for human infections with SFGR at Mudanjiang Forestry Central Hospital of Heilongjiang province in 2012 showed that eight cases were identified by molecular detection and sequence determination, of which five were infected by *Candidatus* R. tarasevichiae, one by *R. sibirica* sp. BJ-90, and two by *R. raoultii*. The SFGR infection was further supported by the presence of IFA antibody against SFGR antigen in sera [36, 37]. In addition, 37 cases were reported to infect uncharacterized species of SFGR, including one in Inner Mongolia, six in Heilongjiang province, 29 in Hainan province, and one in Xinjiang Autonomous Region [127–132]. Patients with SFGR infections were shown these clinical manifestations, mainly included fever, eschar, headache, malaise, asthenia, anorexia, nausea, and lymphadenopathy, and a few patients had rash and neurologic manifestations, for example, coma, neck stiffness, and Kernig's sign [11, 35–37, 57, 59, 127–132].

2.4 Emerging Infections with Agents in the Family Anaplasmataceae

Seven species in the family Anaplasmataceae, including *E. chaffeensis*, *E. canis*, *Ehrlichia* sp. Tibet, *A. phagocytophilum*, "*A. capra*," *A. platys*, and *Candidatus* Neoehrlichia mikurensis, have been identified in China (see Table 2.1).

Tick and Animal Infections

Seven emerging agents in the family Anaplasmataceae were detected from 17 tick species in China (see Fig. 2.1) [4]. *E. chaffeensis* was first identified in *Amblyomma testudinarium* ticks from Yunnan province in 1996 [12]. Several surveys show that it infects various tick species, and is widely dispersed in China [31, 65–69]. It was also identified in dogs from Shandong province, in gerbils and long-tailed ground squirrel from Xinjiang Autonomous Region, in striped field mouse from Heilongjiang province, and in seven species of rodents, including *Rattus (Ra.) norvegicus*, *Ra. losea*, *Ra. flavipectus*, *Ra. niviventer*, *Mus musculus*, *Niviventer confucianus*, and *Ra. edwardsi*, and hares from Zhejiang and Fujian provinces (see Fig. 2.2) [4, 50, 66, 70–73]. *A. phagocytophilum* was first identified in *Ixodes (I.) persulcatus* from Heilongjiang province in 1997 [15], which is the most commonly encountered species in the family Anaplasmataceae located in wide areas with multifarious tick species as its vectors (see Fig. 2.1) [4]. In addition, *A. phagocytophilum* was reported to infect domestic animals, for example, goats, sheep, cattle, horses, dogs, yaks, as well as wild animals including hare and 24 rodent species (see Fig. 2.2) [4, 50, 63, 65, 66, 73, 75–83]. "*A. capra*" was first identified in goats and provisionally nominated by us, and then detected in *I. persulcatus* ticks in Heilongjiang province [17]. Although *Candidatus* Neoehrlichia mikurensis was initially detected in *I. persulcatus* and *H. concinna* ticks [18], and then was found in *D. silvarum* and *H. longicornis* ticks as well as various rodents from many areas in China [18, 87, 88]. The three other species such as *E. canis*, *Ehrlichia* sp. Tibet, and *A. platys* have not been found to infect humans. Data on infected ticks and animal hosts are shown in Figs. 2.1 and 2.2 [4, 13, 14, 16, 68, 74].

Human Infections

Four species of Anaplasmataceae, including *E. chaffeensis*, *A. phagocytophilum*, "*A. capra*," and *Candidatus* Neoehrlichia mikurensis, have been identified to cause human infections in China. The first human monocytic ehrlichiosis (HME) case was reported in Inner Mongolia in 1999 [38], and a total of 12 cases have been diagnosed, with four in Inner Mongolia, two in Beijing, two in Tianjin, and four in Shandong province [38, 66]. A cluster of ten human granulocytic anaplasmosis (HGA) cases was reported in Anhui province in 2006, which was thought to be caused by nosocomial transmission [84]. Additional 94 HGA cases have been reported in China, including 33 in Beijing, six in Tianjin, 41 in Shandong, one in Anhui, and four to five each in Henan, Hubei, and Inner Mongolia [38, 66, 75, 85, 86]. Seven cases infected with *Candidatus*

Neoehrlichia mikurensis were identified from 622 febrile patients in Heilongjiang province in 2010, and a series of 28 cases with "*A. capra*" infection have been reported in the same region [17, 18]. Undifferentiated clinical manifestations were shown in patients with the Anaplasmataceae species infections, for example, fever, malaise, myalgia, arthralgia, and gastrointestinal symptoms including diarrhea, nausea, vomiting, and anorexia. Laboratory abnormalities mainly include leukopenia, thrombocytopenia, elevated hepatic aminopherase, lactate dehydrogenase, and blood urea nitrogen [17, 18, 38, 66, 75, 84–86].

2.5 Emerging Infections with *Borrelia burgdorferi* Sensu Lato

B. burgdorferi sensu lato was first detected in both humans and *I. persulcatus* in Heilongjiang province of northeastern China in 1986 [19], which was later classified as *B. garinii* by molecular biological methods in our laboratory. Five other genospecies, including *B. valaisiana*, *B. sinica*, *B. afzelii*, *B. valaisiana*-related, and *B. burgdorferi* sensu stricto, were subsequently identified (see Table 2.1) [4].

Tick and Animal Infections

B. burgdorferi sensu lato were detected from 26 tick species (see Fig. 2.1) over a wide geographic range of 25 provinces in the mainland of China. *B. garinii* is the most common genospecies, which has been identified from multiple tick species (see Fig. 2.1) [65, 89–96]. It is found in various rodent species from many endemic areas [23, 50, 89, 95, 97, 98], and in dogs, sheep keds (*Melophagus ovinus*), and hares, respectively, from Yunnan, Tibet, and Gansu province (see Fig. 2.2) [99]. *B. afzelii* is the second most common genospecies, which is found in almost the same ticks and rodent species with a similar distribution to *B. garinii* [50, 89, 91, 93–95]. *B. valaisiana*-related, a genetically related but distinct genospecies of *B. valaisiana*, was detected in *I. granulatus* and *H. longicornis* ticks from Guizhou province, and in rodents from Guizhou and Zhejiang provinces [22, 93]. Three other genospecies, including *B. valaisiana, B. sinica,* and *B. burgdorferi* sensu stricto, have not been found to infect humans. Data on infected ticks and animals are shown in Figs. 2.1 and 2.2 [20, 23, 96, 102, 148–156].

Human Infections

Except for Tibet and Shanghai metropolis, Human cases infected with *B. burgdorferi* sensu lato have been reported frequently in almost all provinces in China. *B. garinii*, *B. afzelii*, and *B. valaisiana*-related have been identified to infect humans (see Table 2.2) [4, 19, 21, 23, 39, 100, 101, 133]. The genospecies causing thousands of Lyme disease cases in China have not been characterized [134–139]. We have summarized all the uncharacterized cases regardless of its specific genospecies. Infections caused by different genospecies of *B. burgdorferi* sensu lato may show slightly different clinical manifestations, for example, erythema migrans, arthritis or arthralgia, fever, headache, and fatigue [19, 21, 23, 39, 100, 101, 133–139]. Generally, clinical manifestations of human infections with *B. burgdorferi* sensu lato in China are relatively mild in comparison with those in the USA and Europe [39].

2.6 Emerging *Babesia* Infections

A total of 11 *Babesia* species, including *Ba. ovis*, *Ba. major*, *Ba. ovata*, *Ba. orientalis*, *Ba. motasi*, *Ba. caballi*, *Babesia* sp. Kashi, *Babesia* sp. Xinjiang, *Ba. microti*, *Ba. divergens*, and "*Ba. venatorum*," have been discovered in the mainland of China from 1982 to 2015 (see Table 2.1) [4].

Tick and Animal Infections

The transmission of *Babesia* was found to be associated with 13 tick species in China (see Fig. 2.1). *Ba. microti* was detected in *I. persulcatus* and *H. concinna* and in striped field mice and reed voles (*Microtus fortis*) from Heilongjiang province, in *H. longicornis* and dogs from Henan province, and in rodents from Heilongjiang, Henan, Fujian, and Zhejiangprovinces [32, 50, 69, 114, 115]. *Ba. divergens* was detected in *I. persulcatus*, *H. concinna*, *H. japonica*, and striped field mice in Heilongjiang province [32, 50]. "*Ba. venatorum*" was also detected in *I. persulcatus* from northeastern China [117]. No evidence was shown for the other eight species of *Babesia*, including *Ba. ovis*, *Ba. major*, *Ba. ovata*, *Ba. orientalis*, *Ba. motasi*, *Ba. caballi*, *Babesia* sp. Kashi, and *Babesia* sp. Xinjiang, that they infect humans. Data on their infected ticks and animals are shown in Figs. 2.1 and 2.2 [4, 24–31, 103–113].

Human Infections

The three species of *Babesia*, including *Ba. microti*, *Ba. divergens*, and "*Ba. venatorum*," have been reported to infect humans in the mainland of China (see Fig. 2.1) [4]. In Zhejiang province of eastern China, a case infected with *Ba. microti* was diagnosed by peripheral blood and bone marrow smears as well as PCR assay in 2011 [41]. Additional 10 patients infected with *Ba. microti* were diagnosed by PCR among 449 febrile patients with malaria-like symptoms in Yunnan province from 2012 to 2013 [116]. One case with co-infection with *Plasmodium vivax* and another with *Plasmodium falciparum* were found in these cases. Two cases infected with *Ba. divergens* were detected from 377 anemic patients in Shandong province in 2009 [40]. A pediatric case infected with "*Ba. venatorum*" was found from Xinjiang Autonomous Region [33]. A series of 48 cases infected with "*Ba. venatorum*" were found in our active surveillance at a sentinel hospital in northeastern China from 2011 to 2014, of which 32 were lab-confirmed cases, and 16 were probable cases [117]. This was the first report of endemic human "*Ba. venatorum*" infection anywhere in the world. In addition, two babesiosis cases with uncharacterized *Babesia* species were reported in Yunnan province in 1982 and one case was reported in 2008 [140, 141]. Clinical manifestations and laboratory abnormalities for these patients infected with *Babesia* mainly included fever, fatigue, anemia, and chills, as well as elevated hepatic aminopherase and C-reactive protein [33, 40, 41, 116, 117, 140, 141].

2.7 Emerging SFTSV Infections

SFTSV, a novel member of the genus *Bandavirus* in the Phenuiviridae family, was first identified in China by an enhanced active surveillance in selected provinces of China [34]. Because of a systematic review published [157], we provide only a brief description and some new information of the infection of this virus.

Tick and Animal Infections

SFTSV have been detected in *H. longicornis* and *Rh. microplus*, with a higher prevalence of infection in *H. longicornis* (4–9%) than in *R. microplus* (0–6%) [34, 118]. Various domestic and wild animals, including cattle, goats, pigs, dogs, chickens, and geese, as well as rodents and hedgehogs, may be infected by this virus [118, 119]. Goats and cattle were reported to have the highest seropositive rate in the studies in Shandong, Jiangsu, and Hubei provinces, and big animals usually had higher seropositive rates than small animals [119, 120].

Human Infections

As of 2013, a total of 2543 human SFTS cases have been reported to the China Centers for Disease Control and Prevention (CDC), including 154 deaths [34, 121–126]. The hotspots of incidence are located at the junction of Henan, Hubei, and Anhui provinces, and two areas in Shandong province in the middle-eastern China, as well as coastal area of Liaoning province in northeastern China. Clinical manifestations of SFTS patients are nonspecific, and mainly include a sudden onset of fever up to 38–41 °C, headache, fatigue, myalgia, respiratory tract symptoms, and gastrointestinal symptoms, for example, lack of appetite, nausea, vomiting, and diarrhea. Most patients develop rapidly into multiple organ failure with elevated levels of serum alanine aminotransferase, aspartate aminotransferase, lactate dehydrogenase, and creatine kinase; proteinuria and hematuria; and usually with thrombocytopenia, leukocytopenia, and lymphadenopathy [34, 125].

2.8 Factors Contributing to the Emergence of Tick-Borne Infections

This is no doubt that the progress and application of molecular technologies have led to the discovery of novel agents and facilitated the identification of human infections with pathogens previously identified in ticks. Thus, to some extent, the "emergence" of tick-borne infections has been caused by the application of more sensitive and reliable detection methods. On the other hand, it is likely that various biological and environmental factors causing an increase in the transmission and dissemination of tick-borne diseases might be the main causative factors of this "emergence." [3]

Changes in land use or land cover have affected the emergence of tick-borne diseases by changing the interactions and abundance of ticks, wild and domestic animal hosts, as well as human exposure to pathogens [158]. The emergence of Lyme disease in the northeastern USA is an example. The increased population of white-tailed deer is thought to be associated with the reforestation of this region during the twentieth century, which greatly increased the number of *I. scapularis*. Consequentially, the density of vector ticks grows and expands, contributing significantly to the emergence of Lyme disease in the northeastern USA [159]. In addition, fragmentation of forests in eastern regions of Canada and the USA might play an important role in the increase of the relative abundance of small mammals due to a decrease of predator communities, leading to an elevated infection rate of *B. burgdorferi* sensu lato in *I. scapularis* nymphs. Ultimately, people in these regions are confronted with a higher risk of infection with *B. burgdorferi* sensu lato [160, 161].

A "Greening" program to regain forests and grasslands from former agricultural lands has been initiated by the Chinese central government since the mid-1990s [162]. High-quality vegetative cover that benefited from the reforestation and grass replanting probably increases the abundance and diversity of vector ticks and animal hosts, and then favors the reestablishment of preexisting tick vector enzootic cycles in these regions. Our study of the most severely endemic region of SFTS showed an example, and our findings show that a 10% increase in areas of shrub, forest, and rain-fed cropland causes increased SFTS incidence rates of 51%, 51%, and 90%, respectively, which indicate that high risk of SFTS incidence might be significantly associated with vegetation-rich lands [163].

Urbanization is also associated with the emergence and increasing incidence of tick-borne infections. Studies in Europe indicate that the process of urbanization accompanied by encroachment into forested and uncultivated areas, and the protection of existing green spaces, has created opportunities for ticks to survive in urban areas, especially in suburban environments. In addition, the presence of many pets and domestic animals, which can serve as the hosts of ticks and pathogen reservoirs, might facilitate transmission of various human and animal pathogens by ticks [164, 165]. China has gone through the most rapid urbanization in its history in the past four decades. This rapid urbanization, accompanied by extensive rural-to-urban migration of the human population, intensive long-distance trade, and explosive short-term travel for shopping, has led to substantial health risks resulting from air pollution, occupational and traffic hazards, and altered diets and activity [166]. These changes in human activity, together with the increasing contact between humans, their pets, and nature, might have contributed to the increasing abundance of tick exposure, as observed in other developed countries [164]. Further investigations are needed to examine the relationship between emerging tick-borne infections and urbanization in China.

Less importance was given to global climate change in the recent emergence of most vector-borne zoonotic diseases, including tick-borne diseases, in comparison with changes in land use or land cover, human living conditions, animal host communities, and societal factors [3].

Although climatic factors are thought to have nonlinear effects on the transmission of infectious diseases, and even act in opposing directions in different climatic ecological regions, the seasonal dynamics and abundance of tick vectors are largely determined by climate conditions, which might further influence the species of tick-borne diseases and their seasonal patterns. An increasing temperature in winter has been recognized to be responsible for the northward extension and increased density of *I. ricinus,* which consequently elevated the dissemination risk of tick-borne diseases [167–169]. Although this topic is not settled, climatic change might play a role in the emergence of tick-borne diseases in China. Further studies are needed to better elucidate this issue.

2.9 Perspectives

Ticks are currently thought second only to mosquitoes as vectors of human infectious diseases in the world [170]. More than 120 tick species, including over 100 species in the Ixodidae "hard tick" family and 19 species in Argasidae "soft tick" family, have been reported in China up to 2015 [171]. They transmit a variety of pathogens while feeding on a number of animals, including humans as accidental hosts. In China, approximately 30 tick species have been identified to be able to bite humans [172, 173]. The diverse geographic distribution and abundance of vector ticks mostly depend on optimal environmental conditions and biotopes for each of them, which determine the risk areas for associated tick-borne zoonoses [3]. In addition to emerging tick-borne infections, previously recorded and well-established tick-borne diseases are also an ongoing threat to human health, for example, tick-borne encephalitis in northeastern and northwestern China, tularemia, and North-Asia tick-borne spotted fever in northern China, Crimean-Congo hemorrhagic fever in northwestern China, and Q-fever in wide areas throughout China [174–183].

A major diagnostic challenge was presented due to the nonspecific clinical manifestations caused by these emerging tick-borne pathogens, such as SFGR, *Anaplasma*, *B. burgdorferi* sensu lato, *Babesia*, and SFTSV, and a majority of physicians are unfamiliar with the various tick-borne diseases that have nonspecific symptoms in the early stage of the illness. The wide distributions of the 33 emerging tick-associated agents and their tick vectors, as well as the diversity of tick species throughout China, imply that reported cases might only be the tip of the iceberg, compared with the actual case number of tick-borne diseases. Rapid, convenient, and practical laboratory diagnostic methods are urgently needed for the reasonable differential diagnosis and the identification of specific pathogens of these emerging tick-borne diseases. Although China has made great progress in detecting and identifying various tick-borne pathogens and in diagnosing the infections, most hospitals still do not have the essential technologies. Unfortunately, the importance of tick-borne diseases to human and animal health has not been fully recognized due to the unavailability of etiological diagnosis and inadequate surveillance activities.

As mentioned above, 18 tick-borne agents, including four *Rickettsia* species, two *Ehrlichia* species, an *Anaplasma* species, three genospecies of *B. burgdorferi* sensu lato, and eight *Babesia* species, have been identified in ticks or animals in China, but their pathogenicity to humans is yet to be determined (see Table 2.1). Despite increasing knowledge of their distribution, the natural cycle of them and the natural history of their infections in vector ticks and animal hosts have yet to be elucidated. After the identification of potentially pathogenic agents in ticks, It may take many years to determine human infections, in part because the microbial loads in human blood are much lower than those in arthropods [184]. For example, *R. sibirica* sp. BJ-90 was first found in *D. sinicus* ticks in China in 1990 [7], but not identified to infect humans until 22 years later [36]. Similarly, *A. phagocytophilum* was initially found in China in 1997 [15], but nosocomial transmission of human granulocytic anaplasmosis was recognized 10 years later [84]. Therefore, the 18 tick-associated agents recognized in China in ticks or animals represent potential candidates for new tick-borne diseases. Similarly, the search for potential new pathogens in ticks is still essential for the discovery of emerging tick-borne diseases in humans.

A total of 33 tick species belonging to six genera have been found to be naturally infected with the emerging pathogenic agents described in this chapter. Except for the eight species including *D. abaensis*, *D. daghestanicus*, *H. bispinosa*, *H. flava*, *H. yeni*, *H. sinensis*, *I. myospalacis*, and *Rhipicephalus turanicus*), most tick species carry two or more agents. Conversely, some emerging agents such as *R. heilongjiangensis*, *A. phagocytophilum*, *E. chaffeensis*, and *B. garinii* can infect several tick species (see Fig. 2.1). In addition, tick-borne pathogens that currently infect domestic animals may eventually cause human disease. A representative example is *B. divergens*, which has long been recognized to cause cattle babesiosis in Europe, and was subsequently identified as a human pathogen [185]. In China, a number of emerging tick-borne agents are known to infect various domestic animals (see Fig. 2.2), and their potential to infect human warrants great attention and further investigation. As tick-borne diseases continue to emerge in China, it is critical for China and the rest of the world to improve our understanding of the existence and health burden of these diseases.

2.10 Search Strategy and Selection Criteria

We searched PubMed and ISI Web of Science for literature published in English, and WanFang database, China National Knowledge Infrastructure, and Chinese Scientific Journal Database for literature published in Chinese up to May 31, 2015. We used the following search terms: "tick-borne disease" or "tick-borne zoonotic disease" or "tick-borne zoonosis" or "tick-associated microbe" or "tick-associated agent" and "China," in combination with each of the five genera of tick-borne agents. We also performed a secondary manual search of the references cited in these articles to find relevant articles. We investigated all the articles with regard to detection, identification, or infections of these tick-borne microbes in humans, ticks, and animals. We also contacted the corresponding authors for detailed information such as the time of investigation, location, and origin of tick-borne agents if any of this information was missing in the articles.

References

1. Dantas-Torres F, Chomel BB, Otranto D. Ticks and tick-borne diseases: a one health perspective. Trends Parasitol. 2012;28:437–46.
2. Socolovschi C, Mediannikov O, Raoult D, Parola P. The relationship between spotted fever group rickettsiae and ixodid ticks. Vet Res. 2009;40:34.
3. Kilpatrick AM, Randolph SE. Drivers, dynamics, and control of emerging vector-borne zoonotic diseases. Lancet. 2012;380:1946–55.
4. Fang LQ, Liu K, Li XL, Liang S, Yang Y, Yao HW, et al. Emerging tick-borne infections in mainland China: an increasing public health threat. Lancet Infect Dis. 2015;15:1467–79.
5. Lou D, Wu YM, Wang B. A new specie in *Rickettsia*: isolation and identification of *Rickettsia heilongjiangii*. Chin J Microbiol Immunol. 1985;5:250. (in Chinese)
6. Zhang L, Raoult D, Fournier PE. '*Rickettsia hulinii*' belongs to the *Rickettsia heilongjiangensis* species. Clin Microbiol Infect. 2009;15(Suppl. 2):340–2.
7. Yu X, Jin Y, Fan M, Xu G, Liu Q, Raoult D. Genotypic and antigenic identification of two new strains of spotted fever group rickettsiae isolated from China. J Clin Microbiol. 1993;31:83–8.
8. Li W, Liu L, Jiang X, Guo X, Garnier M, Raoult D, et al. Molecular identification of spotted fever group rickettsiae in ticks collected in Central China. Clin Microbiol Infect Dis. 2008;15:279–80.
9. Tian ZC, Liu GY, Shen H, Xie JR, Luo J, Tian MY. First report on the occurrence of *Rickettsia slovaca* and *Rickettsia raoultii* in *Dermacentor silvarum* in China. Parasit Vectors. 2012;5:19.
10. Zou YX, Wang QY, Fu ZX, Liu PP, Jin HT, Yang HH, et al. Detection of spotted fever group *Rickettsia* in *Haemaphysalis longicornis* from Hebei Province, China. J Parasitol. 2011;97:960–2.
11. Jia N, Zheng YC, Jiang JF, Ma L, Cao WC. Human infection with *Candidatus* Rickettsia tarasevichiae. N Engl J Med. 2013;369:1178–80.
12. Cao WC, Gao YM, Zhang PH, Zhang XT, Dai QH, Dumler JS, et al. Identification of *Ehrlichia chaffeensis* by nested PCR in ticks from southern China. J Clin Microbiol. 2000;38:2778–80.
13. Pan H, Chen XR, Ma YH, SunY YQ, Tong SD, et al. *Ehrlichia canis* DNA found in ticks in the south of China. Chin J Zoonosis. 1999;15:3–6. (in Chinese)
14. Wen BH, Jian R, Zhang YZ, Chen R. Simultaneous detection of *Anaplasma marginale* and a new

Ehrlichia species closely related to *Ehrlichia chaffeensis* by sequence analyses of 16S ribosomal DNA in *Boophilus microplus* ticks from Tibet. J Clin Microbiol. 2002;40:3286–90.

15. Cao WC, Zhao QM, Zhang PH, Dumler JS, Zhang XT, Fang LQ, et al. Granulocytic Ehrlichiae in *Ixodes persulcatus* ticks from an area in China where Lyme disease is endemic. J Clin Microbiol. 2000;38:4208–10.
16. Pan H, Ma YH, Tong SD, Sun Y, Wen BH, Cheng XR. Canine ehrlichiosis caused simultaneously by *Ehrlichia canis* and *Ehrlichia platys*. Microbiol Immunol. 2000;44:737–9.
17. Li H, Zheng YC, Ma L, Jia N, Jiang BG, Jiang RR, et al. Human infections with a novel tick-borne *Anaplasma* species in China: a surveillance study. Lancet Infect Dis. 2015;15:663–70.
18. Li H, Jiang JF, Liu W, Zheng YC, Huo QB, Tang K, et al. Human infection with *Candidatus* Neoehrlichia mikurensis, China. Emerg Infect Dis. 2012;18:1636–9.
19. Ai CX, Wen YX, Zhang YG, Wang SS, Qiu QC, Shi ZX, et al. Clinical manifestations and epidemiological characteristics of Lyme disease in Hailin county, Heilongjiang Province, China. Ann N Y Acad Sci. 1988;539:302–13.
20. Masuzawa T, Takada N, Kudeken M, Fukui T, Yano Y, Ishiguro F, et al. *Borrelia sinica* sp. nov., a Lyme disease-related *Borrelia* species isolated in China. Int J Syst Evol Microbiol. 2001;51:1817–24.
21. Shi CX, Zhang ZF, Wan KL. Analyzing clinical samples of Lyme disease with 5s-23s rRNA gene spacer RFLP analysis. Chin J Zoonoses. 2000;16:21–3. (in Chinese)
22. Chu CY, Liu W, Jiang BG, Wang DM, Jiang WJ, Zhao QM, et al. Novel genospecies of *Borrelia burgdorferi* sensu lato from rodents and ticks in southwestern China. J Clin Microbiol. 2008;46:3130–3.
23. Hao Q, Hou X, Geng Z, Wan K. Distribution of *Borrelia burgdorferi* sensu lato in China. J Clin Microbiol. 2011;49:647–50.
24. Chen DM. Investigation report on sheep babesiosis with *Piroplasma ovis* infection. Chin J Vet Sci Tech. 1982;12:31–2. (in Chinese)
25. Lv WS, Yin H, Lv WX, Yu F, Zhang QC, Dou HF. Detection of *Babesia major* and the identification of its tick vector in the mainland of China. Chin J Vet Sci Tech. 1988;18:11–4. (in Chinese)
26. Bai Q, Liu GY, Zhang L, Zhang JY. Discovery and isolation of *Babesia ovata* in China. Chin J Vet Sci Tech. 1990;20:2–4. (in Chinese)
27. Liu ZL, Zhao JL, Ma LH, Yao BA. *Babesia orientalis* sp. nov. parasitized in buffalo *bubalus bubalis* in China (*Piroplasmida: Babesiidae*). Acta Veterinaria et Zootechnica Sinica. 1997;28:84–9. (in Chinese)
28. Yin H, Luo JX, Lv WS, Lv WX, Zhang QC, Wang YY, et al. Isolation and configuration observation of *Babesia motasi* and *Babesia ovis* inthe mainland of China. Chin J Vet Sci Tech. 1997;27:7–9. (in Chinese)
29. Li YZ, Lu WY, Song JG. Studies on etiology and integrated control measures of difficult equine diseases in Gansu Province, China. J Chin Agric Univ. 1998;S2:130. (in Chinese)
30. Luo JX, Yin H, Liu ZJ, Yang DY, Guan GQ, Liu AH, et al. Molecular phylogenetic studies on an unnamed bovine *Babesia* sp. based on small subunit ribosomal RNA gene sequences. Vet Parasitol. 2005;133:1–6.
31. Liu AH, Yin H, Guan GQ, Schnittger L, Liu ZJ, Ma ML, et al. At least two genetically distinct large *Babesia* species infective to sheep and goats in China. Vet Parasitol. 2007;147:246–51.
32. Yang LW, Hou Y, Li M, Wen ZQ, Yang J, Fan DH. Study of tick-borne pathogens at Heilongjiang Port. Chin Front Health Quar. 2007;30:77–82. (in Chinese)
33. Sun Y, Li SG, Jiang JF, Wang X, Zhang Y, Wang H, et al. *Babesia venatorum* infection in child, China. Emerg Infect Dis. 2014;20:896–7.
34. Yu XJ, Liang MF, Zhang SY, Liu Y, Li JD, Sun YL, et al. Fever with thrombocytopenia associated with a novel bunyavirus in China. N Engl J Med. 2011;364:1523–32.
35. Wu YM, Wei AM, Hu LM, Zhang YG, Zhang JZ, Zhang ZQ, et al. Study on aetiology of *Rickettsia heilongianggii* tick borne spotted fever. Chin Public Health. 2001;7:28–30. (in Chinese)
36. Jia N, Jiang JF, Huo QB, Jiang BG, Cao WC. *Rickettsia sibirica* subspecies *sibirica* BJ-90 as a cause of human disease. N Engl J Med. 2013;369:1176–8.
37. Jia N, Zheng YC, Ma L, Huo QB, Ni XB, Jiang BG, et al. Human infections with *Rickettsia raoultii,* China. Emerg Infect Dis. 2014;20:866–8.
38. Gao DQ, Cao WC, Zhang XT. Investigations on human *Ehrlichia* infectious people in Daxingan Mountains. Chin J Epidemiol. 2001;22:137–41. (in Chinese)
39. Ni XB, Jia N, Jiang BG, Sun T, Zheng YC, Huo QB, et al. Lyme borreliosis caused by diverse genospecies of *Borrelia burgdorferi* sensu lato in northeastern China. Clin Microbiol Infect. 2014;20:808–14.
40. Qi C, Zhou D, Liu J, Cheng Z, Zhang L, Wang L, et al. Detection of *Babesia divergens* using molecular methods in anemic patients in Shandong Province, China. Parasitol Res. 2011;109:241–5.
41. Lei YL, Wang XG, Yao LN, Mei JH, Lan JQ, Zeng CY, et al. Case report of human *Babesia* infections. Chin J Health Lab Tech. 2012;22:651–2. (in Chinese)
42. Kim KH, Yi J, Kim G, Choi SJ, Jun KI, Kim NH, et al. Severe fever with thrombocytopenia syndrome, South Korea, 2012. Emerg Infect Dis. 2013;19:1892–4.
43. Takahashi T, Maeda K, Suzuki T, Ishido A, Shigeoka T, Tominaga T, et al. The first identification and retrospective study of severe fever with thrombocytopenia syndrome in Japan. J Infect Dis. 2014;209:816–27.

44. McMullan LK, Folk SF, Kelly AJ, MacNeil A, Goldsmith CS, Metcalfe MG, et al. A new phlebovirus associated with severe febrile illness in Missouri. N Engl J Med. 2012;367:834–41.
45. Jado I, Oteo JA, Alda'miz M, Gil H, Escudero R, Ibarra V, et al. *Rickettsia monacensis* and human disease, Spain. Emerg Infect Dis. 2007;13:1405–7.
46. Sousa RD, Pereira BI, Nazareth C, Cabral S, Ventura C, Crespo P, et al. *Rickettsia slovaca* infection in humans, Portugal. Emerg Infect Dis. 2013;19:1627–9.
47. Pretorius AM, Birtles RJ. *Rickettsia mongolotimonae* infection in South Africa. Emerg Infect Dis. 2004;10:125–6.
48. Karine RO, Bernard R, Re S, Eric D. Scored antibody reactivity determined by immunoblotting shows an association between clinical manifestations and presence of *Borrelia burgdorferi* sensu stricto, *B. garinii*, *B. afzelii*, and *B. valaisiana* in humans. J Clin Microbiol. 1999;37:4086–92.
49. van Dam AP, Kuiper H, Vos K, Widjojokusumo A, de Jongh BM, Spanjaard L, et al. Different genospecies of *Borrelia burgdorferi* are associated with distinct clinical manifestations of Lyme borreliosis. Clin Infect Dis. 1993;17:708–17.
50. Hu MX, Zhang J, Fan DH, Fu WM, Sun XF, Yang LW. Detection of rodent infected by new tick pathogens in Suifenhe and Dongning Ports. Chin J Vector Bio Control. 2009;20:573–6. (in Chinese)
51. Sun XF, Ding SL, Hu MX, Guo XM, Zhao G. Study on tick-borne *Rickettsia* dermacentroxenus infection at Heilongjiang Port. Chin Front Health Quar. 2007;30:154–6. (in Chinese)
52. Wu YM, Liu GP, Wei AM, Hu LM, Zhang ZQ, Cai ZL, et al. Investigation of spotted fever group *Rickettsia* in the northeastern China. Chin J Public Health. 2003;19:1043–4. (in Chinese)
53. Hao GF, Li H, Sun Y, Ge RP, Qiao GQ, Li B, et al. Detection of tick and tick-borne pathogen in some ports of Inner Mongolia. Chin J Epidemiol. 2009;30:365–7. (in Chinese)
54. Li Y, Li ZK, Chen G, Kang M, Liu DX, Zhang YM. Identification and phylogenetic analysis of spotted fever group *Rickettsia* isolated from Qinghai province. Chin J Vet Sci. 2014;34:1956–61. (in Chinese)
55. Zhang LJ, Zhang JS, Fu XP, Luan MC. First identification of a *Rickettsia* closely related to *R. heilongjiangii* and *R. massilliae* in South China. Infect Dis Inf. 2006;19:65–7. (in Chinese)
56. Liang CW, Li J, Chang LT, Yu HL, Zhang LX, Zhang LJ, et al. Spotted fever group *Rickettsia* in Yunnan Province, China. Vector Borne Zoonotic Dis. 2012;12:281–6.
57. Jin YM, Zhang LJ, Sun LY, Lao SJ, Han J, Huang CH, et al. Epidemiological investigation of emerging spotted fever in Chengmai County, Hainan Province. Dis Surveill. 2011;26:18–22. (in Chinese)
58. Sun JM, Lin JF, Gong ZY, Chang Y, Ye XD, Gu SP, et al. Detection of spotted fever group Rickettsiae in ticks from Zhejiang Province, China. Exp Appl Acarol. 2015;65:403–11.
59. Wu YM, Wei AM, Hu LM, Liu XX, Yang Q, Zhang ZQ, et al. Identification of spotted fever group (SFG) H-5 strain isolated from the patient's blood samples. Chin J Zoonoses. 1998;14:23–6. (in Chinese)
60. Ye XD, Sun Y, Ju WD, Wang X, Cao WC, Wu MY. Vector competence of the tick *Ixodes sinensis* (*Acari: Ixodidae*) for *Rickettsia monacensis*. Parasit Vectors. 2014;7:512–8.
61. Sun X, Zhang GL, Liu R, Liu XM, Zhao Y, Zheng Z. Molecular epidemiological study of *Rickettsia raoultii* in ticks from Xinjiang, China. Chin J Epidemiol. 2013;34:756–7. (in Chinese)
62. Zhuang L, Wang CY, Tong YG, Tang F, Yang H, Liu W, et al. Discovery of *Rickettsia* species in *Dermacentor niveus* Neumann ticks by investigating the diversity of bacterial communities. Ticks Tick Borne Dis. 2014;5:564–8.
63. Dong X, Chen XP, Liu N, Dumler SJ, Zhang YZ. Co-circulation of multiple species of Rickettsiales bacteria in one single species of hard ticks in Shenyang, China. Ticks Tick Borne Dis. 2014;5:727–33.
64. Feng S, Wu H, Zhang LW, Lu ZX, Zhang CL, Li ZP, et al. Molecular epidemiological study of tick-borne spotted fever group *Rickettsia* in western mountain area of Hebei Province, China. Chin J Vector Bio Control. 2013;24:308–12. (in Chinese)
65. Sun X, Zhang GL, Liu XM, Zhao Y, Zheng Z. Investigation of tick species and tick-borne pathogens in Hoxud County of Xinjiang Uyghur Autonomous Region, China. Chin J Vector Biol Control. 2013;24:5–10. (in Chinese)
66. Dong T, Qu ZY, Zhang LJ. Detection of *A. phagocytophilum* and *E. chaffeensis* in patient and mouse blood and ticks by a duplex real-time PCR assay. PLoS One. 2013;8:e74796.
67. Li HM, Jiang BG, He J, Niu JJ, Wang JX, Sun Y, et al. Detection and identification of *Ehrlichia* sp. in *Boophilus microplus* ticks from Xiamen of Fujian Province. J Pathog Biol. 2006;1:174–6. (in Chinese)
68. Meng QL, Qiao J, Sheng JL, Wang JW, Wang WS, Yao N, et al. Survey on tick-borne Anaplasmataceae in the south edge of Gurbantunggut desert. Chin J Vet Sci. 2012;32:1158–63. (in Chinese)
69. Chen Z, Liu Q, Liu JQ, Xu BL, Lv S, Xia S, et al. Tick-borne pathogens and associated co-infections in ticks collected from domestic animals in Central China. Parasit Vectors. 2014;7:237.
70. Zhang LJ, Cui F, Wang LL, Zhang LL, Zhang JS, Wang SW, et al. Investigation of anaplasmosis in Yiyuan County, Shandong Province, China. Asian Pac J Trop Med. 2011;4:568–72.
71. Zhao QL, Huang L, Yang X, Meng QL, Li R, Chen PB, et al. 16s rRNA sequence analysis of *Anaplasma* and *Ehrlichia* in rodents from parts area of Xinjiang. Chin J Zoonoses. 2013;29:743–7. (in Chinese)
72. Gao YM, Zhang XT, Cao WC, Dai QH, Zhang PH, Chen ZG, et al. Detection of *Ehrlichia chaffeensis*

in ticks and rodents using semi-nested PCR. Chin J Zoonoses. 2000;16:25–8. (in Chinese)

73. Xu Z, Xu XH, Zhou YL, Feng L, Hou J, Zhou WQ, et al. Comprehensive surveillance of tick-borne diseases in Jiande, Zhejiang province, China. Chin J Vector Biol Control. 2014;25:350–3. (in Chinese)
74. Li Y, Chen Z, Liu Z, Liu J, Yang J, Li Q, et al. Molecular survey of *Anaplasma* and *Ehrlichia* of red deer and sika deer in Gansu, China in 2013. Transbound Emerg Dis. 2015;63(6):e228–36. https://doi.org/10.1111/tbed.12335.
75. Zhang LJ, Wang GQ, Liu QH, Chen CF, Li J, Long B, et al. Molecular analysis of *Anaplasma phagocytophilum* isolated from patients with febrile diseases of unknown etiology in China. PLoS One. 2013;8:e57155.
76. Zhang LJ, Liu H, Xu BL, Lu QY, Li L, Chang LT, et al. *Anaplasma phagocytophilum* infection in domestic animals in ten provinces/cities of China. Am J Trop Med Hyg. 2012;87:185–9.
77. Li GH, Yu Q, Zhang QX, Pan L, Zhang YN, Yao N, et al. Molecular epidemiology regarding, *Anaplasma phagocytophilum* in *Dermacentor silvarum* in Ningwu County, Shanxi Province. Chin J Epidemiol. 2012;33:642–3. (in Chinese)
78. Jiang JF, Jiang BG, Yu JH, Zhang WY, Gao HW, Zhan L, et al. *Anaplasma phagocytophilum* infection in ticks, China–Russia Border. Emerg Infect Dis. 2011;17:932–3.
79. Li Y, Kang FY, Yang JF, Sun CQ, Liu ZJ, Yin H. Prevalence and coexistence of *Anaplasma phagocytophilum* and *Borrelia burgdorferi* sensu lato in ticks in Gansu, Hunan and Guangdong provinces, China. Chin J Zoonoses. 2013;29:117–21. (in Chinese)
80. Yang JF, Liu ZJ, Guan GQ, Liu Q, Li YQ, Chen Z, et al. Prevalence of *Anaplasma phagocytophilum* in ruminants, rodents and ticks in Gansu, northwestern China. J Med Microbiol. 2013;62:254–8. (in Chinese)
81. Cao WC, Zhao QM, Zhang PH, Yang H, Wu XM, Wen BH, et al. Prevalence of *Anaplasma phagocytophila* and *Borrelia burgdorferi* in *Ixodes persulcatus* ticks from northeastern China. Am J Trop Med Hyg. 2003;68:547–50.
82. Zhang HL, Sun Y, Wang JJ. Investigation on foci severe fever with thrombocytopenia syndrome and human granulocytic anaplasmosis in Lujiang County. Chin J Dis Control Prev. 2015;19:273–6. (in Chinese)
83. Zhang YZ, Wang Y, Yang WH, Zhu XH, Pi ZL, Feng Y, et al. Seroprevalence and molecular biological investigation of commonly known *Rickettsia* species in rodents in Qujing Prefecture, Yunnan Province, China. Chin J Zoonoses. 2015;31:35–40. (in Chinese)
84. Zhang L, Liu Y, Ni D, Li Q, Yu Y, Yu XJ, et al. Nosocomial transmission of human granulocytic anaplasmosis in China. JAMA. 2008;300:2263–70.
85. Wang S, Kou ZQ, Wang M, Ren YY, Hu B, Fang M, et al. A survey and identification of co-infection of *Anaplasma phagocytophilum* and *Ehrlichia chaffeensis* in Shandong. Dis Surveill. 2012;27:642–3. (in Chinese)
86. Li Z, Ding SJ, Lv H, Chen Y, Hou PQ, Wang XJ. Investigation of one case of human granulocytic anaplasmosis in Shandong Province. Infect Dis Inf. 2009;22:165–8. (in Chinese)
87. Li H, Jiang JF, Tang F, Sun Y, Li ZD, Zhang WL, et al. Wide distribution and genetic diversity of "*Candidatus* Neoehrlichia mikurensis" in rodents from China. Appl Environ Microbiol. 2013;79:1024–7.
88. Lu QY, Cheng SY, Peng WL, Zhao JL, Jiang LP, Ge JH. *Candidatus* Neoehrlichia mikurensis infection on animals and related 16S rRNA gene analysis in Zhejiang Province. Chin J Epidemiol. 2012;33:993–4. (in Chinese)
89. Li MQ, Masuzawa T, Takada N, Ishiguro F, Fujita H, Iwaki A, et al. Lyme disease *Borrelia* species in northeastern China resemble those isolated from far eastern Russia and Japan. Appl Environ Microbiol. 1998;64:2705–9.
90. Jiang BG, Yao HW, Tong YG, Yang XF, Huang Y, Jiang JF, et al. Genome sequence of *Borrelia garinii* strain NMJW1, isolated from China. J Bacteriol. 2012;194:6660–1.
91. Chu CY, Jiang BG, He J, Gao Y, Zhang PH, Wu XM, et al. Genetic diversity of *Borrelia burgdorferi* sensu lato isolates from northeastern China. Vector Borne Zoonotic Dis. 2011;11:877–82.
92. Shi SG, Zhang F, Liu ZJ. Molecular epidemiological studies on *Borrelia burgdorferii* in ticks collected from several provinces and autonomous regions of northwestern China. Chin J Zoonoses. 2011;27:461–3. (in Chinese)
93. Chu CY, Jiang BG, Liu W, Zhao QM, Wu XM, Zhang PH, et al. Presence of pathogenic *Borrelia burgdorferi* sensu lato in ticks and rodents in Zhejiang, South-east China. J Med Microbiol. 2008;57:980–5. (in Chinese)
94. Wang HW, He J, Chu CY, Zhang PH, Wu XM, Huang HN, et al. Detection and genotyping of *Borrelia burgdorferi* sensu lato in ticks from some areas of China. J Pathog Biol. 2006;1:81–5. (in Chinese)
95. Zhang JJ, Zhang F, Li L, Liu ZJ. *Borrelia burgdorferi* infection and their genotypes in ticks and rodents collected from Maijishan region, Gansu Province, China. Chin J Zoonoses. 2015;31:357–60. (in Chinese)
96. Hou J, Ling F, Chai CL, Lu Y, Yu XH, Lin JF, et al. Prevalence of *Borrelia burgdorferi* sensu lato in ticks from Eastern China. Am J Trop Med Hyg. 2014;2:262–6.
97. Chu CY, He J, Zhao QM, Zhang PH, Wu XM, Jiang BG, et al. Molecular epidemiological studies on *Borrelia burgdorferi* in rodents collected in the forest area of several provinces and autonomous

regions of China. Chin J Zoonoses. 2006;22:817–20. (in Chinese)
98. Hou XX, Geng Z, Hao Q, Zhang Y, Wan KL. Rats, the primary reservoir hosts of *Borrelia burgdorferi* in six representative provinces, China. Chin J Zoonoses. 2010;26:1034–6. (in Chinese)
99. Zhan L, Chu CY, Zuo SQ, Wu XM, Dumler JS, Jia N, et al. *Anaplasma phagocytophilum* and *Borrelia burgdorferi* in rabbits from southeastern China. Vet Parasitol. 2009;162:354–6.
100. Tan YH, Liu Y, Wan KL, Hao Q, Sun H, Yu LH, et al. Molecular epidemiological study of *Borrelia burgdorferi* infection among population in Xinjiang, China. Chin J Vector Bio Control. 2013;24:297–300. (in Chinese)
101. Zhu X, Zhang L, Hou XB, Geng Z, Chen H, Chen T, et al. Investigation on Lyme disease of patients with arthritis or neurological disorders in Hainan province, China. Chin J Zoonoses. 2015;31:353–6. (in Chinese)
102. Zhang L, Wang ZY, Chen CF, Li YX, Zhang K, Du JY, et al. Isolation of *Borrelia burgdorferi* in *Ixodes* from four counties, in North Xinjiang. Chin J Epidemiol. 2014;35:262–5. (in Chinese)
103. Li W, Peng HS, Li XM. Diagnosis and treatment of a goat infected with *Babesia ovis*. Contemp Ani Hus. 2015;1:12–3. (in Chinese)
104. Luo JX, Yin H, Liu GY, Guan GQ, Liu ZJ, Liu AH, et al. Collection and identification of Piroplasma infected to cattle and sheep in China. Chin J Parasitol Parasit Dis. 2006;24:S48–52. (in Chinese)
105. Bai Q, Liu G, Han G, Hui Y. Isolation and complementary transmission of *Babesia ovata* in Zhangjiachuan of Gansu Province. Chin J Vet Sci Tech. 1994;24:9–10. (in Chinese)
106. He L, Feng HH, Zhang WJ, Zhang QL, Fang R, Xia L, et al. Occurrence of *Theileria* and *Babesia* species in water buffalo (*Bubalus babalis*, Linnaeus, 1758) in the Hubei Province, South China. Vet Parasitol. 2011;186:490–6.
107. Liu Q, Zhou YQ, Zhou DN, Liu EY, Du K, Chen SG, et al. Semi-nested PCR detection of *Babesia orientalis* in its natural hosts *Rhipicephalus haemaphysaloides* and buffalo. Vet Parasitol. 2006;143:260–6.
108. Niu QL, Luo JX, Guan GQ, Ma ML, Liu ZJ, Liu AH, et al. Detection and differentiation of ovine *Theileria* and *Babesia* by reverse line blotting in China. Parasitol Res. 2009;104:1417–23.
109. Sun CQ, Liu ZJ, Gao JL, Guan GQ, Ma ML, Luo JX, et al. Investigations into the natural infection rate of *Haemaphysalis qinghaiensis* with Piroplasma using a nested PCR. Exp Appl Acarol. 2008;44:107–14.
110. He SD, Che FM, Liu WQ. Investigation of *Babesia caballi* in areas around Qinghai Lake, China. Chin Animal Health Insp. 2007;24:28. (in Chinese)
111. Wang XS, Liu JY, Zhang L, Feng LG. Case report of horse *Babesia caballi* infection. J Quacul Feed. 2014;12:56–7. (in Chinese)
112. Yi CY, Guo QY, Xue H, Peng C, Ba YCH. Detection of pathogen DNA of *Babesia caballi* from *Rhipicephalus sanguineus* and *Dermacentor nuttalli*. Heilongjiang Animal Sci Vet Med. 2014;11:38–40. (in Chinese)
113. Guan GQ, Ma ML, Moreau E, Liu JL, Lu BY, Bai Q, et al. A new ovine *Babesia* species transmitted by *Hyalomma anatolicum anatolicum*. Exp Parasit. 2009;122:261–7.
114. Sun Y, Liu GP, Yang LW, Xu RM, Cao WC. *Babesia microti*-like rodent parasites isolated from *Ixodes persulcatus* (*Acari: Ixodidae*) in Heilongjiang Province, China. Vet Parasitol. 2008;156:333–9.
115. Zhao XG, Li H, Sun Y, Zhang YY, Jiang JF, Liu W, et al. Dual infection with *Anaplasma phagocytophilum* and *Babesia microti* in a *Rattus norvegicus,* China. Ticks Tick Borne Dis. 2013;4: 399–402.
116. Zhou X, Li SG, Chen SB, Wang JZ, Xu B, Zhou HJ, et al. Co-infections with *Babesia microti* and *Plasmodium* parasites along the China-Myanmar border. Infect Dis Poverty. 2013;2:24.
117. Jiang JF, Zheng YC, Jiang RR, Li H, Huo QB, Sun Y, et al. Epidemiological, clinical and laboratory characteristics of 48 cases with "*Babesia venatorum*" infection in China: a descriptive study. Lancet Infect Dis. 2015;15:196–203.
118. Zhang YZ, Zhou DJ, Qin XC, Tian JH, Xiong YW, Wang JB, et al. The ecology, genetic diversity, and phylogeny of Huaiyangshan virus in China. J Virol. 2011;86:2864–8.
119. Zhao L, Zhai SY, Wen HL, Cui F, Chi YY, Wang L, et al. Severe fever with thrombocytopenia syndrome virus, Shandong Province, China. Emerg Infect Dis. 2012;18:963–5.
120. Li ZF, Liu JL, Bao CJ, Li PF, Qi X, Qin YF, et al. Seroprevalence of antibodies against SFTS virus infection in farmers and animals, Jiangsu, China. J Clin Virol. 2014;60:185–9.
121. Ding F, Zhang WY, Wang L, Hu W, Soares MR, Sun J, et al. Epidemiologic features of severe fever with thrombocytopenia syndrome in China, 2011–2012. Clin Infect Dis. 2013;56:1682–3.
122. Gai ZT, Liang MF, Zhang Y, Zhang S, Jin C, Wang SW, et al. Person-to-person transmission of severe fever with thrombocytopenia syndrome Bunyavirus through blood contact. Clin Infect Dis. 2012;54:249–52.
123. Yu L, Yu P, Liu DH, Hou J, Chen YF. Surveillance of syndrome of fever with thrombocytopenia in Dalian, 2012–2013. Study Trace Eleme Health. 2014;31:5–6. (in Chinese)
124. Bao CJ, Guo XL, Qi X, Hu JL, Zhou MH, Varma JK, et al. A family cluster of infections by a newly recognized Bunyavirus in eastern China, 2007: further evidence of person-to-person transmission. Clin Infect Dis. 2011;53:1208–14.
125. Gai ZT, Zhang Y, Liang MF, Jin C, Zhang S, Zhu CB, et al. Clinical progress and risk factors for death in severe fever with thrombocytopenia syndrome patients. J Infect Dis. 2012;206:1095–102.
126. Liu K, Zhou H, Sun RX, Yao HW, Yu L, Wang LP, et al. A national assessment of the epidemiology

of severe fever with thrombocytopenia syndrome, China. Sci Rep. 2015;5:9679.
127. Fan MY, Walker DH, Liu QH, Li H, Bai HC, Zhang JK, et al. Rickettsial and serologic evidence for prevalent spotted fever rickettsiosis in Inner Mongolia. Am J Trop Med Hyg. 1987;36:615–20.
128. Lin BH, Sun XJ, Zhan ZN, Lin YZ, Li WG. Serological and etiological studies on undefined rickettsiosis on Hainan Island. J Hainan Med College. 1997;3:97–102. (in Chinese)
129. Lin YZ, Sun XJ, Zhan ZN, Li WG, Wang HM, Lin BH, et al. Serological and etiological studies on rickettsiosis in Hainan Island. Chin J Zoonoses. 1999;15:90–1. (in Chinese)
130. Shi H, Wang Y, Han H, Gao XL, Zhang YM, Zhang WJ, et al. Analysis of 92 patients with tick-borne diseases in Mudanjiang. Chin J Vector Bio Control. 2013;24:295–300. (in Chinese)
131. Fan MY, Wang JG, Jiang YX, Zong DG, Lenz B, Walker DH. Isolation of a spotted fever group *Rickettsia* from a patient and related ecological investigation in Xinjiang Uygur Autonomous Region of China. Am Soc Microbiol. 1987;25:628–32.
132. Wu J, Wang SL, Jin YM, Ma Y, Zeng XJ, Jia PB, et al. Detection of *groEL* gene in spotted fever group *Rickettsia* of patients with fever in Hainan province. Mod Pre Med. 2014;41:2417–9. (in Chinese)
133. Jiang BG, Zheng YC, Tong YG, Jia N, Huo QB, Fan H, et al. Genome sequence of *Borrelia afzelii* strain HLJ01, isolated from a patient in China. J Bacteriol. 2012;194:7014–5.
134. Geng Z, Hou XX, Hao Q, Hu GL, Wan KL. Anti-*borrelia burgdorferi* antibody response in 827 patients with suspected Lyme disease. Chin J Vector Bio Control. 2007;18:219–21. (in Chinese)
135. Zhou XY. The epidemiological and clinical analysis of Lyme disease in Mudanjiang from 1996 to 2003. Chin J Parasit Dis Control. 2005;18:159. (in Chinese)
136. Peng FB, Zhang WF, Zhou GP, Zhang SY, Yuan YM, Wu YY. The detection and clinical study on Lyme disease in Beijing. Chin J Epidemiol. 1994;15:10–3. (in Chinese)
137. Huang ZY, Hou XX, Wan KL. An investigation of Lyme disease in Pingjiang County, Hunan Province, China. Chin J Vector Bio Control. 2001;12:293–4. (in Chinese)
138. Li YL, Hao JG, Zhang ZF, Wan KL, Xia XZ, Zhang JS, et al. The investigation of Lyme disease in Nanchuan County, Sichuan Province, China. Chin J Vector Bio Control. 1991;2:54–6. (in Chinese)
139. Jin SW, Hao Q, Tian Z, Hou XX, Geng Z, Jiang Y, et al. Analysis of surveillance on Lyme disease in Xinjiang prospecting region of Henan oil prospecting bureau. Chin J Zoonoses. 2005;21:501–2. (in Chinese)
140. Li JF, Meng DB, Wang QF, Dong XR, Wang JY. The discovery of human babesiosis. Chin Vet. 1984;6:19–20. (in Chinese)
141. Wang HX. A case of human babesiosis in southwest region of China. Int J Med Parasit Dis. 2012;39:190–2. (in Chinese)
142. Zhang HL, Yang H, Zhang PH, Cao WC, Zhang YZ, Yuan QH, et al. Spotted fever group *Rickettsia* DNA was detected in wild rodents and ticks in Dali, Yunnan Province, China. Chin J Vector Bio Control. 2004;15:461–2. (in Chinese)
143. Huang HN, Ding Z, He J, Wu XM, Jiang BG, Gao Y, et al. Study on the coinfection status of *Borrelia burgdorferi* sensu lato and spotted fever group *Rickettsia* in ticks from Hunchun, Jinlin Province. Chin J Epidemiol. 2006;27:379–83. (in Chinese)
144. Jiang LP, Mo SH, Zheng SG, Meng Z, Chen SY, Xie SY, et al. Spotted fever group rickettsiae DNA was first detected in ticks in Zhejiang Province. Chin J Vector Bio Control. 2006;17:484–5. (in Chinese)
145. Wang Z, Liu XG, Luo Y, Li B, Yu D, Xu P, et al. Investigation of tick-borne spotted fever group *Rickettsia* in northwestern Liaoning Province, China. Animal Husbandry Vet Med. 2015;47:143–4. (in Chinese)
146. Chai CL, Sun JM, Lu QY, Ling F, Jiang LP, Ge JH, et al. A cross-sectional study on tick-borne *Rickettsiae* infections among murine-like animals. Zhejiang Prev Med. 2014;26:659–63. (in Chinese)
147. Wang Z, Yu M, Yang SJ, Qiu GB, Zhai RB, Guo ZY, et al. Epidemiological survey of spotted fever group *Rickettsia* in rodents in northeastern China. Chin Pre Med. 2015;16:184–6. (in Chinese)
148. Wang DM, Hao Q, Cai XH, Wan KL, Wang ZX, Chen J. Study on ribotyping of Lyme borreliosis spirochete in Guizhou Province. Chin J Epidemiol. 2003;24:1129–31. (in Chinese)
149. Yang Y, Zhang XL, Qiao S, Cao XM, Wang L, Hao GF, et al. Investigation on tick-borne pathogens at Ganqimaodu Port between Sino-Mongolia border. Chin Front Health Quar. 2011;34:339–42. (in Chinese)
150. Zuo SY, Tang K, Li Y, Yu JH, Zhang Y, Ni X, et al. DNA detection and sequence analysis of *Borrelia burgdorferi* sensu lato in rodents from Helongjiang forest region. Chin J Epidemiol. 2012;33:643–4. (in Chinese)
151. Yang XF, Wan KL, Lu JP, Temu QH, Zhang ZF, Han XZ, et al. Investigation of geographical epidemiology and etiological studies on Lyme disease in Inner Mongolia. Chin J Zoonosis. 1999;15:98. (in Chinese)
152. Yang XJ, Wan KL, Wang CS, Hao Q, Wang YH, Hou XX, et al. Etiological studies on Lyme disease in Jilin Province. Chin J Health Lab Tech. 2006;16:1355–62. (in Chinese)
153. Zhang DC, Hong Y, Zhang ZQ, Sun GJ, Dong SD, Zhang ZF, et al. Isolation of *Borrelia burgdorferi* in ticks and rodents in Liaoning Province. Chin J Vector Bio Control. 1992;3:19. (in Chinese)
154. Tian WC, Moldenhauer S, Li MQ, Zhang ZK, Guo YX, Wang LN, et al. The first detection of *Borrelia*

burgdorferi in *H. japonica*. Chin J Zoonosis. 1995;11:22–5. (in Chinese)
155. Zhang ZC, Tian WC, Guo YX, Wang LN, Yu QL, Li YP, et al. Investigation of Lyme disease in Hebei Province. Chin J Public Health. 1995;11:253–4. (in Chinese)
156. Wang LJ, Chen ZL, Wan KL, Liu SL, Tao XY, Zhang JS, et al. First isolation and identification of Lyme disease spirochete in Shandong Province. Chin J Vector Bio Control. 1997;8:127–8. (in Chinese)
157. Liu Q, He B, Huang SY, Feng W, Zhou XQ. Severe fever with thrombocytopenia syndrome, an emerging tick-borne zoonosis. Lancet Infect Dis. 2014;14:763–72.
158. Lambin EF, Tran A, Vanwambeke SO, Linard C, Soti V. Pathogenic landscapes: interactions between land, people, disease vectors, and their animal hosts. Int J Health Geogr. 2010;9:54.
159. Barbour AG, Fish D. The biological and social phenomenon of Lyme disease. Science. 1993;260:1610–6.
160. Levi T, Kilpatrick AM, Mangel M, Wilmers CC. Deer, predators, and the emergence of Lyme disease. Proc Natl Acad Sci U S A. 2012;109:10942–7.
161. LoGiudice K, Duerr ST, Newhouse MJ, Schmidt KA, Killilea ME, Ostfeld RS. Impact of host community composition on Lyme disease risk. Ecology. 2008;89:2841–9.
162. Liu JG, Li SX, Ouyang ZY, Tam C, Chen XD. Ecological and socioeconomic effects of China's policies for ecosystem services. Proc Natl Aacd Sci USA. 2008;105:9477–82.
163. Liu K, Cui N, Fang LQ, Wang BJ, Lu QB, Peng W, et al. Epidemiologic features and environmental risk factors of severe fever with thrombocytopenia syndrome, Xinyang, China. PLoS Negl Trop Dis. 2014;8:e2820.
164. Uspensky I. Tick pests and vectors (*Acari: Ixodoidea*) in European towns: introduction, persistence and management. Ticks Tick Borne Dis. 2014;5:41–7.
165. Uspensky I. Ticks (*Acari: Ixodoidea*) as urban pests and vectors with special emphasis on ticks outside their geographical range. Proceedings of the Sixth International Conference on Urban Pests 2008:333–47.
166. Gong P, Liang S, Carlton EJ, Jiang QW, Wu JY, Wang L, et al. Urbanisation and health in China. Lancet. 2012;379:843–52.
167. Parola P. Tick-borne rickettsial diseases: emerging risks in Europe. Comp Immun Microbiol Infect Dis. 2004;27:297–304.
168. Altizer S, Ostfeld RS, Johnson PT, Kutz S, Harvell CD. Climate change and infectious diseases: from evidence to a predictive framework. Science. 2013;341:514–9.
169. Harrus S, Baneth G. Drivers for the emergence and re-emergence of vector-borne protozoal and bacterial diseases. Int J Parasitol. 2005;35:1309–18.
170. Parola P, Raoult D. Ticks and tickborne bacterial diseases in humans: an emerging infectious threat. Clin Infect Dis. 2001;32:897–928.
171. Yang XJ, Chen Z, Liu JZ. Advances in systematics of ticks. Acta Entomol Sin. 2007;50:941–9. (in Chinese)
172. Meng YC. Ticks, acari, and human diseases. 1st ed. Hefei: Chin Sci Tech Press; 1995. p. 43. (in Chinese)
173. Cao WC, Zhang XT, Xu RM. The medical significance of tick and tick-borne disease in public health. Chin J Public Health. 1999;15:221–2. (in Chinese)
174. Wu XB, Na RH, Wei SS, Zhu JS, Peng HJ. Distribution of tick-borne diseases in China. Parasit Vectors. 2013;6:119.
175. Zhao JW, Wang HY, Wang Y. Regional distribution profiles of tick-borne pathogens in China. Chin J Bio Control. 2012;18:45–8. (in Chinese)
176. Zhan L, Cao WC, Jiang JF, Zhang XA, Liu YX, Wu XM, et al. *Anaplasma phagocytophilum* from rodents and sheep, China. Emerg Infect Dis. 2010;16:764–8.
177. Wang YY, Li J, Wang S, Hu M, Lu FL. Tick-borne infectious diseases. Infect Dis Inf. 2011;24:58–61. (in Chinese)
178. Lu Z, Broker M, Liang G. Tick-borne encephalitis inthe mainland of China. Vector Borne Zoonotic Dis. 2008;8:713–20.
179. Xia H, Li P, Yang J, Pan L, Zhao J, Wang Z, et al. Epidemiological survey of Crimean-Congo hemorrhagic fever virus in Yunnan, China, 2008. Int J Infect Dis. 2011;15:e459–63.
180. Wang Y, Peng Y, Hai R, Xia L, Li H, Zhang Z, et al. Diversity of *Francisella tularensis* Subsp. *holarctica* lineages, China. Emerg Infect Dis. 2014;20:1191–4.
181. Chen M, Fan MY. A review on the research of North-Asia tick-borne spotted fever. Chin Public Health. 1997;6:373–6. (in Chinese)
182. Liu YF, Zhang Y. The study progress of Q fever and *Ehrlichiosis*. Med Recap. 2008;6:864–7. (in Chinese)
183. Suss J. Tick-borne encephalitis 2010: epidemiology, risk areas, and virus strains in Europe and Asia–an overview. Ticks Tick Borne Dis. 2011;2:2–15.
184. Philippe P, Paddock CD, Socolovschi C, Labruna MB, Mediannikov O, Kernif T, et al. Update on tick-borne rickettsioses around the world: a geographic approach. Clin Microbiol Rev. 2013;26:657–702.
185. Colwella DD, Dantas-Torresb F, Otranto D. Vector-borne parasitic zoonoses: emerging scenarios and new perspectives. Vet Parasitol. 2011;182:14–21.

Progress on Epidemiology of Influenza A(H1N1) 3

Shigui Yang, Yuqing Zhou, and Lanjuan Li

Abstract

Pandemic influenza A(H1N1) in 2009 is an acute respiratory infectious disease caused by the mutated novel influenza A(H1N1) virus. Patients usually present with influenza-like symptoms, and some may progress to severe cases. Influenza A(H1N1) was once called "human infection" with swine influenza virus, and novel H1N1 influenza in the early stage. Later, it was confirmed that the pathogen of this influenza was not the classical swine influenza virus, but a mutated novel virus. The World Health Organization (WHO) officially named this influenza as pandemic influenza A(H1N1), and the virus was known as human A(H1N1) virus. The virulence of influenza A(H1N1) is strong and can be spread across species. After the outbreak, Chinese scientists developed a safe and effective licensed influenza A(H1N1) vaccine, inoculating 105 million people nationwide, and establishing a large-scale vaccine safety surveillance system. With the further development of the epidemic, the activity and virulence of the virus gradually weakened, and influenza A (H1N1) gradually evolved into a subtype of seasonal influenza. In recent years, the overall global activity of influenza A (H1N1) is low, but it is still active in some tropical regions.

Keywords

Influenza A(H1N1) · Vaccine · Epidemiology

3.1 Etiology of Influenza A(H1N1)

3.1.1 Structure and Biological Characteristics of Influenza A(H1N1) Virus

3.1.1.1 Structure of Influenza A(H1N1) Virus

Influenza A(H1N1) virus belongs to the family of Orthomyxoviridae and is a subtype of influenza virus. Its diameter is 80–120 nm, with a round or slenderness shape. It is a single-stranded negative RNA virus with a genome of about 13.6 k. The virus is composed of three layers. The inner layer is the nucleocapsid of the virus, which is spiral symmetry with a diameter of 10 nm. It contains nucleoprotein (NP), polymerase protein, and RNA. NP is a soluble antigen with type specificity and stable antigenicity. Polymerase protein may be a polymerase required for RNA transcription and replication. The middle layer is a viral envelope, which is composed of bilayer lipid membrane and matrix protein (MP). MP also has

S. Yang (✉) · Y. Zhou · L. Li
State Key Laboratory for Diagnosis and Treatment of Infectious Diseases, The First Affiliated Hospital, Zhejiang University School of Medicine, Hangzhou, China
e-mail: yangshigui@zju.edu.cn

D.-Q. Ye (ed.), *Progress in China Epidemiology*, https://doi.org/10.1007/978-981-19-2199-5_3

stable antigenicity and type specificity. The outer layer is composed of two different glucoproteins, including hemagglutinin (HA) and neuraminidase (NA). Both HA and Na have variation characteristics, so only strain-specific antigenicity is found. HA can cause red blood cell agglutination, which is a tool for virus to attach to the surface of host cells. And NA can hydrolyze sialic acid protein and N-acetylneuraminic acid at the end of cell surface-specific glycoprotein receptor, which is a tool for virus to leave cell surface after virus replication. See Table 3.1.

3.1.1.2 Classification of Influenza Viruses

Influenza viruses are classified into influenza A, influenza B, and influenza C based on the antigenicity of NP. Influenza A virus has the strongest antigenic variability and can infect humans and other animals, causing moderate and severe diseases. Influenza A virus attacks all age groups and has caused several global pandemics. Influenza B virus has weak variability, only infects humans and generally causes mild diseases. Influenza B virus mainly attacks children and can cause local outbreaks. The antigenicity of influenza C virus is relatively stable, only sporadic cases were caused. Influenza A virus is also divided into many subtypes according to different antigens of hemagglutinin (HA) and neuraminidase (NA). HA has 18 subtypes (H1–H18) and N has 11 subtypes (N1–N11). Among them, the three subtypes of H1N1, H2N2, H3N2 mainly infect humans, and the natural hosts of many other subtypes are birds and other animals. But in recent years, highly pathogenic avian influenza viruses such as H5N1, H7N9, and H9N2 have been found to infect humans. In addition, the H17 and H18 subtypes are newly discovered subtypes in recent years. H17 was isolated from fruit bats in 2012, while H18 was discovered from Peruvian bats in 2013. Figure 3.1 shows the five major pandemic influenza viruses originating from cross-species transmission of influenza viruses.

3.1.2 Origin of Influenza A(H1N1) Virus

The swine influenza A(H1N1) strain that caused the global pandemic in April 2009 was not a classic swine influenza virus, but a new strain of

Table 3.1 Gene fragments, corresponding encoded proteins, and functions of Influenza A(H1N1) virus

Gene		Protein	Length	Function
PB2		Polymerase basic protein 2	2341	RNA transcriptase, cutting the mRNA caps of host cells and virus, and capping
PB1		Polymerase basic protein 1	2341	The major component of RNA transcriptase, initiation of transcription and extension of RNA synthesis
PA		Polymerase acidic protein	2233	RNA transcriptase component
HA		Hemagglutinin	1778	Identification and binding of receptors, fusion of host cell membrane, induction of neutralizing antibodies, and the basis of virus subtype typing
NP		Nucleoprotein	1565	Formation transcriptase complex with PB2, PB1 and PA, the structural component of RNA transcriptase, prevention RNA from degradation, and the basis of virus typing
NA		Neuraminidase	1458	Hydrolyzation the terminal sialic acid residue, promotion the release of viruses from the surface of infected cells and the basis of virus subtype typing
M	M1	Matrix protein	1027	Regulation the assembly of progeny virus particles and stabilization the core of virus particles
	M2	Ion channel		Ion channel
NS	NS1	Non-structural protein 1	890	Participation in mRNA synthesis and blocking protein synthesis of host cells
	NS2	Non-structural protein 2		–

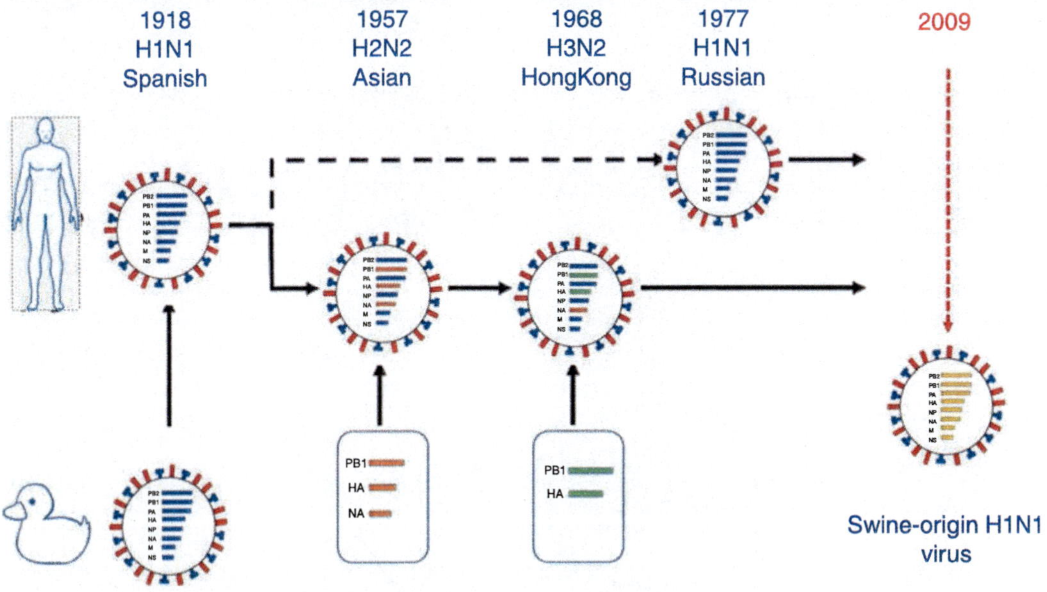

Fig. 3.1 Five major pandemic influenza viruses originating from cross-species transmission of influenza viruses

influenza virus. The nucleocapsid protein of the virus was type A. In 2009, it was isolated from a human host H1N1 influenza virus strain derived from a specimen from California, USA. Its serial number is 04. Therefore, its exact name is A/California/04/2009 (H1N1). Recent studies have systematically described the genetic and antigenic characteristics of influenza A(H1N1) viruses. The new influenza A(H1N1) viruses are eight influenza gene fragments (PB2, PB1, PA, HA, NP, NA, M, NS), of which six fragments (PB2, PB1, PA, HA, NP, NS) are from the triple recombination of avian, swine and human influenza viruses, and the other two fragments (NA, M) originate from swine flu virus in Europe and Asia. Figure 3.2 shows the gene recombination of influenza A (H1N1).

Judging from the origin of the influenza A(H1N1) virus in this epidemic, the HA gene nucleotide sequence of the influenza A(H1N1) virus strain was more than 93% homologous to the H1N2 swine influenza virus strain isolated from the United States earlier. And it has 95% homology with Indiana H1 subtype swine influenza virus (A/Swine/Indiana/P12439/00 (H1N2)). These suggested that the HA gene of the influenza A(H1N1) virus was mutated from the native swine influenza virus in North and Central America. There was no nucleotide deletion in the NA gene, and its sequence had the characteristics of the Eurasian strain of swine influenza virus. Viruses with more than 90% NA gene homology were derived from the H1N1 swine influenza virus in Eurasia, and the nucleotide homology with A/Swine/England/195852/92(H1N1) and A/swine/Spain/WVL6/1991(H1N1) strains was as high as 94%. The nucleotide sequence of the M gene also had the highest homology with the Eurasian strain of swine influenza virus, reaching 96%. It suggested that NA and M genes were derived from swine influenza viruses of Eurasian strains. The nucleotide sequence of PB1, PB2, NP, NS gene had the highest homology with swine influenza viruses isolated from the United States and South Korea, reaching 96%. The nucleotide sequence of the PA gene had the highest homology with swine influenza viruses isolated from the United States, reaching 96%. And the PB2 and PA genes also shared 96% homology with the H3N2 avian influenza virus isolated from South Dakota in 2007.

How this combination of recombinant viruses with typical swine flu virus characteristics came from, how they infected humans, and why they spread only from person to person but not in pigs have not been fully explained. This new type of

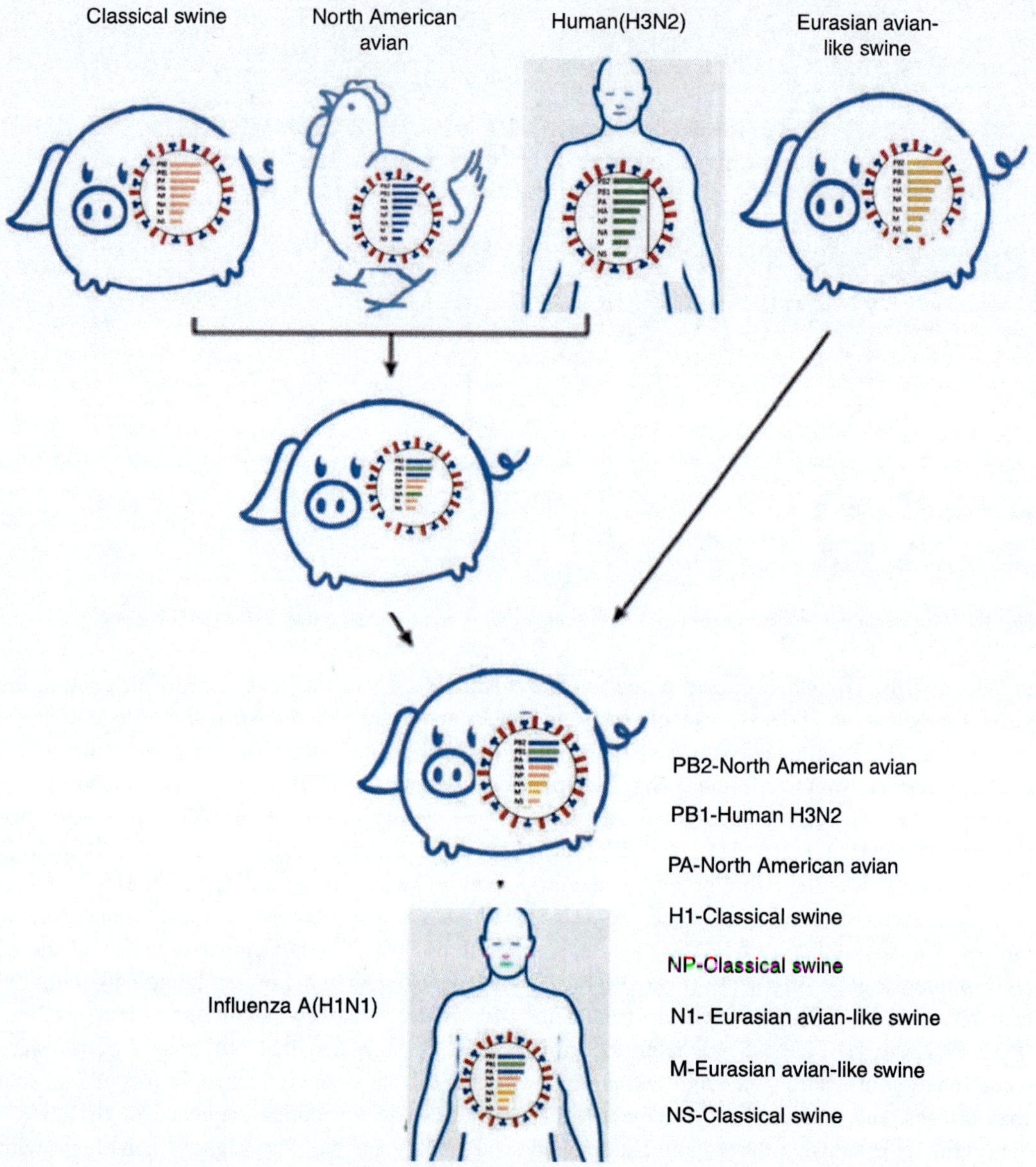

Fig. 3.2 The gene recombination of influenza A (H1N1)

influenza virus was a mixture of two swine flu viruses from North and Central America, Europe, and Asia, which has never been found to infect pigs. And it was never isolated from the swine flu and human flu virus in the United States and other countries and there is no report of virus sequences with similar gene combinations in GenBank. The Eurasian swine flu virus is usually only circulating in Europe and Asia, and it has not been reported to have been found in humans. Humans generally lack immunity to this virus, which may be one of the reasons for the rapid spread of this virus in humans.

Chinese scientists have successfully analyzed the crystal structure of the NA and HA of the new virus for the first time, explained the antigenic similarity between the influenza A(H1N1)pdm09 virus and the 1918 influenza pandemic virus from the three-dimensional structure, and clarified the antigen determinants shared with seasonal influenza virus. At the beginning of the epidemic, in response to the foreign questions about the possible origin of influenza A(H1N1)pdm09 virus in China, tens of thousands of samples of acute respiratory infections collected in the past were screened for influenza A(H1N1) virus, and no positive result was found. At the same time, the level of antibodies against influenza A(H1N1) virus was tested in the population of each age group before the occurrence of the epidemic, which indicated that all-age groups in China were generally susceptible to influenza A(H1N1) virus. The sequence analysis of the virus isolated from the first case showed that the virus was highly similar to the virus isolated from the United States and Mexico. The above research results confirmed that the influenza A(H1N1) pdm09 did not originate in China.

3.1.3 Cross-Species Transmission and Host of Influenza A(H1N1) Virus

3.1.3.1 Cross-Species Transmission of Influenza A(H1N1) Virus

The infection cycle of influenza virus can be divided into several processes: the adsorption of the virus to the receptor, the entry of the virus into the cell, the replication and synthesis of viral genes and proteins, and the packaging and release of the virus. In each link of the infection process, the interaction mechanism between the virus and the host cell determines the replication efficiency of the virus, and the replication efficiency of the virus determines the pathogenicity and transmission of the virus. The highly pathogenic influenza virus is closely related to its rapid replication ability. Therefore, the molecular basis of virus-host interaction during virus infection is the key to cross-species transmission and pathogenicity of viruses.

The adsorption of viruses to cell receptors is the first step of infection. Avian and human influenza viruses recognize different types of cell surface receptors. The avian influenza virus specifically binds to the Sia2, 3Gal receptor, while the human influenza virus specifically binds to the Sia2, 6Gal receptor [1]. The structure of HA of avian influenza and human influenza virus determines the specificity of the receptor, and the distribution of different receptors between avian and human also causes the host restriction of avian influenza and human influenza. Pigs are considered to be a "mixer" of avian and human flu. Its respiratory tract has both poultry and human receptors [2], so these two viruses can infect pigs. When these two viruses infect pigs at the same time, they may recombine to form a new virus. The cross-species infection is limited in the avian and human viruses due to the specificity of their receptors. Certain avian influenza viruses have been able to infect humans to a limited extent, although their specific receptors mainly exist in poultry. The influenza A(H1N1) pdm09 virus was once generally considered to be transmitted from pigs to humans [3]. and effectively spread among people. However, studies have found that the influenza pandemic influenza A(H1N1) virus had dual receptor binding capabilities [4]. Therefore, an in-depth study of the adaptability of influenza viruses in different hosts is very important to assess the possibility of viruses infecting humans. In addition, there are many subtypes of influenza virus and the hemagglutinin binding receptor region of these subtypes has its own uniqueness in sequence. Clarifying the structural requirements of different subtypes on the receptor-binding region and understanding the structural basis that determines the receptor specificity of influenza viruses can help identify the adaptability of influenza viruses in receptor binding.

The combination of virus and receptor is very important for infection, but it cannot determine whether it can successfully cause cross-species transmission. The H9N2 subtype avian influenza virus has been found to infect humans since 1999 [5]. Experimental studies on the binding of the virus to the receptor have found that the H9N2 virus has the ability to bind to the human receptor. At the same time, the H9N2 virus is widespread in poultry [6]. However, current data show that the H9N2 virus infects people only occasionally. These phenomena indicate that in addition to receptor specificity, there are other factors that determine cross-species transmission. After the virus enters the cell, its genome replicates, transcribes, and synthesizes viral proteins in the infected cell. These processes largely depend on the cell's mechanism. Studies have found that certain factors in mammalian cells have a limiting effect on avian influenza viruses which play a role in the replication mechanism of influenza viruses [7]. Influenza virus polymerase complex subunit PB2 and viral nucleoprotein NP have been proved to be the targets of cell limiting factors. These and some undiscovered interactions between cells and viruses are one of the obstacles to the cross-species transmission of influenza viruses. Therefore, studying the role of cell limiting factors in influenza virus replication, transcription and protein synthesis can help determine the functions of those cell limiting factors and provide a scientific basis for the viral targets for new drugs.

Viral infection can induce anti-infective response in the cells, and influenza virus is no exception. The relationship between infection and cell resistance to infection forms another interaction between influenza virus and infected cells, which is also one of the obstacles to the cross-species transmission of influenza virus. During the evolution of mammals, perfect innate immunity has gradually formed to resist viral infections, but many viruses also have mechanisms to evade and fight against the natural immunity of cells. It is known that the non-structural protein NS1 of influenza virus can fight against cellular immunity. NS1 of influenza virus participates in the role of a variety of cellular antiviral signal transduction channels and forms a complex network between infection and the immune system. Recent studies have found that NS1 antagonizes the upstream infection sensing signals in cellular natural immunity, such as RIG-I and OAS. And at the same time, it has direct interaction with cellular antiviral factors such as PKR, PI3K and NF90. The antagonistic mechanism of NS1 with antiviral cell restriction factors and signal transduction is another important part of influenza virus cross-species transmission and host restriction, and it is also a potential target of antiviral drugs.

The release of the virus from the host cell after replication and packaging is one of the keys for the virus to complete the infection cycle. The surface protein of influenza virus and the function of NA are the key to control the release of influenza virus. At present, several major anti-influenza drugs, including Tamiflu and Relenza, all target NA. The adsorption and release of influenza viruses are two opposite processes and are controlled by two surface proteins HA and NA respectively. How these two proteins reach a functional balance during the virus infection process is another important factor for influenza viruses to adapt to new hosts and is also a key part of studying the cross-species transmission of influenza viruses.

3.1.3.2 The Hosts and Receptors of Influenza A Virus

Influenza A virus is a type of animal-derived virus, which can form a variety of serological subtypes through different combinations of surface proteins. Waterfowl are the natural hosts of all influenza viruses, and some avian influenza viruses have gradually adapted to the new hosts including humans through cross-species infection. Since the influenza pandemic in 1918, there have been four pandemics, including the pandemic influenza A(H1N1). Molecular analysis of virus genes indicates that these four influenza pandemics are caused by the new viruses produced by the recombination of the animal-derived virus and the prevailing human influenza virus. The HA of influenza A virus is a major determinant of host restriction. The binding of HA to the receptor on the host cell is a key step for influenza virus to infect the host. The host receptors recognized by HA are divided into two categories: α-2,3-galactoside sialic acid (SA2,3Gal) and α-2,6-galactoside sialic acid (SA2,6Gal). Avian and equine-derived influenza viruses have affinity for SA2,3Gal receptors, while human and swine influenza viruses have the highest affinity for SA2,6Gal receptors. Human respiratory epithelial cells mainly contain SA2, 6Gal receptors, while pig respiratory epithelial cells contain both SA2, 3Gal and SA2, 6Gal receptors. Therefore, both avian and human influenza viruses can infect pigs, which makes it possible for two or more influenza strains of different subtypes to reassort genes in pigs. Pigs are considered to be the intermediate host and gene evolutionary recombination of avian and human influenza viruses. See Fig. 3.3.

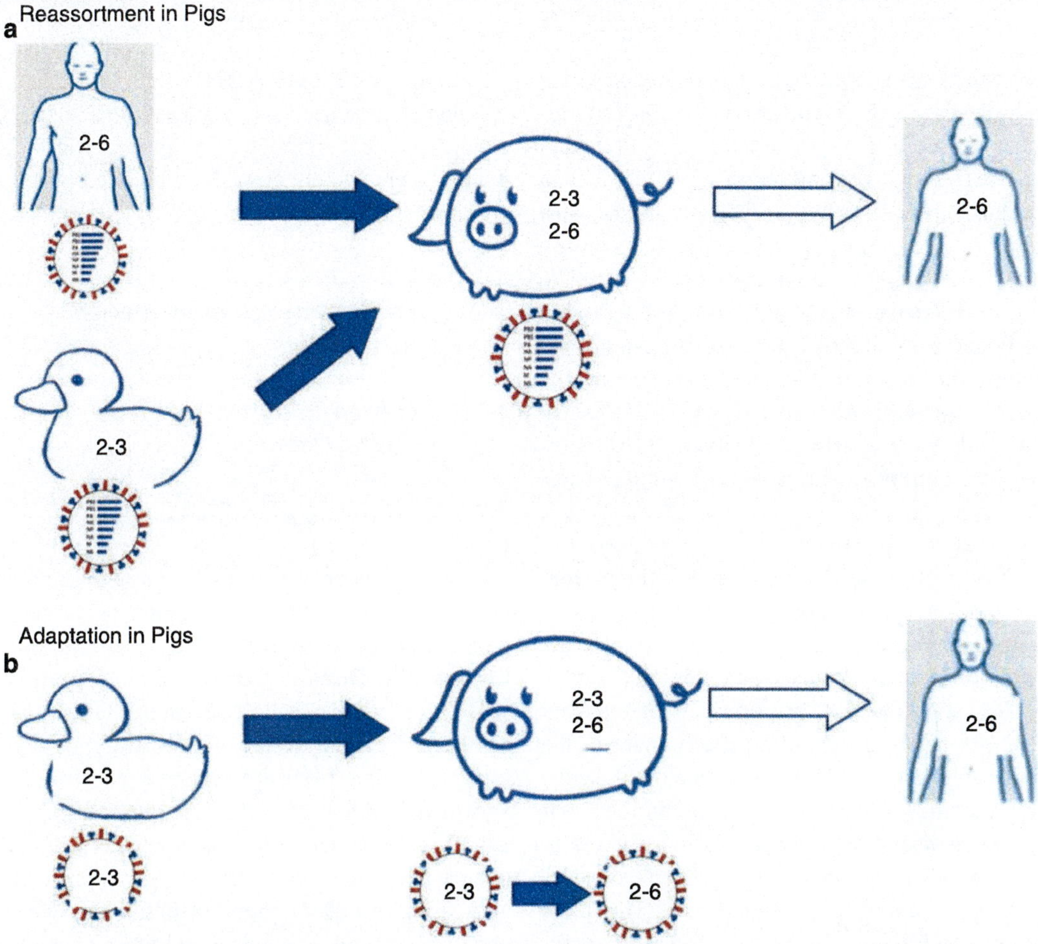

Fig. 3.3 Pig is an intermediate host and gene mixer for avian and human influenza viruses. (**a**) Reassortment in Pigs. (**b**) Adaptation in Pigs

3.1.4 Virulence and Drug Susceptibility of Influenza A(H1N1)

3.1.4.1 Virulence of Influenza A(H1N1)

The glycation of Influenza A(H1N1), especially the increase or decrease of the glycation sites near the head of RBS or the epitopes, has certain effects on the antigenicity and biological characteristics of the virus. The glycation, if happens on receptor binding sites, can affect the ability of virus to bind to receptors; if glycation appears on cleavage sites, it can make direct impact upon the cleavage of HA proteins; while the glycation of antigen-determining sites can lead to the production of protective neutralizing antibodies. Amino acids at positions 98, 153, 183, 190, 194, and 225 in the HA gene of Influenza A(H1N1) are Phe, Trp, His, Asp and Leu respectively, which are highly conserved like other influenza viruses, ensuring the structural stability of the reception-binding region. There are eight glycation sites on the HA protein sequence of Influenza A(H1N1), among which six were located at positions13, 14, 26, 90, 279, and 290 of N in HA1 region, and two were located at positions 154 and 213 of N in HA2 region. If no additional glycation sites exist in the 158th position of HA protein of Influenza A(H1N1), and meanwhile, no amino acid is absent on the neck of NA protein, evidence has suggested that this combination reveals increasingly strong virulence among H5N1 subtype of avian influenza virus.

The cleavage site sequence of Influenza A(H1N1) HA is PSIQSR↓GLFGAI, which is consistent with the amino acid sequence at the HA cleavage site of typical H1N1 subtype influenza viruses. This characteristic can only be recognized and lysed by certain proteases and certain bacterial enzymes present in the host respiratory or digestive tract cells, thus causing local infection of the respiratory or digestive tract. Molecular characteristics of the highly pathogenic strain (RXR/KR↓GLF) have not yet appeared. The cleavage site sequence of the H1N1 virus strain discovered in the 1918 Spanish flu pandemic was also PSIQSR↓GLFGAI, without insertion of a number of basic amino acids. However, the pathogenicity of the strain was extremely strong, which was possibly linked with its NA protein and HA cleavage but the mechanism was still ambiguous. So low-pathogenicity influenza viruses can be virulent not only by HA mutations but also by NA mutations.

The amino acid at position 627 of the viral PB2 protein is an important determinant of the host range and virulence of influenza A virus: when the 627th position was K, the virulence of the virus was strong and it was more likely to infect humans; the pathogenicity of the strain was weak when the 627th position was E. The 627th position of PB2 of influenza A(H1N1) still retains the less virulent E. Moreover, influenza A(H1N1) is a mix of two kinds of swine flu viruses from North America and Eurasia, with which human has never been infected. Therefore, human bodies lack immunity protection against this novel virus, which reveals strong pathogenicity of the virus. However, no super transmission of influenza A(H1N1) has been seen so far, suggesting that the transmission capacity of this virus may be limited and can be effectively controlled.

3.1.4.2 Analysis of Drug Susceptibility

At present, antiviral drugs against influenza A(H1N1) are mainly neuraminidase inhibitors. The generation of NA inhibitor resistance reported clinically varies with the drugs used. After treatment with Tamiflu, mutations including R292K, E119V, D198N, and H274Y were discovered. While only R152K mutation occurred after treatment with zanamivir, and the occurrence of mutations at different sites had type specificity. The analysis of influenza A(H1N1) found that there was no mutation from H to Y at position 274, indicating that neuraminidase inhibitors such as Tamiflu were still effective, which was consistent with the clinical therapeutic effect.

3.2 Epidemiology of Influenza A(H1N1)

3.2.1 Epidemiological Characteristics

3.2.1.1 Discovery of Influenza A(H1N1)

Influenza A(H1N1) was first detected in a 10-year-old patient in California through routine clinical tests for influenza, and the result suggested a novel human virus. Two days later, the Centers for Disease Control and Prevention (CDC) confirmed a second case of this virus from another patient, an 8-year-old in California who lived 130 miles from the first case and had no known connection with the first one. The CDC analyzed the samples of virus obtained from the two patients and discovered that the viruses were very similar to each other, but unlike any virus previously found in humans and other animals. Studies showed that the virus was resistant to amantadine and rimantadine- two antiviral drugs, but sensitive to oseltamivir and zanamivir.

Between December 2005 and January 2009, a total of 12 human cases of swine flu were reported, of which five were from direct exposure to pigs, six were infected through close contact with pigs, and the source of infection of the remaining one was still unknown. Before this, human-to-human transmission of swine influenza was seldom reported and was not anticipated to break out in the population. Nevertheless, these two patients of swine influenza without epidemiologic connection stroked a concern that swine influenza virus had entered human society and had spread among populations.

As the outbreak unfolded, the CDC maintained close ties with the international health community. On April 18, 2009, according to the

International Health Regulations, the United States reported cases of the novel influenza A(H1N1) to WHO and, at the same time, to the Pan American Health Organization (PAHO), Canada and Mexico.

To uncover the origin of influenza A(H1N1), research teams at Hong Kong University conducted an evolutionary analysis of the virus. With support from the NIAID Centre for Virus Research and Surveillance, Professor Gavin Smith's team found that the virus originated in pigs that had already been infected and that its first transmission had occurred months earlier. In addition, due to inadequate surveillance, the evolutionary recombination of porcine viruses may occur years before the virus is detected in humans [8].

3.2.1.2 Profile of Influenza A(H1N1) Epidemic

The influenza A(H1N1) epidemic originated from Mexico in 2009, followed by a significant increase of influenza-like cases in March and a confirmation of a new strain of influenza A(H1N1) virus to which the majority of people in the world have no immunity in April. This disease quickly spread to countries and regions in Europe and Asia. On May 11, 2009, the first case was detected in China. From April 2009 ever since the outbreak in North America, to June 2009, within the merely 2 months, WHO claimed that a total of 74 countries had reported laboratory-confirmed cases; and by the day of December 4, 2009, more than 8768 deaths were reported, according to WHO. China's Ministry of Health announced that in the week from November 23 to November 29, 2009, 31 provinces in China reported 12,500 confirmed cases of influenza A(H1N1), among them 3765 cases were hospitalized and 74 people died. Given the rapid spread of the epidemic, WHO increased the influenza pandemic alert to phase 5 on April 29; with the further spreading, WHO raised the level of influenza pandemic alert to the highest phase 6 on June 11, 2009, which meant an official declaration that a novel influenza pandemic was under way. The descriptions of epidemic phases by WHO are displayed in Table 3.2.

3.2.1.3 Epidemiological Characteristics of Influenza A(H1N1)

With the further raging of the pandemic, the activity and virulence of the virus weakened, and influenza A(H1N1) gradually evolved into a subtype of seasonal influenza. In recent years, influenza A(H1N1) epidemic has been less active in the world as a whole, with a consistently low level in temperate regions of the southern Hemisphere in winter, but a relatively higher level in tropical areas, particularly in South and Southeast Asia, the Caribbean and West Africa.

In the surveillance for influenza-like cases in Australia and New Zealand, influenza A(H1N1) detected was only a small proportion. In Chile in late June 2010, respiratory samples tested less than 5% positive for influenza, mostly influenza A(H1N1) virus, with a small proportion of seasonal influenza H3N2 and B viruses. In Argentina, the overall level of influenza-like cases was also low and meanwhile, lower than that of the past three winter flu seasons.

Table 3.2 WHO influenza pandemic phases

Phase	Description[a]
1	No animal influenza virus circulating among animals has been reported to cause infection in humans.
2	An animal influenza virus circulating in domesticated or wild animals is known to have caused infection in humans and is therefore considered a specific potential pandemic threat.
3	An animal or human-animal influenza reassortant virus has caused sporadic cases or small clusters of disease in people but has not resulted in human-to-human transmission sufficient to sustain community-level outbreaks.
4	Verified human-to-human transmission of an animal or human-animal influenza reassortant virus able to sustain community-level outbreaks.
5	The same identified virus has caused sustained community-level outbreaks in two or more countries in one WHO region.
6	The pandemic phase is characterized by community-level outbreaks in at least one other country in another WHO region in addition to the criteria defined in Phase 5.

[a]Source: http://english.cctv.com/20090612/105352.shtml

Overall, influenza A was not active in Asia, except India, Malaysia, Singapore, etc. In India, the spread of influenza A(H1N1) was relatively active, but with the exception of the southern state of Kerala where the influenza was relatively stable. Since mid-June 2010, weekly reports of new, severe and fatal cases had increased. A small rise in influenza A(H1N1) outbreaks had also been detected in other southern and western parts of India. In Singapore, the spread of acute respiratory infections and influenza A(H1N1) peaked in May 2010 but began to decline in June 2010, with a positive rate of influenza A-H1N1 virus testing around 16% in the first week of July 2010. In Malaysia, the number of new cases of influenza A(H1N1) began to decline in June 2010 after peaking from mid-April to mid-May 2010 and continued to drop since then. In the mainland of China, Hong Kong (China), Taipei (China), and South Korea, very small amounts of seasonal influenza B kept circulating after June 2010.

After the 2009 pandemic, influenza A(H1N1) and seasonal influenza were not vigorous in the tropical regions of the Americas, except in parts of Central America. Mixed influenza A(H1N1) and seasonal influenza H3N2 were detected in some areas of Central America. In Panama, influenza A epidemic was on the rise in June 2010, mainly H3N2 with a few H1N1 strains. In Nicaragua, the seasonal influenza H3N2 began circulating in late May 2010 and peaked in mid-June, but soon subsided significantly.

In sub-Saharan Africa, the influenza A(H1N1) pandemic has not changed much, with influenza A and seasonal flu being monitored in many countries. The influenza A(H1N1) epidemic remained raging after peaking in early April 2010 in Ghana (West Africa), and seasonal influenza B kept spreading in parts of central and southern Africa, especially Cameroon. In Eastern Africa, influenza activity is dominated by a small number of seasonal influenza H3N2 viruses.

In general, influenza A(H1N1) and seasonal influenza were found sporadically or at very low levels in temperate regions of the northern Hemisphere (North America and Europe) during the post-pandemic period.

3.2.1.4 Epidemic Characteristics under China's Effective Intervention in Pandemic Influenza A(H1N1)

China made a rapid response to pandemic influenza A(H1N1) in the early stage. Strict inspection and quarantine measures at ports were deployed; prevention and control strategy of "blocking overseas imports" was implemented; and real-time screening and monitoring of the influenza A(H1N1) epidemic trend was carried out, through which the positive rate was much higher than that of other WHO member states adopting inspection and quarantine measures at ports. Meanwhile, all confirmed cases caught by the port screening and surveillance system were isolated and treated in designated hospitals, and their close contacts were placed under careful medical observation, which effectively alleviated the spreading velocity and epidemic intensity in China. The monitoring results suggested that the early containment measures limited the epidemic at a low level in the first 3 months when the pandemic was raging across the world and did not reach the peak until September 2009, when compared with the peak in the summer seen in countries such as the United States. This characteristic was called "China's flat platform". Without high intensity of cases and community-level transmission, China gained valuable time and advantage in preparing for the research, development, production, and storage of drugs and vaccines to confront bigger challenges that may arise.

3.2.2 Epidemic Relevant Parameters

The sources of influenza A(H1N1) are mainly patients and asymptomatic carriers. The route of transmission is similar to previous human influenza, namely through droplets from human to human or from human to pigs [9]. But there is no evidence suggesting transmission from animals to human beings. The whole population is considered as susceptible to influenza A(H1N1). When compared with seasonal influenza, the infective period and detoxification duration of influenza A were longer.

Detoxification lasts from 1 day before symptoms until 8 days after illness [10]. The rate of symptomatic infection and asymptomatic infection among close contacts of confirmed cases of influenza A(H1N1) was about 2.4% and 17.2%, respectively [11]. The researchers analyzed data from confirmed cases reported in Ontario, Canada, assessed the incubation period, duration of symptoms, and their distribution, and used a competitive risk model to estimate the risk of fatality in hospitalized cases. Markov chain Monte Carlo model was used to simulate disease transmission and it was found that the median incubation period was 4 days, that the symptom duration was 7 days, and that patients younger than 18 years recovered faster than those older than 18 years (hazard ratio 1.23, 95% confidence interval 1.06–1.44). The risk of admission was 4.5% (95% CI: 3.8–5.2%) and the case-fatality rate was 0.3% (95% CI: 0.1–0.5%). Patients younger than 1 year and older than 65 years were the highest risk groups for admission. Cases over the age of 50 account for 7% of the total. With the simulation model, researchers discovered that the average basic reproductive number (R_0, the number of new cases that a single case among a susceptible population can create) was 1.31 (95% CI: 1.25–1.38), the average incubation period was 2.62 days (95% CI: 2.28–3.12), the infection duration was 3.38 days (95% CI: 2.06–4.69). Based on the above data, the infectious period (the average time between the onset of symptom in one case and infection in another from the former) was assessed as 4 to 5 days [12].

3.3 Progress in Clinical Diagnosis and Treatment of Influenza A(H1N1)

3.3.1 Clinical Feature

3.3.1.1 Clinical Manifestation

Symptoms of influenza A(H1N1) are similar to those of previous seasonal influenza and usually present with Flu-like symptoms, including fever, cough, sore throat, headache, body aches, chills, and fatigue. Some may also have vomiting and diarrhea, muscle pain or fatigue, and red eyes. A few cases have only mild upper respiratory symptoms without fever. The main signs include pharynx congestion, tonsil enlargement. The condition of some patients can progress rapidly, with sudden high fever and body temperature exceeding 39 °C, and may even be followed by severe pneumonia, acute respiratory distress syndrome, pulmonary hemorrhage, pleural effusion, renal failure, septicemia, shock and Reye syndrome, respiratory failure and multi-organ failure. Severe illness can lead to death.

3.3.1.2 Risk Factors for Severe Illness of Influenza A(H1N1)

Studies have reported that pregnant women, especially pregnant women in the first 3 months of pregnancy, children younger than 2 years of age, and chronic lung diseases are high-risk groups for severe influenza A(H1N1). Another study found that 30–35% of hospitalized patients with H1N1 influenza are obese (BMI $\geq$ 30) or morbidly obese (BMI > 40), suggesting that obesity is also a high-risk factor. In addition, it is reported that 117 of the 179 hospitalized cases have chronic diseases or immunosuppressive agents, suggesting that chronic diseases or immunosuppressive agents have also increased the risk of severe illness.

The "The influenza A(H1N1). Diagnosis and Treatment Plan (2009 Third Edition)" issued by the General Office of the Ministry of Health of China proposes that five categories of people are more likely to become severe cases after flu-like symptoms, namely: (1) pregnant women; (2) associated with the following diseases or conditions: chronic respiratory diseases, cardiovascular diseases (except hypertension), kidney diseases, liver diseases, blood system diseases, nervous system and neuromuscular diseases, metabolic and endocrine system diseases, immune function suppression (including the application of immunosuppression or HIV infection), and those who are under 19 years old and take aspirin for a long time; (3) obese people (the risk of body mass index ≥40 is high, and a body mass index of 30–39 may be a high risk factor); (4) children younger than 5 years old (severe complications are more likely to occur if the age is less than 2 years); (5) elderly people ≥65 years old. Once these five types of people show flu-like symptoms, great attention should be given to them, and the nucleic acid test of influenza A(H1N1) virus and other necessary inspections should be carried out as soon as possible.

3.3.2 Laboratory Findings

3.3.2.1 Peripheral Hemogram

The total number of white blood cells in peripheral blood is generally not high or low. Most severely ill patients have a decrease in the total number of white blood cells and lymphocytes, accompanied by a decrease in platelets. When combined with bacterial infection, white blood cells or neutrophils may increase.

3.3.2.2 Biochemical Examination of Blood

Some patients have hypokalemia, and a few patients have elevated creatine kinase, aspartate aminotransferase, alanine aminotransferase, and lactate dehydrogenase.

3.3.2.3 Etiological Examinations

Viral nucleic acid detection: RT-PCR (preferably real-time RT-PCR) is used to detect the nucleic acid of influenza A(H1N1) virus in respiratory tract samples (throat swabs, nasal swabs, nasopharyngeal or tracheal extracts, sputum). The results may be positive. Virus isolation: influenza A(H1N1) virus can be isolated from respiratory specimens. Serological testing: dynamic detection of double sera, the level of influenza A(H1N1) virus-specific antibodies is 4 times or more than 4 times increase in blood sera collected from the acute and convalescent stages of illness.

3.3.2.4 Chest Radiological Examinations

Patchy shadows can be seen in the lungs with pneumonia.

3.3.3 Diagnosis and Classification

3.3.3.1 Diagnostic Criteria

Diagnosis mainly combines epidemiological history, clinical features, and pathogenic examinations. Early detection and early diagnosis are the keys to prevention and effective treatment.

3.3.3.1.1 Suspected Case

A suspected case can be diagnosed if one of the following conditions is met: (1) Close contact with a confirmed case of infectious influenza A(H1N1) within 7 days before the onset of illness, and influenza-like clinical manifestations. Close contact refers to the diagnosis, treatment, and care of patients with influenza A(H1N1) during the infectious period without effective protection; living with the patient; contact with the respiratory secretions and body fluids of the patient. (2) Have been to areas where influenza A(H1N1) has been prevalent (continuous human-to-human transmission of influenza A(H1N1)and epidemics and outbreaks based on the community level) within 7 days before the onset of illness, and have influenza-like clinical manifestations. (3) Influenza-like clinical manifestations, positive for influenza A virus and no further virus subtypes have been tested. If possible, further pathogenic inspections for influenza A(H1N1) can be done in the above situations.

3.3.3.1.2 Clinically Diagnosed Cases

In the outbreak of influenza A(H1N1), a case of influenza-like symptoms that has not been confirmed by the laboratory can be diagnosed as a clinically diagnosed case when other diseases that cause influenza-like symptoms are excluded. Influenza A(H1N1) outbreak refers to an abnormal increase in flu-like cases in a region or unit in a short period of time, which is confirmed as influenza A(H1N1) by laboratory testing. If possible, the clinically diagnosed cases can be further tested for etiology.

3.3.3.1.3 Confirmed Cases

With flu-like clinical manifestations, and one or more of the following laboratory test results: (1) Nucleic acid test of influenza A(H1N1) virus is positive (real-time RT-PCR and RT-PCR methods can be used); (2) Influenza A(H1N1) virus is isolated; (3) The specific antibody level of influenza A(H1N1) virus coming from double sera is 4 times or more than 4 times increase.

3.3.3.2 Diagnosis of Severe and Critical Influenza A(H1N1)

The patient with one of the following conditions is a severe case: (1) Continuous high fever>3 days; (2) Strong cough, coughing up purulent sputum, bloody sputum, or chest pain; (3) Rapid breathing, difficulty breathing, and cyanotic lips; (4) Consciousness changes: slow response, hypersomnia, mania, convulsions; (5) Severe vomiting, diarrhea, and dehydration; (6) Image examination shows signs of pneumonia; (7) The levels of myocardial enzymes such as creatine kinase (CK) and creatine kinase isoenzyme (CK-MB) increase rapidly; (8) The original underlying disease has significantly worsened. With one of the following conditions is a critical case: (1) respiratory failure; (2) toxic shock due to infection; (3) multiple organ dysfunction; (4) other serious clinical conditions that require monitoring and treatment.

3.3.4 Complications

The condition of some patients may progress rapidly, with sudden high fever and body temperature exceeding 39 °C. Patients may die of secondary severe pneumonia, acute respiratory distress syndrome, pulmonary hemorrhage, pleural effusion, pancytopenia, renal failure, sepsis, shock, Reye syndrome, Respiratory failure and multiple organ damage.

3.3.5 Treatment

3.3.5.1 Isolation

In November 2013, the National Health and Family Planning Commission of the People's Republic of China posted a notice that influenza A (H1N1) was adjusted from class B infectious diseases to Class C, and classified as seasonal influenza. Isolation was not compulsory for every case since then. When medical agencies find patients of influenza A(H1N1), they shall take necessary measures for treatment and for control of their spread according to the patients' conditions.

3.3.5.2 Symptomatic Treatment

Pay attention to rest, drink plenty of water, strengthen nutrition, and closely observe changes in the condition; antipyretic treatment can be given to cases of high fever. The best treatment period is within 48 hours after the onset of onset. Chest X-ray should be taken to check blood gas for patients with obvious clinical symptoms.

3.3.5.3 Antiviral Therapy

Studies have shown that the influenza A(H1N1) virus is currently sensitive to neuraminidase inhibitors oseltamivir and zanamivir, and resistant to amantadine and rimantadine.

For cases of influenza A(H1N1) with mild clinical manifestations, no comorbidities, and the conditions tend to be self-limiting, there is no need to actively apply neuraminidase inhibitors. For cases with severe illness, dynamic deterioration after the onset, and high-risk groups of influenza A(H1N1), neuraminidase inhibitors should be given antiviral treatment in time. Antiviral therapy should be started within 48 hours of the onset of disease (36 hours is the best). For high-risk groups who are more likely to develop into severe cases, once flu-like symptoms appear, antiviral treatment can be started without waiting for the virus nucleic acid test results. Pregnant women should be treated with neuraminidase inhibitors as soon as possible after flu-like symptoms appear.

Oseltamivir: 75 mg for adults, twice a day, treatment for 5 days. For severe or critical cases, the dose of oseltamivir can be increased to 150 mg, twice a day. For protracted cases, the medication time can be extended appropriately. Children who are 1 year old and older should be administered according to their body weight: those who weigh less than 15 kg, 30 mg, twice a day; those who weigh 15–23 kg, 45 mg, twice a day; those who weigh 23–40 kg, 60 mg, twice a day for those who weigh more than 40 kg, 75 mg twice a day. For children who have difficulty swallowing capsules, oseltamivir suspension can be used.

Zanamivir: For adults and children over 7 years old. Adult dosage is 10 mg inhalation, twice a day, the course of treatment is 5 days. The usage for children aged 7 and above is the same as that for adults.

China has established the world's largest clinical database containing 4110 cases of influenza

A(H1N1), and analysis reveals that antiviral therapy can significantly reduce the case fatality rate of patients with influenza A(H1N1). Antiviral therapy has a higher protective effect for men, patients aged 14–60 years, and whose baseline oxygenation index is less than 200. But the double dose of oseltamivir has no additional protective effect for cases weighing less than 78 kg.

3.3.5.4 Other Treatment

If hypoxemia or respiratory failure occurs, appropriate treatment measures should be given in time, including oxygen therapy or mechanical ventilation. When combined with shock, give corresponding anti-shock treatment. When other organ dysfunction occurs, give corresponding supportive treatment. When combined with bacterial and/or fungal infections, give the corresponding antibacterial and/or antifungal drugs. Analysis of the neutralizing antibody titers in the plasma of convalescent patients suggests that the convalescent plasma can treat critically ill patients, effectively reducing the mortality rate. Therefore, for severe and critical cases, convalescent plasma from recently recovered influenza A(H1N1) patients or immunological plasma from vaccinators can also be considered for treatment. Patients with recovery period plasma or vaccinated immune plasma for treatment. Furthermore, for severe and critical cases within 1 week of onset, early usage would be better under the premise of ensuring medical safety. Generally, 100–200 ml for adults, 50 ml for children (or adjust dosage according to the specificity of plasma antibody titer), intravenous infusion, can be reused if necessary, pay attention to allergic reactions during use.

3.3.5.5 Discharge Standard

Normal body temperature for 3 days, other flu-like symptoms disappeared basically, the clinical situation is stable, can be discharged. In cases of influenza A(H1N1) that require long-term hospitalization due to underlying diseases or severe complications and further treatment can be transferred from the isolation ward to the corresponding ward after the nucleic acid of influenza A(H1N1) is negatively detected by a throat swab.

3.4 Progress of Influenza A(H1N1) Vaccine

3.4.1 Comparison of Influenza A(H1N1) Virus Strain and Seasonal Influenza Vaccine Strain

Influenza A(H1N1) is a new influenza virus, which belongs to the mixture of swine influenza viruses from North, Central America, and Eurasia. In history, swine influenza viruses that infect these two strains have rarely been found in humans. Therefore, the human body lacks protective immunity against influenza A(H1N1) virus. At that time, seasonal influenza vaccines were screened from known influenza virus strains. However, due to the large differences in antigenic and genetic between human seasonal influenza vaccines and swine influenza viruses, influenza vaccines at that time could not effectively prevent influenza A(H1N1). By comparing the amino acid sequence homology of HA antigenic determinant between vaccine candidate strains and influenza A(H1N1) virus strains and evaluating their cross-protection, it was found that the spherical head of HA protein of common H1 subtype influenza virus had five antigenic sites, namely Cb, Sa, Sb, Ca1, and Ca2. A/Solomon Islands/3/2006 was recommended by WHO as the candidate strain of influenza vaccine H1N1 subtype for 2008–2009. By comparing the amino acid sequence similarity of HA antigenic locus of influenza A(H1N1) virus with that of influenza A(H1N1) virus, it was found that there were great differences in the amino acid sequences of the five antigenic sites between the two strains, indicating that the conventional influenza vaccine strains at that time had limited protection against new influenza A(H1N1) virus.

3.4.2 Research Progress of Influenza A(H1N1) Vaccine in China

Since the outbreak of influenza A(H1N1), the number of confirmed cases has increased rapidly worldwide. In order to effectively deal with the outbreak of influenza A(H1N1), Chinese scientists took the lead in the development of new influenza A(H1N1) vaccine in the world in the shortest time, and China became the world's first country approved a listing, and first announced to the world: The influenza A(H1N1) vaccine has a significant memory immune protection response after 2 weeks of vaccination at 15 μg/dose. It can effectively prevent influenza A(H1N1) and provide an important and basic scientific basis for the global production and use of influenza A(H1N1) vaccine. The protective effect of the new vaccine is confirmed for the first time to reach 87%. In the course of the study, Chinese scientists firstly established the ferret models of influenza A(H1N1) and used it for preclinical study of influenza A(H1N1) vaccine. Since the vaccine strain was obtained, the establishment and verification of a three-level seed bank of vaccine strain, optimization and determination of virus passage and amplification conditions, establishment of virus purification and lysis process, establishment of vaccine quality verification system, animal experiments, and other vaccine development processes have been rapidly completed, and the lysis vaccine of influenza A(H1N1) virus conforming to international standards has been successfully developed. A large-scale clinical trial was carried out on the spot on the new influenza A(H1N1) vaccine strain, and a double-blind, randomized, controlled clinical trial was organized and implemented with the largest scale (12,691 people), the earliest time (July 22, 2009), and the most varieties (seven varieties with different doses, adjuvants and without adjuvants, lysis and whole virus). The results confirmed the safety and efficacy of a single dose of adjuvant-free 15-ug influenza A(H1N1) vaccine, provided an important scientific basis for global vaccine production and use, greatly improved the availability of vaccine supply, and made it possible to vaccinate more people. At the same time, in less than 3 months (87 days), it has created a way to achieve the transcendence of pandemic influenza vaccine from scratch, which has been highly evaluated by WHO and relevant institutions at home and abroad. The production of influenza A(H1N1) vaccine has also promoted the rapid increase in the production capacity of influenza vaccine in China, from 126 million doses in origin to 285 million doses, which has improved the production capacity of vaccine against influenza pandemic.

During the global influenza A(H1N1) epidemic, China's health sector used the self-developed influenza A(H1N1) vaccine to vaccinate 105 million people throughout the country and established the world's largest vaccine safety monitoring system, including 70 million people, which proved that the new vaccine was safe. It was proposed that the Green-Barre syndrome had nothing to do with the vaccination of influenza A(H1N1) vaccine, which provided a scientific basis for the safety of large-scale vaccination in the world, and also enabled China to pass WHO vaccine regulatory certification, ending the history that Chinese vaccine was not recognized by international organizations [13, 14].

3.4.3 Influenza A(H1N1) Vaccine Approved by the United States and the European Union

The US Food and Drug Administration (FDA) approved four influenza A(H1N1) monovalent vaccines on September 15, 2009, and another monovalent vaccine on November 10, 2009. The registration procedures were all based on the procedures for replacing strains with seasonal influenza vaccines that have been listed. The dose and vaccination procedures were also based on the clinical trials of influenza monovalent vaccines. On September 25, 2009, and October 6, 2009, the European Union approved Focetria, Pandemrix, Celvapan three pandemic influenza A(H1N1) vaccine, registration procedures using H5N1 influenza vaccine replacement program, dose and vaccination procedures based on the H5N1 influenza vaccine existing clinical trial data and preliminary incomplete clinical trials of pandemic influenza A(H1N1) vaccine. Due to the H5N1 influenza vaccine approval recommended procedures for two shots, the corresponding A H1N1 vaccine product recommended procedures for two shots, with the continuous supplement of clinical trial data, the EU implementation of a needle immunization program (see Table 3.3).

Table 3.3 Types of pandemic influenza A(H1N1) vaccine

Manufacturer	Packaged form	Dose (Strain)	Thimerosal (mercury content)	Vaccination procedure, dosage	Applicable population	Route
Baxter	5 ml vial 10 servings	7.5 μg/0.5 ml A/California/7/2009 (H1N1)v-like virus	No	Two shots, 0.5 ml/shot, 3 weeks interval	>6 months, including children, adults, pregnant women	Upper arm intramuscular injection
CSL	5 ml vial 10 servings	15 μg/0.5 ml	Yes (preservative) 24.5 mg/0.5 ml	One shot, 0.5 ml/shot	>18 years	Intramuscular injection
CSL	5 ml vial 10 servings	15 μg/0.5 ml	Yes (preservative) 24.5 mg/0.5 ml	One shot, 0.5 ml/shot	>18 years	Intramuscular injection
GSK	Vaccines and adjuvants for separate packaging, on-site mixing, 2.5 ml vaccine, vial, 2.5 ml adjuvant, vial, mixed for 10 people	3.75 μg/0.5 ml A/California/7/2009 (H1N1)v-like virus (XX-179A)	Yes(excipient) 0.005 mg/0.5 ml	10–60 years, >60 years old, two shots, 0.5 ml/shot, 3 weeks interval	>6 months, including children, adults, pregnant women	Upper arm intramuscular injection
GSK	Vaccines and adjuvants for separate packaging, on-site mixing, 2.5 ml vaccine, vial, 2.5 ml adjuvant, vial, mixed for 10 people	3.75 μg/0.5 ml A/California/7/2009 (H1N1)v-like virus (XX-179A)	Yes(excipient) 0.005 mg/0.5 ml	6 months-9 years, two shots, 0.25 ml/shots, 3 weeks interval	>6 months, including children, adults, pregnant women	Upper arm intramuscular injection
ID Biomedical Corporation of Quebec	5 ml vial 10 servings	NA	Yes(preservative) 25 mg/0.5 ml	One shot	≥18 years	Intramuscular injection
Medimmune	Prefilled nasal sprayer	10FFU/0.2 ml	No	Two shots, 1 month interval	2–9 years	Intranasal inoculation
Medimmune	Prefilled nasal sprayer	10FFU/0.2 ml	No	One shot	10–49 years	Intranasal inoculation
Novartis	0.5 ml prefilled syringe single serving	7.5 μg/0.5 ml	Yes(excipient) 0.05 mg/0.5 ml	10–60 years, one shot, 0.5 ml/shot	>6 months, including children, adults, pregnant women	Upper arm intramuscular injection
Novartis	0.5 ml prefilled syringe single serving	15 μg/0.5 ml	Yes (process residue) ≤ 1 mg/0.5 ml	Two shots, 1 month interval	4–9 years	Intramuscular injection

Novartis	5 ml vial 10 servings	7.5 μg/0.5 ml	Yes (preservative)	6 months-9 years, >60 years, 0.5 ml/shot, two shots, 3 weeks interval	>6 months, including children, adults, pregnant women	Upper arm intramuscular injection
Novartis	5 ml vial 10 servings	15 μg/0.5 ml	Yes(preservative) 25 mg/0.5 ml	One shot	≥10 years	Intramuscular injection
Pasteur	0.25 ml prefilled syringe single serving	15 μg/0.5 ml	No	Two shots, 1 month interval	6–35 months	Intramuscular injection
Pasteur	0.5 ml prefilled syringe single serving	15 μg/0.5 ml	No	Two shots, 1 month interval	36 months-9 years	Intramuscular injection
Pasteur	0.5 ml vial single serving	15 μg/0.5 ml	No	One shot	≥10 years	Intramuscular injection
Pasteur	5 ml vial 10 servings	15 μg/0.5 ml	Yes(preservative) 25 mg/0.5 ml	One shot	≥10 years	Intramuscular injection

References

1. Skehel JJ, Wiley DC. Receptor binding and membrane fusion in virus entry: the influenza hemagglutinin. Annu Rev Biochem. 2000;69:531–69.
2. Webster RG, Bean WJ, Gorman OT, et al. Evolution and ecology of influenza a viruses. Microbiol Rev. 1992;56:152–79.
3. Garten RJ, Davis CT, Russell CA, et al. Antigenic and genetic characteristics of swine-origin 2009 A(H1N1) influenza viruses circulating in humans. Science. 2009;325:197–201.
4. Childs RA, Palma AS, Wharton S, et al. Receptor-binding specificity of pandemic influenza A(H1N1) 2009 virus determined by carbohydrate microarray. Nat Biotechnol. 2009;27:797–9.
5. Peiris M, Yuen KY, Leung CW, et al. Human infection with influenza H9N2. Lancet. 1999;354(9182):916–7.
6. Xu KM, Smith GJ, Bahl J, et al. The genesis and evolution of H9N2 influenza viruses in poultry from southern China, 2000 to 2005. J Virol. 2007;81(19):10389–401.
7. Konig R, Stertz S, Zhou Y, et al. Human host factors required for influenza virus replication. Nature. 2010;463(7282):813–7.
8. Smith GJ, Vijaykrishna D, Bahl J, et al. Origins and evolutionary genomics of the 2009 swine-origin H1N1 influenza A epidemic. Nature. 2009;459(7250):1122–5.
9. Zhou K, He HX. Avian and swine flu viruses: new insights into transspecies transmission. Prog Biochem Biophys. 2009;36(05):523–9.
10. Yu HJ, Liao QH, Yuan Y, et al. Effectiveness of oseltamivir on disease progression and viral RNA shedding in patients with mild pandemic 2009 influenza a H1N1: opportunistic retrospective study of medical charts in China. Br Med J. 2010;341:c4779.
11. Pang XH, Yang P, Li S, et al. Pandemic(H1N1) 2009 among quarantined close contacts, Beijing, People's Republic of China. Emerg Infect Dis. 2011;17(10):1824–30.
12. Tuite AR, Greer AL, Whelan M, et al. Estimated epidemiologic parameters and morbidity associated with pandemic H1N1 influenza. CMAJ. 2010;182(2):131–6.
13. Liang XF, Li L, Liu DW, et al. Safety of influenza a (H1N1) vaccine in postmarketing surveillance in China. N Engl J Med. 2011;364(7):638–47.
14. http://scitech.people.com.cn/n/2015/0216/c1007-26573909.html. people.cn. 8 world-first research results: made a significant contribution to the global epidemic prevention and control[JB/OL]. http://scitech.people.com.cn/n/2015/0216/c1007-26573909.html 2015-2-16).

4 Progress in Novel Vaccine Clinical Epidemiology Research in China

Jingxin Li, Siyue Jia, and Fengcai Zhu

Abstract

China has developed quickly in almost every field of science and technology, including biotechnology and novel vaccine development, which promote the rapid development of vaccine clinical research. Vaccine clinical epidemiology researches are a series of clinical studies that scientifically evaluate the safety, immunogenicity, and efficacy of vaccines in humans, including pre-licensure and post-licensure clinical research. In this chapter, we reviewed the three most representative vaccine clinical epidemiology types of research in recent years, including the studies on the Recombined hepatitis E vaccine, Enterovirus 71 vaccine, and Ebola vaccine. We aimed to summarize and refine the key technologies of vaccine clinical research and provide the "Chinese experience" for other countries.

Keywords

Recombined hepatitis E vaccine · Enterovirus 71 vaccine · Ebola vaccine · Vaccination schedule · Safety · Immunogenicity · Protective efficacy

Vaccine clinical epidemiology researches are a series of clinical studies that scientifically evaluate the safety, immunogenicity, and efficacy of vaccines in humans, including pre-licensure and post-licensure clinical research. Pre-licensure researches of novel vaccines contain phase 1 to 3 clinical trials, which can provide key evidence for the approval of vaccines for marketing. While post-licensure research is referred to as phase 4 clinical trials, epidemical research or surveillance studies after the marketing of vaccines,

J. Li
NHC Key Laboratory of Enteric Pathogenic Microbiology, Jiangsu Provincial Center for Disease Control and Prevention,
Nanjing, Jiangsu, People's Republic of China

Institute of Global Public Health and Emergency Pharmacy, China Pharmaceutical University,
Nanjing, Jiangsu, People's Republic of China

S. Jia
NHC Key Laboratory of Enteric Pathogenic Microbiology, Jiangsu Provincial Center for Disease Control and Prevention,
Nanjing, Jiangsu, People's Republic of China

F. Zhu (✉)
NHC Key Laboratory of Enteric Pathogenic Microbiology, Jiangsu Provincial Center for Disease Control and Prevention,
Nanjing, Jiangsu, People's Republic of China

Institute of Global Public Health and Emergency Pharmacy, China Pharmaceutical University,
Nanjing, Jiangsu, People's Republic of China

Center for Global Health, Nanjing Medical University,
Nanjing, Jiangsu, People's Republic of China

D.-Q. Ye (ed.), *Progress in China Epidemiology*, https://doi.org/10.1007/978-981-19-2199-5_4

generally focus on further evaluation of the safety and effectiveness of vaccines in a mass-scale vaccination campaign in the population.

In the past several decades, Chinese vaccine companies mainly imitated the vaccines that have been on the foreign market for many years, so the vaccine clinical trials conducted in China mainly followed the experiences and the studies already done previously in foreign countries. However, during the recent ten years, biotechnology in China has developed rapidly and started to lead in the development and clinical research of some novel vaccines in the world. For these novel vaccines, there is no existing route and known tracks to follow, the clinical evaluations of the vaccines are full of challenges and evidence-based decisions are needed to make. The selection of the optimal dose formulation and immunization regimen, and determination of the dose-response relationship of specific antibody responses are important. In addition, the clinical evaluation of efficacy is the most core and critical research to determine the protection of a novel vaccine. With the increasing demand for clinical evaluation of novel vaccines, both the quality and quantities of vaccine clinical research in China have been gradually improved, contributing valuable scientific evidence to the world. Here, we shared the most representative epidemiology research of novel recombined hepatitis E vaccine, inactive enterovirus type 71 vaccine, and SARS-CoV-2 vaccines conducted in China in recent years.

4.1 Recombined Hepatitis E Vaccine

4.1.1 Background and Rational

Hepatitis E is an inflammation of the liver caused by hepatitis E virus (HEV) infection, which is transmitted through the fecal-oral route. This disease is mainly circulating in developing countries, including Asia, Africa, and Latin America [1]. There are eight genotypes of HEV, of which types 1, 2, 3, and 4 have been found to spread in humans, with epidemics in Asia and Africa mainly caused by type 1 and 2 [2], and in western countries mainly associated with type 3 and 4 from ingestion of contaminated animal products and liver transplant [3–5]. World Health Organization (WHO) estimated that 20 million people worldwide were infected with HEV each year and hepatitis E caused about 44,000 deaths in 2015, representing 3.3 percent of deaths from viral hepatitis [6].

Hepatitis E causes self-limiting acute hepatitis and in rare cases leads to acute liver failure (ALF) and even cirrhosis. Pregnant women infected with HEV in the last trimester have a significantly increased risk of ALF [7]. There is no established treatment for HEV in pregnant women, only symptomatic treatment can be provided, and the associated maternal mortality rate is as high as 30% [8].

China is recognized as an area with a high prevalence of hepatitis E [9]. From 2004 to 2017, reported cases of hepatitis E in China increased from 16,444 to 29,014, with Jiangsu, Guangdong, and Zhejiang leading the list of reported cases. The reported incidence of hepatitis E in eastern China was higher than that in central and western China and increased with age, and that in males was higher than in females [10].

There are two candidate vaccines for hepatitis E, one is the vaccine expressed in insect cells (AA112-AA607), and the other is the vaccine expressed in bacteria (HEV 239). The HEV 239 vaccine (Hecolin™) is the first licensed hepatitis E vaccine worldwide, which was developed in China, and is currently not available in other countries. HEV 239 vaccine developed by Xiamen Innovax Biotech CO., LTD contains an active antigen which is a recombinant peptide corresponding to aa 368–aa 606 of HEV ORF2 of a genotype 1 strain of HEV, and adjuvanted with aluminum hydroxide [11].

4.1.2 Methods

4.1.2.1 Participants and Study Site

In the early stage, a randomized-controlled study was conducted in a rural area of southern China with a low prevalence of hepatitis E from January 2005 to June 2006 to evaluate the safety and immunogenicity of the HEV 239 vaccine [12]. This trial included the dose scheduling and dose-escalation components, healthy people aged 16–55 years who were seronegative for HEV are eligible to participate, and the appropriate immunization regimen and optimal dosage were ultimately determined.

Subsequently, a large-scale randomized, double-blind, placebo-controlled phase 3 clinical trial including over 110,000 participants was done to evaluate the efficacy of the HEV 239 vaccine between August 2007 and June 2009 in Dongtai County, Jiangsu Province, China, which is a region with a relatively high prevalence of hepatitis E [13]. Healthy participants aged 16–55 years who understood the study procedures were recruited and observed for cases of laboratory-confirmed HEV for 1 year.

After completing the phase 3 clinical trial of the HEV 239 vaccine, an extended follow-up study based on the original phase 3 trial was designed, in which the treatment assignment remained double-blinded, and the follow-up lasted for 4.5 years [14].

4.1.2.2 Design of Optimal Dosage, Formulation, and Immunization Schedule

In the phase 2 clinical trial, adults were randomly assigned to three groups at a ratio of 1:1:1. Group A and B received three doses (month 0, 1, 6) and two doses (month 0, 6) of 20 μg HEV 239 vaccine, respectively, group C received three doses (month 0, 1, 6) of 5 μg commercial hepatitis B vaccine. Participants in groups A and C were taken blood samples for serum separation on months 0, 2, 6, 7, and 13, and those in group B were taken blood samples on months 0, 1, 6, 7, and 13 (Fig. 4.1). Similarly, high school students were randomly assigned to 4 groups at a ratio of 2:2:2:1 in a dose-escalation manner. The participants in each group were given three doses of HEV 239 vaccine at 10 μg (group E), 20 μg (group F), 30 μg (group G), or 40 μg (group H), with a schedule of 0, 1, and 6 months. Blood samples were taken from all participants on months 0, 2, 6, 7, and 13 (Fig. 4.2).

4.1.2.3 Study Design of Vaccine Efficacy

In the phase 3 clinical trial, adults were randomly divided into two groups at a ratio of 1:1 to receive

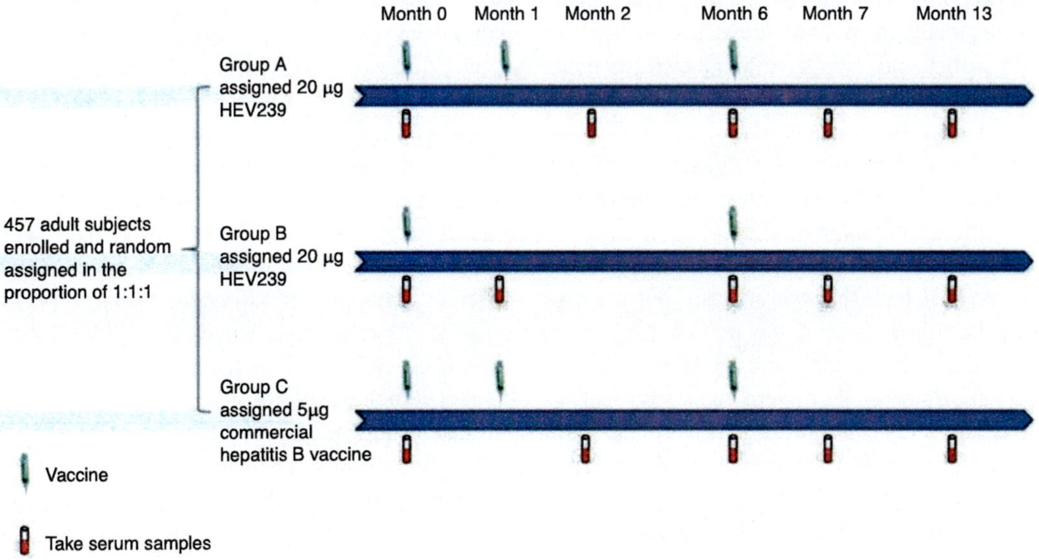

Fig. 4.1 Study design of the dose and regimen exploration for the HEV 239 vaccine

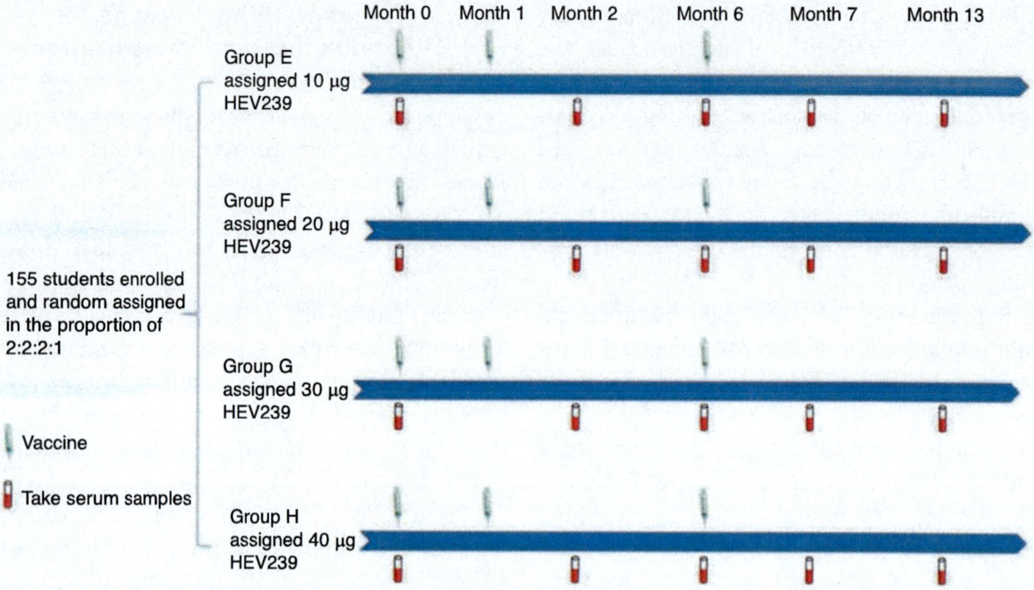

Fig. 4.2 Study design of the dosage escalation for the HEV 239 vaccine

three doses of HEV 239 (30 μg) or licensed hepatitis B vaccine intramuscularly at a schedule of 0, 1, and 6 months. In the immunogenicity subset, serum samples were taken before the first dose vaccination and 1 month after the third dose vaccination for detecting the concentration of IgG against the hepatitis E virus. All participants were followed up till month 19 (Fig. 4.3). The primary efficacy endpoint was the prevention of hepatitis E in participants who have completed the entire study within 1 year from the 31st day after receiving the third dose. In the extended follow-up study after month 19, the treatment allocation of all participants remained double-blind, and the follow-up continued to month 55 (Fig. 4.4).

Acute hepatitis cases were defined as patients with an ALT level that was at least 2.5 times high than the upper limit of the normal range (i.e., 40 U per liter for men and 31 U per liter for women). These patients were taken with sequential serum samples for testing in central laboratories. Cases with HEV infection were diagnosed if at least two of the following three markers were present. First, the positive testing result of IgM antibody against HEV. Second, the positive testing result of HEV RNA. Third, a level of IgG antibody against HEV that was at least four times higher than that measured previously at any time during the same illness.

4.1.2.4 Statistical Analysis

OpenEpi (version 2) calculators were used to compute the 95% CI for specificity or sensitivity of the data in the phase 2 trial. The percentages of participants with AEs among groups were compared using a two-sided Fisher's exact test. The geometric mean titers (GMTs) of different groups were compared using two sample independent t-tests. All participants completing the full-course vaccination and being collected serum samples at the given time points were included in the vaccine efficacy cohort in the phase 3 trial. The person-time rates of new hepatitis E infection in different groups were compared using a two-sided Mid-P exact test. A two-sided 95% CI for vaccine efficacy (1 minus the rate ratio) was calculated with the conditional maximum likelihood estimate using OpenEpi (version 2) calculators.

Vaccine efficacy and 95% CIs were calculated based on the observed difference and the accrued person-years between the vaccine and control groups. And considering that the number of hepatitis E cases in both groups are independent Poisson random variables, a precise conditional

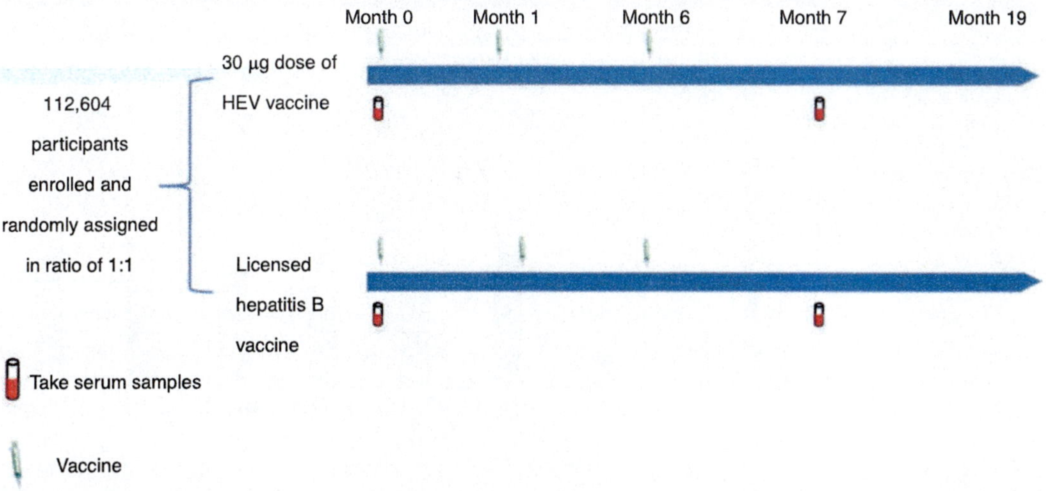

Fig. 4.3 Study design of the efficacy study for the HEV 239 vaccine

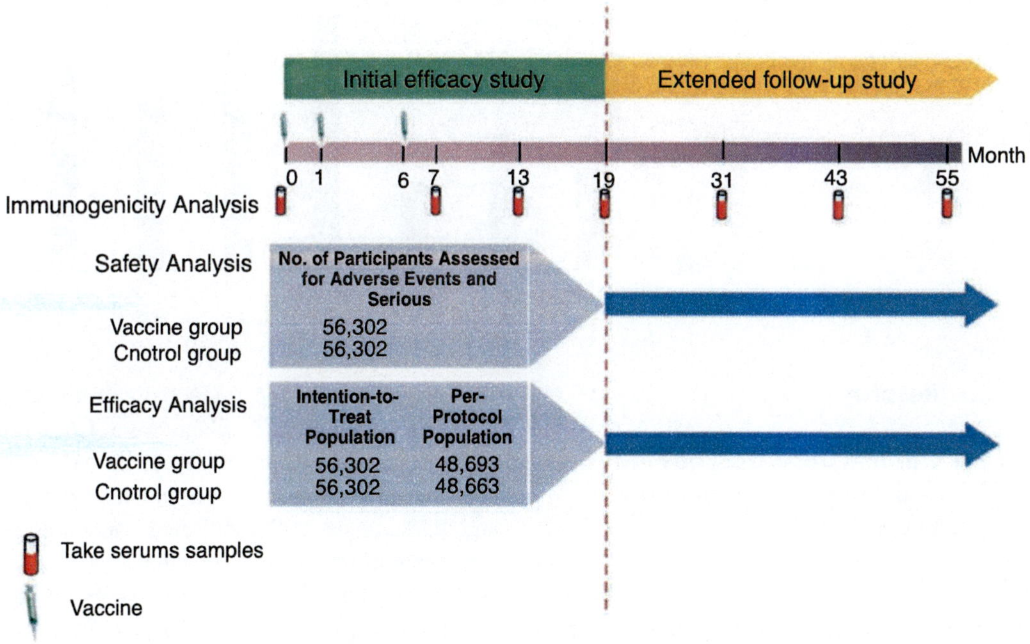

Fig. 4.4 Study design of the long-term efficacy study for the HEV 239 vaccine

procedure is used to evaluate the efficacy. For the robustness of the results, the Cox proportional hazards model was used to evaluate the efficacy, and the log-rank test was used to compare the cumulative incidence of hepatitis E between groups. Besides, long-term safety was assessed according to the rate of serious adverse events in the intention-to-treat set, the rates, and 95% CIs were compared between groups using a two-sided Fisher's exact test.

SAS software was used for data analysis. All reported *p*-values are two-sided, and values of less than 0.05 were considered to be statistically significant. An independent third-party statistician performed the efficacy analysis to keep the blindness.

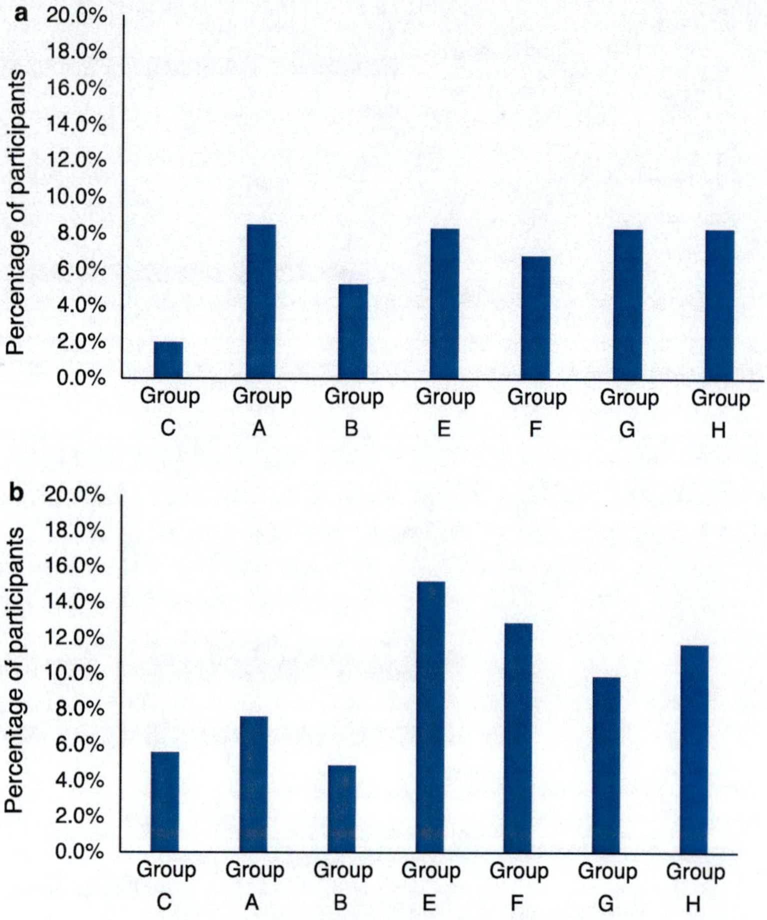

Fig. 4.5 Adverse events were reported within 30 days after each vaccination. (**a**) Total injection site adverse events reported within 30 days after each vaccination. (**b**) Total systemic adverse events were reported within 30 days after each vaccination

4.1.3 Results

4.1.3.1 Optimal Dose, Dosage Form, and Vaccination Schedule of HEV Vaccine

Safety

In the phase 2 trial, in terms of the rate of reporting at least one AE at the injection site within 30 days after each vaccination, group C (2.0%) was much lower than group A (8.5%) or group B (5.2%) ($p < 0.05$), and group E (8.3%), F (6.8%), G (8.3%) and H (8.3%) were similar (Fig. 4.5a). Itch (4.2%) is the most common injection site AE. The proportion of reporting at least one systemic AE within 30 days after each vaccination in groups A, B, C, E, F, G, and H was 7.6%, 4.9%, 5.6%, 15.2%, 12.9%, 9.9%, and 8.3%, respectively (Fig. 4.5b). Fever (4.3%) is the most common systemic AE. There were no AEs of > Grade 3 severity. Grade 3 local AEs were observed in group A and group H, which were 1.6% and 1.7%, respectively. Grade 3 systemic AEs were observed in groups E and H, which were 0.8% and 1.7%, respectively. However, there was no significant difference in the incidence of local or systemic events between group E and group H.

Immunogenicity

The seroconversion rate and the geometric mean antibody concentration (GMC) and 95% CI 1 month after completing all immunization schedules were used to assess the immunogenicity of the vaccine (Fig. 4.6). Vaccination can cause seroconversion in nearly all participants, except for the two participants in group B, who only received two doses of 20 μg of HEV 239 vaccine in month 0 and month 6. 8% of the participants in the control group were seropositive.

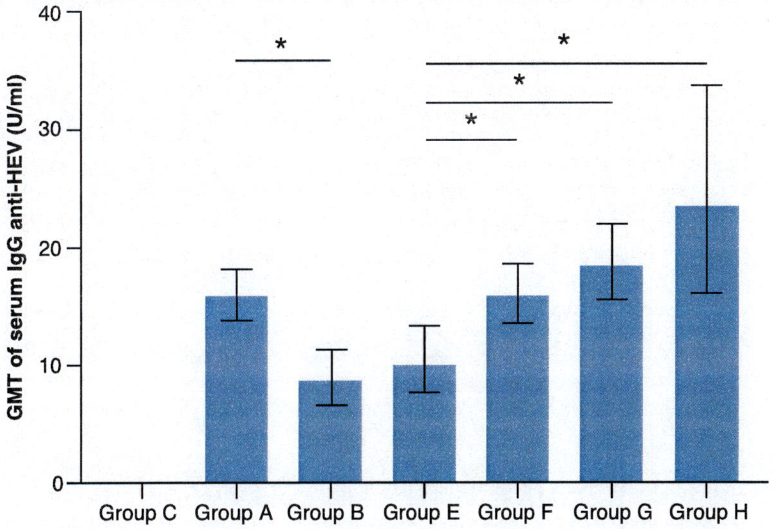

Fig. 4.6 The geometric mean titers of serum IgG anti-HEV after completion of the vaccination courses. * *p*-value <0.05

In the dose scheduling study, the GMC induced by three doses of 20 μg HEV vaccine was higher than that of two doses, and the difference between the two groups was statistically significant ($p < 0.05$). In the dose-escalation study, the vaccine-induced GMC increased with the increase of the dosage, and the difference between the groups was statistically significant. The GMC value of the participant after vaccination was between the antibody level of the mixed serum samples of hepatitis E patients (43 U/ml) and the HEV seropositive participants (0.76 U/ml).

In participants receiving three doses of 20 μg HEV 239 vaccine on months 0, 1, and 6, the GMC rose to 5.95 U/ml 1 month after receiving the second dose, declined to 3.12 U/ml before the third dose, further rose to 15.88 U/ml 1 month after receiving the third dose, and then declined to 3.73 U/ml 7 months after receiving the third dose (Fig. 4.7). The GMC of participants who received two doses of HEV 239 vaccine at 20 μg doses on months 0 and 6 rose to 0.8 U/ml 1 month after receiving the first dose, declined to 0.5 U/ml before the second dose, further rose to 8.62 U/ml 1 month after receiving the second dose, and then declined to 3.01 U/ml 7 months after receiving the second dose.

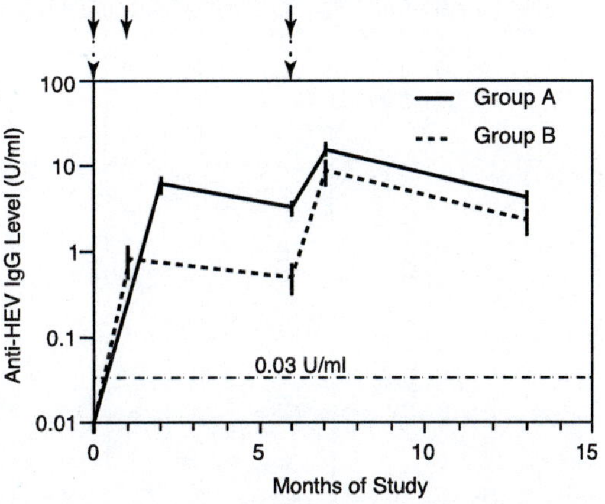

Fig. 4.7 The geometric mean titers of serum IgG anti-HEV during the study. (Reprinted with permission from Fig. 3, Zhang J, Liu CB, Li RC, et al. Randomized-controlled phase II clinical trial of a bacterially expressed recombinant hepatitis E vaccine. *Vaccine* 2009; 27(12): 1869–74)

4.1.3.2 Efficacy of HEV Vaccine

In the phase 3 trial, 122,179 people were enrolled and screened for eligibility. 112,604 eligible participants aged 16–65 years were randomized for at least one dose vaccination, and 97,356 participants completed all three doses and were included in the analysis of the primary endpoint.

In the primary analysis population who completed all three doses, 15 participants in the placebo group developed hepatitis E within 13 months after receiving the third dose, and no participant who developed hepatitis E in the vaccine group developed hepatitis E (Table 4.1). The efficacy of the hepatitis E vaccine after three doses was 100.0% (95% CI, 72.1–100.0), and the

Table 4.1 Efficacy of recombinant hepatitis E vaccine in the initial phase 3 study

	Follow-up (month of study)	Vaccine group			Placebo group			Vaccine efficacy (95% Cl)	p-value
		Number of participants/ person-years at risk	Number of cases	Incidence (per 10,000 person-years)	Number of participants/ person-years at risk	Number of cases	Incidence (per 10,000 person-years)		
Pre-protocol									
The whole group (three doses)	7–19	48,693/48,594.6	0	0.0	48,663/48,555.1	15	3.1	100.0% (72.1–100.0)	<0.0001
First 6 months of follow-up	7–13	48,693/23,981.9	0	0.0	48,663/23,965.8	6	2.5	100.0% (15.12–100.0)	0.014
Second 6 months of follow-up	14–19	48,693/24,612.8	0	0.0	48,663/24,589.3	9	3.7	100.0% (49.4–100.0)	0.003
First two doses subset	1.5–5	54,986/20,202.1	0	0.0	54,973/20,196.8	5	2.5	100.0% (9.1–100.0)	<0.0001
Population receiving at least one dose	7–19	56,302/56,104.7	1	0.2	56,302/56,081.2	16	2.9	93.8% (59.8–99.9)	0.0001
Modified subset one (all participants received at least one dose)	0–19	56,302/87,354.2	1	0.1	56,302/87,323.2	22	2.5	95.5% (66.3–99.4)	<0.0001
Modified subset two (participants in the reactogenicity subset were excluded because of lacking follow-up data during 0–6 months)	0–19	54,986/86,040.4	1	0.1	54,973/86,003.4	21	2.4	95.2% (64.6–99.4)	<0.0001

Person-years at risk are the cumulative follow-up years of at-risk participants at the indicated timepoint. The number of at-risk participants is the initial number of participants entered in the study–(cumulative hepatitis E cases + participants who had dropped out of the study)

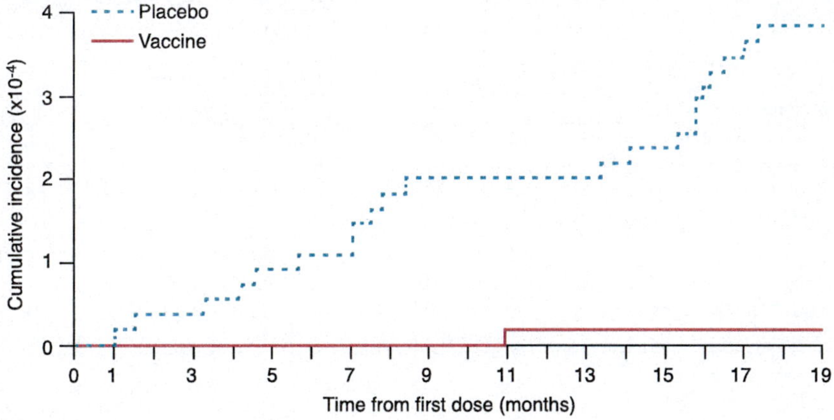

Number at risk											
Placebo	54973	54964	54942	54917	54885	54852	54794	54761	54716	54679	54661
Vaccine	54986	54979	54957	54925	54899	54868	54813	54790	54758	54728	54709
Cumulative number of participants with hepatitis E											
Placebo	0	0	2	5	6	11	11	11	13	19	21
Vaccine	0	0	0	0	0	0	0	1	1	1	1

Fig. 4.8 Cumulative incidence of hepatitis E in the initial phase 3 study. (Reprinted with permission from Fig. 3, Zhu FC, Zhang J, Zhang XF, et al. Efficacy and safety of a recombinant hepatitis E vaccine in healthy adults: a large-scale, randomized, double-blind placebo-controlled, phase 3 trial. *Lancet (London, England)* 2010; 376(9744): 895–902.). Cumulative incidence in each group at an indicated time = (cumulative number of cases/cumulated following-up time for at-risk participants × 10,000). The number at risk = initial number of participants who entered the study − (cumulative hepatitis E cases + participants who had subsequently dropped out of the study). The difference between the groups was significant ($p < 0.001$ by log-rank test)

protection for all participants lasted up to over 1 year. Besides, 5 participants in the placebo group developed hepatitis E between 14 days after the second dose and before the third dose, and the vaccine efficacy after two doses was also 100.0% (95% CI, 9.1–100.0).

Most participants who received at least one dose of vaccination were followed up for 19 months, and a small number of participants were followed up from the seventh month of the study. During the follow-up period, 23 hepatitis E cases were obtained, with 1 case in the vaccine group (at least one dose) and 22 cases in the placebo group (Table 4.1). In participants who received at least one dose of vaccination, the vaccine efficacy was 95.5% (95% CI, 66.3–99.4). Within 12 months from the 31st day after receiving the final dose (which could be the first, second, or third dose), 17 hepatitis E cases were founded, one in the vaccine group and 16 in the placebo group, with the efficacy of 93.8% (95% CI, 59.8–99.9%).

As shown the cumulative incidence of hepatitis E followed up for 19 months from the beginning (Fig. 4.8), and the two groups were significantly different.

The severity of most AEs in the phase 3 trial was mild. The incidence of serious adverse events during the study was similar between the vaccine group and placebo group, and none of them were vaccine-related (Table 4.2). In the reactogenicity subset, the incidence of solicited injection-site AEs within 72 h after each dose in the vaccine group was significantly higher than that in the placebo group (13.5% vs. 7.1%, $p < 0.0001$). The most common injection-site AEs were pain, swelling, and itching, and the incidence of them was higher in the vaccine group compared with the placebo group. The proportion of systemic AEs was similar in the two groups (20.3% vs. 19.8%). In the participants not in the reactogenicity subset, the incidence of solicited injection-site AEs in the vaccine group was significantly higher

Table 4.2 Safety outcomes

	Number of adverse events (rate, 95% CI)		
	Vaccine group	Placebo group	*p*-value
Reactogenicity subset			
Number of participants who received more than one dose	1316	1329	–
Solicited local adverse events within 72 h after each dose			
Local adverse events	177 (13.5%, 11.65–15.41)	94 (7.1%, 5.75–8.59)	<0.0001
Local adverse events ≥ grade 3	2 (0.2%, 0.02–0.55)	0 (0.0%, 0.00–0.28)	0.248
Solicited systemic adverse events within 72 h after each dose			
Systemic adverse events	267 (20.3%, 18.15–22.56)	263 (19.8%, 17.68–22.03)	0.748
Systemic adverse events ≥ grade 3	7 (0.5%, 0.21–1.09)	4 (0.3%, 0.08–0.77)	0.356
Total vaccinated cohort minus the reactogenicity subset			
Number of participants who received more than one dose	54,986	54,973	–
Solicited local adverse events within 72 h after each dose			
Local adverse events	1532 (2.8%, 2.65–2.93)	1051 (1.9%, 1.80–2.03)	<0.0001
Local adverse events ≥grade 3	61 (0.1%, 0.08–0.14)	27 (0.1%, 0.03–0.07)	<0.0001
Solicited systemic adverse events within 72 h after each dose			
Systemic adverse events	1068 (1.9%, 1.83–2.06)	1045 (1.9%, 1.79–2.02)	0.617
Systemic adverse events ≥ grade 3	60 (0.1%, 0.08–0.14)	63 (0.1%, 0.09–0.15)	0.786

Symptoms with a frequency of more than 1% in any group are listed. **p*-values are two-sided and were calculated by Fisher's exact test

than that in the placebo group (2.8% vs. 1.9%, $p < 0.0001$) and there was no significant difference in the proportion of solicited systemic AEs between the two groups.

Serum samples were collected from 11,165 participants before vaccination and 1 month after receiving the third dose, with 5567 in the vaccine group and 5598 in the placebo group. The proportion of participants who had four times or more increase in antibody concentration after vaccination in the vaccine group was 98.7%, whose GMC increased from 0.14 Wu/mL to 19.0 Wu/mL (95% CI, 18.6–19.4). In the placebo group, 2.1% of the participants had an antibody response and the episodes were all subclinical infections.

The overall follow-up period of the participants who were enrolled in the initial efficacy study was 54 months. Together with the 37 hepatitis E cases in the extended study, a total of 60 cases were founded. The cumulative incidence of hepatitis E in the vaccine group was significantly lower than that in the control group, with 53 cases in the control group, and 7 in the vaccine group (Table 4.3). In the vaccine group, the number of cases who received three doses, two doses, and one dose were 3, 1, and 3, respectively. There was no significant difference in clinical disease manifestations between the vaccine group and the placebo group. Laboratory test results of the cases were generally similar between the two groups, but there were differences in the affinities of antibodies in patients in the acute phase. The high affinity of antibodies in the vaccine group was consistent with the recall response of previously immunized patients. In contrast, the low affinity

Table 4.3 Incidence of Hepatitis E and vaccine efficacy in the extended phase 3 study

	Vaccine group		Control group		Vaccine efficacy	
	Cases of Hepatitis E	Incidence	Cases of Hepatitis E	Incidence		
		No./10,000 person-year (95% cl)		No./10,000 person-year (95% cl)	% (95% Cl)	*p*-value
Modified intention-to-treat						
0–18 months	1	0.1 (0.0–0.6)	22	2.5 (1.6–3.8)	95.5 (66.3–99.4)	<0.001
0–30 months	4	0.3 (0.1–0.7)	38	2.7 (1.9–3.6)	89.5 (70.5–96.2)	<0.001
0–42 months	5	0.3 (0.1–0.6)	45	2.3 (1.7–3.0)	88.9 (72.0–95.6)	<0.001
0–54 months	7	0.3 (0.1–0.6)	53	2.1 (1.6–2.7)	86.8 (71.0–94.0)	<0.001
Intention-to-treat						
7–18 months	1	0.2 (0.0–1.0)	16	2.8 (1.6–4.6)	93.8 (52.9–99.2)	<0.001
7–30 months	4	0.4 (0.1–0.9)	32	2.9 (2.0–4.0)	87.5 (64.7–95.6)	<0.001
7–42 months	5	0.3 (0.1–0.7)	39	2.3 (1.7–3.2)	87.2 (67.5–95.0)	<0.001
7–54 months	7	0.3 (0.1–0.6)	47	2.1 (1.5–2.8)	85.1 (67.1–93.3)	<0.001
19–54 months	6	0.4 (0.1–0.8)	31	1.9 (1.3–2.6)	80.1 (53.7–91.9)	<0.001
Per-protocol						
7–18 months	0	0.0 (0.0–0.0)	15	3.1 (1.7–5.1)	100.0 (72.1–100.0)	<0.001
7–30 months	1	0.1 (0.0–0.6)	30	3.1 (2.1–4.4)	96.7 (75.6–99.6)	<0.001
7–42 months	1	0.1 (0.0–0.4)	37	2.6 (1.8–3.5)	97.3 (80.3–99.6)	<0.001
7–54 months	3	0.2 (0.0–0.5)	45	2.3 (1.7–3.1)	93.3 (78.6–97.9)	<0.001
19–54 months	3	0.2 (0.0–0.6)	30	2.1 (1.4–3.0)	90.0 (67.3–97.0)	<0.001

The cumulative incidence in the two study groups at an indicated time was calculated in the following way: the cumulative number of cases/cumulative follow-up time for at-risk participants × 10,000 of antibodies in most patients in the control group was consistent with the antibody response of people who had no previous immunity. Among the hepatitis E cases, twenty-nine were sequenced with virus isolates, of which 26 were infected with HEV genotype 4 and 3 were infected with HEV genotype 1.

The extended follow-up study showed that the efficacy of the hepatitis E vaccine did not decrease, and there was still significant efficacy at the 54th month (Table 4.3). Vaccine efficacy in the modified intention-to-treat set, the intention-to-treat set, and the per-protocol set was 86.8% (95% CI, 71.0–94.0), 85.1% (95% CI, 67.1–93.3), and 93.3% (95% CI, 78.6–97.9), respectively.

4.1.4 Conclusions

4.1.4.1 Safety

Studies have shown that the safety of the HEV 239 vaccine is good. The most common reported injection-site AEs were pain, itching, and swelling. The proportion of injection-site AEs in the vaccine group is significantly higher than that in the placebo group, which may be because the protein content of the HEV vaccine is higher than that of the HBV vaccine. The proportion of systemic AEs in the two groups was similar, and the most common systemic AE reported was fever. The proportions of injection-site and systemic AEs with severity level 3 or higher caused by the vaccine between the vaccine group and the placebo group were similar and small, but they were both deemed unrelated to vaccination.

4.1.4.2 Immunogenicity

The HEV 239 vaccine induced a robust and persistent immune response. Participants in the phase 2 trial had 100% seroconversion after three doses, and 98% seroconversion after two doses. The mean antibody level induced by the vaccine was lower than that of the pooled serum from hepatitis E patients but markedly higher than that of the pooled sera from seropositive participants. The extended follow-up efficacy study showed that 87% of participants who received three doses of 30 μg vaccine remained seropositive at month 55.

4.1.4.3 Efficacy

The HEV 239 vaccine is effective for the population over 16 years old and the efficacy can last for a long time. In the primary analysis population of the phase 3 trial, HEV 239 vaccine recipients were not infected with hepatitis E. Participants who are infected with hepatitis E were all vaccinated with HBV. The efficacy of the three-doses and two-doses HEV 239 vaccine were both 100%. The extended follow-up study confirmed the long-term efficacy of the HEV 239 vaccine.

4.1.4.4 Post-Licensure Surveillance

The WHO Strategic Advisory Group of Experts on Immunization issued a position paper in 2015 that reviewed the existing evidence on the safety, immunogenicity, and effectiveness of the hepatitis E vaccine that was first licensed in China [15]. It stated that many experimental hepatitis E vaccines have been evaluated in non-human primate virus attack studies, other animal models, or clinical trials, but only China's HEV 239 has been approved for use as of 2018. Phase 4 clinical studies have shown that patients with chronic hepatitis B can induce anti-HEV antibodies at 11.89 (95% CI, 9.86–14.35) Wu/ml, and healthy people can induce anti-HEV antibodies at 17.35 (95% CI, 15.57–19.34) Wu/ml after receiving HEV 239 vaccine [16].

The HEV 239 vaccine has attracted widespread attention from the international community after it went on the market. In 2017, Bangladesh started the first overseas clinical trial of the HEV 239 vaccine, and a total of 19,000 people were vaccinated. In 2019, the U.S. Food and Drug Administration (FDA) approved the application for clinical trials of the HEV 239 vaccine in the United States. This is the first clinical trial of a Chinese vaccine in the United States. In 2019, the Pakistani government approved the marketing registration of the HEV 239 vaccine.

4.2 Enterovirus 71 Vaccine

4.2.1 Background and Rational

Enterovirus 71 (EV71) is a small, single-stranded, positive-sense RNA virus from the Enterovirus genus of the *Picornaviridae* family that is highly infectious and was first isolated in California in 1969 [17, 18]. The main diseases caused by EV71 infection are hand, foot, and mouth disease (HFMD), and herpes angina (HA), a few severe cases can be complicated with encephalitis, aseptic meningitis, pulmonary edema, severe brain failure, etc. [19, 20].

EV71 is one of the main pathogens of HFMD, and EV71-associated HFMD has been reported worldwide [21]. For the past few years, the prevalence of HFMD caused by EV71 mainly occurred in the Asia-Pacific region and has become a significant public health problem [22–24]. In 2008, a large-scale HFMD epidemic broke out in Fuyang City, Anhui Province in China, which attracted great attention from the government and health authorities [25]. In the same year, the Ministry of Health of China put HFMD under the management of the "C" class infectious disease.

Diverse vaccine platforms were used for the research and development of EV71 vaccines, including the inactivated vaccine which is the primary platform in mainland China, live attenuated vaccine, DNA vaccine, subunit vaccine, virus-like particle vaccine, and so on. The Phase III clinical trials of the EV71 vaccine developed in 2003 by Kunming Institute, Sinovac, Sinopharm, and Wuhan Biologics were completed in 2013 [26]. The EV71 vaccines from Kunming Institute and Sinovac were approved for marketing by the National Food and Drug Administration in December 2015 [27].

4.2.2 Methods

4.2.2.1 Participants and Study Sites

Previous epidemiological data indicated that infants aged 6–35 months are the population most susceptible to EV71 infection, due to the lack of protective antibodies against EV71. In consequence, infants aged 6–35 months are considered to be the target population for inactivated EV71 vaccine. Healthy children aged from 6 to 35 months with no history of HFMD, no vaccine contraindications, and signed inform consent forms were recruited [28, 29].

Epidemiological surveillance showed that a large-scale HFMD epidemic occurring every 2 or 3 years on account of EV71 was periodically prevalent. In the study of determining the optimal vaccine dosage, formulation, and regime, to avoid the great interference of excessive natural epidemic of EV71 on the vaccine-induced antibody, areas with epidemics of HFMD in the past 2 years were selected as EV71 prevalence was likely to be low during the study period. In the study of evaluating vaccine efficacy, EV71-associated diseases needed to be monitored, so areas with low epidemic levels of HFMD in the past 2 years and that a large-scale epidemic of EV71 may occur during the study period were selected.

4.2.2.2 Design of Optimal Dosage, Formulation, and Immunization Schedule

The inactivated EV71 vaccine developed by Beijing Vigoo Biological (Beijing, China) used EV71 strain FY7VP5/AH/CHN/2008 as the seed virus (GenBank accession number JX025561).

In the randomized, double-blind, placebo-controlled, phase 2 trial, healthy infants aged 6–11 months and children aged 12–36 months were recruited and screened for eligibility [28]. Eligible participants were sequentially and randomly allocated to be vaccinated with the EV71 vaccine of 160 U with adjuvant, 320 U with adjuvant, 640 U with adjuvant, and 640 U without adjuvant or placebo at a ratio of 1:1:1:1:1. A total of 1200 participants were involved, with 120 participants in each dose group in both age groups.

Fourteen months after completing the first dose vaccination in the phase 2 trial, participants who had received two-dose EV71 vaccines regardless of dosage or adjuvant were re-recruited for a booster vaccination [30]. In the booster study, participants were classified into four dose groups, including the EV71 antigen of 160 U with adjuvant, 320 U with adjuvant, 640 U with adjuvant, and 640 U without adjuvant. In each dose group, participants were booster vaccinated with the priming dose of EV71 vaccine or placebo in a ratio of 2:1, and blood samples were taken 28 days after booster vaccination (Fig. 4.9).

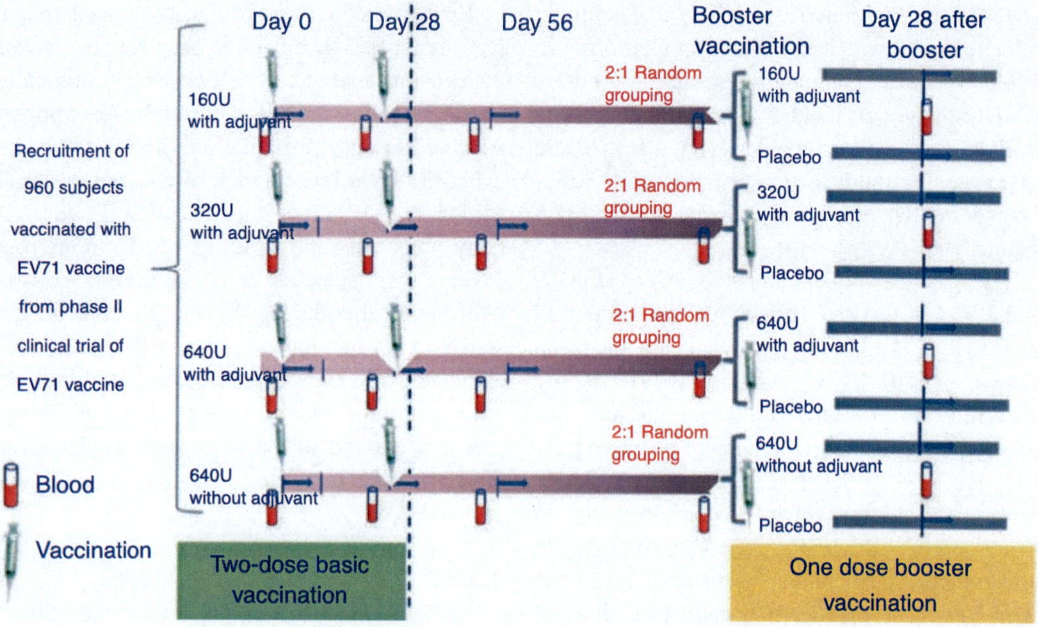

Fig. 4.9 Vaccine formulation, immunization regimen, and prime-boost immunization design

4.2.2.3 Study Design of Vaccine Efficacy

There were reported two phase III trials with similar study designs but different vaccines. One of the experimental vaccines was developed by Sinovac using EV71 strain H07 (subgenotype C4) containing 400 U of EV71 antigen including alum-adjuvant, and the other was developed by Beijing Vigoo Biological using EV71 strain FY7VP5/AH/CHN/2008 (genotype C4) containing 320 U of antigen and 0.18 mg of alum. The placebo used in both trials contained the same adjuvant as the corresponding vaccine and did not contain the EV71 antigen [31, 32].

Both studies were multicenter, randomized, double-blind, placebo-controlled clinical trials. Children aged 6–35 months are recruited from multiple towns or villages in several centers. Participants with a history of HFMD and previous EV71 vaccination were excluded through medical history inquiry and physical examination. Eligible participants were randomly assigned 1:1 to receive two doses of EV71 vaccine or placebo on days 0 and 28. All vaccinated individuals achieved surveillance of EV71-associated disease for 1 year (from day 56 through month 14). Blood samples were collected before the first dose (day 0) and 28 days after the second dose (day 56). Additionally, at months 8 and 14, blood samples were taken from a subset of participants (immunogenicity cohort). Neutralizing antibodies against EV71 were measured with a modified cytopathogenic effect assay. Participants were visited at home or came to the clinic at 5, 8, 11, and 14 months to record any medically significant events. All potential cases were reported by the clinics or hospitals. Throat or rectal swabs or both were taken from them within 24 h and sent to the central laboratories for pathogen detection. Real-time PCR (fluorescence assay) was used to test for EV71, Coxsackie A virus 16, and other enteroviruses. Participants who were positive for EV71-specific RNA were considered suspected cases. Then throat and anal swabs and stool samples from them were collected every 3 days in the acute phase and every week in the convalescence phase. All specimens as well as blood samples in the acute phase were transferred to the laboratory to confirm cases. Virological confirmation of EV71-associated disease was defined as two consecutive PCR tests positive for EV71RNA or virus isolation with positive VP1 sequence in the throat and anal swabs or stool samples.

The primary endpoint of the trial was the efficacy of EV71-related HFMD from 14 days after completion of vaccination to 1 year after the first dose. The secondary endpoints were efficacy for severe HFMD during the same study period and seropositive rates for serum EV71-neutralizing antibodies at 56 and 180 days after the first dose.

Based on the efficacy study cohort, a nested case-control study was designed [31, 32]. Confirmed cases of EV71-related disease were matched to a control group without EV71-related disease by location and age in a ratio of 1:5. At day 56, sensitivity was calculated by dividing the number of EV71-associated cases with neutralizing antibody titers below the cutoff value by all cases, and specificity was calculated by dividing the number of controls with neutralizing antibody titers equal to or above the cutoff value by all controls. When the sum of sensitivity and specificity reached the peak, the corresponding lowest titer was the possible alternative endpoint for protection.

However, in phase 3 clinical trial of the CAMS vaccine, the age range of children recruited was extended to 6–71 months. Unlike the two Vero cell-based vaccines, the CAMS vaccine was cultured in human diploid cells and then purified and inactivated, containing 100 U of inactivated EV71 virus antigen, adsorbed in 0.5 mg aluminum hydroxide, and suspended in 0.5 mL buffered saline. The placebo contained equal volumes of aluminum hydroxide and buffered saline and without EV71 antigen. Two doses of vaccine or placebo are given 28 days apart. Eligible participants were divided into two groups of 6–23 months and 24–71 months for analysis. Immunogenicity was also evaluated in a subgroup of participants, whose blood samples were collected at 56 and 180 days to assess neutralizing antibody levels.

4.2.2.4 Statistical Analysis

The baseline characteristics of the participants in the EV71 vaccine group and placebo group were described, and the balance between groups was compared. We used the χ^2 test or Fisher's exact test to analyze categorical data, and ANOVA to analyze continuous data. If it did not meet normal distribution, the rank-sum test was used.

Unless otherwise stated, all statistical tests were two-sided, and statistical significance was defined as $p < 0.05$. If there is a significant difference in the χ^2 test, the pairwise comparison is carried out, and the test level α is adjusted to: $\alpha' = 1 - \sqrt[m]{1-\alpha}$, m is the number of pairwise comparisons. If there are significant differences among multiple groups in ANOVA, it is necessary to use the Student-Newman-Keuls test to make a pairwise comparison among multiple groups.

The immunogenicity data include the study of optimal immune dose and dosage form, immune procedure, immune persistence and booster immunity, batch consistency, and immunogenicity in cross-immunization with poliomyelitis.

The seroconversion rate and positive rate were calculated as follows: the seroconversion rate (%) = the number of people whose serum antibody turned positive after immunization/the number of people in this group who were randomized and vaccinated; the positive rate (%) = the number of people whose serum antibody level was positive after immunization/the number of people in this group who were randomized and vaccinated.

The geometric mean titer (GMT) is the inverse log conversion value of the average log conversion value of neutralizing antibody titer in EV71. The geometric mean titer growth multiple (GMFI) is the inverse log conversion value of the average log conversion value of neutralizing antibody titer growth multiple in EV71.

The analysis of the antibody seroconversion rate of the participants after vaccination refers to the comparison of the antibody level and the average increase times of the antibody titer between the vaccine group and the control group after immunization compared with that before immunization. The qualitative data were tested by the χ^2 test, and the quantitative data obeyed the approximately normal distribution after logarithmic conversion. The converted data were compared between groups by u-test or ANOVA.

Protection efficacy data mainly includes protection efficacy monitoring data and cross-protection monitoring data. Main statistical indicators:

Incidence density rate = (Number of years of patients/Observation number of years) *100%;

Observation number of years

$$= \sum_{i=1}^{n} \frac{\text{each number of days}}{365.25};$$

Each number of days = End date-Observation begin date + 1;

Number of days of patients = Onset date-Observation begins date + 1;

The protection rate of the vaccine was calculated according to the following formula:

Vaccine efficacy was defined as 100 × (1 − vaccine incidence density rate/placebo incidence density rate).

Vaccine efficacy was estimated by a Cox proportional hazard model. If no participant in the vaccine group had EV71 disease, the 95% CI for efficacy was assessed by an exact conditional procedure dependent on a Poisson distribution. We used the Kaplan-Meier method to estimate event-free survival.

The serum anti-EV71 neutralizing antibodies of the participants in this subgroup on the 56th day were analyzed, and the sensitivity and specificity of distinguishing cases from non-cases were calculated when different levels of neutralizing antibodies were used as cutoff [33, 34]. The cutoff with the maximum Youden index could be thought of as a surrogate of protection for it could provide the clearest distinction between cases and controls.

Sensitivity: on the 56th day, the proportion of diseases caused by EV71 infection in all cases caused by EV71 infection when the level of serum neutralization antibody was lower than the threshold.

Specificity: the proportion of participants whose serum antibody levels were equal to or higher than the threshold on the 56th day among the participants (non-cases) who did not develop diseases caused by EV71 infection.

Youden index ([sensitivity + specificity] − 1).

4.2.3 Results

4.2.3.1 Immune Program for Optimal Immune Dose Form

In the phase 2 trial of the Vigoo EV71 vaccine, a total of 1200 eligible participants were enrolled, half infants and half children. All participants received their first dose of vaccine or placebo and completed a 28-day follow-up. One thousand one hundred fifty of them received a second dose on day 28, and 1148 accomplished the 56-day follow-up to evaluate safety. According-to-protocol immunogenic analysis consists of 1106 participants, whose three blood samples were collected consecutively on days 0, 28, and 56 (Fig. 4.10).

The seropositive rate at baseline ranged from 33.3% to 45.0% in the children group, and from 18.3% to 26.7% in the infants' group. GMTs at baseline were low and did not differ significantly between groups (Table 4.4). GMT, serum conversion rate, and GMFI after vaccination were significantly higher in participants in the vaccine group than those in the placebo group ($p < 0.0001$). Of the four vaccine groups, the GMT value on day 56 was the lowest in the adjuvant-free vaccine group. The GMT was significantly higher in the adjuvanted vaccine group than in the adjuvant-free vaccine group. However, the placebo elicits very little antibody response.

In the seronegative subgroup of participants at baseline, GMT, serum conversion rate, and GMFI slightly increased after immunization with the first dose and greatly increased after immunization with the second dose. Dose-dependent immunogenicity was observed in the three adjuvant formulations, with GMT and GMFI increasing from low dose to high (Table 4.5). But seroconversion rates were higher in all four groups than in the placebo group.

Blood samples were collected from 461 (76.8%) infants and 505 (84.2%) children at 8 months to analyze immune persistence. The GMTs declined to 86.3 (160 U adjuvant vaccine), 96.3 (320 U adjuvant vaccine), 177.4 (640 U adjuvant vaccine), and 58.8 (640 U adjuvant-free vaccine). However, seroconversion rates in infants and children were almost identical at 8 months and 56 days.

One year later, a booster immunization study included 844 participants from the phase 2 trial. They were then classified into four groups by their primary doses. Each group was randomly divided into two groups in a ratio of 2:1 and received one booster vaccine in compliance with the primary dose or placebo (Fig. 4.11). A total of 773 booster recipients completed the 28-day safety follow-up, of whom 707 were included in

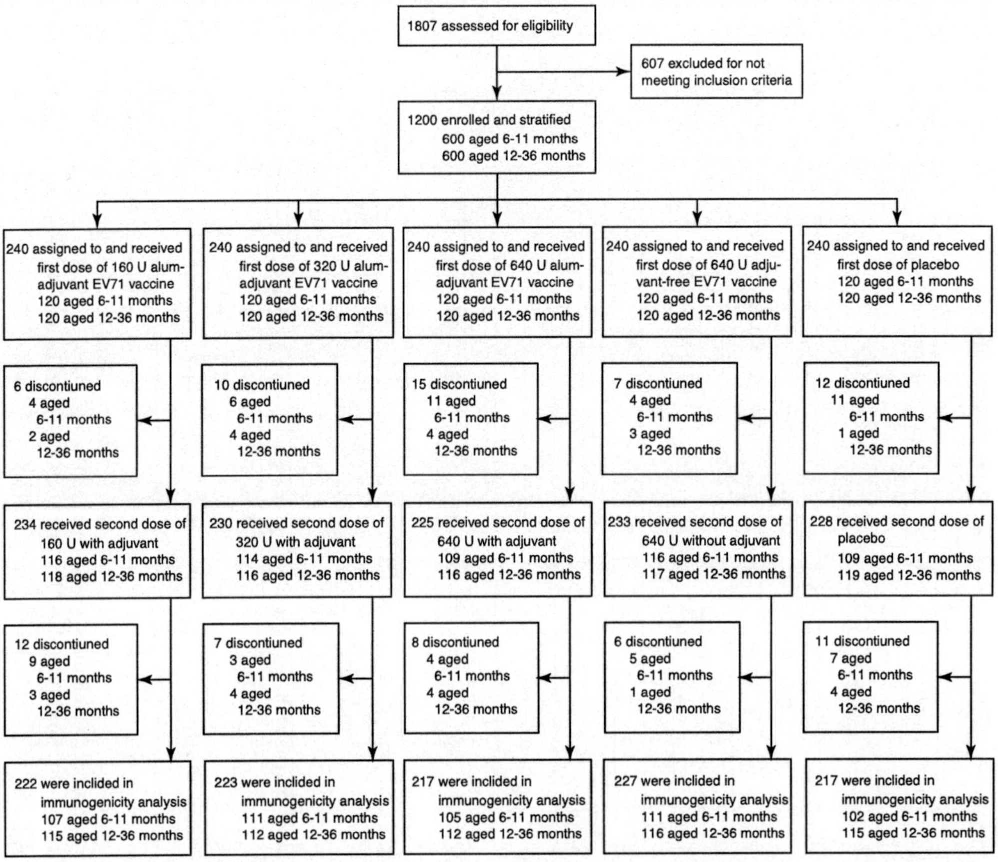

Fig. 4.10 Trial profile. (Reprinted with permission from Zhu FC, Liang ZL, Li XL, et al. Immunogenicity and safety of an enterovirus 71 vaccine in healthy Chinese children and infants: a randomized, double-blind, placebo-controlled phase 2 clinical trial. *Lancet (London, England)* 2013; 381(9871): 1037–45)

the according-to-protocol cohort for immunogenicity analysis.

The GMTs of EV71 antibody in four groups were fairly high (>138.2) before the booster injection. But the booster immunization with the 320 U and 640 U with adjuvant-induced substantial antibody response as shown of GMTs than with 640 U without adjuvant. The 640 U with the adjuvant formulation group has the highest GMTs (4410.7; 95% CI, 3565.6–5456.1) after the booster dose, followed by 320 U with the adjuvant formulation group (3352.5; 95% CI, 2779.1–4044.0), the 160 U with adjuvant formulation group (2352.6; 95% CI, 1959.0–2825.4) and 640 U without an adjuvant group (2214.8; 95% CI, 1844.2–2659.8) (Table 4.6).

The proportion of participants with a titer of ≥1:32 numerically increased after the booster vaccination, but only significantly in the groups that received 160 U with adjuvant ($p = 0.001$) or 640 U without adjuvant ($p = 0.0006$). GMFIs ranged from 12.0 to 16.7 in all formulation groups, whereas almost no change was in placebo ($p < 0.01$). A similar trend was observed concerning seroconversion rates, with the highest (92.1%) in the 640 U With the adjuvant group. Similar results were also observed in the intention-to-treat cohort for the evaluation of the immunogenicity of the booster dose.

After 28 days of booster immunization, the higher proposition of participants with antibody titer ≥cutoff values in each vaccine group, showed a strong immune response, while almost no increase was observed among those who received placebo (Fig. 4.12).

In phase 2 of the Sinovac EV71 vaccine, a total of 480 participants were enrolled and ran-

Table 4.4 GMT, seroconversion rate, and GMFI of neutralizing antibody against EV71. (Reprinted with permission from Table 2, Zhu FC, Liang ZL, Li XL, et al. Immunogenicity and safety of an enterovirus 71 vaccine in healthy Chinese children and infants: a randomized, double-blind, placebo-controlled phase 2 clinical trial. *Lancet (London, England)* 2013; 381(9871): 1037–45.)

	160 U with adjuvant	320 U with adjuvant	640 U with adjuvant	640 U without adjuvant	Placebo	*p*-value
6–11 months						
n	107	111	105	111	102	
Day 0						
GMT	9.0 (6.4–12.7)	7.9 (5.8–10.8)	11.6 (7.9–17.2)	9.9 (7.0–14.0)	10.0 (7.0–14.3)	–
Day 28						
GMT	21.2 (14.8–30.4)[c]	28.5 (20.4–39.7)[bc]	67.3 (47.5–95.4)[a]	43.3 (30.0–62.3)[ab]	10.7 (7.3–15.5)[d]	<0.0001
Seroconversion	18 (16.8%,10.3–25.3)	28 (25.2%, 17.5–34.4)	48 (45.7%, 36.0–55.7)	38 (34.2%, 25.5–43.8)	5 (4.9%, 1.6–11.1)	<0.0001
GMFI	2.4 (1.9–2.9)[c]	3.6 (2.9–4.5)[bc]	5.8 (4.7–7.2)[a]	4.4 (3.4–5.7)[ab]	1.1 (0.9–1.2)[d]	<0.0001
Day 56						
GMT	357.0 (270.1–471.9)[b]	497.9 (383.1–647.0)[ab]	742.2 (577.3–954.3)[a]	210.3 (161.5–273.9)[c]	11.8 (7.9–17.6)[d]	<0.0001
Seroconversion	93 (86.9%, 79.0–92.7)	105 (94.6%, 88.6–98.0)	100 (95.2%, 89.2–98.4)	93 (83.8%, 75.6–90.1)	5 (4.9%, 1.6–11.1)	<0.0001
GMFI	39.6 (28.1–55.9)[a]	62.8 (48.0–82.4)[a]	63.9 (46.0–88.9)[a]	21.2 (15.9–28.3)[b]	1.2 (1.0–1.5)[c]	<0.0001
12–36 months						
n	115*	112	112	116	115	
Day 0						
GMT	20.1 (13.3–30.4)	26.7 (17.6–40.6)	15.0 (10.3–21.8)	23.9 (15.5–36.8)	21.4 (14.3–32.1)	–
Day 28						
GMT	61.8 (41.0–93.1)[b]	139.0 (91.4–211.2)[a]	99.6 (66.8–148.7)[ab]	113.4 (74.6–172.3)[ab]	28.6 (18.6–44.2)[c]	<0.0001
Seroconversion	33 (28.7%, 20.7–37.9)	53 (47.3%, 37.8–57.0)	63 (56.3%, 46.6–65.6)	45 (38.8%, 29.9–48.3)	8 (7.0%, 3.1–13.3)	<0.0001
GMFI	3.1 (2.5–3.7)[b]	5.2 (4.1–6.6)[a]	6.6 (5.4–8.2)[a]	4.8 (3.7–6.1)[a]	1.3 (1.1–1.7)[c]	<0.0001
Day 56						
GMT	731.4 (536.2–997.8)[b]	1383.2 (1037.3–1844.5)[a]	1330.2 (1000.9–1767.7)[a]	509.0 (372.8–694.8)[b]	37.0 (22.9–59.7)[c]	<0.0001
Seroconversion	103 (89.6%, 82.5–94.5)	107 (95.5%, 89.9–98.5)	109 (97.3%, 92.4–99.4)	98 (84.5%, 76.6–90.5)	16 (13.9%, 8.2–21.6)	<0.0001
GMFI	36.4 (26.3–50.2)[b]	51.7 (38.6–69.4)[a]	88.7 (65.7–119.7)[a]	21.3 (16.1–28.4)[c]	1.7 (1.3–2.3)[d]	<0.0001

Data are GMT (95% CI), number of participants (%, 95% CI), or GMFI (95% CI). n = total participants included in immunogenic according-to-protocol analysis. The p-values are the result of a comparison between the five treatment groups. Multi comparisons were applied based on an adjusted $\alpha = 0.005$ for seroconversion rate. The Student-Newman-Keuls test was used for the multicomparison of GMTs and GMFIs. a, b, c, and d (where a > b > c > d) mark statistically significant differences between each treatment group. Measurements on day 0 were taken immediately before vaccination. GMT = geometric mean titer. GMFI = geometric mean fold increase

*One participant in this group had a prevaccination antibody titre of 1:8192 and a postvaccination titre of 1:16 384 (upper end of assay) so was classed as not having had seroconversion after vaccination because he had only had a two-fold increase; however, it is possible that his post-vaccination titre was higher than 1:16 384

Table 4.5 GMT, seroconversion rate, and GMFI of neutralizing antibody against EV71 in the subgroup of participants with a baseline antibody titer of <1:8. (Reprinted with permission from Table 3, Zhu FC, Liang ZL, Li XL, et al. Immunogenicity and safety of an enterovirus 71 vaccine in healthy Chinese children and infants: a randomized, double-blind, placebo-controlled phase 2 clinical trial. *Lancet (London, England)* 2013; 381(9871): 1037–45.)

	160 U with adjuvant	320 U with adjuvant	640 U with adjuvant	640 U without adjuvant	Placebo	*p*-value
6–11 months						
n	85	93	80	85	78	
Day 28						
GMT	10.5 (8.3–13.2)[c]	16.1 (12.9–20.1)[b]	30.4 (24.0–38.5)[a]	21.2 (16.2–27.8)[b]	4.4 (3.9–4.8)[d]	<0.0001
Seroconversion	13 (15.3%, 8.4–24.7)	22 (23.7%, 15.5–33.6)	38 (47.5%, 36.2–59.0)	28 (32.9%, 23.1–44.0)	1 (1.3%, 0.0–6.9)	<0.0001
GMFI	2.6 (2.1–3.3)[c]	4.0 (3.2–5.0)[b]	7.6 (6.0–9.6)[a]	5.3 (4.0–7.0)[b]	1.1 (1.0–1.2)[d]	<0.0001
Day 56						
GMT	280.9 (207.4–380.6)[b]	358.2 (280.5–457.5)[b]	522.8 (403.9–676.6)[a]	141.0 (111.2–178.8)[c]	4.8 (3.8–6.0)[d]	<0.0001
Seroconversion	80 (94.1%, 86.8–98.1)	91 (97.9%, 92.5–99.7)	79 (98.8%, 93.2–100.0)	79 (92.9%, 85.3–97.4)	2 (2.6%, 0.3–9.0)	<0.0001
GMFI	70.2 (51.8–95.2)[b]	89.6 (70.1–114.4)[b]	130.7 (101.0–169.2)[a]	35.3 (27.8–44.7)[c]	1.2 (1.0–1.5)[d]	<0.0001
12–36 months						
n	71	59	74	69	70	
Day 28						
GMT	14.5 (11.5–18.4)[b]	24.3 (17.6–33.6)[a]	28.0 (21.8–35.8)[a]	22.5 (17.3–29.4)[a]	6.4 (4.4–9.3)[c]	<0.0001
Seroconversion	15 (21.1%, 12.3–32.4)	24 (40.7%, 28.1–54.3)	34 (46.0%, 34.3–57.9)	26 (37.7%, 26.3–50.2)	6 (8.6%, 3.2–17.7)	<0.0001
GMFI	3.6 (2.9–4.6)[b]	6.1 (4.4–8.4)[a]	7.0 (5.5–8.9)[a]	5.6 (4.3–7.4)[a]	1.6 (1.1–2.3)[c]	<0.0001
Day 56						
GMT	372.7 (277.9–499.9)[b]	498.0 (383.4–646.9)[ab]	708.4 (524.1–957.6)[a]	171.9 (133.9–220.7)[c]	7.3 (4.8–11.1)[d]	<0.0001
Seroconversion	71 (100.0%, 94.9–100.0)	59 (100.0%, 93.9–100.0)	73 (98.7%, 92.7–100.0)	67 (97.1%, 89.9–99.7)	7 (10.0%, 4.1–19.5)	<0.0001
GMFI	93.2 (69.5–125.0)[b]	124.5 (95.9–161.7)[ab]	177.1 (131.0–239.4)[a]	43.0 (33.5–55.2)[c]	1.8 (1.2–2.8)[d]	<0.0001

Data are GMT (95% CI), number of participants (%, 95% CI), or GMFI (95% CI). *n* = total participants with a baseline antibody titer of <1:8 included in immunogenic according-to-protocol analysis. The *p*-values are the result of a comparison between the five treatment groups. Multi comparisons were applied based on an adjusted $\alpha = 0.005$ for seroconversion rate. The Student-Newman-Keuls test was used for the multicomparison of GMTs and GMFIs. a, b, c, and d (where a > b > c > d) mark statistically significant differences between each treatment group. Measurements on day 0 were taken immediately before vaccination

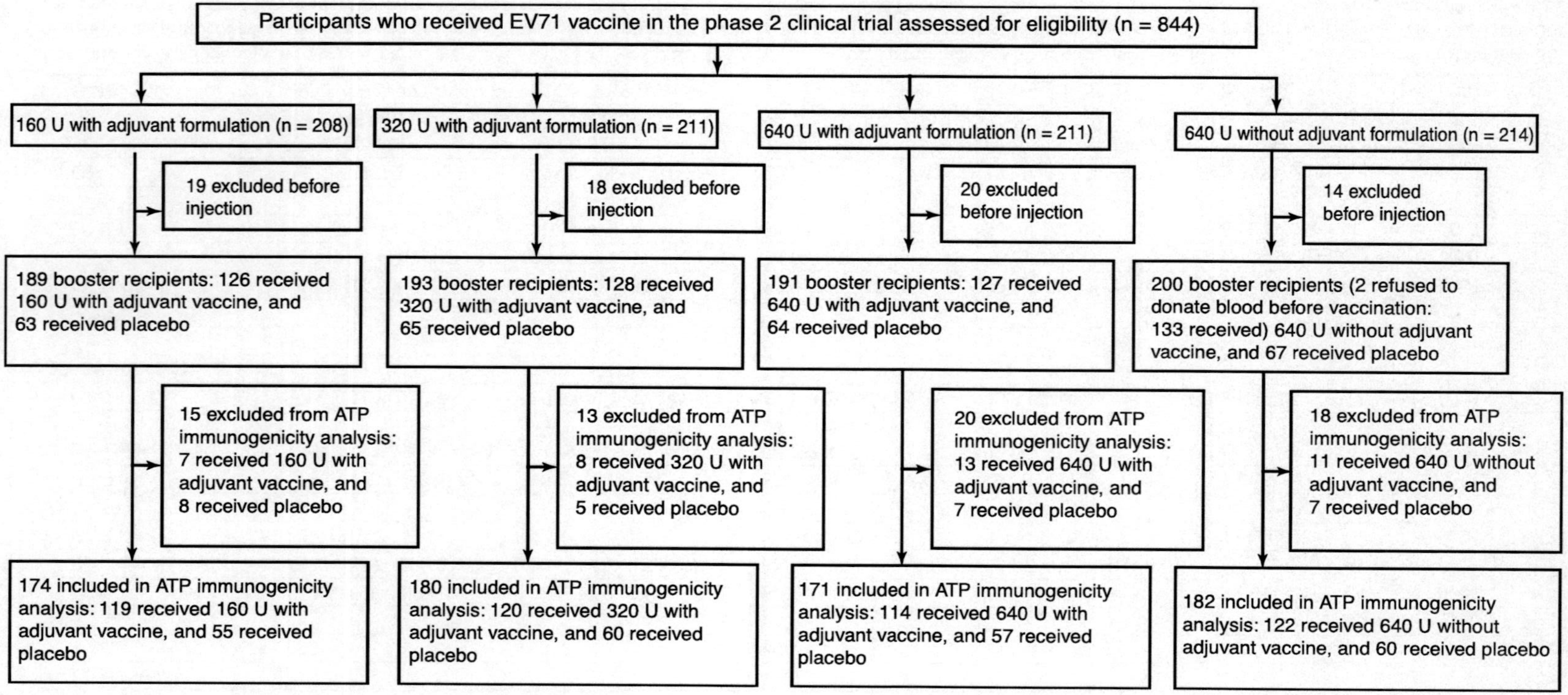

Fig. 4.11 Trial profile. (Reprinted with permission from Fig. 1, Shenyu W, Jingxin L, Zhenglun L, et al. A booster dose of an inactivated enterovirus 71 vaccine in Chinese young children: a randomized, double-blind, placebo-controlled clinical trial. *The Journal of infectious diseases* 2014; 210(7): 1073–82)

Table 4.6 Immune response to a booster dose of EV71 vaccine or placebo in the according-to-protocol Population (Reprinted with permission from Table 2, Shenyu W, Jingxin L, Zhenglun L, et al. A booster dose of an inactivated enterovirus 71 vaccine in Chinese young children: a randomized, double-blind, placebo-controlled clinical trial. *The Journal of infectious diseases* 2014; 210(7): 1073–82.)

Variable	160 U with adjuvant formulation			320 U with adjuvant formulation			640 U with adjuvant formulation			640 U without adjuvant formulation			p^a value
	160 U with adjuvant vaccine (n = 119)	Placebo (n = 55)	p-value	320 U with adjuvant vaccine (n = 120)	Placebo (n = 60)	p-value	640 U with adjuvant vaccine (n = 114)	Placebo (n = 57)	p-value	640 U without adjuvant vaccine (n = 122)	Placebo (n = 60)	p-value	
Before vaccination													
GMT (95% CI)	185.6 (145.0–237.6[bc])	221.8 (154.8–317.7)	.37	209.1 (168.4–259.7[b])	309.6 (231.9–413.3)	.28	264.3 (209.1–334.0[b])	303.3 (230.3–399.5)	.90	138.2 (108.3–176.4[c])	170.1 (124.0–233.4)	.69	<.01
Titer ≥1:32													
Children, No.	109	52	.71	116	59	.87	109	57	.26	104	57	.05	<.01
Children, % (95% CI)	91.6 (85.1–95.9[bc])	94.6 (84.9–98.9)		96.7 (91.7–99.1[b])	98.3 (91.1–100.0)		95.6 (90.1–98.6[b])	100.0 (93.7–100.0)		85.3 (77.7–91.0[c])	95.0 (86.1–99.0)		
After vaccination													
GMT (95% CI)	2352.6 (1959.0–2825.4[d])	164.5 (111.9–241.7)	<.01	3352.5 (2779.1–4044.0[c])	264.9 (187.4–374.4)	<.01	4410.7 (3565.6–5456.1[b])	250.8 (180.1–349.3)	<.01	2214.8 (1844.2–2659.8[d])	132.7 (97.3–181.1)	<.01	<.01
Titer ≥1:32													
Children, No.	119	49	<.01	120	59	.33	113	54	.21	122	53	<.01	.24
Children, % (95% CI)	100.0 (97.0–100.0)	89.1 (77.8–95.9)		100.0 (97.0–100.00	98.3 (91.1–100.0)		99.1 (95.2–100.0)	94.7 (85.4–98.9)		100.0 (97.0–100.0)	88.3 (77.4–95.2)		
Seroconversion													
Children, No.	95	1	<.01	102	6	<.01	105	3	<.01	97	1	<.01	.03
Children, % (95% CI)	79.8 (71.5–86.6[c])	1.8 (0.0–9.7)		85.0 (77.3–90.9[bc])	10.0 (3.8–20.5)		92.1 (85.5–96.3[b])	5.3 (1.1–14.6)		79.5 (71.3–86.3[c])	1.7 (0.0–8.9)		
GMFI (95% CI)	12.7 (9.6–16.7)	0.7 (0.6–0.9)	<.01	16.0 (12.3–20.8)	0.9 (0.6–1.1)	<.01	16.7 (12.6–22.2)	0.8 (0.6–1.1)	<.01	16.0 (12.1–21.2)	0.8 (0.6–1.0)	<.01	.49

Seroconversion was defined as either a ≥ fourfold increase in titer or a change from a negative baseline titer (with a titer of less than 1:8) to a titer of 1:32 or more. The ATP population was defined as participants who had correctly received the priming 2-dose vaccinations in the previous phase 2 trial, who received the booster dose in this complementary clinical trial 1 year later (±30 days), and for whom antibody titers in serum both before and after booster injection were available. From multiple comparisons analysis between participants who received booster EV71 vaccine within each formulation group. Multiple comparisons were used based on an adjusted $\alpha = 0.0083$ for rate or proportion. The Student-Newman-Keuls test was used for multiple comparison analyses of GMTs and GMFIs. Different characters (i.e., b, c, and d, after the 95% CIs of each group) were used to mark the differences (b > c > d) between each treatment group by multiple comparison analyses

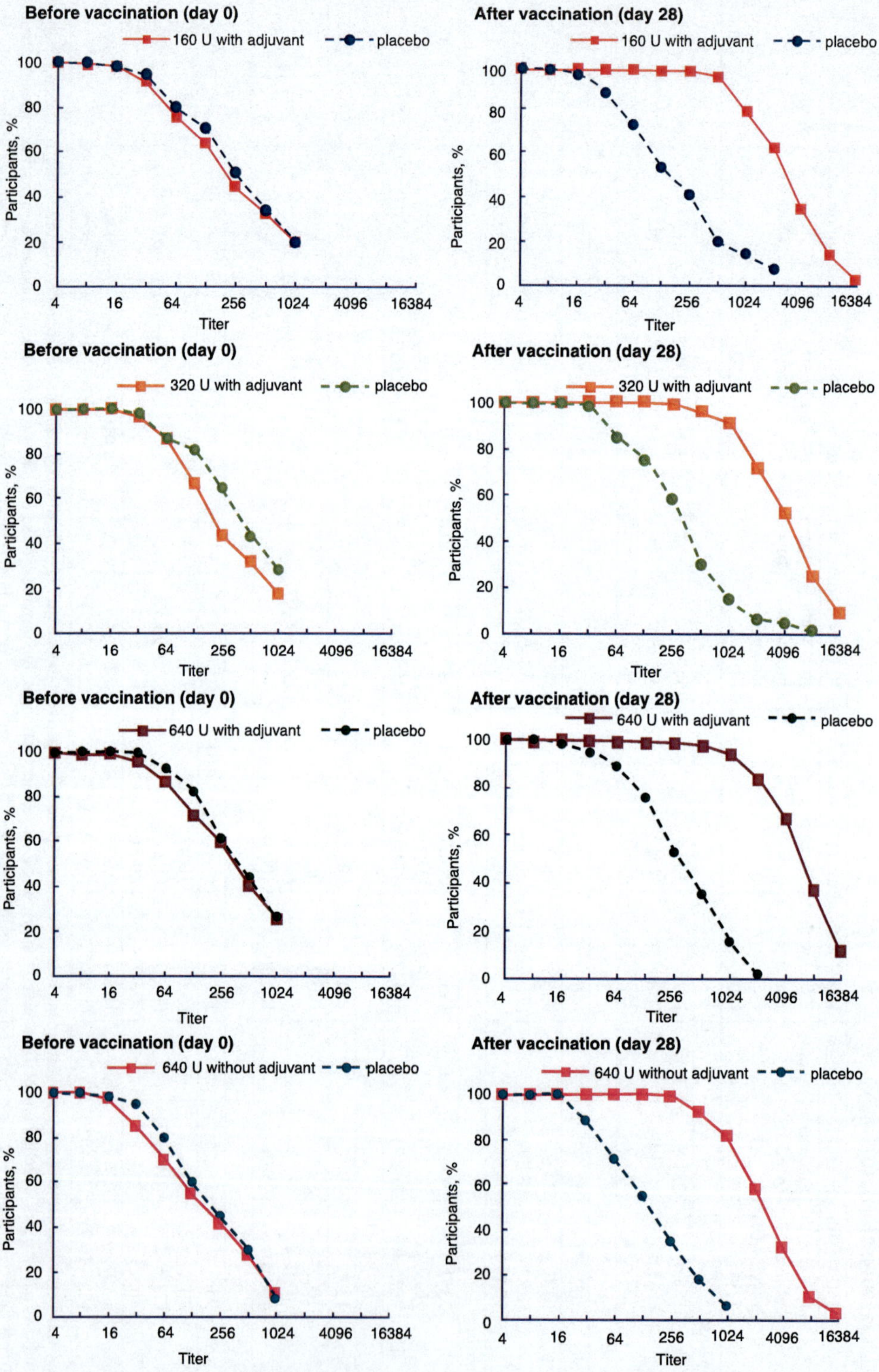

Fig. 4.12 Reverse cumulative curves for EV71 neutralizing antibody titers of participants included in the according-to-protocol cohort before (on day 0) and after (on day 28) booster vaccination, by formulation groups and treatment groups. (Reprinted with permission from Fig. 2, Shenyu W, Jingxin L, Zhenglun L, et al. A booster dose of an inactivated enterovirus 71 vaccine in Chinese young children: a randomized, double-blind, placebo-controlled clinical trial. *The Journal of infectious diseases* 2014; 210(7): 1073–82)

domly assigned to receive at least 1 dose of the EV71 vaccine or placebo [35]. Four hundred and four participants were included in the according-to-protocol cohort for immunogenicity analysis. Two hundred and thirty-two participants were included in the according-to-protocol cohort for antibody persistence analysis. Twenty-eight days after the second dose, there were 92.3%, 95.9%, and 99.0% seropositive participants (with titers ≥ 1:8) in the 100 U, 200 U, and 400 U groups, respectively (Table 4.7). GMT measured by neutralizing antibody assay increased to 60.2 (95% CI, 41.9–86.4), 72.8 (95% CI, 50.8–104.3), and 252.1 (95% CI, 180.8–351.6) for the 100 U, 200 U, and 400 U groups, respectively. A dose-response relationship was observed till 13 months after the second vaccination, although antibody levels decreased.

4.2.3.2 Efficacy

In the phase 3 trial of Vigoo EV71 vaccine, 10,245 eligible participants were randomly assigned to either the vaccine ($n = 5120$) or placebo group ($n = 5125$) (Fig. 4.13). 9858 (96.2%) participants received two doses of vaccine ($n = 4915$) or placebo ($n = 4943$). Ten thousand and two hundred twenty-six participants who received at least one dose of vaccine and completed 12 follow-up months were enrolled for modified intention-to-treat analysis ($n = 5111$ in the vaccine group, $n = 5115$ participants in the placebo group). Then participants were classified according to age into infants aged 6–11 months ($n = 2496$) and children aged 12–35 months ($n = 7730$). The proportion of participants who withdrew from the study between days 0 and 56 was similar between the vaccine and placebo groups.

A Protection Rate of HFMD Caused by EV71 Infection

During the 12-month monitoring period, 36 cases of HFMD caused by EV71 were confirmed, including 3 cases in the vaccine group and 33 cases in the placebo group in the modified intention-to-treat population. According to the different time points of follow-up, the HFMD protection rates of EV71 vaccine against EV71 infection at 3 months, 6 months, 9 months and 12 months were 86.39% (95% CI, 54.53%–95.93%), 88.91% (95% CI, 63.46%–96.64%), 90.65% (95%CI, 69.45%–97.14%) and 90.93% (95%CI, 70.42%–97.22%), respectively (Table 4.8). The density of HFMD induced by EV71 in the EV71 vaccine group was significantly lower than that in the placebo group, and the difference was statistically significant.

Protection Rate Against Diseases Caused by EV71 Infection

During the 12-month surveillance period, 8 cases of diseases caused by EV71 infection were diagnosed in the EV71 vaccine group, including 3 cases of HFMD, 3 cases of upper respiratory tract infection, and 2 cases of diarrhea, while 44 cases of diseases caused by EV71 infection were diagnosed in the placebo control group, including 33 cases of HFMD and 11 cases of upper respiratory tract infection. The incidence densities of diseases caused by EV71 infection in the EV71 vaccine group and placebo group were 1.63 and 8.97 max 1000 person-years, respectively, and there was a significant difference between the two groups. The protection rate of the vaccine against diseases caused by EV71 infection was 81.85% (95% CI, 61.46%–91.46%) (Table 4.9).

During the 12-month monitoring period, there were 1 case of disease caused by EV71 infection in the EV71 vaccine group and 11 cases in the placebo group of infant group, 7 cases in the EV71 vaccine group, and 33 cases in the placebo group of children group (modified intention-to-treat population). The protection rate of the EV71 vaccine against diseases caused by EV71 in the infant group was 90.87% (95% CI, 29.29%–98.82%), and that of the EV71 vaccine in the children group against diseases caused by EV71 was 78.87% (95% CI, 52.23%–90.65%) (Table 4.10).

A Protection Rate of HFMD Hospitalized Cases Caused by EV71 Infection

Eight patients in the placebo group (modified intention-to-treat population) were admitted to the hospital for EV71-associated HFMD (including one severe case of HFMD accompanied by

Table 4.7 Immune response after each vaccination and 1-year antibody persistency

	100 U	200 U	400 U	Placebo	*p*-value
Before vaccination					
n	104	98	95	107	
GMT	7.5 (5.5–10.2)	6.6 (4.9–9.0)	6.7 (5.1–9.0)	6.3 (4.8–8.2)	0.86
Seroconversion	16 (15.4%, 9.3–24.1)	12 (12.2%, 6.8–20.8)	13 (13.7%, 7.8–22.7)	12 (11.2%, 6.2–19.2)	0.83
28 days after dose 1					
n	91	85	88	94	
GMT	11.2 (7.9–16.0)	11.8 (8.3–16.7)	23.1 (16.0–33.2)	6.4 (4.8–8.5)	<0.001
GMFI	1.59 (1.4–1.9)	1.93 (1.6–2.3)	3.78 (3.0–4.7)	1.02 (1.0–1.1)	<0.001
Seroconversion	44 (48.4%, 37.8–59.1)	47 (55.3%, 44.1–66.1)	75 (85.2%, 75.7–91.9)	9 (9.6%, 4.7–17.9)	<0.001
28 days after dose 2					
n	104	98	95	107	
GMT	60.2 (41.9–86.4)	72.8 (50.8–104.3)	252.1 (180.8–351.6)	7.3 (5.3–10.0)	<0.001
GMFI	8.0 (6.3–10.4)	11.0 (8.5–14.1)	37.5 (28.9–48.5)	1.2 (1.0–1.3)	<0.001
Seroconversion	96 (92.3%, 85.4–96.6)	94 (95.9%, 89.9–98.9)	94 (99.0%, 94.3–100.0)	17 (15.9%, 9.5–24.2)	<0.001
7 months after dose 2					
n	80	80	72	–	
GMT	23.2 (15.6–34.5)	61.7 (38.3–99.4)	93.1 (65.4–132.4)	–	<0.001
GMFI	3.21 (2.4–4.3)	8.78 (5.8–13.2)	14.55 (10.6–20.0)	–	<0.001
Seroconversion	59 (73.8%, 62.5–82.9)	76 (95.0%, 87.0–98.9)	72 (100.0%,93.7–101.3)	–	<0.001
13 months after dose 2					
n	80	80	72	–	
GMT	59.9 (37.8–95.0)	67.6 (43.3–105.7)	94.7 (66.0–136.0)	–	0.002
GMFI	8.28 (5.3–12.9)	9.63 (6.3–14.7)	14.81 (10.4–21.2)	–	0.133
Seroconversion	64 (80.0%, 69.3–88.1)	70 (87.5%, 77.8–93.9)	69 (95.8%, 87.5–99.6)	–	0.017

Data are GMT (95% CI), number of participants (%, 95% CI), or GMFI (95% CI). *n* = total participants included in immunogenic according-to-protocol analysis. GMT = geometric mean titer. GMFI = geometric mean fold increase. Seroconversion was defined as either a ≥ fourfold increase in titer or a change from a negative baseline titer (with a titer of less than 1:8) to a titer of 1:32 or more. The *p*-values are the result of a comparison between the four treatment groups

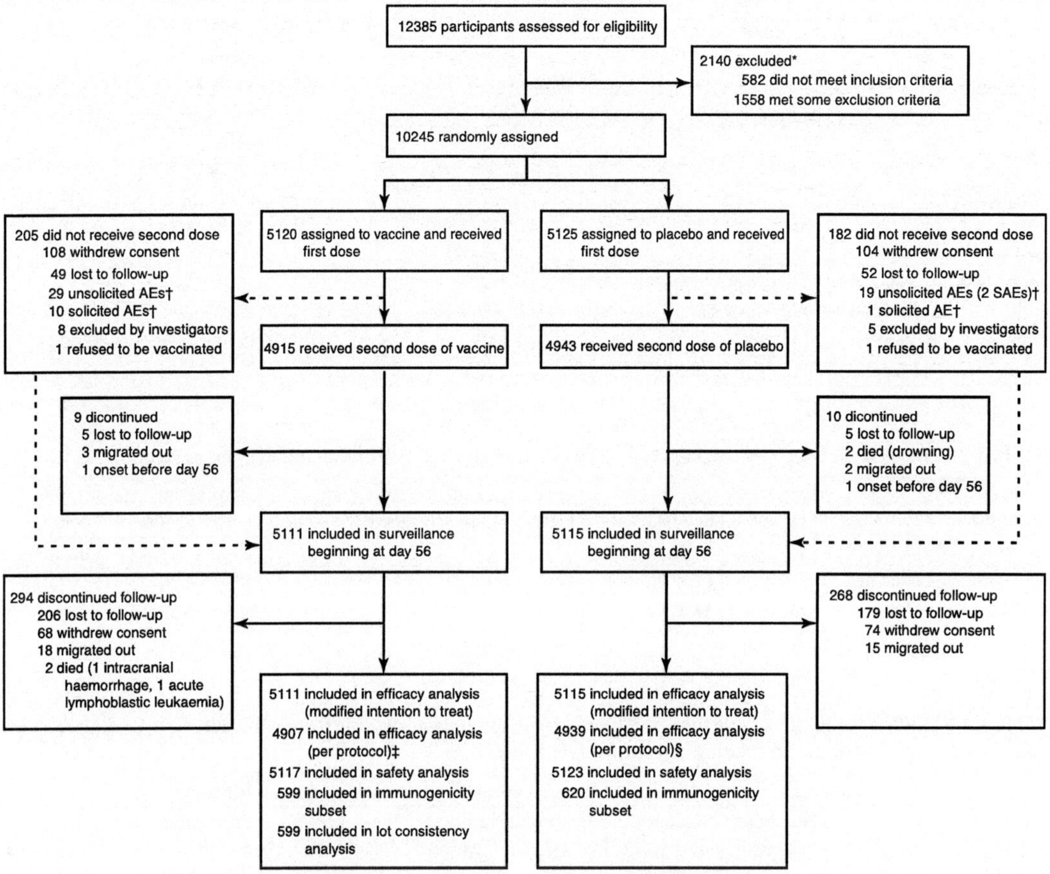

Fig. 4.13 Trial profile (Reprinted with permission from Fig. 1, Zhu FC, Meng FY, Li JX, et al. Efficacy, safety, and immunology of an inactivated alum-adjuvant enterovirus 71 vaccine in children in China: a multicenter, randomized, double-blind, placebo-controlled, phase 3 trial. *Lancet* 2013; 381(9882): 2024–32.). The modified intention-to-treat analysis included all participants who received at least one dose and entered surveillance on day 56. AE = adverse event. SAE = serious adverse event. ‡204 participants were excluded because they received only the first dose. §175 participants received only the first dose and one participant received the vaccine at the second dose in the placebo group, so were excluded from the per-protocol analysis

Table 4.8 The protective rate of the EV71 vaccine against HFMD caused by EV71 infection at different times

Time	Group	Person	Person-years	Case	Incidence density rate (cases/1000 person-years)	Protection rate(95%CI)/%	*p*-value
3 months	Vaccine	5111	1255.23	3	2.39	86.39 (54.53,95.93)	0.0012
	Placebo	5115	1253.31	22	17.55		
6 months	Vaccine	5111	2503.84	3	1.20	88.91 (63.46,96.64)	0.0003
	Placebo	5115	2496.46	27	10.82		
9 months	Vaccine	5111	3740.73	3	0.80	90.65 (69.45,97.14)	0.0001
	Placebo	5115	3730.41	32	8.58		
12 months	Vaccine	5111	4915.50	3	0.61	90.93 (70.42,97.22)	0.0001
	Placebo	5115	4903.50	33	6.73		

Table 4.9 Protection rate of EV71 vaccine against diseases caused by EV71 infection

Diagnosis	Group	Person	Person-years	Case	Incidence density rate (cases/1000 person-years)	Protection rate (95%CI)/%	*p*-value
HFMD	Vaccine	5111	4915.50	3	0.61	90.93 (70.42, 97.22)	0.0001
	Placebo	5115	4903.50	33	6.73		
Upper respiratory tract infection	Vaccine	5111	4915.50	3	0.61	72.78 (2.43, 92.41)	0.0458
	Placebo	5115	4903.50	11	2.24		
Diarrhea	Vaccine	5111	4915.50	2	0.41	–	–
	Placebo	5115	4903.50	0	0.00		
Total	Vaccine	5111	4915.50	8	1.63	81.85 (61.46, 91.46)	<0.0001
	Placebo	5115	4903.50	44	8.97		

Table 4.10 Analysis of the protective effect of diseases caused by EV71 infection in different age groups

Age group	Group	Person	Person-years	Case	Incidence density rate (cases/1000 person-years)	Protection rate (95%CI)/%	*p*-value
Infant	Vaccine	1245	1195.36	1	0.84	90.87 (29.29, 98.82)	0.0219
	Placebo	1251	1199.81	11	9.17		
Children	Vaccine	3866	3720.14	7	1.88	78.87 (52.23, 90.65)	0.0002
	Placebo	3864	3703.69	33	8.91		

Table 4.11 EV71 vaccine efficacy against EV71-associated hospitalized cases in the modified intention-to-treat cohort and according-to-protocol cohort during 1 year of surveillance

	Vaccine group			Placebo group			Efficacy	
	Person-years	Numbers of cases	Incidence density rate (cases/1000 person-years)	Person-years	Numbers of cases	Incidence density rate (cases/1000 person-years)	Protection rate (95%CI)/%	*p*
Modified intention-to-treat cohort	4915.5	0	0.0	4903.5	8	1.6	100.0 (41.6–100.0)	0.0078
According-to-protocol cohort	4725.4	0	0.0	4742.9	7	1.5	100.0 (30.4–100.0)	0.0156

encephalitis and oral herpes) compared with none in the vaccine group, suggesting a vaccine efficacy of 100% (95% CI, 41.6–100.0) for potential severe (admitted to hospital) or severe cases (Table 4.11).

To evaluate the correlation between immunogenicity and efficacy, 51 cases of disease caused by EV71 infection and 254 matched controls were assessed (one in each group was excluded because a blood sample at day 56 was unavailable). When the titer value is 1:8, the Youden index reaches the peak. Combined with sensitivity, specificity, and the Jordon index, neutralizing antibodies with titers between 1:16 and 1:32 appear to offer maximum protection against EV71-related diseases (Table 4.12).

The phase 3 trial of the Sinovac EV71 vaccine enrolled 10,077 participants in total who received at least one dose of EV71 vaccine or placebo. Of them, 5041 in the vaccine group and 5028 in the placebo group entered surveillance beginning at day 57 and were included in the primary efficacy analysis (intention-to-treat). A total of 119 cases of EV71-associate disease (13 [0.3%] in the vaccine group and 106 [2.1%] in the placebo group) were identified during the 12-month surveillance period in the intention-to-treat cohort. The vaccine efficacy against EV71-associated HFMD or

Table 4.12 Sensitivity and specificity of different neutralizing antibody levels to distinguish between cases and non-cases caused by EV71 infection

Neutralizing antibody	Sensitivity (95%CI)%	Specificity (95%CI)%	Youden index (sensitivity + specificity − 1)
1:4	1.9 (0.0,10.3)	99.6 (97.8,100.0)	0.0150
1:8	73.1 (59.0,84.4)	74.3 (68.5,79.6)	0.4740
1:16	84.6 (71.9,93.1)	70.8 (64.7,76.3)	0.5540
1:32	88.5 (76.6,95.6)	66.0 (59.8,71.8)	0.5450
1:64	88.5 (76.6,95.6)	63.2 (57.0,69.2)	0.5170
1:128	90.4 (79.0,96.8)	57.3 (51.0,63.5)	0.4770
1:256	90.4 (79.0,96.8)	49.4 (43.1,55.7)	0.3980
1:512	94.2 (84.1,98.8)	41.9 (35.7,48.2)	0.3610
1:1024	100.0 (93.2,100.0)	31.2 (25.6,37.3)	0.3120

herpangina was 94.8% (95% CI, 87.2–97.9; $p < 0.001$) in this cohort. Vaccine efficacies against EV71-associated hospitalization (0 cases vs. 24 cases) and hand, foot, and mouth disease with neurologic complications (0 cases vs. 8 cases) were both 100% (95% CI, 83.7–100 and 42.6–100, respectively). Neutralizing antibodies with titers between 1:16 appear to offer maximum protection against EV71-associated HFMD or herpangina in vaccinated children.

The phase 3 trial of CAMS EV71 vaccine enrolled 12,000 participants in total who received at least one dose of EV71 vaccine or placebo [36]. Of them, 5481 children in the vaccine group and 5499 in the placebo group were included in the per-protocol analysis. A total of 594 cases of EV71-associate disease (202 [3.7%] in the vaccine group and 392 [7.1%] in the placebo group) were reported during the 11-month surveillance period in the per-protocol cohort. The vaccine efficacy against EV71-associated HFMD was 97.4% (95% CI, 92.9–99.0) in the intention-to-treat analysis and 97.3% (95% CI, 92.6–99.0) in the per-protocol analysis. Vaccine efficacies against EV71-associated HFMD hospitalization (0 cases vs. 23 cases) and severe HFMD (0 cases vs. 8 cases) were both 100% (95% CI, 82.9–100, and 42.3–100, respectively).

4.2.4 Conclusion and Evaluation

4.2.4.1 Safety

Generally, all three EV71 vaccines showed acceptable safety in clinical trials. The most common adverse reaction was fever, followed by diarrhea. It is noteworthy that the incidence of induration in the alum-adjuvant formulation was significantly higher than that in the adjuvant-free group. In addition, in the phase 3 trial, there were more adverse events associated with withdrawal in the vaccine group than in the placebo group, mainly due to fever.

4.2.4.2 Immunogenicity

In terms of antibody level and antibody growth after immunization, the immunogenicity of the EV71 vaccine with adjuvant was better than that of the EV71 vaccine without adjuvant, and the antibody response level of two doses was significantly higher than that of one dose. A certain dose-response relationship was observed in the three doses of EV71 vaccine groups with adjuvant. Finally, 320 U EV71 vaccine with adjuvant and two-dose immunization program of 0, 28 days were selected.

Although the level of anti-EV71 neutralizing antibody at the 14th month may not need to be boosted, studies have confirmed that booster immunization can quickly stimulate the body to produce a recall response and induce a high level of neutralizing antibody. The level of GMT after booster immunization was 6–10 times higher than that of GMT 28 days after two doses of basic immunization. However, the current immune persistence is observed under the condition that there is a natural epidemic of EV71. If large-scale population vaccination is carried out after the EV71 vaccine is put on the market in the future, the epidemic rule and cycle of EV71 may be changed, while the anti-EV71 neutralizing antibody in the vaccinated population will continue to decline due to the lack of "natural enhancement" formed by natural infection. In this case, enhanced immunization of the EV71 vaccine may become a demand. At present, most countries have adopted three doses of basic immunization followed by one dose to maintain a long-term level of protection [37].

4.2.4.3 Efficacy

Within 1 year after immunization with the experimental vaccine, the protective rate against HFMD caused by EV71 infection was 90.93%, and against diseases caused by EV71 infection was 81.85%. It is worth noting that in the study, the protective rate of the EV71 vaccine against HFMD hospitalized cases caused by EV71 infection was 100.00%.

Studies have confirmed that the EV71 experimental vaccine has a high protection rate against HFMD caused by EV71 infection, especially for hospitalized or severe cases caused by EV71. Most cases of severe HFMD with complications and even death are caused by EV71 infection, so from this point of view, the vaccine is of great public health significance [38].

4.2.4.4 Post-Licensure Surveillance

A phase 4 post-marketing control study was conducted in Xiangyang, Hubei province, due to its representativeness of the incidence in mainland China [39]. The large population of 155,995 children aged 6–71 months was included, 40,724 of whom received two doses of vaccine 1 month apart, and the remainder were considered a control group. EV71-related HFMD was observed in all participants for up to 14 months from 28 days after the second dose using the local infectious disease surveillance system. The results showed that there were 30 cases of EV71-related HFMD in 106,818 per protocol, including 1 in the vaccine group and 29 in the control group, as a result of the overall effectiveness level of 89.7% (95% CI, 24.0–98.6) against EV71 infection. Only one of the 26 EV71-related HFMD hospitalizations was in the vaccine group, resulting in a protective efficacy of 88% against EV71-related HFMD hospitalizations. There was only one severe case of EV71-related HFMD (control group), therefore vaccine effectiveness against severe cases of EV71-related HFMD is almost 100%. The cumulative incidence of EV71-related HFMD in the control group increased over time, compared with a total of 1 case in the vaccine group, which occurred shortly after the completion of the vaccination program, again demonstrating the efficacy of the vaccine against EV71.

During the active surveillance period of 28 days after each vaccination, there were 1865 adverse events (AEs) (4.58%) in the vaccine group. The passive surveillance recorded 180 AEs (0.44%), of which 30 were severe, mainly allergic reactions. Local adverse reactions were mainly redness at the injection site, and systemic adverse reactions were mainly fever, which was similar to phase 2 and 3 trials. Of note, the age-stratified analysis showed that children aged 6–11 months had the highest incidence of systemic and local adverse reactions. In addition, the incidence of adverse reactions was lower in the older subgroup during both active and passive monitoring periods. This trend again highlights the importance of post-marketing safety monitoring, especially for vulnerable populations.

Another post-marketing study evaluated the immunogenicity and safety of EV71 vaccines developed by different manufacturers [40]. Eligible children aged 6–35 months were randomly assigned (1:1:1:1) to receive two doses of Sinovac EV71 vaccine, two doses of CAMS EV71, the first dose of Sinovac EV71 vaccine, and the second dose of CAMS EV71 vaccine or the first dose of CAMS EV71 vaccine and the second dose of CAMS EV71 vaccine, in 1 month. The immunogenicity analysis in the per-protocol cohort showed that 98.4%–100% of the participants in each group were positive for anti-EV71 neutralizing antibody 60 days after the first vaccination with no significant difference between groups. The GMT of participants with CAMS vaccine followed by Sinovac vaccine was the highest (460.5; 95% CI, 356.0–595.7) among all four groups, while the GMT in another group with a sequence of vaccine exchanged is lowest (211.4; 95% CI, 155.1–288.1). It requires further exploration and research to determine the impact of interchanging vaccination schedules on immune responses. Safety profiles were similar among the four groups and no serious adverse events related to the vaccination were reported.

To increase vaccine coverage among infants, trials have been conducted to assess the safety and immunogenicity of the licensed EV71 vaccine administered simultaneously with other Expand Program of Immunization (EPI) vaccines. Simultaneous administration is defined as the administration of more than one recommended vaccine on the same day, at different anatomical sites, and in separate syringes. A published study of concomitant immunization of EV71 vaccine with recombinant hepatitis B vaccine and group A meningococcal polysaccharide vaccine versus either vaccine alone showed that simultaneous administration achieved non-inferiority in immunogenicity and safety compared with separate administration [41], which provided the first evidence on simultaneous vaccination of EV71 vaccine and EPI vaccines.

4.2.4.5 Evaluation

The characteristic clinical symptom of EV71 infection is HFMD, but HFMD can also be caused by multiple or single other pathogens. What is more, EV71 infection can also lead to a variety of non-specific diseases. Therefore, the causal relation between EV71 and HFMD was complicated, which was shown in the phase 3 study of the Vigoo vaccine with higher protective efficacy against EV71-associated HFMD than against EV71-associated with non-specific symptoms. HFMD, especially severe HFMD, is usually passively monitored using the National Infectious Disease Reporting Surveillance Management System. However, the sensitivity and specificity of the system are low. In these studies, several steps were taken to improve the specificity of case diagnosis. All participants diagnosed with suspected cases should be sampled for Real-time PCR EV71-specific nucleic acid detection, and the first positive cases should be re-sampled and re-tested to avoid false positives, and the samples should be cultured and isolated. However, it is very difficult to evaluate the efficacy of the new EV71 vaccine by carrying out the kind of clinical studies with the clinical endpoint as the evaluation index, including long-term follow-up of large sample populations and onerous disease surveillance. Therefore, it is very important to determine a suitable immunological surrogate endpoint for the evaluation of the efficacy of new EV71 vaccines in the future. In phase 3 clinical trials of the Vigoo vaccine and Sinovac vaccine, additional subgroup studies for immunogenicity were performed to preliminarily identify the immune markers for optimal protection. Both studies showed that a serum antibody titer of 1:32 could be used as a proxy for clinical endpoints. More post-marketing studies to determine immunology will be necessary to replace the endpoint since it is more economical and faster than the clinical study of observing the protective effect.

4.3 Ebola Vaccine

4.3.1 Background

Ebola virus is an enveloped, single-stranded, negative-sense RNA virus that was discovered in 1976 in southern Sudan and the Ebola River region of the DRC (formerly known as Zaire) [42]. It causes Ebola hemorrhagic fever (EBHF) or Ebola diseases, the most deadly viral hemorrhagic fever in the world today, with symptoms including nausea, vomiting, diarrhea, changes in skin color, general aches and pains, internal bleeding, external bleeding, and fever [43–45]. Mortality rates for people infected with the Ebola virus range from 50% to 90%, with the leading causes of death being stroked, myocardial infarction, hypovolemic shock, or multiple organ failure [46].

The 2014 epidemic in West Africa was the largest and most severe Ebola outbreak in history, with a total of approximately 28,646 reported cases and 11,323 deaths as of 27 March 2016 [46, 47]. As there is no specific drug or treatment for Ebola virus disease, vaccination is considered to be the most effective way to control the spread of the Ebola virus [48, 49].

Ebola virus disease used to be considered regional and with few cases, and as a result, vaccine development did not receive sufficient attention and progress was slow, with most research still at the animal study stage [50, 51]. However, since the outbreak in 2014, the development of an Ebola vaccine has accelerated significantly and clinical trials of various Ebola vaccine candidates have been initiated as an urgent response to the crisis, including cAd3-EBOV, rVSVΔG-EBOVGP, cAd3-EBO, et al. [52]. A recombinant human Ad5 vector Ebola vaccine (Ad5-EBOV), which expresses the glycoprotein of the 2014 epidemic Ebola strain, was developed by the Beijing Institute of Biotechnology and Tianjin Casino Biotechnology, in China. First-in-human study of the vaccine was carried out in Jiangsu Province in China in late December 2014, and the phase 2 trial was conducted in Sierra Leone.

4.3.2 Methods

4.3.2.1 Participants and Locations

The entire population is susceptible to Ebola infection. However, as a novel vaccine, the first-in-human phase 1 clinical trial of the recombinant human Ad5 vector Ebola vaccine (Ad5-EBOV) was conducted in healthy adults aged 18–60 years [53]. One hundred and twenty eligible healthy adults, who were free of HIV infection, and with no liver or kidney dysfunction were included in the study. The trial aimed to evaluate the preliminary safety and immunogenicity of the Ad5-EBOV.

For the Phase 2 clinical trial, which was conducted at the Sierra Leone-China Friendship Hospital in Freetown, Sierra Leone, 500 healthy participants aged 18–50 years were recruited who were HIV-free, had no history of Ebola infection, and had not previously received other Ebola vaccine candidates [54]. The trial was designed to assess the safety and immunogenicity of this vaccine in healthy adults in Sierra Leone, who was at the center of the Ebola risk, to determine the optimal dose.

4.3.2.2 Design of Optimal Dosage, Formulation, and Immunization Schedule

The Phase 1 trial was a randomized, double-blind, placebo-controlled study. Participants were recruited and randomized at a 2:1 ratio to receive either the low-dose vaccine or placebo (Group 1) or the high-dose vaccine or placebo (Group 2). The low-dose Ad5-EBOV containing 4.0×10^{10} viral particles(vp) and the high-dose Ad5-EBOV containing 1.6×10^{11} vp per dose (Fig. 4.14). All participants who received the vaccination were evaluated for safety and provided blood samples for testing on days 3, 7, 14, and 28 after vaccination.

Since the durability of a single dose of Ad5-EBOV remains unknown, it was necessary to assess the need for a booster dose vaccination to establish adequate long-term immunity [55]. Six months after the prime dose, all the participants were recruited again for a booster dose study. Participants received the same dose as their initial prime vaccination, and blood samples were collected for antibody testing at days 0, 28, and 12 months.

For the phase 2 trial in Sierra Leone, participants were enrolled and randomly assigned (2:1:1) to receive either the high-dose vaccine (1.6×10^{11} vp/dose), the low-dose vaccine (8.0×10^{10} vp/dose), or the placebo (Fig. 4.15). Blood samples were collected from participants before and on days 14, 28, and 168 post-vaccination to assess Ebola-specific antibody responses against vaccine-matched glycoproteins.

4.3.2.3 Statistical Analysis

Baseline characteristics of participants in the Ad5-EBOV vaccine and placebo groups are described and the balance between groups is compared. Categorical data were analyzed using the χ^2 test or Fisher's exact test, and comparisons were made according to Bonferroni-adjusted alpha when there were significant differences between treatment groups. Analysis of variance was used for log-transformed antibody titers, while the Wilcoxon rank-sum test was used for non-normal data. The Student-Newman-Keuls test was used for some comparisons when relevant. The effect of pre-existing adenovirus type-5 neutralizing antibody titers on the immune response to Ebola glycoprotein was assessed using the

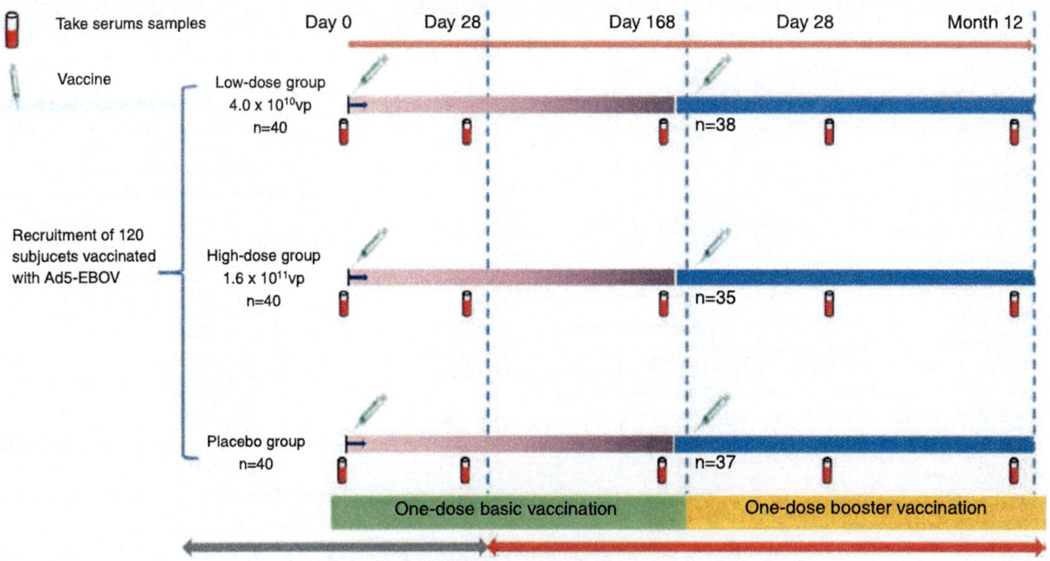

Fig. 4.14 Study design for the prime dose and booster dose immunization for Ad5-EBOV

Fig. 4.15 Study design for the dose selection for Ad5-EBOV

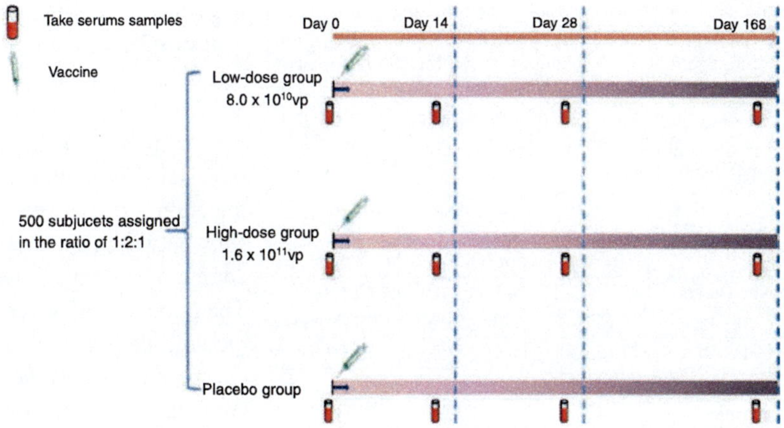

Spearman rank correlation method. Immune responses were analyzed and stratified according to participants' baseline adenovirus-5 neutralizing antibody titers (low or negative ≤1:200 or high >1:200) after the original dose up to day 168, while booster responses were stratified according to adenovirus-5 neutralizing antibody titers (low or negative ≤1:200 or high >1:200) on day 168 before the booster injection. All statistical tests were two-sided, $\alpha = 0.05$, and performed by independent statisticians using SAS (version 9.3).

4.3.3 Results

4.3.3.1 The Target Vaccine Dose, or Formulations and Regimen for Primary Immunization

In the Phase 1 trial, 120 participants were recruited and randomly allocated to receive either a placebo ($n = 40$), low-dose Ad5-EBOV vaccine 4.0×10^{10} vp/dose ($n = 40$), or high-dose Ad5-EBOV vaccine 1.6×10^{11} vp/dose ($n = 40$; Fig. 4.16). All participants completed their scheduled visit within 28 days of vaccina-

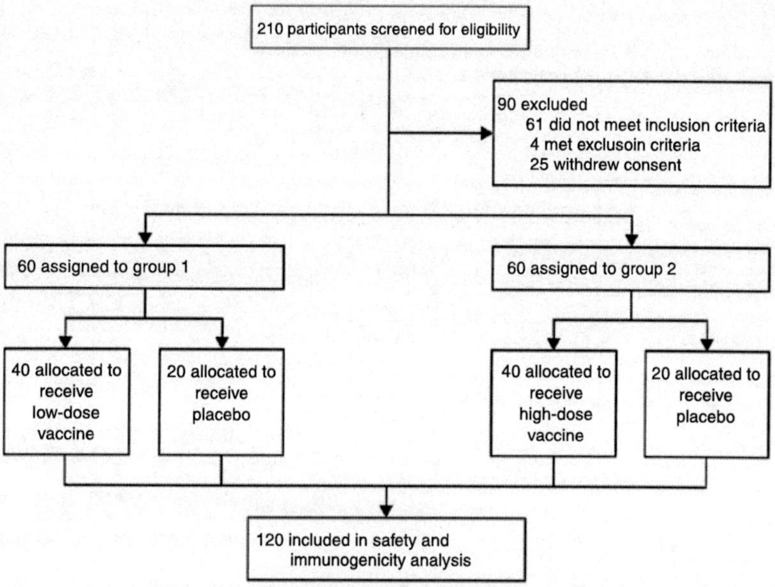

Fig. 4.16 Trial profile of the phase 1 first-in-human study of the Ad5-EBOV vaccine. (Reprinted from Figure 1, Zhu, F.C., et al., Safety and immunogenicity of a novel recombinant adenovirus type-5 vector-based Ebola vaccine in healthy adults in China: preliminary report of a randomised, double-blind, placebo-controlled, phase 1 trial. *Lancet*, 2015. **385**(9984): p. 2272–9)

Table 4.13 Baseline characteristics and titers of pre-existing adenovirus type-5 neutralizing antibodies. (Reprinted from Table 1, Zhu, F.C., et al., Safety and immunogenicity of a novel recombinant adenovirus type-5 vector-based Ebola vaccine in healthy adults in China: preliminary report of a randomised, double-blind, placebo-controlled, phase 1 trial. *Lancet*, 2015. **385**(9984): p. 2272–9)

	Placebo group (*n* = 40)	Low-dose group (*n* = 40)	High-dose group (*n* = 40)
Age (years)	42.4 (12.1)	43.6 (10.0)	43.2 (10.1)
18–44	19 (47%)	21 (53%)	20 (50%)
45–60	21 (53%)	19 (47%)	20 (50%)
Sex			
Male	18 (45%)	20 (50%)	21 (53%)
Female	22 (55%)	20 (50%)	19 (47%)
BMI (kg/m^2)	24.2 (2.3)	23.7 (2.6)	24.4 (2.8)
<18.5	0	1 (3%)	1 (3%)
18.5–24.9	26 (65%)	28 (70%)	24 (60%)
25–29.9	14 (35%)	10 (25%)	14 (35%)
≥30.0	0	1 (3%)	1 (3%)
Pre-existing adenovirus type-5 antibody titers[a]			
>1:12	34 (85%)	30 (75%)	32 (80%)
>1:200	24 (60%)	22 (55%)	25 (63%)

Data are mean (SD) or n (%). BMI = body-mass index
[a]No significant difference between treatment groups

tion. Baseline demographic characteristics of the participants were similar between groups (Table 4.13).

Overall, 82 (68%) participants reported at least one vaccine-induced adverse reaction within 7 days of vaccination (Table 4.14). There were significant differences in the incidence of adverse reactions between the treatment groups. The most common reaction was mild pain at the injection site. The incidence of mild redness at the injection site showed a dose-response relationship between the treatment groups. The most common systemic adverse reaction was fever. The frequency of adverse reactions was higher in the high-dose group than in the low-dose group, except that most of the adverse reactions were in Grade 1. No serious adverse events were recorded at the 28-day follow-up. Pre-existing immunity to adenovirus type-5 did not affect the incidence of adverse events (Table 4.15).

Ebola glycoprotein-specific ELISA titers were measured on days 3, 7, 14, and 28 after vaccination. No specific antibody response was detected during the first 7 days. In the low and high-dose vaccine groups, ELISA EC_{90} titers increased significantly on day 14 and continued to increase until day 28, whereas no specific responses were recorded in the placebo group (Table 4.16). All participants in the high-dose group had a positive antibody response on day 28 except for two participants in the low-dose group. Participants in the high-dose group had higher ELISA EC_{90}

Table 4.14 Summary of solicited adverse reactions and unsolicited adverse reactions occurring within 28 days of vaccination. (Reprinted from Table 2, Zhu, F.C., et al., Safety and immunogenicity of a novel recombinant adenovirus type-5 vector-based Ebola vaccine in healthy adults in China: preliminary report of a randomised, double-blind, placebo-controlled, phase 1 trial. **Lancet**, 2015. **385**(9984): p. 2272–9)

	Placebo group ($n = 40$)	Low-dose group ($n = 40$)	High-dose group ($n = 40$)	p-value
Solicited adverse reactions within 7 days				
Any	19 (48%)	27 (68%)	36 (90%)	0.0002
				0.002[a]
Grade 1	18 (45%)	26 (65%)	28 (70%)	0.0541
Grade 2	1 (3%)	0	8 (20%)	0.0018[b]
Grade 3	0	1 (3%)	0	1.0000
Injection-site adverse reactions				
Pain				
Grade 1	8 (20%)	14 (35%)	29 (73%)	<0.0001[c]
Grade 2	0	0	1 (3%)	1.0000
Induration				
Grade 1	0	1 (3%)	0	1.0000
Redness				
Grade 1	5 (13%)	8 (20%)	14 (35%)	0.0493[d]
Grade 3	0	1 (3%)	0	1.0000
Swelling				
Grade 1	0	2 (5%)	2 (5%)	0.5442
Grade 2	0	0	1 (3%)	1.0000
Itch				
Grade 1	0	0	1 (3%)	1.0000
Systemic adverse reactions				
Fever				
Grade 1	9 (23%)	6 (15%)	6 (15%)	0.5948
Grade 2	1 (3%)	0	7 (18%)	0.0056[e]
Headache				
Grade 1	1 (3%)	2 (5%)	1 (3%)	1.0000
Fatigue				
Grade 1	3 (8%)	6 (15%)	5 (13%)	0.6790
Grade 2	0	0	1 (3%)	1.0000
Vomiting				
Grade 1	0	1 (3%)	3 (8%)	0.3220
Diarrhea				
Grade 1	1 (3%)	0	2 (5%)	0.7721
Muscle pain				
Grade 1	2 (5%)	0	1 (3%)	0.7721
Grade 2	0	0	1 (3%)	1.0000
Joint pain				
Grade 1	1 (3%)	0	1 (3%)	1.0000
Throat pain				
Grade 1	1 (3%)	1 (3%)	1 (3%)	1.0000
Cough				
Grade 1	3 (8%)	2 (5%)	1 (3%)	0.8701
Unsolicited adverse events within 0–28 days				

Table 4.14 (continued)

	Placebo group ($n = 40$)	Low-dose group ($n = 40$)	High-dose group ($n = 40$)	p-value
Any	17 (43%)	15 (38%)	22 (55%)	0.2690
Grade 1	9 (23%)	10 (25%)	17 (43%)	0.1042
Grade 2	8 (20%)	4 (10%)	5 (13%)	0.4103
Grade 3	0	1 (3%)	0	1.0000

Data are n (%). Grade 1 was a mild reaction, grade 2 was a moderate reaction, and grade 3 was a severe reaction (i.e., prevented activity). We applied multiple comparisons based on an adjusted $\alpha = 0.017$ when incidence differed significantly between treatment groups. [a]$p = 0.0139$ for high-dose group versus low-dose group, $p < 0.0001$ for high-dose group versus the placebo group, and $p = 0.0704$ for low-dose group versus placebo group; [b]$p = 0.0053$ for high-dose group versus low-dose group, $p = 0.0289$ for high-dose group versus the placebo group, and $p = 1.0000$ for low-dose group versus placebo group; [c]$p = 0.0008$ for the high-dose group versus the low-dose group, $p < 0.0001$ for the high-dose group versus the placebo group, and $p = 0.1330$ for the low-dose group versus placebo group; [d]$p = 0.1330$ for high-dose group versus low-dose group, $p = 0.0181$ for high-dose group versus the placebo group, $p = 0.3632$ for low-dose group versus placebo group; [e]$p = 0.0117$ for the high-dose group versus the low-dose group, $p = 0.0568$ for the high-dose group versus the placebo group, and $p = 1.0000$ for the low-dose group versus the placebo group

titers than those in the low-dose group (geometric mean antibody titer 1305.7 [95% CI 970.1–1757.2] vs. 682.7 [424.3–1098.5]).

There was an inverse relationship between baseline adenovirus-5 neutralizing antibody titers and vaccine-elicited Ebola glycoprotein-specific antibody titers after log-transformation, independent of vaccine dose.

ELISpot T-cell responses at baseline were undetectable, with near zero spot-forming cells in the different treatment groups (Fig. 4.17). On day 14, specific T-cell responses reached a median of 465.0 spot-forming cells (IQR 180.0–1202.5) for participants in the low-dose group and 765.0 spot-forming cells (400.0–1460.0) for participants in the high-dose group, before decreasing to 95 spot-forming cells (40.0–250.0) on day 28 and 210 spot-forming cells (80.0–525.0). Participants in the high-dose group had significantly higher T-cell responses than the low-dose group on both day 14 and day 28. Although baseline adenovirus-5 neutralizing antibodies significantly reduced post-vaccination T-cell responses in both vaccine groups, T-cell responses were still increasing in participants receiving the high-dose vaccine in the presence of pre-existing high levels of neutralizing antibodies.

In addition, T-cell responses were assessed by intracellular cytokine staining analysis to determine the proportion of specific CD^4 and CD^8 T-cell populations based on IFN-γ, TNF-α, or IL-2 secreted at different time points. Both CD^4 and CD^8 T-cell responses increased significantly after vaccination, independent of the vaccine dose, and peaked at day 14 (Fig. 4.18). Participants in the high-dose vaccine group responded to a greater extent than those in the low-dose group, and those with low or negative pre-existing adenovirus type-5 neutralizing antibodies responded to a greater extent than those with high pre-existing antibodies.

For specific CD^4 and CD^8 T-cell responses with CD69 expression, similar dose-response associations were found between participants in the low and high-dose groups (Fig. 4.19). Specific T-cell responses with double or triple cytokine positivity were recorded after vaccination in both groups. The multifunctional phenotype was predominantly detected in memory CD^4 T-cells, whereas the monofunctional phenotype was predominant in memory CD^8 T-cells. Pre-existing adenovirus type-5 neutralizing antibodies also hurt the pattern of T-cell responses. Adenovirus type-5 neutralizing antibodies were significantly increased in vaccinated individuals after vaccination.

4.3.3.2 A Homologous Boost After the Primary Immunization

One hundred and twenty participants received either 4.0×10^{10} viral particles of Ebola virus type 5 adenovirus vaccine, 1.6×10^{11} viral particles of Ebola virus type 5 adenovirus vaccine, or placebo as primary immunization in the ini-

Table 4.15 Adverse reactions occurred within 28 days after vaccination in stratified subgroups according to the pre-existing Ad5 neutralizing antibody level. (Reprinted from Appendix 1, Zhu, F.C., et al., Safety and immunogenicity of a novel recombinant adenovirus type-5 vector-based Ebola vaccine in healthy adults in China: preliminary report of a randomised, double-blind, placebo-controlled, phase 1 trial. *Lancet*, 2015. **385**(9984): p. 2272–9)

		Placebo group ($n = 40$)			Low-dose group ($n = 40$)			High-dose group ($n = 40$)		
		Pre-Ad5 ≤ 1:200	Pre-Ad5 > 1:200		Pre-Ad5 ≤ 1:200	Pre-Ad5 > 1:200		Pre-Ad5 ≤ 1:200	Pre-Ad5 > 1:200	
		($n = 16$)	($n = 24$)	*p*-value	($n = 18$)	($n = 22$)	*p*-value	($n = 15$)	($n = 25$)	*p*-value
Solicited adverse reactions within 0–7 days										
	Any	7(43.8)	12(50.0)	0.6982	13(72.2)	14(63.6)	0.5641	13(86.7)	23(92.0)	1.0000
	Grade 3	0(0.0)	0(0.0)	–	1(5.6)	0(0.0)	0.4500	0(0.0)	0(0.0)	–
Injection-site adverse reactions										
Pain	Any	2(12.5)	6(25.0)	0.5722	8(44.4)	6(27.3)	0.2573	11(73.3)	19(76.0)	1.0000
Induration	Any	0(0.0)	0(0.0)	–	1(5.6)	0(0.0)	0.4500	0(0.0)	0(0.0)	–
Redness	Any	1(6.3)	4(16.7)	0.6256	4(22.2)	5(22.7)	1.0000	7(46.7)	7(28.0)	0.2308
	Grade 3	0(0.0)	0(0.0)	–	1(5.6)	0(0.0)	0.4500	0(0.0)	0(0.0)	–
Swelling	Any	0(0.0)	0(0.0)	–	1(5.6)	1(4.6)	1.0000	2(13.3)	1(4.0)	0.6419
Itch	Any	0(0.0)	0(0.0)	–	0(0.0)	0(0.0)	–	1(6.7)	0(0.0)	0.3750
Systemic adverse reactions										
Fever	Any	6(37.5)	4(16.7)	0.2636	4(22.2)	2(9.1)	0.4764	7(46.7)	6(24.0)	0.2572
Headache	Any	0(0.0)	1(4.2)	1.0000	2(11.1)	0(0.0)	0.1962	1(6.7)	0(0.0)	0.3750
Fatigue	Any	2(12.5)	1(4.2)	0.7132	3(16.7)	3(13.6)	1.0000	3(20.0)	3(12.0)	0.8191
Vomiting	Any	0(0.0)	0(0.0)	–	0(0.0)	1(4.6)	1.0000	3(20.0)	0(0.0)	0.0882
Diarrhea	Any	1(6.3)	0(0.0)	0.4000	0(0.0)	0(0.0)	–	2(13.3)	0(0.0)	0.1346
Muscle pain	Any	1(6.3)	1(4.2)	1.0000	0(0.0)	0(0.0)	–	1(6.7)	1(4.0)	1.0000
Joint pain	Any	0(0.0)	1(4.2)	1.0000	0(0.0)	0(0.0)	–	0(0.0)	0(0.0)	–
Throat pain	Any	0(0.0)	1(4.2)	1.0000	1(5.6)	0(0.0)	0.4500	0(0.0)	0(0.0)	–
Cough	Any	2(12.5)	1(4.2)	0.7132	0(0.0)	2(9.1)	0.4923	2(9.1)	1(4.0)	0.6419
Unsolicited adverse events within 0–28 days										
	Any	7(43.8)	10(41.7)	0.8961	7(38.9)	8(36.4)	0.8696	8(53.3)	14(56.0)	0.8696
	Grade3	0(0.0)	0(0.0)	–	0(0.0)	1(4.6)	1.0000	0(0.0)	0(0.0)	–

Pre-Ad5 = pre-existing Ad5 neutralizing antibody

Table 4.16 Antibody responses to the 2014 Zaire Ebola virus glycoprotein. Table 3, Zhu, F.C., et al., Safety and immunogenicity of a novel recombinant adenovirus type-5 vector-based Ebola vaccine in healthy adults in China: preliminary report of a randomised, double-blind, placebo-controlled, phase 1 trial. *Lancet*, 2015. **385**(9984): p. 2272–9)

		Day 14				Day 28			
		Placebo group (n = 40)	Low-dose group (n = 40)	High-dose group (n = 40)	p-value	Placebo group (n = 40)	Low-dose group (n = 40)	High-dose group (n = 40)	p-value
GMT (95% CI)		5.0 (..)	421.4 (249.7–711.3)	820.5 (598.9–1124.0)	<0.0001	5.0 (..)	682.7 (424.3–1098.5)	1305.7 (970.1–1757.2)	<0.0001
Responders		0	37 (93%)	40 (100%)	<0.0001	0	38 (95%)	40 (100%)	<0.0001
Pre-existing adenovirus type-5 antibody titers ≤1:200									
	N	16	18		15	16	18	15	
	GMT (95% CI)	5.0 (..)	842.3 (460.7–1539.7)	1493.4 (888.5–2510.1)	<0.0001	5.0 (..)	1592.5 (1029.4–2463.6)	2231.8 (1268.6–3926.2)	<0.0001
	Responders	0	18 (100%)	15 (100%)	<0.0001	0 (0.0–20.6)	18 (100%, 81.5–100.0)	15 (100%)	<0.0001
Pre-existing adenovirus type-5 antibody titers>1:200									
	N	24	22	25		24	22	25	
	GMT (95% CI)	5.0 (..)	239.2 (110.5–517.9)	572.8 (405.3–809.6)	<0.0001	5.0 (..)	341.4 (172.6–675.3)	946.5 (705.4–1270.1)	<0.0001
	Responders	0	19 (86%)	25 (100%)	<0.0001	0	20 (91%)	25 (100%)	<0.0001

Data are n (%) unless otherwise indicated. Optical density was read at 450 nm. Positive Ebola-specific antibody response was defined as an ELISA antibody 90% effective concentration (EC_{90}) of 10 or more; for concentrations less than 10 we used a value of 5 for GMT calculation. GMT = geometric mean titer

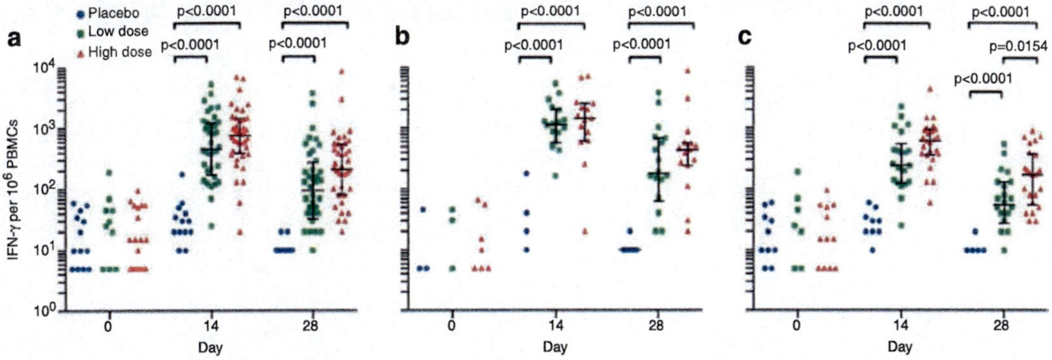

Fig. 4.17 Glycoprotein-specific T-cell response in all participants (**a**) and those with pre-existing adenovirus type-5 neutralizing antibody titers ≤1:200 (**b**) or >1:200 (**c**). IFN = interferon. PBMC = peripheral blood mononuclear cells. (Reprinted from Figure 2, Zhu, F.C., et al., Safety and immunogenicity of a novel recombinant adenovirus type-5 vector-based Ebola vaccine in healthy adults in China: preliminary report of a randomised, double-blind, placebo-controlled, phase 1 trial. *Lancet*, 2015. **385**(9984): p. 2272–9)

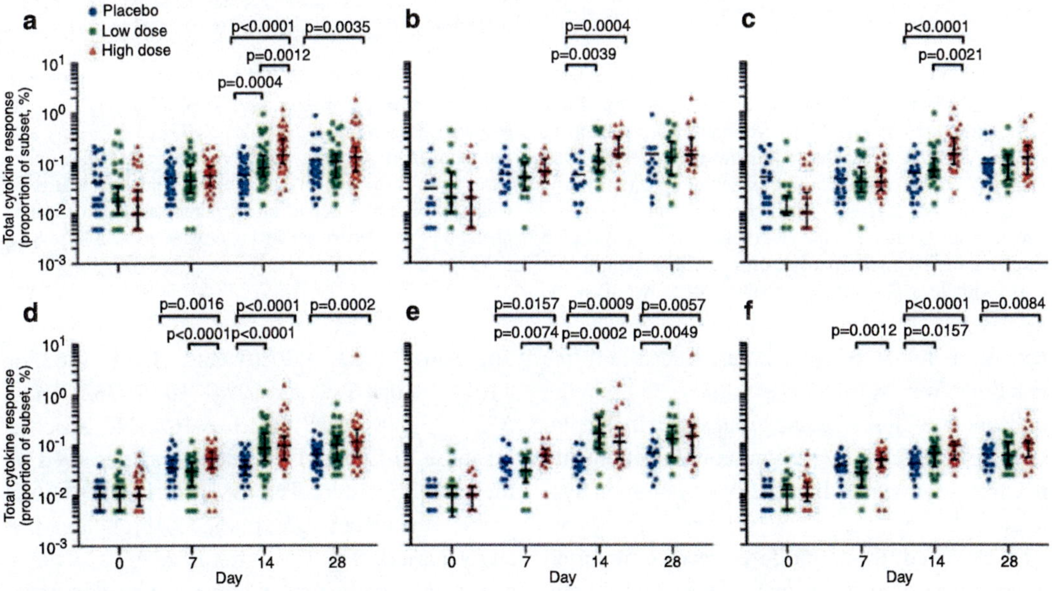

Fig. 4.18 CD4 and CD8 T-cell response. CD4 T-cell response in all participants (**a**) and those with pre-existing adenovirus type-5 neutralizing antibody titres ≤1:200 (**b**) or >1:200 (**c**), and CD8 T-cell response in all participants (**d**) and those with pre-existing-adenovirus-type-5--antibody titres ≤1:200 (**e**) or >1:200 (**f**). (Reprinted from Figure 3, Zhu, F.C., et al., Safety and immunogenicity of a novel recombinant adenovirus type-5 vector-based Ebola vaccine in healthy adults in China: preliminary report of a randomised, double-blind, placebo-controlled, phase 1 trial. *Lancet*, 2015. **385**(9984): p. 2272–9)

tial study, with 40 participants in each group. This was done until the end of the 6-month follow-up on day 168 (Fig. 4.20). All 120 participants were then invited to a booster study 6 months after the primary vaccination, of which 110 agreed to participate. Ten participants declined to receive the booster, two in the low-dose group, five in the high-dose group, and three in the placebo group.

On day 56, only a small number of adverse events were detected that were mildly symptomatic and clinically insignificant. The overall incidence of adverse reactions was similar to that observed after the initial vaccination. The inci-

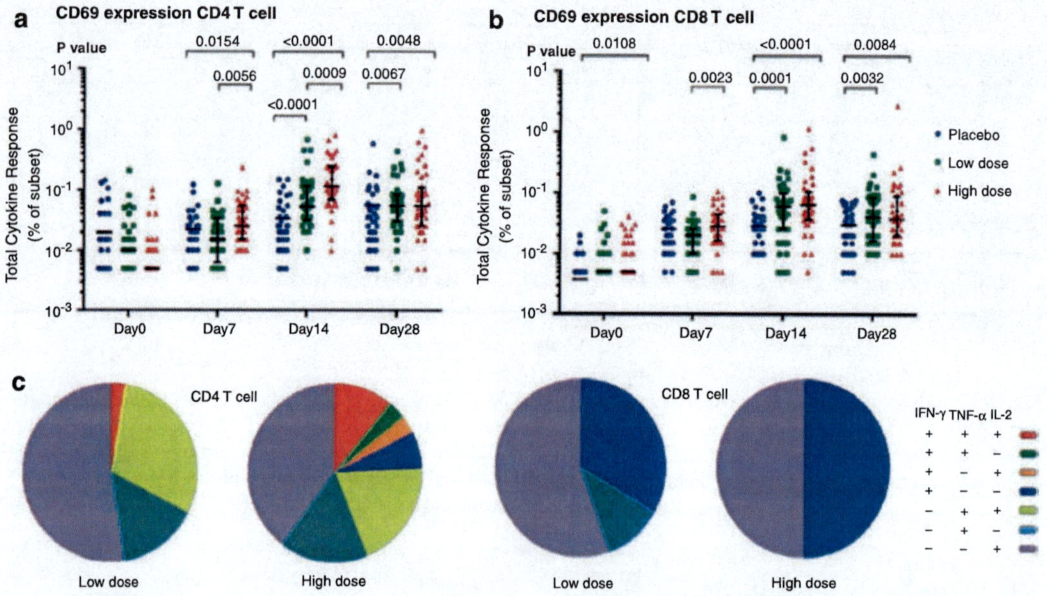

Fig. 4.19 Ebola glycoprotein-specific CD69 expression CD^4 and CD^8 T-cell response measured by Flow Cytometry with intracellular cytokine staining method. Panels A and B show the individual response of CD69 expression CD^4 and CD^8 T-cells secreting interferon-γ, tumor necrosis factor-*α*, or interleukin-2 in all participants, respectively. Each symbol represents a positive response of one participant at different time points, and those with zero T-cells responses are not shown. Panel C shows the proportions of CD4 and CD^8 T-cells producing any combination of the three cytokines, on day 14. (Reprinted from Appendix 8, Zhu, F.C., et al., Safety and immunogenicity of a novel recombinant adenovirus type-5 vector-based Ebola vaccine in healthy adults in China: preliminary report of a randomised, double-blind, placebo-controlled, phase 1 trial. *Lancet*, 2015. **385**(9984): p. 2272–9)

dence of mild- or moderate-induced adverse reactions was significantly higher in both the high and low-dose vaccine groups than in the placebo group. The most common injection site reaction was pain, while the most common systemic adverse reaction was fever. Participants who received the high-dose vaccine reported higher rates of pain, atrophy, fever, and fatigue than those who received a placebo.

Following adenovirus-5 Ebola vaccination, we found a significant increase in ELISA EC_{90} titers on day 14 and a peak on day 28 in the high and low-dose vaccine groups (682.7 [95% CI 424.3–1098.5] in the low-dose vaccine group and 1305.7 [970.1–1757.2] in the high dose vaccine group), while the placebo group, no specific reactions were recorded (Table 4.17 and Fig. 4.21). ELISA EC_{90} titers of the low-dose and high-dose vaccine groups gradually decreased, with a geometric mean titer (GMT) of 489.8 (95% CI 295.3–812.3) and 1282.9 (998.6–1648.3) at day 56, 386.4 (252.7–591.0) and 856.8 (662.9–1107.4) at day 112, and 197.9 (107.9–362.7) and 575.5 (394.8–838.8) at day 168. No specific response to Ebola glycoprotein was observed in the placebo group. The GMT for ELISA EC_{90} titers in the placebo group was 5.0 throughout the study period. The GMT for ELISA EC_{90} titers was significantly higher and more persistent in the high-dose group than in the low-dose group throughout the 6-month follow-up period. However, no difference in the proportion of positive responders was found between the high and low-dose groups. The preexistence of higher adenovirus type-5 neutralizing antibodies not only attenuated the vaccine-elicited glycoprotein-specific antibody response but also accelerated the decay of ELISA EC_{90} titers, particularly in participants receiving low doses. In contrast, participants with naive or low baseline anti-adenovirus 5 neutralizing antibodies showed only a slight attenuation of antibody titers, sug-

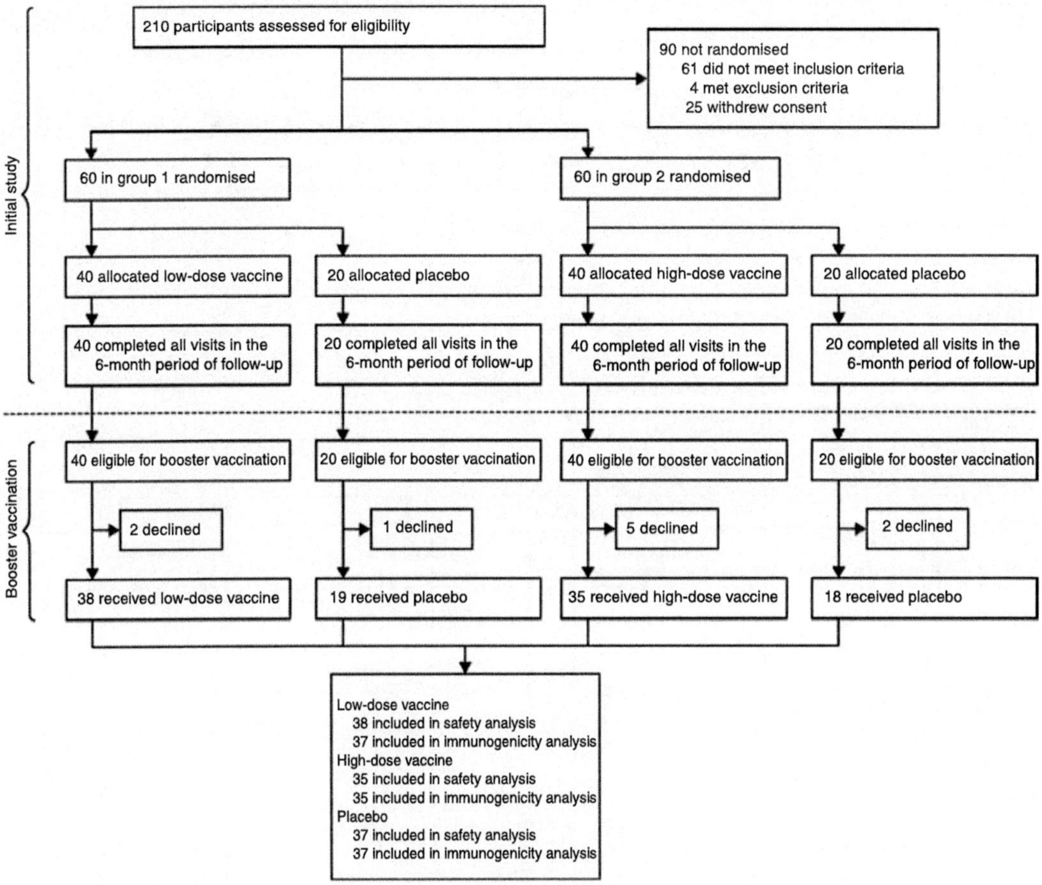

Fig. 4.20 Trial profiles of the initial study and the booster study. High-dose vaccine = adenovirus type-5 Ebola virus vaccines of 1.6×10^{11} vp/dose. Low-dose vaccine = adenovirus type-5 Ebola virus vaccines of 4.0×10^{10} vp/dose. (Reprinted from Figure 1, Li, J.X., et al., Immunity duration of a recombinant adenovirus type-5 vector-based Ebola vaccine and a homologous prime-boost immunisation in healthy adults in China: final report of a randomised, double-blind, placebo-controlled, phase 1 trial. *Lancet Glob Health*, 2017. **5**(3): p. e324–e334)

Table 4.17 ELISA antibody responses to the Ebola glycoprotein after initial and boost vaccination. (Reprinted from Table 3, Li, J.X., et al., Immunity duration of a recombinant adenovirus type-5 vector-based Ebola vaccine and a homologous prime-boost immunisation in healthy adults in China: final report of a randomised, double-blind, placebo-controlled, phase 1 trial. *Lancet Glob Health*, 2017. **5**(3): p. e324–e334)

	Overall			Pre-existing adenovirus type-5 antibody titers ≤ 1:200[a]			Pre-existing adenovirus type-5 antibody titers > 1:200[a]		
	n	GMT	Responders	*n*	GMT	Responders	*n*	GMT	Responders
Day 56									
Placebo group	40	5.0	0	16	5.0	0	24	5.0	0
Low-dose group	40	489.8 (295.3–812.3)	37	18	1163.3 (303.0–5283.0)	18	22	241.3 (5.0–3465.0)	19
High-dose group	40	1282.9 (998.6–1648.3)	40	15	2290.1 (1268.0–7220.0)	15	25	906.2 (305.4–5802.0)	25
p-value		<0.0001[b]	<0.0001[c]		<0.0001[b]	<0.0001[b]		<0.0001[b]	<0.0001[c]

(continued)

Table 4.17 (continued)

	Overall			Pre-existing adenovirus type-5 antibody titers ≤ 1:200[a]			Pre-existing adenovirus type-5 antibody titers > 1:200[a]		
	n	GMT	Responders	*n*	GMT	Responders	*n*	GMT	Responders
Day 112									
Placebo group	40	5.0	0	16	5.0	0	24	5.0	0
Low-dose group	40	386.4 (252.7–591.0)	38	18	780.3 (189.9–4227.0)	18	22	217.4 (5.0–3159.0)	20
High-dose group	40	856.8 (662.9–1107.4)	40	15	1538.2 (720.5–6010.0)	15	25	603.1 (142.4–4576.0)	25
p-value		<0.0001[b]	<0.0001[c]		<0.0001[b]	<0.0001[b]		<0.0001[b]	<0.0001[c]
Day 168									
Placebo group	40	5.0	0	16	5.0	0	24	5.0	0
Low-dose group	40	197.9 (107.9–362.7)	34	18	539.2 (262.5–1107.8)	17	22	87.1 (38.4–197.4)	17
High-dose group	40	575.5 (394.8–838.8)	39	15	1216.2 (978.6–1511.4)	15	25	367.3 (217.7–619.7)	24
p-value		<0.0001[b]	<0.0001[b]		<0.0001[b]	<0.0001[c]		<0.0001[b]	<0.0001[c]
Day 28 after boost									
Placebo group	37	5.0	0	16	5.0	0	21	5.0	0
Low-dose group	37	6110.3 (4705.4–7934.6)	37	17	7553.3 (5090.6–11,207.4)	17	20	5102.7 (3558.6–7316.7)	20
High-dose group	35	11,824.9 (8903.6–15,704.8)	35	14	15,680.0 (11,041.5–22,267.0)	14	21	9797.1 (6475.8–14,821.9)	21
p-value		<0.0001[b]	<0.0001[b]		<0.0001[b]	<0.0001[b]		<0.0001[b]	<0.0001[b]
Month 12 after boost									
Placebo group	34	5.0	0	14	5.0	0	20	5.0	0
Low-dose group	33	674.1 (505.9–898.2)	33	16	840.1 (555.5–1270.4)	16	17	547.9 (361.8–829.8)	17
High-dose group	35	856.8 (573.8–1279.2)	34	14	1314.5 (1022.3–1690.2)	14	21	644.0 (339.6–1221.5)	20
p-value		<0.0001[c]	<0.0001[c]		<0.0001[b]	<0.0001[b]		<0.0001[c]	<0.0001[c]

GMT = geometric mean titer. *N* = number of participants. Ebola antibody EC_{90} was measured by ELISA, according to treatment groups and time points. Optical density was read at 450 nm. Positive Ebola-specific antibody response was defined as the EC_{90} 10 or more. For Ebola ELISA antibody EC_{90} less than 10, a value of 5 was used for GMT calculation

[a]The stratified analyses of the immune responses were performed according to the baseline adenovirus type-5 neutralizing antibody titers of participants before the prime injection

[b]The pairwise comparisons showed a significantly higher response level in the high-dose group compared with that in the low-dose group, and both the high-dose and low-dose groups showed significantly higher responses than did the placebo group

[c]Both the high-dose and low-dose groups showed significantly higher responses than did the placebo group, but no significant difference was noted between the high-dose and low-dose groups

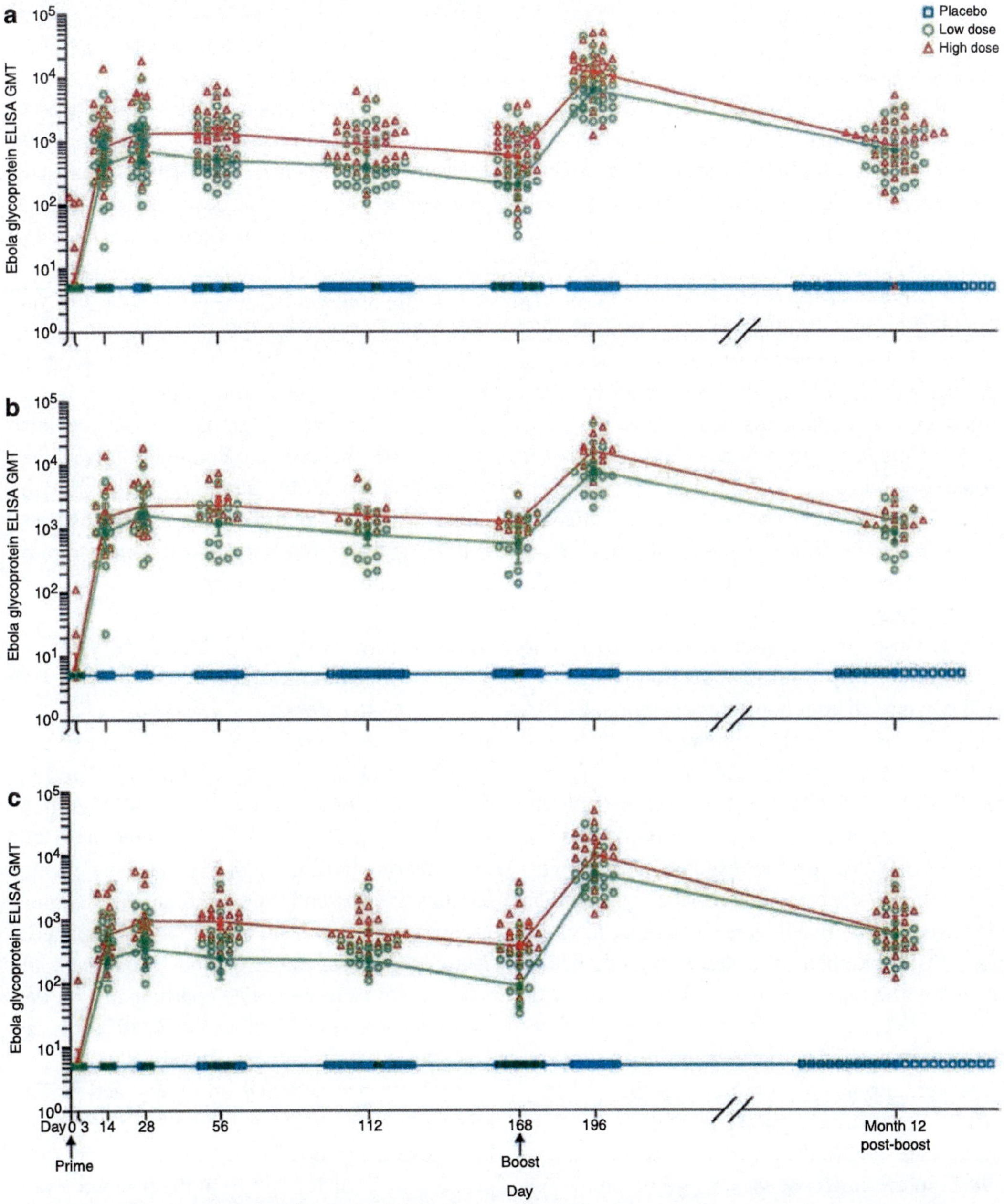

Fig. 4.21 Ebola-specific ELISA EC_{90} titers to glycoprotein. GMT = geometric mean titer (**a**) all participants, (**b**) patients with baseline adenovirus type-5 neutralizing antibody titers, (**c**) patients with baseline adenovirus type-5 neutralizing antibody titers > 1:200. (Reprinted from Figure 2, Li, J.X., et al., Immunity duration of a recombinant adenovirus type-5 vector-based Ebola vaccine and a homologous prime-boost immunisation in healthy adults in China: final report of a randomised, double-blind, placebo-controlled, phase 1 trial. *Lancet Glob Health*, 2017. **5**(3): p. e324–e334)

gesting a good persistence of antibody responses following single-dose vaccination. In individuals with high baseline anti-adenovirus type-5 neutralizing antibodies, the Ebola glycoprotein-specific ELISA titers observed following high-dose vaccination were similar to those observed following low-dose vaccination in those with low baseline anti-adenovirus type-5 neutralizing antibodies.

Positive responses for specific CD^4 and CD^8 T-cells in participants who received the vaccine peaked on day 14 after the primary vaccination and then gradually decreased over the next study period. On day 168, there was no significant difference in CD^4 and CD^8 T-cell responses between the vaccine and placebo groups (Fig. 4.19). Double or triple cytokine-positive specific CD^4 and CD^8 T-cell responses also decreased but remained detectable in both vaccine groups until 168 days after the primary vaccination.

A strong humoral immune response to the Ebola glycoprotein was induced by a booster dose of homologous vaccine at month 6 after the initial immunization, regardless of pre-existing immunity to adenovirus type 5 at the time of the booster (Fig. 4.21). Antibodies specific to the booster dose of glycoprotein were superior to those induced by a single induction of the vaccine. On day 28 after booster vaccination, ELISA EC_{90} titers rose rapidly by more than 30-fold to 6110 (95% CI 4705–7935) in the low-dose group and 20-fold to 11,825 (8904–15,705) in the high-dose group compared with the pre-booster period (Table 4.17). No specific response to Ebola glycoprotein was observed in the placebo group. The GMT for ELISA EC90 titers in the placebo group was 5.0 throughout the study period. Those receiving the high dose of 1.6×10^{11} viral particles showed stronger post-booster antibody titers than those receiving the low dose of vaccine. However, Ebola glycoprotein-specific ELISA EC_{90} titers declined gradually after reaching a peak, with a GMT of 674.1 (95% CI 505.9–898.2) in the low-dose vaccine group and 856.8 (573.8–1279.2) in the high-dose vaccine group at month 12 post-boost, levels that were significantly higher than those at month 6 post-initial vaccination. In contrast, the three high-dose participants who did not receive a booster injection in the initial primary study showed ELISA EC_{90} titers ranging from 152 to 610 at the same time point, with a mean of 285.5.

Specific T-cell responses quantified with interferon-γ (IFN-γ) showed a modest increase following booster injection, with 23.3 spot-forming cells in the low-dose group (IQR 16.7–90.0) and 95.0 spot-forming cells in the high-dose group (63.3–196.7), significantly higher than in the placebo group (Fig. 4.22). Although the booster induced greater T-cell IFN-γ expression than on day 168 before the booster, the magnitude of the response was significantly lower than that observed on day 28 after the initial vaccination.

Neutralizing antibody titers against the vaccine vector adenovirus type 5 peaked on day 14 after primary vaccination and then tapered off over the next 6 months. Although booster immunization with the homologous vaccine also increased the neutralizing antibody titers against adenovirus type 5, the antibody titers following booster immunization were not as high as those following the initial dose and declined rapidly over the following 12 months.

4.3.3.3 Immunogenicity and Safety for Optimal Doses of the Vaccine

In the phase 2 trial, 618 healthy adults were recruited and screened, of whom 500 were randomly allocated to receive either the high-dose vaccine ($n = 250$), the low-dose vaccine ($n = 125$), or placebo ($n = 125$; Fig. 4.23). Baseline characteristics were essentially similar across treatment groups (Table 4.18). All participants completed a 7-day safety observation period. Blood samples were drawn from 496 (99%) participants on day 14, 497 (99%) on day 28, and 493 (99%) on day 168.

At least one solicited adverse reaction was reported by 132 of 250 participants (53%) in the high-dose group, 60 of 125 (48%) in the low-dose group, and 54 of 125 (43%) in the placebo group within 7 days of vaccination (Table 4.19). Most adverse reactions were mild and self-limiting, occurring within the first 24 h after injection and lasting no longer than 48 h. However, in the post-hoc analysis, there was a significant difference in the incidence of injection site adverse reactions between the three groups ($p = 0.0169$). In multiple comparisons based on an adjusted alpha of 0.017, the difference between the high and low-dose groups was not significant ($p = 0.9002$),

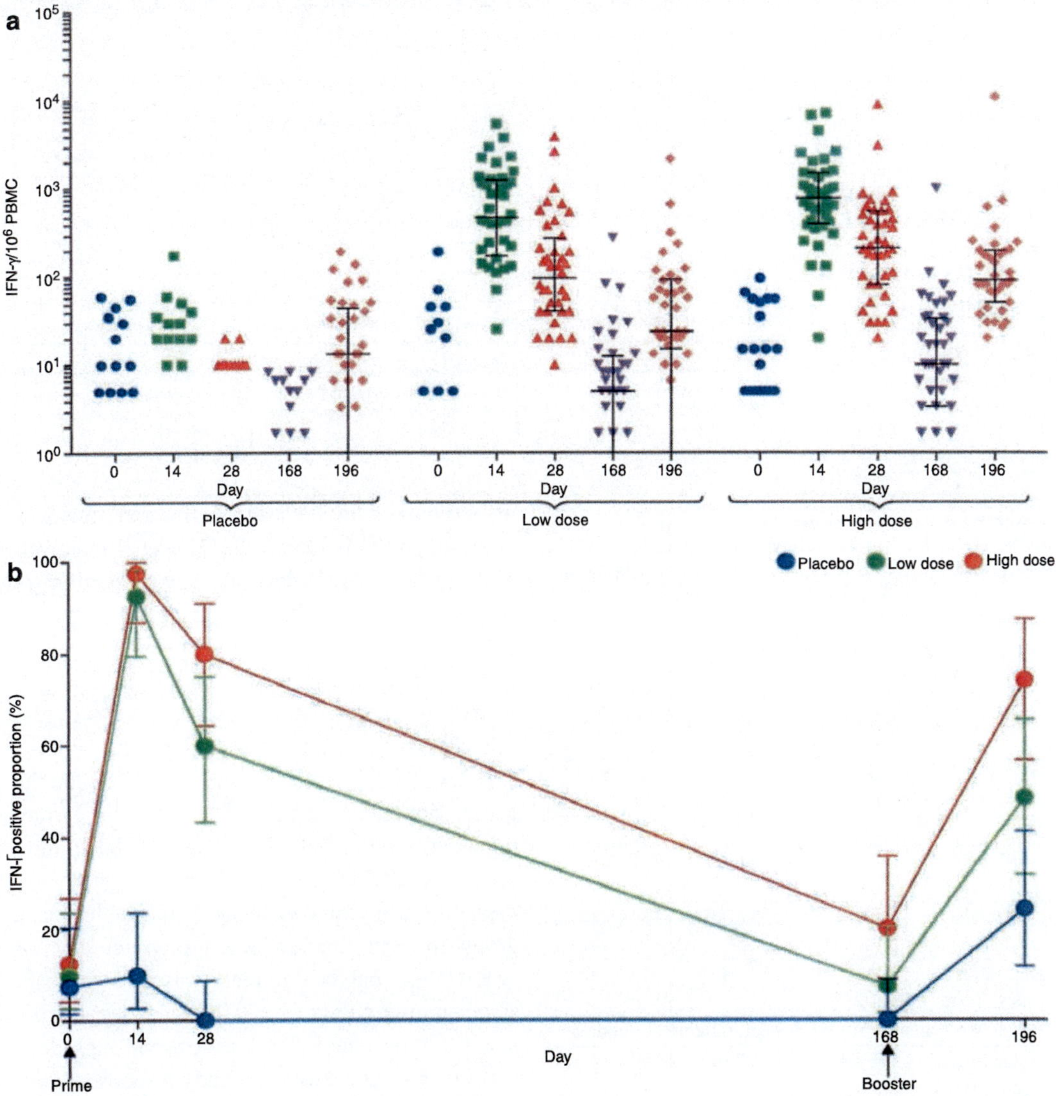

Fig. 4.22 Glycoprotein-specific T-cell response measured by Enzyme-Linked ImmunoSpot at different time points before and after prime and boost vaccination. (**a**) IFN-γ expressing T-cells per 10^6 PBMC. (**b**) The proportion of participants with a positive response of IFN-γ expressing T-cells. IFN = interferon. PBMC = peripheral blood mononuclear cells. (Reprinted from Figure 3, Li, J.X., et al., Immunity duration of a recombinant adenovirus type-5 vector-based Ebola vaccine and a homologous prime-boost immunisation in healthy adults in China: final report of a randomised, double-blind, placebo-controlled, phase 1 trial. *Lancet Glob Health*, 2017. **5**(3): p. e324–e334)

while both the high and low-dose groups had significantly more solicited injection site adverse reactions than the placebo group ($p = 0.0077$ for the high dose group versus the placebo group and $p = 0.0361$ for the low-dose group versus the placebo group). The most common injection site adverse reaction was pain and the most common systemic adverse reactions were headache and fever (Table 4.19). At least one or more unsolicited adverse reactions were reported by 147 (59%) participants in the high-dose group, 81 (65%) participants in the low-dose group, and 67 (54%) participants in the placebo group within 28 days of vaccination. This paragraph is reused from Zhu, F.C., et al, Lancet, 2017. 389(10069): p. 621–628.

Although all participants included in the study had negative HIV screening results at enrolment,

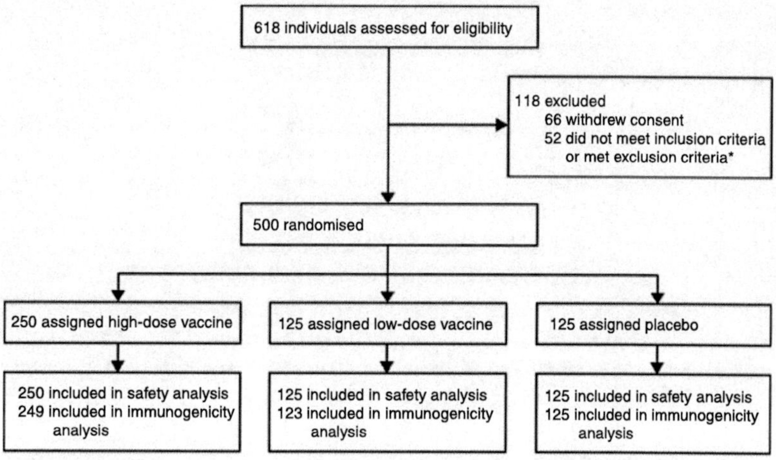

Fig. 4.23 Trial profile. (Reprinted from Figure 1, Zhu, F.C., et al., Safety and immunogenicity of a recombinant adenovirus type-5 vector-based Ebola vaccine in healthy adults in Sierra Leone: a single-centre, randomised, double-blind, placebo-controlled, phase 2 trial. *Lancet*, 2017. **389**(10069): p. 621–628)

Table 4.18 Baseline characteristics. (Reprinted from Table 1, Zhu, F.C., et al., Safety and immunogenicity of a recombinant adenovirus type-5 vector-based Ebola vaccine in healthy adults in Sierra Leone: a single-centre, randomised, double-blind, placebo-controlled, phase 2 trial. *Lancet*, 2017. **389**(10069): p. 621–628)

	Placebo (*n* = 125)	Low-dose vaccine (*n* = 125)	High-dose vaccine (*n* = 250)
Age, years	32.4 (8.4)	32.7 (9.2)	32.2 (8.8)
Sex			
Male	72 (58%)	70 (56%)	126 (50%)
Female	53 (42%)	55 (44%)	124 (50%)
Body-mass index, kg/m^2	24.9 (4.2)	24.9 (4.7)	24.7 (4.6)
Pre-existing adenovirus type-5 neutralizing antibodies			
Geometric mean titer	109.4 (5.4)	136.7 (4.8)	150.6 (4.4)
>1:12	104 (83%)	105 (84%)	221 (88%)
>1:200	49 (39%)	58 (46%)	117 (47%)

Data are mean (SD) or *n* (%)

six participants (five in the high-dose group and one in the placebo group) were confirmed to be HIV-positive on day 168. The incidence of HIV infection during follow-up was not significantly different between treatment groups ($p = 0.3223$). This paragraph is reused from Zhu, F.C., et al, Lancet, 2017. 389(10069): p. 621–628.

Glycoprotein-specific antibody responses were detected from day 14 onwards, with at least 96% of responders in both the high- and low-dose groups on day 14 (Table 4.20). However, there was no significant difference in the proportion of responders between the low and high-dose groups at all three-time points. The glycoprotein-specific antibody response peaked at day 28 with a geometric mean titer of 1471.8 (95% CI 1151.0–1881.8) in the low-dose group and 2043.1 (1762.4–2368.4) in the high-dose group, while the geometric mean titer in the placebo group remained around 6.0–6.8 throughout the follow-up period (Table 4.20). Notably, the geometric mean titer was temporarily higher in the high-dose group than in the low-dose group on day 28 ($p = 0.0495$), but the difference was not significant at other time points ($p = 0.0671$ on day 14 and $p = 1.000$ on day 168). Both low and high-dose vaccines induced strong antibody responses (geometric mean titers > 1000) within 28 days post-vaccination, regardless of pre-existing adenovirus type 5 neutralizing antibody titers (Fig. 4.24). This paragraph is reused from Zhu, F.C., et al, Lancet, 2017. 389(10069): p. 621--628.

Furthermore, the vaccine-induced antibody response declined significantly after the peak: on day 168, the geometric mean titers were 223.3 (148.2–336.4) in the low-dose group and 254–2 (185.0–349.5) in the high-dose group.

Before vaccination, most participants had neutralizing antibodies against adenovirus type 5 and the geometric mean titers were well balanced across treatment groups at baseline (Table 4.18). On day 14, the geometric mean titers of these

Table 4.19 Solicited and unsolicited adverse reactions. (Reprinted from Table 2, Zhu, F.C., et al., Safety and immunogenicity of a recombinant adenovirus type-5 vector-based Ebola vaccine in healthy adults in Sierra Leone: a single-centre, randomised, double-blind, placebo-controlled, phase 2 trial. **Lancet**, 2017. **389**(10069): p. 621–628)

		Placebo (n = 125)	Low-dose vaccine (n = 125)	High-dose vaccine (n = 250)	p-value[a]
Solicited adverse reactions within 7 days					
Any		54 (43%)	60 (48%)	132 (53%)	0.2093
Grade 1		49 (39%)	56 (45%)	121 (48%)	0.2449
Grade 2		10 (8%)	12 (10%)	33 (13%)	0.3039
Grade 3		1 (1%)	0	3 (1%)	0.8110
Solicited injection-site adverse reactions within 7 days					
Any		17 (14%)	31 (25%)	65 (26%)	0.0169
Pain					
	Grade 1	14 (11%)	25 (20%)	48 (19%)	0.1009
	Grade 2	1 (1%)	1 (1%)	6 (2%)	0.4542
Induration					
	Grade 1	0	1 (1%)	3 (1%)	0.8110
	Grade 2	0	1 (1%)	2 (1%)	0.8114
	Grade 3	0	0	1 (<1%)	1.0000
Redness					
	Grade 1	2 (2%)	2 (2%)	4 (2%)	1.0000
	Grade 2	0	0	5 (2%)	0.0802
Swelling					
	Grade 1	0	2 (2%)	5 (2%)	0.3660
	Grade 2	0	1 (1%)	1 (<1%)	1.0000
	Grade 3	0	0	1 (<1%)	1.0000
Rash					
	Grade 1	1 (1%)	0	0	0.5000
Itch					
	Grade 1	2 (2%)	6 (5%)	12 (5%)	0.3138
	Grade 2	0	0	1 (<1%)	1.0000
Solicited systemic adverse reactions within 7 days					
Any		45 (36%)	45 (36%)	105 (42%)	0.3954
Fever					
	Grade 1	11 (9%)	11 (9%)	20 (8%)	0.9328
	Grade 2	2 (2%)	3 (2%)	8 (3%)	0.7158
Headache					
	Grade 1	21 (17%)	22 (18%)	56 (22%)	0.3618
	Grade 2	6 (5%)	4 (3%)	11 (4%)	0.8778
	Grade 3	1 (1%)	0	1 (<1%)	1.0000
Fatigue					
	Grade 1	8 (6%)	10 (8%)	22 (9%)	0.7685
	Grade 2	0	1 (1%)	3 (1%)	0.8110
Vomiting					
	Grade 1	0	2 (2%)	2 (1%)	0.3727
Diarrhea					
	Grade 1	3 (2%)	3 (2%)	3 (1%)	0.5023
	Grade 2	1 (1%)	0	1 (<1%)	1.0000
Muscle pain					
	Grade 1	4 (3%)	7 (6%)	12 (5%)	0.6696
	Grade 2	1 (1%)	1 (1%)	3 (1%)	1.0000

(continued)

Table 4.19 (continued)

		Placebo (n = 125)	Low-dose vaccine (n = 125)	High-dose vaccine (n = 250)	p-value[a]
Joint pain					
	Grade 1	2 (2%)	7 (6%)	18 (7%)	0.0577
	Grade 2	1 (1%)	2 (2%)	1 (<1%)	0.5610
Throat pain					
	Grade 1	0	1 (1%)	2 (1%)	0.8114
	Grade 2	0	0	1 (<1%)	1.0000
Cough					
	Grade 1	1 (1%)	0	4 (2%)	0.4500
	Grade 2	0	0	1 (<1%)	1.0000
Unsolicited adverse reactions within 28 days					
Any		67 (54%)	81 (65%)	147 (59%)	0.1938
	Grade 1	63 (50%)	78 (62%)	143 (57%)	0.1617
	Grade 2	10 (8%)	8 (6%)	14 (6%)	0.6421

Data are n (%) unless indicated otherwise. Grade 1 was a mild reaction, grade 2 was a moderate reaction, and grade 3 was a severe reaction (i.e., prevented activity)

[a]Calculated with χ^2 test or Fisher's exact test

Table 4.20 Glycoprotein-specific antibody responses. (Reprinted from Table 3, Zhu, F.C., et al., Safety and immunogenicity of a recombinant adenovirus type-5 vector-based Ebola vaccine in healthy adults in Sierra Leone: a single-centre, randomised, double-blind, placebo-controlled, phase 2 trial. *Lancet*, 2017. **389**(10069): p. 621–628)

	Day 14			Day 28			Day 168		
	Placebo (n = 125)	Low-dose vaccine (n = 123)	High-dose vaccine (n = 248)	Placebo (n = 125)	Low-dose vaccine (n = 123)	High-dose vaccine (n = 249)	Placebo (n = 124)	Low-dose vaccine (n = 123)	High-dose vaccine (n = 246)
Geometric mean titer (95% CI)*	6.2 (5.2–7.3)	1251.0 (976.6–1602.5)	1728.4 (1459.4–2047.0)	6.8 (5.5–8.3)	1471.8 (1151.0–1881.8)	2043.1 (1762.4–2368.4)	6.0 (5.1–7.0)	223.3 (148.2–336.4)	254.2 (185.0–349.5)
Number of responders (%; 95% CI)[a]	6 (5%; 2–10)	118 (96%; 91–99)	241 (97%; 94–99)	8 (6%; 3–12)	118 (96%; 91–99)	244 (98%; 95–99)	5 (4%; 1–9)	93 (76%; 67–83)	179 (73%; 67–78)

[a]Significant differences were noted across the treatment groups, with $p < 0.0001$ at all three-time points

neutralizing antibodies increased more than tenfold in both the low and high-dose groups. Despite a rapid decline in titers thereafter, antibody titers at day 168 were still threefold–fivefold higher than at baseline in both low and high-dose vaccine recipients.

4.3.4 Conclusion

4.3.4.1 Safety

Based on the results of these studies, it was shown that the Ad5-EBOV has a good safety profile in healthy adults. The incidence of adverse reactions was consistent with previous studies of other viral vector Ebola vaccines. The incidence of injection site pain was significantly higher in participants in the high-dose vaccine group, possibly due to the higher dose of viral particles. However, almost all reported adverse reactions or events were mild or moderate, and the high-dose vaccine remained well tolerated.

4.3.4.2 Immunogenicity

Notably, the adenovirus type 5 vaccine elicited a significantly higher immune response than the placebo. The magnitude of the immune response to the vaccine was dose-dependent. Ebola glycoprotein-specific antibodies increased significantly on day 14 and continued to increase until day 28 post-vaccination, while Ebola glycoprotein-specific T-cell responses peaked on

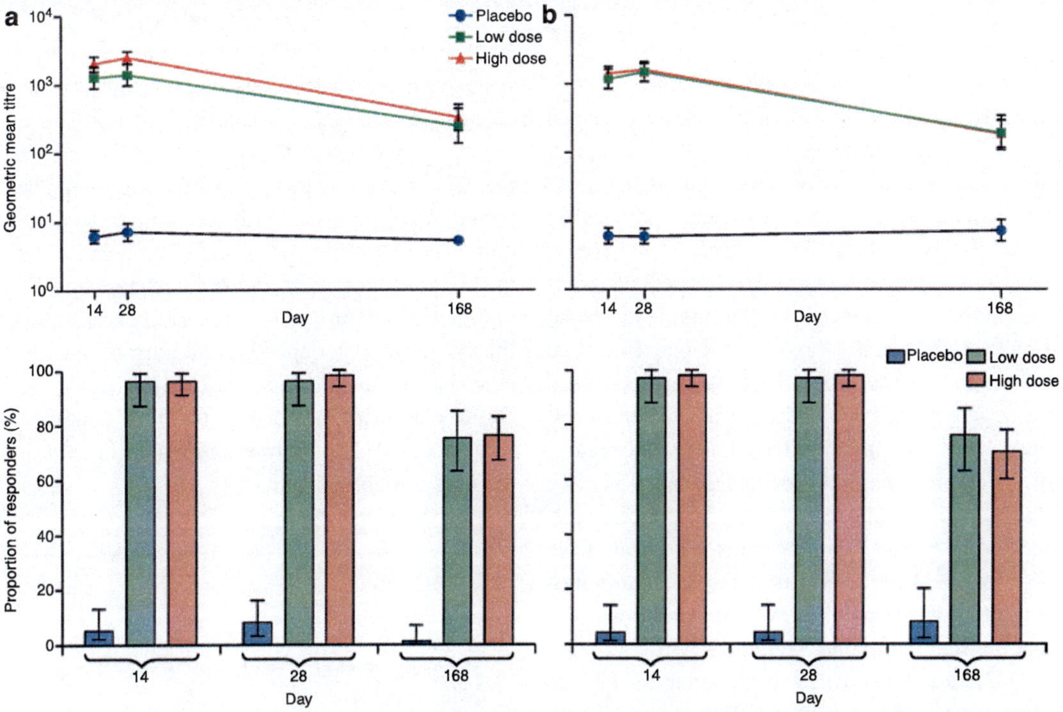

Fig. 4.24 Glycoprotein-specific antibody responses, by titers of adenovirus type-5 neutralizing antibodies at baseline. (**a**) Low titer (≤1:200). (**b**) High titer (>1:200). Error bars indicate 95% CIs. (Reprinted from Figure 2, Zhu, F.C., et al., Safety and immunogenicity of a recombinant adenovirus type-5 vector-based Ebola vaccine in healthy adults in Sierra Leone: a single-centre, randomised, double-blind, placebo-controlled, phase 2 trial. *Lancet*, 2017. **389**(10069): p. 621–628)

day 14. However, both vaccine-elicited Ebola glycoprotein-specific antibody responses and T-cell responses were partially attenuated by pre-existing anti-Ebola virus type 5 immunity, particularly in participants in the low-dose group. The high-dose vaccine overcame the negative effects of pre-existing immunity and still induced robust Ebola glycoprotein-specific antibody and T-cell responses in participants with high baseline neutralizing antibody concentrations. Since a large proportion of adults have pre-existing immunity to adenovirus type 5, particularly in developing countries, high doses of viral particles appear to be necessary. Data from the trial showed that on day 14, the concentration of vaccine-elicited Ebola glycoprotein-specific antibodies was within the range of concentrations associated with protection in non-human primate studies. However, the generalizability of this finding is likely to be low, particularly since the proportion of adults with baseline adenovirus type 5 neutralizing antibodies is even higher in African populations.

Considering that the booster effect of the homologous vaccine may be affected by the high anti-adenovirus type 5 neutralizing antibodies induced by the first dose, the booster dose was administered at 6-month intervals to avoid the peak in antibodies against the vaccine vector induced by the initial vaccination. Following booster vaccination, a significant immune memory response was found, with glycoprotein-specific antibodies being greatly enhanced and significantly higher than the invested response. However, there was relatively little enhancement of T-cell immunogenicity.

4.3.4.3 Efficacy

After phase 1 and phase 2 clinical trials (skipping Phase 3 clinical trials), the Ebola vaccine was approved in China [56]. Ebola vaccine efficacy studies have not been conducted in the country because the disease is rare and geographically limited and not prevalent in the country.

Although Phase 1 and Phase 2 clinical trials have been completed to demonstrate the safety of the human adenovirus type 5 (rAd5) Ebola vaccine, there are still some shortcomings that need to be addressed. The most advanced vaccines are cAd3-EBOV, an Ebola vaccine based on a replication-deficient chimpanzee type 3 adenovirus vector, developed by the National Institutes of Health (NIH) and GlaxoSmithKline, Inc., and "rVSVΔG-EBOVGP", an Ebola vaccine based on an attenuated stomatitis virus vector developed by the National Microbiology Laboratory of the Public Health Agency of Canada [57, 58]. These two vaccine candidates have been fast-tracked to Phase 1 clinical trials. The trials have demonstrated the excellent safety and immunogenicity of "cAd3-EBOV." In addition, the recombinant vesicular stomatitis virus vaccine (rVSVΔG-EBOVGP) is considered to be the most promising vaccine candidate and has shown significant protection against Ebola virus disease in phase 3 clinical trials in Guinea [59].

4.4 Summary

China has developed quickly in almost every field of science and technology, including biotechnology and novel vaccine development. The vaccine industry Vaccine research and development have transformed imitation into innovation, changing from traditional technological vaccines such as live attenuated vaccines and inactivated vaccines to a new generation of vaccines. Such as genetic engineering vaccines, recombinant subunit vaccines, vector vaccines, virus-like particle vaccines, and so on. The vaccine epidemiology research has also been transferred from the clinical evaluation of vaccine has shifted from epidemiological surveillance based on observational research to a randomized-controlled double-blind clinical study, from a single serological evaluation index to the compound multi-index evaluation endpoint; from the study of immunization strategy of the general population to personalized and refined immunization strategy.

At present, the research and development of traditional vaccines with simple antigen components have been completed. In the future, vaccine companies will face more and more difficulties in novel vaccine research and development, and at the same time, vaccine clinical research will also face more challenges. With the continuous deepening and innovation of vaccine clinical research in China, summarizing and refining the key technologies of vaccine clinical research and forming the "Chinese experience" at the core of the vaccine research and development will help promote China's innovative vaccines to other countries, and enhance China's international influence in the field of public health.

References

1. Khuroo MS, Khuroo MS, Khuroo NS. Transmission of hepatitis E virus in developing countries. Viruses. 2016;8(9):253.
2. Asrani SK, et al. Burden of liver diseases in the world. J Hepatol. 2019;70(1):151–71.
3. Lee GH, et al. Chronic infection with camelid Hepatitis E virus in a liver transplant recipient who regularly consumes camel meat and milk. Gastroenterology. 2016;150(2):355–7.e3.
4. Woo PC, et al. New hepatitis E virus genotype in Bactrian camels, Xinjiang, China, 2013. Emerg Infect Dis. 2016;22(12):2219–21.
5. European Association for the Study of the Liver. EASL clinical practice guidelines on hepatitis E virus infection. J Hepatol. 2018;68(6):1256–71.
6. WHO. Hepatitis E. 24 June 2022. Available from https://www.who.int/news-room/fact-sheets/detail/hepatitis-e.
7. Bhatia V, et al. A 20-year single-center experience with acute liver failure during pregnancy: is the prognosis really worse? Hepatology. 2008;48(5):1577–85.
8. Nimgaonkar I, et al. Hepatitis E virus: advances and challenges. Nat Rev Gastroenterol Hepatol. 2018;15(2):96–110.
9. Zhu FC, et al. Epidemiology of zoonotic hepatitis E: a community-based surveillance study in a rural population in China. PLoS One. 2014;9(1):e87154.
10. Sun XJ, et al. Epidemiological analysis of viral hepatitis E in China, 2004-2017. Zhonghua Yu Fang Yi Xue Za Zhi. 2019;53(4):382–7.
11. Li SW, et al. A bacterially expressed particulate hepatitis E vaccine: antigenicity, immunogenicity and protectivity on primates. Vaccine. 2005;23(22):2893–901.
12. Zhang J, et al. Randomized-controlled phase II clinical trial of a bacterially expressed recombinant hepatitis E vaccine. Vaccine. 2009;27(12):1869–74.

13. Zhu FC, et al. Efficacy and safety of a recombinant hepatitis E vaccine in healthy adults: a large-scale, randomised, double-blind placebo-controlled, phase 3 trial. Lancet. 2010;376(9744):895–902.
14. Zhang J, et al. Long-term efficacy of a hepatitis E vaccine. N Engl J Med. 2015;372(10):914–22.
15. WHO. Recommendations to assure the quality, safety and efficacy of recombinant Hepatitis E vaccines. 25 May 2019. Available from https://www.who.int/publications/m/item/recombinant-hepatitis-e-vaccines-annex-2-trs-1016.
16. ClinicalTrial. A phase IV clinical trial of the recombinant Hepatitis E vaccine (Escherichia Coli)(the chronic Hepatitis B patients). Available from https://clinicaltrials.gov/ct2/show/NCT02964910.
17. Orenstein WA, Bernier RH, Hinman AR. Assessing vaccine efficacy in the field. Further observations. Epidemiol Rev. 1988;10:212–41.
18. Solomon T, et al. Virology, epidemiology, pathogenesis, and control of enterovirus 71. Lancet Infect Dis. 2010;10(11):778–90.
19. Wang SM, Liu CC. Update of enterovirus 71 infection: epidemiology, pathogenesis and vaccine. Expert Rev Anti-Infect Ther. 2014;12(4):447–56.
20. Bible JM, et al. Genetic evolution of enterovirus 71: epidemiological and pathological implications. Rev Med Virol. 2007;17(6):371–9.
21. McMinn PC. Enterovirus vaccines for an emerging cause of brain-stem encephalitis. N Engl J Med. 2014;370(9):792–4.
22. Xing W, et al. Hand, foot, and mouth disease in China, 2008-12: an epidemiological study. Lancet Infect Dis. 2014;14(4):308–18.
23. McMinn P, et al. Neurological manifestations of enterovirus 71 infection in children during an outbreak of hand, foot, and mouth disease in Western Australia. Clin Infect Dis. 2001;32(2):236–42.
24. Chua KB, Kasri AR. Hand foot and mouth disease due to enterovirus 71 in Malaysia. Virol Sin. 2011;26(4):221–8.
25. Pallansch MA, Oberste MS. Enterovirus 71 encephalitis: a new vaccine on the horizon? Lancet. 2013;381(9871):976–7.
26. Prevention, CCfDCa. Technical guidelines for the use of enterovirus 71 inactivated vaccines issued by the Chinese Center for Disease Control and Prevention. 2016-06-08. Available from https://www.chinacdc.cn/zxdt/201606/t20160608_131032.html.
27. NMP, A. The marketing of enterovirus 71 inactivated vaccine approved by National Medical Products Administration. 2015. Available from https://www.nmpa.gov.cn/directory/web/nmpa/yaopin/ypjgdt/20151203164201285.html.
28. Zhu FC, et al. Immunogenicity and safety of an enterovirus 71 vaccine in healthy Chinese children and infants: a randomised, double-blind, placebo-controlled phase 2 clinical trial. Lancet. 2013;381(9871):1037–45.
29. Zhu FC, et al. Reactogenicity and immunogenicity of an enterovirus 71 vaccine in Chinese healthy children and infants. Pediatr Infect Dis J. 2012;31(11):1158–65.
30. Shenyu W, et al. A booster dose of an inactivated enterovirus 71 vaccine in Chinese young children: a randomized, double-blind, placebo-controlled clinical trial. J Infect Dis. 2014;210(7):1073–82.
31. Zhu F, et al. Efficacy, safety, and immunogenicity of an enterovirus 71 vaccine in China. N Engl J Med. 2014;370(9):818–28.
32. Zhu FC, et al. Efficacy, safety, and immunology of an inactivated alum-adjuvant enterovirus 71 vaccine in children in China: a multicentre, randomised, double-blind, placebo-controlled, phase 3 trial. Lancet. 2013;381(9882):2024–32.
33. Jin P, et al. Validation and evaluation of serological correlates of protection for inactivated enterovirus 71 vaccine in children aged 6-35 months. Hum Vaccin Immunother. 2016;12(4):916–21.
34. Zhu W, et al. Correlates of protection for inactivated enterovirus 71 vaccine: the analysis of immunological surrogate endpoints. Expert Rev Vaccines. 2017;16(9):945–9.
35. Li YP, et al. Immunogenicity, safety, and immune persistence of a novel inactivated human enterovirus 71 vaccine: a phase II, randomized, double-blind, placebo-controlled trial. J Infect Dis. 2014;209(1):46–55.
36. Rubin LG, et al. 2013 IDSA clinical practice guideline for vaccination of the immunocompromised host. Clin Infect Dis. 2014;58(3):e44–100.
37. Hu Y, et al. Five-year immunity persistence following immunization with inactivated enterovirus 71 type (EV71) vaccine in healthy children: a further observation. Hum Vaccin Immunother. 2018;14(6):1517–23.
38. Badell ML, et al. Risks associated with smallpox vaccination in pregnancy: a systematic review and meta-analysis. Obstet Gynecol. 2015;125(6):1439–51.
39. Guan X, et al. Effectiveness and safety of an inactivated enterovirus 71 vaccine in children aged 6-71 months in a phase IV study. Clin Infect Dis. 2020;71(9):2421–7.
40. Xu Q, et al. Interchangeability of two enterovirus 71 inactivated vaccines in Chinese children: a phase IV, open-label, and randomized controlled trial. Vaccine. 2020;38(12):2671–7.
41. Zhang Z, et al. Immunogenicity and safety of an inactivated enterovirus 71 vaccine administered simultaneously with Hepatitis B vaccine and group A meningococcal polysaccharide vaccine: a phase 4, open-label, single-center, randomized, noninferiority trial. J Infect Dis. 2019;220(3):392–9.
42. Malvy D, et al. Ebola virus disease. Lancet. 2019;393(10174):936–48.
43. Nicastri E, et al. Ebola virus disease: epidemiology, clinical features, management, and prevention. Infect Dis Clin N Am. 2019;33(4):953–76.
44. Baseler L, et al. The pathogenesis of Ebola virus disease. Annu Rev Pathol. 2017;12:387–418.

45. Rojas M, et al. Ebola virus disease: an emerging and re-emerging viral threat. J Autoimmun. 2020;106:102375.
46. WHO. Ebola virus disease. 23 February 2021. Available from https://www.who.int/news-room/fact-sheets/detail/ebola-virus-disease.
47. Wang Y, et al. Ebola vaccines in clinical trial: the promising candidates. Hum Vaccin Immunother. 2017;13(1):153–68.
48. Furuyama W, Marzi A. Ebola virus: pathogenesis and countermeasure development. Annu Rev Virol. 2019;6(1):435–58.
49. Tomori O, Kolawole MO. Ebola virus disease: current vaccine solutions. Curr Opin Immunol. 2021;71:27–33.
50. Keshwara R, Johnson RF, Schnell MJ. Toward an effective Ebola virus vaccine. Annu Rev Med. 2017;68:371–86.
51. Matz KM, Marzi A, Feldmann H. Ebola vaccine trials: progress in vaccine safety and immunogenicity. Expert Rev Vaccines. 2019;18(12):1229–42.
52. Higgs ES, et al. Accelerating vaccine development during the 2013-2016 west African Ebola virus disease outbreak. Curr Top Microbiol Immunol. 2017;411:229–61.
53. Zhu FC, et al. Safety and immunogenicity of a novel recombinant adenovirus type-5 vector-based Ebola vaccine in healthy adults in China: preliminary report of a randomised, double-blind, placebo-controlled, phase 1 trial. Lancet. 2015;385(9984):2272–9.
54. Zhu FC, et al. Safety and immunogenicity of a recombinant adenovirus type-5 vector-based Ebola vaccine in healthy adults in Sierra Leone: a single-centre, randomised, double-blind, placebo-controlled, phase 2 trial. Lancet. 2017;389(10069):621–8.
55. Li JX, et al. Immunity duration of a recombinant adenovirus type-5 vector-based Ebola vaccine and a homologous prime-boost immunisation in healthy adults in China: final report of a randomised, double-blind, placebo-controlled, phase 1 trial. Lancet Glob Health. 2017;5(3):e324–34.
56. China, TNMPAo. First recombinant Ebola virus disease vaccine receives new drug registration approval. 2017-10-20. Available from https://www.nmpa.gov.cn/yaopin/ypjgdt/20171020094701899.html.
57. Kennedy SB, et al. Phase 2 placebo-controlled trial of two vaccines to prevent Ebola in Liberia. N Engl J Med. 2017;377(15):1438–47.
58. Heppner DG Jr, et al. Safety and immunogenicity of the rVSVΔG-ZEBOV-GP Ebola virus vaccine candidate in healthy adults: a phase 1b randomised, multicentre, double-blind, placebo-controlled, dose-response study. Lancet Infect Dis. 2017;17(8):854–66.
59. Halperin SA, et al. Immunogenicity, lot consistency, and extended safety of rVSVΔG-ZEBOV-GP vaccine: a phase 3 randomized, double-blind, placebo-controlled study in healthy adults. J Infect Dis. 2019;220(7):1127–35.

5 Progress in Epidemiology of Ebola Virus Disease

Hong-Wu Yao, Li-Qun Fang, Ji-Jiang Suo, Yun-Xi Liu, and Wu-Chun Cao

Abstract

Ebola virus disease (EVD) is a zoonotic disease caused by Ebola virus. It has become one of the most harmful diseases in humans for its high mortality and strong infectivity. Since entering the twenty-first century, the repetition and abruptness of EVD outbreaks in Africa, especially the unprecedented and huge EVD outbreaks in West Africa from 2013 to 2016, has attracted much attention from the global media and public, and made EVD an urgent public health threat worldwide. EVD not only causes serious casualties and leads to heavy economic losses, but also affects the normal operation of the public health system and triggers more social problems. China is one of the earliest countries that assisted EVD epidemic areas in West Africa, and has not only provided financial support and material equipment and dispatched epidemic prevention experts and medical staffs in multiple batches to participate in the prevention and control of EVD epidemic in West Africa, but also made outstanding contributions to researches of EVD etiology, clinical symptoms, pathological changes, pathogenesis, diagnostic and therapeutic drugs, epidemiology, and vaccine development. With the development and acceleration of economic globalization, the more convenient transportation and frequent personnel flow have greatly promoted the cross-regional transmission of EVD, and countries around the world are at risk of EVD importation and transmission; however, there still exist many key scientific issues regarding EVD global prevention and control that are not clear. In order to provide basic information for the development of global prevention and response strategies for the disease, this chapter focuses on EVD transmission dynamics, distribution characteristics, influencing factors, and prevention and control measures to comprehensively and systematically understand the epidemiology and current challenges of EVD, which helps guide the formulation of global public health crisis policies, and provides a scientific basis for the development in the ability to effectively respond to the impact of EVD outbreaks.

Keywords

Ebola virus · Ebola virus disease Transmission · Distribution · Influencing factors · Prevention and control

H.-W. Yao · J.-J. Suo · Y.-X. Liu
Department of Disease Prevention and Control, The First Medical Center, Chinese PLA General Hospital, Beijing, People's Republic of China

L.-Q. Fang · W.-C. Cao (✉)
The State Key Laboratory of Pathogen and Biosecurity, Beijing Institute of Microbiology and Epidemiology, Beijing, People's Republic of China
e-mail: caowc@bmi.ac.cn

D.-Q. Ye (ed.), *Progress in China Epidemiology*, https://doi.org/10.1007/978-981-19-2199-5_5

5.1 Introduction

Ebola virus disease (EVD) is an infectious disease caused by Ebola virus with symptoms such as acute onset of fever, myalgia, bleeding, rash, and liver and kidney function impairment, which is mainly transmitted by contact with body fluids, excreta, and secretions of patients or infected animals [1–4]. EVD was previously called Ebola hemorrhagic fever, while in the outbreaks in recent years, infected individuals experienced relatively few clinical symptoms of hemorrhagic fever, so this disease is now renamed EVD [3]. The Ebola virus was first discovered in Sudan and Zaire [now the Democratic Republic of the Congo (DRC)] in central Africa in 1976, and endemic areas were mainly distributed in the African region and classified by the World Health Organization (WHO) as one of the most harmful viruses to humans because of their extremely high mortality [4–6]. DRC, as the country with the highest frequency of EVD outbreaks, had four EVD outbreaks during 2014–2018 alone. The most recent two occurred in 2018. In May 2018, the province of Equateur in the DRC experienced the ninth EVD outbreak in the history of the country, which was not declared to end until July. It caused a total of 54 cases and 33 deaths; however, only a few days later, a new EVD outbreak was confirmed in the province of North Kivu in the country, which was still ongoing as of December 27, 2018, with a cumulative incidence of 591 cases and 357 deaths [4, 7, 8].

EVD outbreaks in the African region have become more frequent since entering the twenty-first century. The most alarming and panicky outbreak of EVD occurred in West Africa [9]. In late 2013, a small-scale EVD outbreak in Guinea turned into an unprecedented global public health emergency in a few months, with epidemic areas spreading rapidly to adjacent countries of Sierra Leone and Liberia. The outbreak was declared to end on June 9, 2016, with a total of 28,652 cases and 11,325 deaths reported - with the highest number of morbidity and mortality, the widest impact, and the longest duration in history [4]. Repeated outbreaks of EVD not only bring a lot of casualties, but also lead to heavy economic losses [10]. The World Bank estimates that the West African EVD epidemic has brought economic losses between 2014 and 2015 to $2 billion in West African countries. When the reduction of fiscal revenue, the cost of fighting the epidemic, and the reduction of foreign investment are considered comprehensively, the overall economic loss is about 3.8 billion US dollars [11]. Furthermore, EVD outbreaks in West Africa were different from those in the past; the previous outbreaks often appeared in remote areas or villages with sparse population density and less population movement, so the epidemic could be effectively controlled in a short period. In contrast, EVD outbreaks in West Africa, although they first appeared in rural areas of southeast Guinea, were imported into densely populated urban areas in just a few weeks and transmitted to Liberia and Sierra Leone across borders. Coupled with the scarcity of health resources and backward security systems in West African countries, the lack of EVD prevention and control experience in national health departments, the lack of early identification and diagnostic ability of EVD, as well as the lack of awareness of EVD in the population, large-scale EVD outbreaks in West Africa occurred.

The EVD epidemic in West Africa had spread rapidly and was characterized by a rapid increase in the number of patients, high mortality rate, and deficiency of effective vaccine and therapeutic drug during the epidemic period. The WHO announced this epidemic as a "Public Health Emergency of International Concern" on August 8, 2014 [12], and issued a crisis warning to the world. The three countries in West Africa (Sierra Leone, Liberia, and Guinea) also requested assistance from all countries in the world. The WHO, China, the USA, Médecins Sans Frontières (Doctors Without Borders, MSF), and other countries and organizations subsequently responded to the call to provide materials and equipment and personnel to assist West African countries for carrying out Ebola virus disease epidemic prevention and control. China has close cooperation with African countries in the fields of labor, commerce, education, tourism, etc., and close personnel contacts, and the foreign aid medical team is resident in African countries, which is one of the earliest countries to respond to assistance. In order to help West African countries better control the EVD epidemic, apart from the aid medical team in Liberia and the established EVD diagnosis and treatment center [13], the Chinese government also dispatched the China Mobile Lab Testing Team to Sierra Leone to carry out the "anti-Ebola and assist Sierra Leone" task, and dispatched experts and medical staffs in multiple batches to participate in the prevention and control of the Ebola epidemic in West Africa, including providing masses of rescue materials, assisting protective equipment vehicles and funds, establishing infrastructures such as EVD observation treatment centers and testing laboratories, and dispatching professionals to help establish a prevention and control system [14, 15]. In addition, like the USA and the UK [1, 16–19], Chinese scientists have also been continuously committed to EVD-related scientific research in recent years. It has contributed a lot to the solution of key scientific problems in EVD prevention and control and made outstanding contributions to the study of EVD etiology, clinical symptoms, molecular evolution, diagnosis and treatment, and vaccine research and development. It mainly includes describing and analyzing the clinical characteristics of the disease and risk factors for poor prognosis [20–23]; providing valuable Ebola virus sequencing data and elaborating the molecular evolution of Ebola virus [24–27]; analyzing the transmission dynamic and intervention efficacy of EVD [28–30]; carrying out the study of early diagnosis and detection reagents of EVD [31–34]; developing new drugs and vaccines [31, 35–38]; and elaborating the prevention and control strategies of the disease [15, 39–41]. China's action to help Africa fight Ebola is a huge step forward for China to truly participate in global public health action.

China closely cooperates with African countries, with nearly 600,000 people coming to Africa each year [42]. Similar to most countries, China is also at risk of importation of virulent infectious diseases such as EVD, Marburg virus disease, and Rift Valley fever. To better master the epidemic regularity of EVD and promote the global prevention and control of EVD, this chapter mainly systematically reviews the research on the transmission regularity, distribution characteristics, and prevention and control of EVD. This will assist us comprehensively and systematically to understand the transmission process, epidemic characteristics, and existing challenges of EVD and provide basic information and scientific basis for the development of EVD prevention and response strategies.

5.2 Etiology and Animal Host

Ebola virus belongs to the order Mononegavirales and Filoviridae, and belongs to the same family as Marburg virus and encode a total of seven structural proteins and one non-structural protein: 3′ -nucleoprotein (NP), polymerase cofactor (VP35), matrix protein (VP40), glycoprotein (GP), transcription activator VP30, matrix protein (VP24), and RNA-dependent RNA polymerase (L) and one non-structural small glycoprotein—sGP [43]. The nucleocapsid with replicase and transcriptase function is composed of genomic RNA encapsidated by the NP and together with polymerase L, VP35, and VP30. VP30 is important for the reinitiation of transcription of subsequent genes, and is a potentially interesting candidate as an antiviral therapy target. Mutations in the sequences encoding the VP40 might lead to inhibition of virus release from the infected cell. Other structural nucleocapsid proteins (VP35 and polymerase L) participate in the synthesis of the viral genome. GP spikes are known to involve in the entry of virions into the host cell and are used in the mechanisms similar to macropinocytosis. It is known that VP24 and VP35 are important virulence factors, because they act as type I interferon (IFN) antagonists. The gene arrangement order is 3′-NP-VP35-VP40-GP/sGP-VP30-VP24-L-5′, which belongs to biosafety level 4 class I pathogens, and the leader and trailer at the 3′- and 5′-ends carry important signals to control transcription, replication, and packaging of the viral genomes into new capsids [43].

At present, six Ebola virus subtypes have been found and named according to their discovery sites, Zaire ebolavirus (EBOV) was discovered in towns in northern Zaire, 1976, Sudan ebolavirus (SUDV) was in southern Sudan, 1976, Reston ebolavirus (RESTV) in cynomolgus monkeys in Leston, Virginia, USA, 1989, Tai Forest ebolavirus (TAFV) in forests in Côte d'Ivoire, 1994, Bundibugyo ebolavirus (BDBV) in western Uganda, 2007, and Bombali ebolavirus (BOMV) in Bombali District in Sierra Leone, 2018, with complete genome sequence differences of less than 30% for the same subtype of Ebola virus. Except for RESTV (which causes only latent infection but not a disease in humans) and BOMV (while BOMV has the potential to infect human cells, there is currently no evidence that the virus causes disease), the other four viral subtypes are pathogenic in humans [2, 4, 44, 45] and vary in virulence, with EBOV being the most virulent, followed by SUDV. After the outbreak in West Africa, scientists found that the sequences of the circulating strains were quite different from those of the previous circulating strains, the mutation rate was getting faster, and there were many accumulated mutation sites. It suggested that the Ebola virus may have been introduced into West Africa from Central Africa long ago and continuously mutated and evolved with the expansion of the epidemic size [24, 27, 46].

Nonhuman primates take an extremely high mortality rate after infection with Ebola virus and are therefore unlikely to be a natural reservoir of Ebola virus. Some scientists believe that rodents and arthropods may be the natural hosts of Ebola virus, and laboratory animals (such as mice, guinea pigs, and rabbits), as well as domestic animals (such as horses, cattle, and pigs), can also be infected with Ebola virus under laboratory conditions [47], and even experimentally infected pigs can transmit Ebola virus to monkeys, but this assumption was quickly denied [48, 49]. Between 1976 and 1998, researchers detected Ebola virus in samples from only six mice and one shrew in Central Africa among approximately 30,000 specimens collected by investigating mammals, birds, reptiles, amphibians, and arthropods in endemic areas [9]. The researchers used the EBOV to infect 24 plant and 19 vertebrate and invertebrate species and found that only bats (including insectivorous and frugivorous bats) supported the replication of EBOV and showed no obvious symptoms, thus speculating that bats may be the natural reservoir of EBOV [50]. The prevalence of Ebola virus was found to be temporally related to bat migration, infection, and death, such as the overlap of migration time and route between DRC EVD outbreak time and location and franquet's epauletted fruit bat and hammerhead fruit bats in 2007 [51]. Moreover, the detection of RNA and antibodies to Ebola virus from the bodies of three African fruit bats suggests that fruit bats are likely to be natural reservoir hosts for Ebola virus, while the rate of Ebola virus infection in bats is very low and Ebola virus can rarely be isolated or detected in bats; therefore, the issue of natural reservoir hosts for Ebola virus has been controversial [16, 52–54].

At present, although great progress has been made in the study of the etiology and host of Ebola virus, it is still a necessity to explore the molecular evolutionary characteristics and infection and transmission mechanism of Ebola virus in more depth to better provide useful information on the origin of Ebola virus and the research and development of drugs and vaccines.

5.3 Clinical Features and Prognosis

The incubation period of EVD is 2–21 days, generally 5–12 days. The more viral load, the shorter incubation period and the more severe the disease. The nonspecific symptoms of EVD include fever, malaise, fear of cold, headache, myalgia, anorexia, nausea, vomiting, chest pain, shortness of breath, runny nose, diarrhea, pharyngitis, dysphagia, rash, conjunctival congestion, and edema [1, 55, 56]. However, the nonspecific nature of these early symptoms prevents EVD from being well separated from other infectious diseases, such as malaria, leptospirosis, influenza, and other respiratory viral infections, as well as yellow fever, dengue, and many other arboviruses or enteroviruses or bacterial infections [16, 57]. During the 2013–2016 outbreak in West Africa, through investigation and research, the WHO Emergency Prevention and Control Group found before the epidemic that the vast majority of cases had symptoms such as fever, fatigue, loss of appetite, vomiting, diarrhea, and headache. Of all patients, 95% presented an incubation period within 21 days, 11.4 days of the mean incubation period, 5.0 ± 4.7 days of the mean time from the onset of symptoms to hospital stay, 6.4 days of the mean hospital stay, and 4.2 ± 6.4 days of the time from the onset of symptoms to death [58, 59]. There are also a few reports of asymptomatic or mildly symptomatic [60, 61] and Akerlund et al. even reported that the initial symptoms of EVD infection in pregnant women were limited to mild abdominal pain and uterine contractions without febrile symptoms [62].

Surviving cases of EVD generally begin to improve in 6–11 days after a few days of fever, but may undergo a rehabilitation period with sequelae such as myelitis, recurrent hepatitis, psychosis, and uveitis, and pregnant women are also at risk of miscarriage [2, 59]. Lotsch et al. found that depression, insomnia, fatigue, anxiety, and posttraumatic stress were common sequelae in patients with EVD, although there were litter data from high-quality studies [63]. EVD dead cases generally present with severe symptoms early in the course of the disease and often die from complications such as multiple organ failure and septic shock between 6 and 16 days [2], and factors or indicators associated with EVD death or poor prognosis have also been reported in recent years. For example, Hunt et al. conducted a study of factors associated with EVD mortality and poor prognosis in the diagnosis and treatment of 150 EVD patients in Sierra Leone and found that early hospitalization of EVD patients contributed to a good prognosis, with Ebola virus RT-PCR Ct values less than 20 (OR 6.7, 95% CI 1.5–30.1), and acute kidney injury (OR 5.8, 95% CI 1.2–29.6) is an independent risk factor for death in infected patients; creatinine levels more than 115 mmol/L and respiratory distress on admission are also factors for poor prognosis [3, 64, 65]; Jiang et al. found that viral load and cytokine and chemokine levels were significantly higher in dead cases than in the early stages of infection [22]; Li et al. found that viral load, age, and diarrhea patients were associated with mortality [20]; Smit et al. reviewed the treatment of 122 children with EVD in West Africa and found that their overall mortality rate was 57%, with factors such as viral load and under 5 years of age associated with mortality in children with EVD [66]; in a study of 2310 adult cases of EVD in Guinea, univariate analysis revealed that patient age, history of visiting or close contact with suspected or confirmed EVD and presence of seven admission symptoms (fever, hiccups, vomiting, diarrhea, cough, sore throat, and unexplained bleeding) were closely related to EVD patients mortality Multivariate analysis showed that patient age was independently associated with EVD mortality (OR 1.06, 95% CI 1.03–1.09), while clinical symptoms at admission were not significantly associated with death, and older age was a factor in the death of EVD patients, which was similar to the conclusions drawn from several studies in Sierra Leone [67]. In addition, Bebell et al. found that pregnancy was also significantly associated with the severity of the disease and the risk of death, but the difference in the course of EVD between pregnant and nonpregnant women is a scientific issue that has not yet been systematically addressed [68].

The nonspecific clinical characteristics of EVD have always been the main bottleneck affecting the accurate diagnosis of EVD. To truly achieve early detection, diagnosis, treatment, and control, scientists worldwide still need to deepen and make breakthroughs in the differences in clinical symptoms between non-EVD patients and EVD patients and in the research of rapid and convenient diagnostic and detection reagents in the early stage of EVD.

5.4 Transmission

Humans and nonhuman primates infected with Ebola virus are the sources of EVD infection, and EVD outbreaks are usually sporadic, and the sources of many outbreaks that have occurred point to wild animals such as gorillas, chimpanzees, and monkeys that die in tropical rainforests in Africa, but also point the source of infection to fruit bats [69]. There are mainly two ways for the transmission of Ebola virus [1]: "animal–human" transmission and "human–human" transmission. "Animal–human" transmission occurs when humans are infected by handling animal carcasses or by direct contact with infected nonhuman primates, and scientists believe that the index patient in each EVD outbreak is infected by contact, handling, or consumption of animals infected by Ebola virus (e.g., chimpanzees, gorillas, fruit bats, monkeys, forest antelopes) [2, 70–73]. The type of human–human transmission is the main route of transmission of outbreaks, which is mainly transmitted by intimate contact between people and infected individuals (including sexual behavior), handling of infected individuals' carcasses, exposure to contaminated environments with body fluids of infected individuals, and exposure of medical staff to patient blood and other body fluids [74]. The primary cases (index cases) of most human outbreaks are hunters, gold seekers, felling workers, and other populations operating in forest areas, while the secondary infected population is the patient's family members or medical staffs who have close contact with them, and the outbreak is basically spread centered on the family of the index case and the hospital where they live [75].

5.4.1 Contact Transmission

Blood, saliva, sweat, secretions, feces, vomitus, semen, and milk from patients with EVD all contain viruses and are infectious [76, 77]. Although Ebola virus has been detected in breast milk, there is no significant evidence to support transmission routes such as breastfeeding, mosquito and insect bites, and aerosol transmission [73, 77]. Contact transmission is the most important mode of transmission for outbreaks of EVD. In EVD outbreaks, the risk of EVD transmission is mainly closely related to three behaviors: close contact during the later stages of the disease, caring for the patient, and preparing the deceased for burial matters [78]. There are many ways of contact, including face-to-face conversation, eating and sleeping, unprotected bedside care, sharing syringes, and cleaning corpses. In the presence of an EVD patient, the virus in the blood or body fluids of an EVD patient can be transmitted through broken skin or mucous membranes to contacts such as family members, physicians, etc., and people can also be infected by contact with objects contaminated with the patient's body fluids. In addition, Ebola virus can also be transmitted from mother to infant in utero, during delivery, or through contact with maternal body fluids including breast milk [4]. Direct contact with infected body fluids, including vomitus, diarrheal material, and blood, has been shown to increase the risk of transmission at least threefold during EVD outbreaks [3, 79]. Therefore, the high-risk group of EVD epidemic is mainly the medical staff who contact and accompany the patients in the family, fail to take correct and effective protective measures to provide treatment for the patients, have contact with the corpses, and participate in the funeral of the patients.

5.4.2 Household Transmission

In the 2014–2015 Sierra Leone EVD outbreak, Ajelli et al. found that 74% of transmission events occurred between family members or extended family members, 18% between friends and other community contacts, and 8% within hospitals [80]. Fang et al., by including the data analysis of 634 families in Sierra Leone, showed that the household transmission force (i.e., the probability that an indicator case infects a family member during its infection period) was 0.056–0.062, and it was found that males were less likely to be infected by family members than females, with an odds ratio (OR) between them of 0.62 (95% CI 0.44–0.88), and juvenile females belonged to the group most susceptible to Ebola virus infection at home, with a household transmission force of 0.11 (95% CI 0.063–0.18) [30]. Another study showed that 32% (95% CI 26–38%) of household contacts who reported direct contact cases had a low risk of disease transmission (OR 1%, 95% CI 0–5%) between household members who did not have direct contact. In addition, the higher the risk of acquiring EVD, the higher the risk of taking care of EVD cases (especially deaths) in the community and participating in behaviors such as traditional funerals [78].

5.4.3 Nosocomial Transmission

Contact transmission within families or communities is often confined to small areas or families, but iatrogenic transmission often causes large-scale and cross-regional outbreaks, such as 85 (26.7%) of the 318 patients in the 1976 Zaire EVD outbreak who were infected with Ebola virus due to the use of contaminated syringes [5]. The basic reproduction number (R0) of EVD epidemic in Uganda in 2000 was 2.7 (95% CI 2.5–4.1), including 2.6 (95% CI 0.3–2.8), 0.01 (95% CI 0.0–3.5), and 0.1 (95% CI 0.0–3.2) for regional transmission, nosocomial transmission, and funeral transmission, respectively, which decreased to 0.3 (95% CI 0.2–0.4) after considering intervention parameters. In addition, studies have compared the two types of outbreaks, "small area-centered" and "hospital-centered," and found that when the epidemic spreads in a small village, the epidemic will eventually end spontaneously due to geographical and patient range of motion restrictions, such as the Zaire EVD epidemic that occurred in 55 villages in the Yambuku area of Zaire (now DRC) in 1976 and 25 villages in the Kikwit area in 1995, with basically less than 10 cases per village, and similar situations have occurred in the outbreak that occurred in the Ekata area of Gabon in 2001. However, when the epidemic occurred in hospitals, due to backward sanitary conditions and medical equipment and lack of awareness of protection among the medical staffs, the epidemic could easily spread among medical staff and cause high mortality, such as the outbreak in Kikwit Hospital in Zaire (DRC) in 1995, which caused more deaths of medical staff [81–83]; studies related to the epidemic in West Africa found that as of May 20, 2015, a total of 869 medical staffs were infected, of which 507 died [84], and during May 23 to October 31, 2014, the incidence of EVD in the medical population was 103 times that in the general population [85].

5.4.4 Sexual Transmission

Ebola virus can persist in the host, and the virus can still be detected in semen and eye fluid for a certain period (e.g., within three months) in cases after recovery [86–88]. A follow-up survey of EVD rehabilitation patients found that the virus can be detected in the semen of rehabilitation patients for a long time: RNA of the virus was detected in the semen of 65% and 26% of surviving patients tested at 4–6 and 7–9 months after the onset of infection, respectively [89]. In addition, Mate et al. conducted an epideiological investigation and molecular epidemiological study, suggesting that Ebola virus can indeed be sexually transmitted. The source of infection was an EVD patient who recovered for 500 days. Through this mode of transmission, 10 new cases occurred in Guinea in March 2016 [86], which also supported the statement that Ebola virus can remain in the body for a long time. Due to the possibility of sexual transmission of Ebola virus, the WHO and the US CDC recommend that all male survivors of EVD do have safe sex until 12 months after EVD onset or after two consecutive virus-negative tests of semen samples [3, 90].

5.4.5 Other Possible Transmission

At present, it has not been confirmed whether Ebola virus can be transmitted by aerosol. However, the scientific community generally believes that Ebola virus has the possibility and potential for airborne transmission. The International Convention on the Prohibition of Biological Weapons had classified the Ebola virus as a potentially lethal biological warfare agent. In 2004, Leffel et al.'s article published in *Biosecurity and Bioterrorism* and, in the same year, Salvaggio et al.'s article published in *Dermatologic Clinics* were highlighting the risk of Ebola virus as a potential biological warfare agent, especially in the form of aerosol transmission [91–93]. In recent years, scientists have constructed animal models of aerosol infection of Ebola virus including macaques, rhesus monkeys, and African green monkeys in the laboratory, which can infect nonhuman primates through aerosols, and can cause fatal infections at very low doses. The successful establishment of these animal models not only confirms that Ebola virus can infect experimental animals by aerosol under existing experimental conditions, but also lays a foundation for future in-depth studies on the mechanism of this viral infection. In the future, we can use such animal models to carry out studies on Ebola virus infection and transmission under simulated natural environmental conditions [4, 93].

The Ebola virus can also be detected in patients' breast milk and body fluids, which suggests the risk of mother-to-child transmission or vertical transmission [77]. One study revealed that four out of the five breastfed infants with EBOV-positive breast milk were found positive for Ebola virus infection, and all of these Ebola virus-positive infants died [94]. With the current evidence, there is no certainty that mother-to-child transmission or vertical transmission is the main route of EBOV transmission.

The current mainstream hypothesis on the natural history of Ebola virus disease is [44]: Ebola virus is mainly transmitted naturally and circularly among fruit bats, and humans are infected with the disease by contact with animals such as infected bats, chimpanzees, gorillas, forest antelopes, and porcupines, and then close contact between human leads to outbreaks of the disease [2]. However, the circulation mode, infection mechanism, and cross-species transmission mechanism of Ebola virus in nature are still undefined scientific problems, and only by solving these scientific problems can spillover transmission of Ebola virus be prevented from the source.

5.5 Overview of EVD Epidemic Distribution

During 1976–2018, a total of 28 human EVD outbreaks have occurred in the African region (Figs. 5.1 and 5.2), including 24 epidemic outbreaks and 4 sporadic outbreaks [see Fig. 5.1, (3), (5), (10), (21)]; no primary cases of EVD have been found outside Africa, except imported or laboratory infection cases [4, 8, 95, 96]. In addition, nine outbreaks of animal EVD caused by RESTV infection occurred outside of Africa, of which seven occurred in non-primates and two in pigs, and three of these outbreaks detected RESTV antibodies in the relevant population (Table 5.1). By 2014, the EVD epidemic was confined to the Central African rainforest and savannah of southeast Africa, mainly five countries: Gabon, Republic of the Congo, the DRC, Uganda, and Sudan (see Fig. 5.2), and EVD patients were mainly from relatively closed remote rural areas, with sporadic cases also occurring in Côte d'Ivoire in western Africa and South Africa in southern Africa. The EVD outbreak from 2013 to 2016 in West Africa was the largest and most widespread outbreak in history, mainly in three countries in West Africa: Guinea, Liberia, and Sierra Leone, and most of the EVD patients came from densely populated large cities, such as Conakry, Monrovia, and Freetown. In the second half of 2014, the West African outbreak also spread to seven countries: Nigeria, Senegal, the USA, Spain, Mali, the UK, and Italy (see Figs. 5.1 and 5.2) [16, 49]. The reported number of cases in this outbreak had exceeded the total number of cases in previous outbreaks.

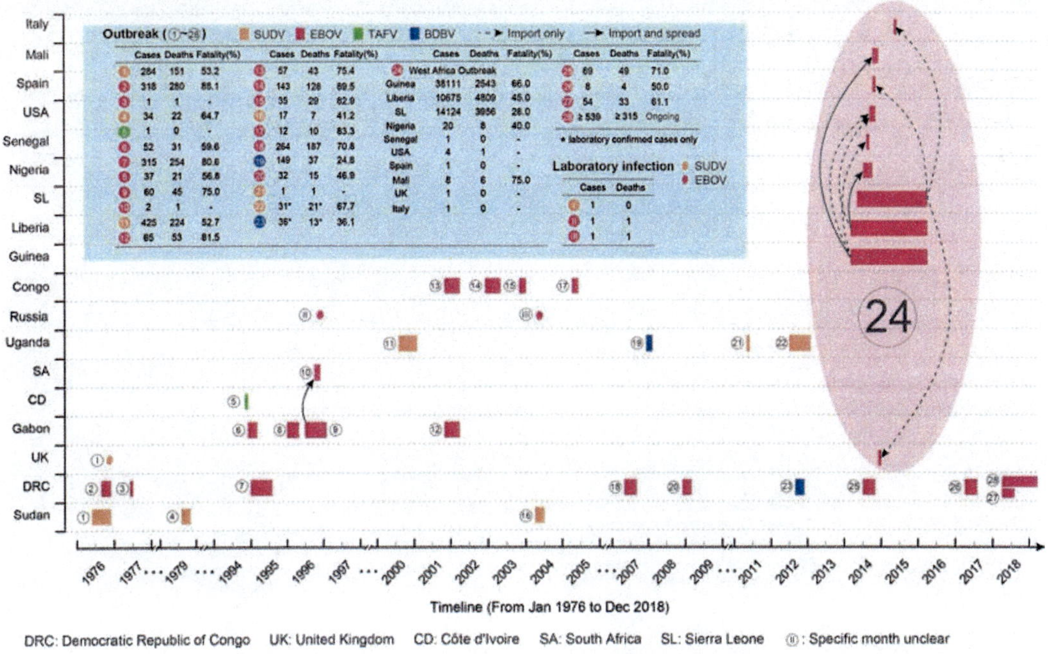

Fig. 5.1 The timeline and situation of human EVD outbreaks from January 1976 to December 2018

5.5.1 Seasonal, Population, and Regional Distribution Characteristics

The epidemic time of EVD covers the whole year, does not show specific seasonal characteristics, and shows no significant correlation between outbreak years [49]. For example, the outbreak in Sudan in 1976 occurred from June to November; the four outbreaks in Gabon mainly occurred around January; the outbreak in Gabon in 1996 occurred from January to April; and the outbreak in the border area between Gabon and Congo occurred from October 2001 to March 2002; the three outbreaks in Uganda mainly occurred around October, while the four outbreaks in Congo and the outbreaks in DRC were distributed in all months of the year [4]. The population is generally susceptible to Ebola virus, which affects people of all ages, from infancy to old age [5, 16], with a lower incidence in children and the elderly and a higher incidence in women and healthcare workers, which may be related to the frequent exposure of women and healthcare workers accompanying EVD patients.

As shown in Figs. 5.1 and 5.2, as of December 2018, DRC had a total of 10 EVD outbreaks, the most recent one still continuing [4]; Sudan had three EVD outbreaks during 1976–2004, mainly in the southern region; Gabon had four EVD outbreaks, mainly in the northern region; Uganda had four EVD outbreaks, mainly in the northwestern region; and the Republic of the Congo had four EVD outbreaks, mainly in the northwestern region. The emergence of Ebola virus subtypes in Côte d'Ivoire differs from the past, and only one case has been found. Sporadic cases in South Africa came mainly from the importation of the EVD epidemic in Gabon [97]. The 2013–2016 EVD outbreak in West Africa, Guinea, Liberia, and Sierra Leone had EVD cases spread throughout the country, while Nigeria and Mali had local transmission due to the importation of EVD cases, but were limited to transmission in small areas, and Senegal had only imported cases and no local transmission [16].

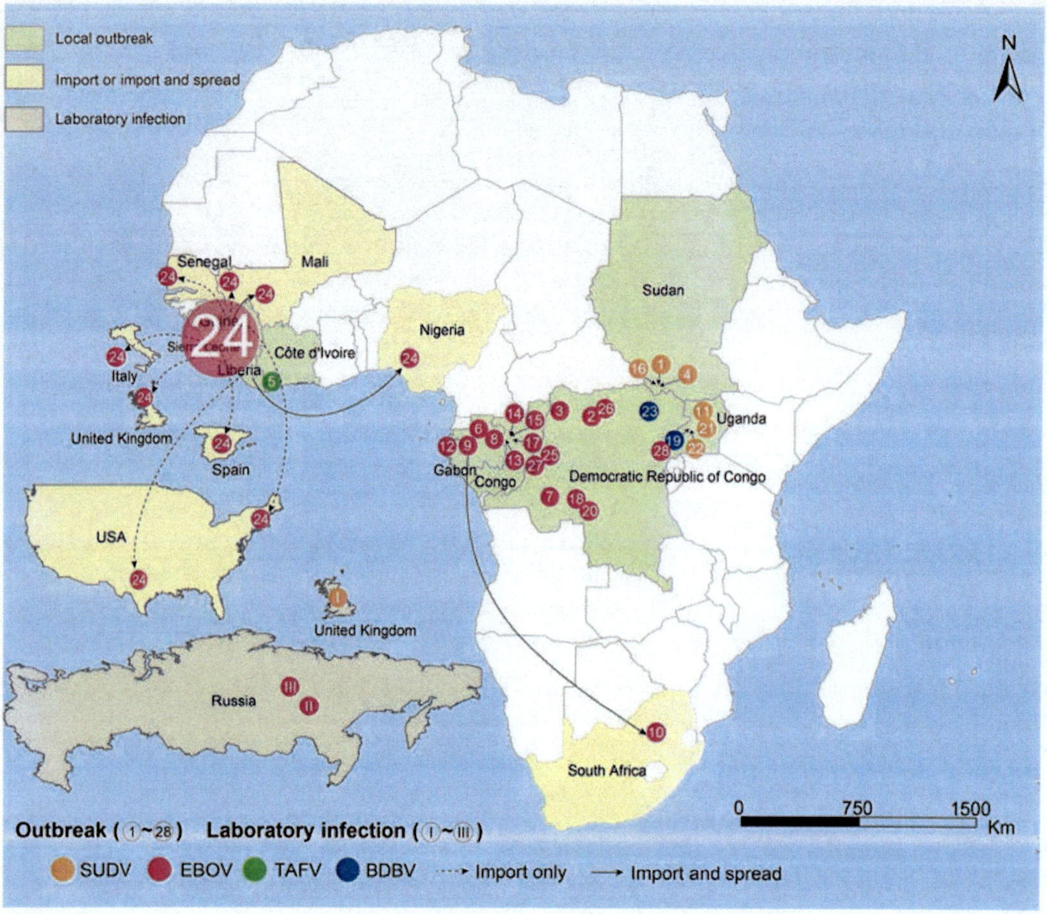

Fig. 5.2 The geographical distribution of human EVD outbreaks from January 1976 to December 2018. The boundaries and names shown and the designations used on this map do not imply the expression of any opinion concerning the legal status of any country, territory, city, or area or of its authorities, or concerning the delimitation of its frontiers or boundaries

In the EVD outbreak in West Africa, imported cases of EVD occurred in the USA, the UK, Spain, and Italy, but did not cause local transmission [16]. The incidence of infection in laboratory workers was reported three times in the UK and Russia (see Figs 5.1 and 5.2) [8, 44, 95]. As shown in Table 5.1, EVD outbreaks in macaques have also been reported in the UA, Italy, and the Philippines, in which infected macaques in both the USA and Italy were from the Philippines; the virus was first isolated from pigs in 2008 in the Philippines and pigs in 2011 in China; Ebola virus antibodies have been detected in the sera of people who have been exposed to macaques and pigs in the USA and the Philippines, but none of them developed clinical symptoms of EVD [98–102]. Apart from laboratory infections, no locally infected cases of EVD have been identified outside Africa, but antibodies to Ebola virus can be detected in residents of some African regions without EVD outbreak [83, 103].

5.5.2 Distribution Characteristics of Virus Subtypes

Among the 28 EVD outbreaks, there were 19 EBOV outbreaks, six SUDV outbreaks, two BDBV outbreaks, and one TAFV outbreak (see Fig. 5.1), EBOV outbreaks were most common in

Table 5.1 List of RESTV outbreaks occurred outside of Africa

Date(year)	Country	Number of outbreaks of human seropositive antibody	Animal outbreaks
1989–1990	Philippines	3	Crab-eating macaques
1989	United States	0	Monkeys from Philippines
1990	United States	4	Monkeys from Philippines
1992	Italy	0	Monkeys from Philippines
1996	Philippines	0	Monkeys from Philippines
1996	United States	0	Monkeys from Philippines
2008	Philippines	6	Pigs
2011	China	0	Pigs
2015	Philippines	0	Monkeys

western Central Africa and West Africa, and SUDV and BDBV outbreaks were most common in eastern Central Africa [16]. EBOV was mainly distributed in Liberia, Guinea, Sierra Leone, Nigeria, and Mali of West Africa, and also in Gabon, DRC, and Congo; SUDV was mainly distributed in Sudan and Uganda; BDBV was distributed in Uganda and Congo; TAFV was isolated from only one patient in Côte d'Ivoire, and RESTV was mainly distributed in the Philippines, the USA, Italy, and China. Each human EVD outbreak has its specific viral subtype, and outbreaks caused by EBOV are the most frequent, except for Uganda and DRC, where outbreaks of different viral subtypes have occurred; other countries in Africa are limited to outbreaks of only one viral subtype. In terms of virulence and mortality, the case fatality rate of BDBV infection is about 40% and that of SUDV infection is about 50%, while the case fatality rate of EBOV infection is the highest, approximately 70–90%, and the case fatality rate of TAFV infection is still unclear, with only one case reported historically, while RESTV causes disease and death only in nonhuman primates [2].

It is a fact that outbreaks and transnational, cross-continental transmission of EVD had repeatedly occurred in Africa. Understanding the distribution pattern of natural foci of EVD and mastering the occurrence and dynamic development trend of outbreaks are helpful for targeted disease entry surveillance and follow-up investigation, which is of great significance to prevent the imported transmission of EVD.

5.6 Influencing Factors

The mechanism by which Ebola virus is transmitted from host animals to humans is not clear, but large-scale outbreaks of EVD are inseparable from the influence of factors such as the natural environment, human behavior and cultural customs, and socioeconomic and political factors [49]. Fang et al. evaluated the efficacy of Sierra Leone's national strategic prevention and control program (including isolation of patients, increasing beds, and performing safe funerals) in controlling EVD, and systematically explored the nonlinear relationship between meteorological, socioeconomic factors and EVD transmission. The study found that interventions such as the National Strategic Prevention and Control Program were confirmed to effectively reduce the risk of EVD transmission by 43–65%, and the results of univariate analysis showed that the distribution of primary roads, secondary roads and railways, population density, and building area had a significant positive correlation with the spread of EVD; three factors, including the distance to the nearest hospital, the distance to the nearest Ebola treatment center (ETC), and the forest coverage area, had a significant negative correlation with the spread of EVD; through further multivariate analysis, the optimal model showed that the spread of EVD was closely related to the distribution of primary roads, secondary roads, and hospitals. The study also showed that these influencing factors, such as religion, temperature, humidity, population density, farmland distribution, and healthcare facility distribution, had a significant nonlinear relationship with EVD epidemics [30]. The results of a study on the risk factors associated with the Sudanese EVD outbreak in Uganda in 2000 showed that 20 of 83 contacts in this area were affected, and through epidemiological investigation and univariate analysis of these 83 contacts, it was found that direct contact with patients was more dangerous than indirect contact with patients, and the more routes of contact, the higher risk of infection [79]. Other similar studies had also found that the prevalence and spread of EVD were associated with indicators such as agricultural production, income, road density, hospital bed density, number of unsafe funerals, and days from onset to hospitalization [104, 105].

5.6.1 Natural Environmental Factors

Before 2014, EVD occurred mainly in five Central African countries near the equator, and forests and mines in endemic areas belonged to high-risk sites for this disease source. A study conducted a serological survey of rural residents in Gabon, randomly selected 4349 adults and 362 children, and conducted a correlation study for factors such as EBOV serum antibodies and type of residence in the study population, and logistic regression analysis revealed that the positive rate of IgG antibodies in the serum of people near forest areas (32.4%) was higher than that of the general population (15.3%) [103]. In addition, the typical tropical rainforest climate in central Africa has created lush and dense forests and vast grasslands, making the animals and plants in this area have good natural growth sites. Central African regions are divided into two dry seasons and two rainy seasons throughout the year, and some studies suggest that multiple outbreaks in this region begin at the end of the rainy season or transition to the dry season, and researchers believe that at the end of the rainy season, the sudden dry ecological environment may be a trigger point for the emergence of outbreaks [97, 106]. By studying the location of each outbreak and the corresponding ecological environment, the results of niche model analysis showed that EVD outbreak may be associated with factors such as altitude, temperature, and humidity [107–109].

5.6.2 Factors of Human Behavior and Cultural Practices

The evidence for the correlation between EVD outbreak and human behavior is not yet complete, and some factors are even contradictory between regions [16], but both etiological surveys and epidemiological data have shown that outbreaks of EVD are closely related to forest operation activities of the population, and activities such as going to deep forest, cutting trees, reclaiming agricultural land, hunting and trafficking, and mining gold mines have greatly increased the chance of infection in humans in contact with virus-carrying animal hosts or infected animals [49, 110]. African residents have the habit of hunting animals, trafficking animals, and eating raw animals, such as bats and monkeys, and often have direct or indirect contact with wild animals, increasing their exposure to the Ebola virus; in addition, some local generations of customs, such as injecting monkey blood into humans to treat diseases and removing the clothing and jewelry of the deceased before funerals, have the potential to cause the local spread and prevalence of diseases [49]. Besides, the lack of awareness of prevention and traditional customs of people in some parts of Africa have also promoted the spread of EVD, such as the lack of scientific understanding of EVD, the belief that it is a disease caused by evil or devil, misunderstanding, fear, and exclusion of social and public health services associated with it; for example, residents of the Sadialu village in Sierra Leone who still choose to live with patients, refuse to go to the hospital, believe that the hospital is the place of death sentencing, and some even avoid local healthcare institutions [111].

5.6.3 Socioeconomic and Political Factors

Poverty (e.g., continuous expansion of the range of activities such as hunting, felling, and mining for survival), unsound systems in hospitals (e.g., lack of medical gloves, disposable injection needles), lack of awareness of protection by healthcare workers (lack of awareness of EVD), inefficiency of local government in epidemic prevention and control, and socioeconomic and political factors such as lack of resources, civil conflicts, and civil wars have a decisive impact on the spread and prevalence of EVD [49]. Larger outbreaks often last for months, which is closely related to the backward local medical and health conditions and technical means. Since there is no good diagnostic technique, they usually misdiagnose the epidemic as the infection of other tropical diseases at the early stage, thus misjudging the transmission and risk of the disease, resulting in the spread of the epidemic. For example, the Zaire EVD outbreak in Gabon in 1994 was considered yellow fever at the early stage. Some people also believe that the outbreak area of EVD has been in a state of economic backwardness and imperfect public health system for a long time due to many years of folk conflicts and failure policies, resulting in that the epidemic situation cannot be effectively controlled and even aggravating the spread of EVD. For example, Liberia and Sierra Leone have been devastated by civil war among the three countries with the most severe epidemic in West Africa from 2013 to 2016, while Guinea is a very poor country, and these socioeconomic and political reasons have greatly reduced the effectiveness of government departments in epidemic prevention and control [106].

Small-scale local outbreaks of EVD are inseparable from the results of a combination of natural environment and human production behavior, but large-scale outbreaks often expose the socioeconomic and political factors existing in the country in response to public health crises, which also suggests that countries should pay attention to strengthening the construction of national infectious disease epidemic response mechanisms and emergency response prevention and control systems.

5.7 Prevention and Control

The strong infectivity and incubation period up to 3 weeks of EVD make the disease easy to spread across borders, regions, and even cause local epidemics, posing a serious threat to human health and socioeconomic sustainable development. Therefore, preventing and controlling outbreaks and epidemics of EVD has become a global public health problem that must be faced by countries around the world [49, 112] and has also prompted continuous strengthening of relevant research efforts in this field internationally.

5.7.1 Drugs and Vaccines

There is no specific treatment for EVD worldwide, and there is no specific drug approved for marketing. Although some antiviral drugs have obtained good therapeutic effects in animal experiments, their safety and effectiveness in clinical trials still need to be confirmed by scientific research. At present, the treatment is based on symptomatic and supportive treatment to minimize viral replication and slow down the disease process and gain time for eliminating infections through natural and adaptive immunity, and the main measures include general treatment, antiviral therapy, monoclonal antibody therapy, and symptomatic treatment against cytokine storms and multiple organ failure [1, 2, 16, 19, 59]. The outbreak of EVD in West Africa has rapidly driven clinical research on multiple EVD drugs with good results; for example, the USA urgently approved the entry of two drugs, ZMapp and TKM-Ebola, into clinical trials, and ZMapp was also used in two American patients and one Spanish patient, two of whom in the USA improved [113]; a case report from January 2017 showed that the first newborn with EVD successfully survived a combination of the three drugs [114]. Chinese investigators used the favipiravir (T-705) for the first time in Sierra Leone for the treatment of EVD and achieved good efficacy [35]. Chen and other Chinese researchers have developed the world's first ebola virus vaccine with recombinant adenovirus type 5 Ebola virus vector to enter the clinic and completed a phase 2 clinical trial, which has made a breakthrough [38]; the rVSV-ZEBOV recombinant vesicular stomatitis virus vector vaccine developed by US researchers is currently the most effective vaccine confirmed, which has carried out clinical trials in Guinean epidemic areas, and the efficacy rate of the vaccine is as high as 100% (95% CI 74.7–100) [115]. The immune response induced by this type of vaccine has the advantages of rapid response, high level, and long duration, and has a good prospect, which has been demonstrated to have a good protective effect in EVD outbreaks in West Africa and EVD outbreaks in the Congo in the past two years after ring vaccination intervention [116–118]. However, it has also been pointed out that vaccine-induced immunity is still not rapid enough to prevent EVD in humans, even when the vaccine is administered as soon as possible after exposure [119].

5.7.2 Control and Intervention

To control the spread of EVD, prevention and control measures are mainly used to control the source of infection and cut off the route of transmission and protect the population, including emergency isolation, national education, judicial intervention, and monitoring and tracking [15]. It has been shown that the spread of EVD can be effectively prevented by early diagnosis, patient isolation and care, infection control, safe and dignified burial of those who die of EVD, strict tracking of contacts, and the use of targeted vaccines [58, 96, 115, 117, 119]. Key elements of EVD prevention and control have also been published by US CDC experts, involving monitoring, isolation, investigation, tracking, education, reporting, training, etc. [73, 120]. When the EVD epidemic occurs, early detection and confirmation of cases; implementation of strict isolation measures for patients and infected individuals; blockade of epidemic areas and strict control of population movement in epidemic areas; close observation of contacts and timely follow-up investigation and handling; necessary ideological communication and publicity work to strengthen effective personal protection from high-risk exposures, especially self-protection of staff such as hospitals and laboratories; maintenance of daily case reports; prohibition of holding clustered activities such as traditional funerals; and strengthening effective hospital and community infection control and other measures, including improving personal protective equipment, self-protection skills training, strict disinfection measures, and strengthening laboratory biosafety, can play an important role in controlling the spread of EVD [49, 121, 122]. Muoghalu et al. showed that the transmission rate of EVD in the community declined to a rather low level as EVD cases were removed from the community and entered the community EVD care center. In addition, with the implementation of comprehensive measures for prevention and control, the transmission caused by iatrogenic infection has also been further reduced [104].

The prevention and control of EVD have always been the focus of global attention, and the emergence of EVD has challenged the fragile health and epidemic prevention system in African underdeveloped countries and also reminded other countries to remain vigilant in responding to the threat of infectious diseases. With the acceleration of globalization, cooperation and exchanges in the fields of trade, labor, education, tourism, etc. are becoming more and more frequent among countries around the world, and convenient transportation and frequent personnel movement greatly increase the risk of cross-regional spread of EVD, and countries outside Africa are facing the potential threat of EVD importation. Therefore, international, national, and regional cooperation should be strengthened to establish an effective international quarantine, monitoring, and sharing system to effectively block the export of EVD from natural foci and local outbreak [123, 124].

5.8 Prospects and Challenges

Ebola virus is a type of zoonotic virus, and although related studies on Ebola virus emerge endlessly, some scientific questions remain unsolved, including (1) What is the natural host? (2) Can it be transmitted through aerosols? (3) How does the rate of virus mutation change? (4) How to assess the risk dynamics of its cross-species, cross-regional transmission? (5) What are the exact causes of Ebola virus spillover of wild animals infecting humans and causing outbreaks? (6) How does the change in the physical geographical ecological environment, ecological behavior of host animals, and human production behavior exacerbate the spread of Ebola virus in nature? Answering these questions still needs further in-depth study. To effectively prevent and control the spread of EVD worldwide, it is necessary not only to develop appropriate and effective diagnosis and treatment specifications and anti-EVD drugs and vaccines, but also to further carry out EVD-related social ecology, epidemiology, and molecular biology research, which can help us to more deeply understand the epidemiological characteristics of the epidemic that has occurred, to predict and prevent the epidemic that will occur, including determining the risk area, affected population, and risk factors, and to explore its transmission mechanism. Although the focus of attention is more on how to quickly and effectively eliminate the epidemic in the short term, attention and research on the above scientific issues will be conducive to guiding effective prevention and control.

Since entering the twenty-first century, the EVD epidemic in Africa has become more and more frequent and involves more and more extensive regions. It suggests that in recent years, the contact between humans and wild animals has been increasing, the cross-regional spread of EVD epidemic has occurred continuously, the impact of EVD far exceeds the number of reported EVD cases and deaths, and the economic burden caused by large-scale outbreaks of EVD epidemic and the negative impact on other public healthcare services in the affected area countries have also become a tragic lesson [125]. Therefore, the global public health and safety situation is still not optimistic in the future, and improving the ability to effectively prevent and control and cope with public health crises should be a key area that needs to be focused on by each country. EVD outbreaks are closely related to the limited and fragile public health system in West Africa, especially related to the old public health infrastructure of countries in affected areas and the lack of public knowledge about Ebola virus and its transmission [49]. In the future, the international community should seek reform in emergency response capacity, international financing, budget allocation and human resource construction, and timely transfer of the focus of work to the recovery and reconstruction of countries in epidemic areas. Besides, the key is to help countries in epidemic areas establish a stronger public health system and actively carry out assistance and cooperation in the fields of disease prevention and control, personnel training, and drug research and development.

For China, global public health events are frequent, and putting forward the gateway of infectious disease prevention and control is the overall trend. Although China sets a good example for global EVD prevention and control and promotes the global understanding of the key scientific problems of EVD with valuable experience in assisting local governments to fight the Ebola epidemic in Africa, together with the existing EVD research results, due to the wide region, large population movement, and high population density, there are still many challenges in EVD prevention and control in China, and many scientific problems still need to make breakthroughs [14, 15, 126, 127]. It includes technical reserves in EVD detection, treatment, and prevention; the gap of the construction of emergency detection forces such as "virus detection technology, biosafety protection, laboratory capacity and mobile capacity construction" compared with Europe and the USA; the shortcomings in biosafety protection and team management; further breakthroughs in vaccines and drugs in clinical trials; the participation of international cooperation, the establishment of foreign research platforms; the trial site carrying out epidemiological prospective studies; and the scientific establishment of emergency response organization command system and mechanism. In addition, the WHO has issued some guidelines related to EVD prevention and control involving virus detection, storage and transportation of experimental samples, clinical nursing, prevention of medical staff, and prevention and control of inbound and outbound infectious diseases. China should share rights and interests and resource allocation with the international community, strengthen the capacity level of international rescue teams, and reflect the image and style of large countries. Furthermore, on the basis of existing results, it should improve the relevant guidelines for EVD prevention and control, diagnosis, and treatment adapted to China's national conditions and with guiding significance and further strengthen the emergency response capacity of public health incidents in China to effectively respond to its cross-border transmission.

5.9 Conflict of Interest

All authors declare no conflict of interest.

References

1. Khalafallah MT, Aboshady OA, Moawed SA, Ramadan MS. Ebola virus disease: essential clinical knowledge. Avicenna J Med. 2017;7(3):96–102.
2. Feldmann H, Geisbert TW. Ebola haemorrhagic fever. Lancet. 2011;377(9768):849–62.
3. Caswell RJ, Manavi K. Emerging sexually transmitted viral infections: 1. Review of Ebola virus disease. Int J STD AIDS. 2017;28(13):1352–9.
4. WHO. Ebola virus disease. https://www.who.int/zh/news-room/fact-sheets/detail/ebola-virus-disease.
5. WHO. Ebola haemorrhagic fever in Zaire, 1976. Bull World Health Organ. 1978;56(2):271–93.
6. WHO. Ebola haemorrhagic fever in Sudan, 1976. Bull World Health Organ. 1978;56(2):247–70.
7. WHO. Ebola situation reports: Democratic Republic of the Congo. [cited Dec 31, 2018]. https://www.who.int/ebola/situation-reports/drc-2018/en/.
8. CDC. Years of Ebola virus disease outbreaks. [cited Dec 31, 2018]. https://www.cdc.gov/vhf/ebola/history/chronology.html.
9. Pourrut X, Kumulungui B, Wittmann T, Moussavou G, Delicat A, Yaba P, et al. The natural history of Ebola virus in Africa. Microbes Infect. 2005;7(7–8):1005–14.
10. Gatiso TT, Ordaz-Nemeth I, Grimes T, Lormie M, Tweh C, Kuhl HS, et al. The impact of the Ebola virus disease (EVD) epidemic on agricultural production and livelihoods in Liberia. PLoS Negl Trop Dis. 2018;12(8):e0006580.
11. World Bank Group. Update on the economic impact of the 2014 Ebola epidemic on Liberia, Sierra Leone, and Guinea. [cited Dec 31, 2018]. http://www.worldbank.org/content/dam/Worldbank/document/Economic%20Impact%20Ebola%20Update%202%20Dec%202014.pdf.
12. WHO. WHO statement on the meeting of the International Health Regulations Emergency Committee regarding the 2014 Ebola outbreak in West Africa. [cited Dec 31, 2018]. http://www.antarpath.com/wp-content/uploads/2018/12/whoStatement-Ebola.pdf.
13. You J, Mao Q. An improved word architecture for treatment of patients with Ebola virus disease in Liberia. Am J Trop Med Hyg. 2016;94(4):701–3.
14. Li C, Tong Y, Jiang T, Sun Y, Fang T. The role of international cooperation in the prevention and control of Ebola virus disease epidemic in Sierra Leone. Chin J Epidemiol. 2015;36(9):1026–8. (in Chinese)
15. Tong Y, Li C, Tan Y, He J, Gao B, Fang T. Ebola virus disease emergency response organization and command system in Sierra Leone. Chin J Epidemiol. 2015;36(9):1029–30. (in Chinese)
16. Baseler L, Chertow DS, Johnson KM, Feldmann H, Morens DM. The pathogenesis of Ebola virus disease. Annu Rev Pathol. 2017;12:387–418.
17. Merens A, Bigaillon C, Delaune D. Ebola virus disease: biological and diagnostic evolution from 2014 to 2017. Med Mal Infect. 2018;48(2):83–94.
18. Broadhurst MJ, Brooks TJ, Pollock NR. Diagnosis of Ebola virus disease: past, present, and future. Clin Microbiol Rev. 2016;29(4):773–93.
19. Zeitlin L, Whaley KJ, Olinger GG, Jacobs M, Gopal R, Qiu X, et al. Antibody therapeutics for Ebola virus disease. Curr Opin Virol. 2016;17:45–9.
20. Li J, Duan HJ, Chen HY, Ji YJ, Zhang X, Rong YH, et al. Age and Ebola viral load correlate with mortality and survival time in 288 Ebola virus disease patients. Int J Infect Dis. 2016;42:34–9.
21. Qin E, Bi J, Zhao M, Wang Y, Guo T, Yan T, et al. Clinical features of patients with Ebola virus disease in Sierra Leone. Clin Infect Dis. 2015;61(4):491–5.
22. Jiang T, Jiang JF, Deng YQ, Jiang BG, Fan H, Han JF, et al. Features of Ebola virus disease at the late outbreak stage in Sierra Leone: clinical, virological, immunological, and evolutionary analyses. J Infect Dis. 2017;215(7):1107–10.
23. Zhang X, Rong Y, Sun L, Liu L, Su H, Zhang J, et al. Prognostic analysis of patients with Ebola virus disease. PLoS Negl Trop Dis. 2015;9(9):e0004113.
24. Tong YG, Shi WF, Liu D, Qian J, Liang L, Bo XC, et al. Genetic diversity and evolutionary

dynamics of Ebola virus in Sierra Leone. Nature. 2015;524(7563):93–6.
25. Ni M, Chen C, Qian J, Xiao HX, Shi WF, Luo Y, et al. Intra-host dynamics of Ebola virus during 2014. Nat Microbiol. 2016;1(11):16151.
26. Li T, Yao HW, Liu D, Ren HG, Hu Y, Kargbo D, et al. Mapping the clinical outcomes and genetic evolution of Ebola virus in Sierra Leone. JCI. Insight. 2017;2(15)
27. Deng L, Liu M, Hua S, Peng Y, Wu A, Qin FX, et al. Network of co-mutations in Ebola virus genome predicts the disease lethality. Cell Res. 2015;25(6):753–6.
28. Jiang S, Wang K, Li C, Hong G, Zhang X, Shan M, et al. Mathematical models for devising the optimal Ebola virus disease eradication. J Transl Med. 2017;15(1):124.
29. Xia ZQ, Wang SF, Li SL, Huang LY, Zhang WY, Sun GQ, et al. Modeling the transmission dynamics of Ebola virus disease in Liberia. Sci Rep. 2015;5:13857.
30. Fang LQ, Yang Y, Jiang JF, Yao HW, Kargbo D, Li XL, et al. Transmission dynamics of Ebola virus disease and intervention effectiveness in Sierra Leone. Proc Natl Acad Sci USA. 2016;113(16):4488–93.
31. Liu G, Wong G, Su S, Bi Y, Plummer F, Gao GF, et al. Clinical evaluation of Ebola virus disease therapeutics. Trends Mol Med. 2017;23(9):820–30.
32. Yang M, Ke Y, Wang X, Ren H, Liu W, Lu H, et al. Development and evaluation of a rapid and sensitive EBOV-RPA test for rapid diagnosis of Ebola virus disease. Sci Rep. 2016;6:26943.
33. Chen Z, Liang H, Chen X, Ke Y, Zhou Z, Yang M, et al. An Ebola virus-encoded microRNA-like fragment serves as a biomarker for early diagnosis of Ebola virus disease. Cell Res. 2016;26(3):380–3.
34. Li WG, Chen WW, Li L, Ji D, Ji YJ, Li C, et al. The etiology of Ebola virus disease-like illnesses in Ebola virus negative patients from Sierra Leone. Oncotarget. 2016;7(19):27910–5.
35. Bai CQ, Mu JS, Kargbo D, Song YB, Niu WK, Nie WM, et al. Clinical and Virological characteristics of Ebola virus disease patients treated with favipiravir (T-705)-Sierra Leone, 2014. Clin Infect Dis. 2016;63(10):1288–94.
36. Wang H, Wong G, Zhu W, He S, Zhao Y, Yan F, et al. Equine-origin immunoglobulin fragments protects nonhuman primates from Ebola virus disease. J Virol. 2018;
37. Shuai L, Wang X, Wen Z, Ge J, Wang J, Zhao D, et al. Genetically modified rabies virus-vectored Ebola virus disease vaccines are safe and induce efficacious immune responses in mice and dogs. Antivir Res. 2017;146:36–44.
38. Zhu FC, Wurie AH, Hou LH, Liang Q, Li YH, Russell JB, et al. Safety and immunogenicity of a recombinant adenovirus type-5 vector-based Ebola vaccine in healthy adults in Sierra Leone: a single-centre, randomised, double-blind, placebo-controlled, phase 2 trial. Lancet. 2017;389(10069):621–8.
39. Gao R, Chen C, Wang F, Wang H, Jiang T, Sun Y, Fang T. Analysis of mechanism for international joint prevention and control of Ebola virus disease in Sierra Leone. Chin J Epidemiol. 2015;36(9):1031–3. (in Chinese)
40. Huang Q, Fu WL, You JP, Mao Q. Laboratory diagnosis of Ebola virus disease and corresponding biosafety considerations in the China Ebola treatment center. Crit Rev Clin Lab Sci. 2016;53(5):326–40.
41. Jiang H, Shi GQ, Tu WX, Zheng CJ, Lai XH, Li XX, et al. Rapid assessment of knowledge, attitudes, practices, and risk perception related to the prevention and control of Ebola virus disease in three communities of Sierra Leone. Infect Dis Poverty. 2016;5(1):53.
42. Chen T, Ka-Kit Leung R, Liu R, Chen F, Zhang X, et al. Risk of imported Ebola virus disease in China. Travel Med Infect Dis. 2014;12(6 Pt A):650–8.
43. Zawilińska B, Kosz-Vnenchak M. General introduction into the Ebola virus biology and disease. Folia Med Cracov. 2014;54(3):57–65.
44. Li Y, Ren X, Li D, Cheng Y, Gao F, Yu HJ. Ebola virus disease: epidemiology, ecology, diagnosis, treatment, and control. Sci Technol Rev. 2014;32(24):15–24. (in Chinese)
45. Goldstein T, Anthony SJ, Gbakima A, Bird BH, Bangura J, Tremeau-Bravard A, et al. The discovery of Bombali virus adds further support for bats as hosts of ebolaviruses. Nat Microbiol. 2018;3(10):1084–9.
46. Gire SK, Goba A, Andersen KG, Sealfon RS, Park DJ, Kanneh L, et al. Genomic surveillance elucidates Ebola virus origin and transmission during the 2014 outbreak. Science. 2014;345(6202):1369–72.
47. Nakayama E, Saijo M. Animal models for Ebola and Marburg virus infections. Front Microbiol. 2013;4:267.
48. Weingartl HM, Embury-Hyatt C, Nfon C, Leung A, Smith G, Kobinger G. Transmission of Ebola virus from pigs to non-human primates. Sci Rep. 2012;2:811.
49. Yang XL, Ge XY, Hu B, Shi ZL, Zhang YZ, Fang LQ, et al. The epidemiology of Ebola virus disease. J ZheJiang U (Med Sci). 2014;43(06):621–45. (in Chinese)
50. Swanepoel R, Leman PA, Burt FJ, Zachariades NA, Braack LE, Ksiazek TG, et al. Experimental inoculation of plants and animals with Ebola virus. Emerg Infect Dis. 1996;2(4):321–5.
51. Leroy EM, Epelboin A, Mondonge V, Pourrut X, Gonzalez JP, Muyembe-Tamfum JJ, et al. Human Ebola outbreak resulting from direct exposure to fruit bats in Luebo, Democratic Republic of Congo, 2007. Vector Borne Zoonotic Dis. 2009;9(6):723–8.
52. Pourrut X, Delicat A, Rollin PE, Ksiazek TG, Gonzalez JP, Leroy EM. Spatial and temporal patterns of Zaire ebolavirus antibody prevalence in the possible reservoir bat species. J Infect Dis. 2007;196(Suppl 2):S176–83.
53. Towner JS, Amman BR, Sealy TK, Carroll SA, Comer JA, Kemp A, et al. Isolation of genetically

diverse Marburg viruses from Egyptian fruit bats. PLoS Pathog. 2009;5(7):e1000536.
54. Leroy EM, Kumulungui B, Pourrut X, Rouquet P, Hassanin A, Yaba P, et al. Fruit bats as reservoirs of Ebola virus. Nature. 2005;438(7068):575–6.
55. Ansumana R, Jacobsen KH, Sahr F, Idris M, Bangura H, Boie-Jalloh M, et al. Ebola in Freetown area, Sierra Leone—a case study of 581 patients. N Engl J Med. 2015;372(6):587–8.
56. Schieffelin JS, Shaffer JG, Goba A, Gbakie M, Gire SK, Colubri A, et al. Clinical illness and outcomes in patients with Ebola in Sierra Leone. N Engl J Med. 2014;371(22):2092–100.
57. Bwaka MA, Bonnet MJ, Calain P, Colebunders R, De Roo A, Guimard Y, et al. Ebola hemorrhagic fever in Kikwit, Democratic Republic of the Congo: clinical observations in 103 patients. J Infect Dis. 1999;179(Suppl 1):S1–7.
58. WHO Ebola Response Team. Ebola virus disease in West Africa—the first 9 months of the epidemic and forward projections. N Engl J Med. 2014;371(16):1481–95.
59. Li LJ, Xu JG, Gao F. Ebola virus disease. Zhejiang: Zhejiang University Press; 2015. (in Chinese)
60. Heffernan RT, Pambo B, Hatchett RJ, Leman PA, Swanepoel R, Ryder RW. Low seroprevalence of IgG antibodies to Ebola virus in an epidemic zone: Ogooue-Ivindo region, northeastern Gabon, 1997. J Infect Dis. 2005;191(6):964–8.
61. Leroy EM, Baize S, Volchkov VE, Fisher-Hoch SP, Georges-Courbot MC, Lansoud-Soukate J, et al. Human asymptomatic Ebola infection and strong inflammatory response. Lancet. 2000;355(9222):2210–5.
62. Akerlund E, Prescott J, Tampellini L. Shedding of Ebola virus in an asymptomatic pregnant woman. N Engl J Med. 2015;372(25):2467–9.
63. Lotsch F, Schnyder J, Goorhuis A, Grobusch MP. Neuropsychological long-term sequelae of Ebola virus disease survivors - a systematic review. Travel Med Infect Dis. 2017;18:18–23.
64. Uyeki TM, Mehta AK, Davey RT Jr, Liddell AM, Wolf T, et al. Clinical management of Ebola virus disease in the United States and Europe. N Engl J Med. 2016;374(7):636–46.
65. Hunt L, Gupta-Wright A, Simms V, Tamba F, Knott V, Tamba K, et al. Clinical presentation, biochemical, and haematological parameters and their association with outcome in patients with Ebola virus disease: an observational cohort study. Lancet Infect Dis. 2015;15(11):1292–9.
66. Smit MA, Michelow IC, Glavis-Bloom J, Wolfman V, Levine AC. Characteristics and outcomes of pediatric patients with Ebola virus disease admitted to treatment units in Liberia and Sierra Leone: a retrospective cohort study. Clin Infect Dis. 2017;64(3):243–9.
67. Cherif MS, Koonrungsesomboon N, Diallo MP, Le Gall E, Kasse D, Cherif F, et al. The predictor of mortality outcome in adult patients with Ebola virus disease during the 2014–2015 outbreak in Guinea. Eur J Clin Microbiol Infect Dis. 2017;36(4):689–95.
68. Bebell LM, Oduyebo T, Riley LE. Ebola virus disease and pregnancy: a review of the current knowledge of Ebola virus pathogenesis, maternal, and neonatal outcomes. Birth Defects Res. 2017;109(5):353–62.
69. Feldmann H, Jones S, Klenk HD, Schnittler HJ. Ebola virus: from discovery to vaccine. Nat Rev Immunol. 2003;3(8):677–85.
70. Osterholm MT, Moore KA, Kelley NS, Brosseau LM, Wong G, Murphy FA, et al. Transmission of Ebola viruses: what we know and what we do not know. MBio. 2015;6(2):e00137.
71. Leroy EM, Rouquet P, Formenty P, Souquiere S, Kilbourne A, Froment JM, et al. Multiple Ebola virus transmission events and rapid decline of central African wildlife. Science. 2004;303(5656):387–90.
72. Olival KJ, Hayman DT. Filoviruses in bats: current knowledge and future directions. Viruses. 2014;6(4):1759–88.
73. Dixon MG, Schafer IJ, CDC. Ebola viral disease outbreak—West Africa, 2014. MMWR Morb Mortal Wkly Rep. 2014;63(25):548–51.
74. Baize S, Pannetier D, Oestereich L, Rieger T, Koivogui L, Magassouba N, et al. Emergence of Zaire Ebola virus disease in Guinea. N Engl J Med. 2014;371(15):1418–25.
75. Larsen T, Stevens EL, Davis KJ, Geisbert JB, Daddario-DiCaprio KM, Jahrling PB, et al. Pathologic findings associated with delayed death in nonhuman primates experimentally infected with Zaire Ebola virus. J Infect Dis. 2007;196(Suppl 2):S323–8.
76. WHO. What we know about transmission of the Ebola virus among humans. [cited Dec 31, 2018]. https://www.who.int/mediacentre/news/ebola/06-october-2014/en/.
77. Bausch DG, Towner JS, Dowell SF, Kaducu F, Lukwiya M, Sanchez A, et al. Assessment of the risk of Ebola virus transmission from bodily fluids and fomites. J Infect Dis. 2007;196(Suppl 2):S142–7.
78. Brainard J, Hooper L, Pond K, Edmunds K, Hunter PR. Risk factors for transmission of Ebola or Marburg virus disease: a systematic review and meta-analysis. Int J Epidemiol. 2016;45(1):102–16.
79. Francesconi P, Yoti Z, Declich S, Onek PA, Fabiani M, Olango J, et al. Ebola hemorrhagic fever transmission and risk factors of contacts. Uganda Emerg Infect Dis. 2003;9(11):1430–7.
80. Ajelli M, Parlamento S, Bome D, Kebbi A, Atzori A, Frasson C, et al. The 2014 Ebola virus disease outbreak in Pujehun, Sierra Leone: epidemiology and impact of interventions. BMC Med. 2015;13:281.
81. Busico KM, Marshall KL, Ksiazek TG, Roels TH, Fleerackers Y, Feldmann H, et al. Prevalence of IgG antibodies to Ebola virus in individuals during an Ebola outbreak, Democratic Republic of the Congo, 1995. J Infect Dis. 1999;179(Suppl 1):S102–7.
82. Becquart P, Wauquier N, Mahlakoiv T, Nkoghe D, Padilla C, Souris M, et al. High prevalence of both

humoral and cellular immunity to Zaire ebolavirus among rural populations in Gabon. PLoS One. 2010;5(2):e9126.
83. Gonzalez JP, Nakoune E, Slenczka W, Vidal P, Morvan JM. Ebola and Marburg virus antibody prevalence in selected populations of the Central African Republic. Microbes Infect. 2000;2(1):39–44.
84. Hogardt M, Wolf T, Kann G, Brodt HR, Brandt C, Keppler OT, et al. Management of microbiological samples in a confirmed case of Ebola virus disease: constraints and limitations. J Clin Microbiol. 2015;53(11):3396–400.
85. Lancet T. Ebola: protection of health-care workers. Lancet. 2014;384(9961):2174.
86. Mate SE, Kugelman JR, Nyenswah TG, Ladner JT, Wiley MR, Cordier-Lassalle T, et al. Molecular evidence of sexual transmission of Ebola virus. N Engl J Med. 2015;373(25):2448–54.
87. Colebunders R, Borchert M. Ebola haemorrhagic fever—a review. J Infect. 2000;40(1):16–20.
88. Rowe AK, Bertolli J, Khan AS, Mukunu R, Muyembe-Tamfum JJ, Bressler D, et al. Clinical, virologic, and immunologic follow-up of convalescent Ebola hemorrhagic fever patients and their household contacts, Kikwit, Democratic Republic of the Congo. Commission de Lutte contre les Epidemies a Kikwit. J Infect Dis. 1999;179(Suppl 1):S28–35.
89. Deen GF, Broutet N, Xu W, Knust B, Sesay FR, McDonald SLR, et al. Ebola RNA persistence in semen of Ebola virus disease survivors—final report. N Engl J Med. 2017;377(15):1428–37.
90. WHO. Sexual and reproductive health interim advice on the sexual transmission of the Ebola virus disease. [cited Dec 31, 2018]. https://www.who.int/reproductivehealth/topics/rtis/ebola-virus-semen/en/.
91. Salvaggio MR, Baddley JW. Other viral bioweapons: Ebola and Marburg hemorrhagic fever. Dermatol Clin. 2004;22(3):291–302.
92. Leffel E, Reed D. Marburg and Ebola viruses as aerosol threats. 2004.
93. Wang ZY, Nie X, Guo ZD, Li JJ, Cheng HL, et al. Advances in research on the aerosol infection and transmission of Eboa virus. J Pathog Biol. 2018;13(08):914–6. (in Chinese)
94. Medina-Rivera M, Centeno-Tablante E, Finkelstein JL, Rayco-Solon P, Peña-Rosas JP, Garcia-Casal MN, et al. Presence of Ebola virus in breast milk and risk of mother-to-child transmission: synthesis of evidence. Ann N Y Acad Sci. 2021;1488(1):33–43.
95. Wikipedia. List of Ebola outbreaks. [cited Dec 31, 2018]. https://en.wikipedia.org/wiki/List_of_Ebola_outbreaks#cite_note-77.
96. Ebola Outbreak Epidemiology Team. Outbreak of Ebola virus disease in the Democratic Republic of the Congo, April–May, 2018: an epidemiological study. Lancet. 2018;392(10143):213–21.
97. Murray MJ. Ebola virus disease: a review of its past and present. Anesth Analg. 2015;121(3):798–809.
98. Pan Y, Zhang W, Cui L, Hua X, Wang M, Zeng Q. Reston virus in domestic pigs in China. Arch Virol. 2014;159(5):1129–32.
99. Jahrling PB, Geisbert TW, Dalgard DW, Johnson ED, Ksiazek TG, Hall WC, et al. Preliminary report: isolation of Ebola virus from monkeys imported to USA. Lancet. 1990;335(8688):502–5.
100. Philippine monkeys infected with Ebola not lethal to humans. [cited Dec 31, 2018]. https://www.philstar.com/headlines/2015/09/05/1496305/philippine-monkeys-infected-ebola-not-lethal-humans.
101. Hayes CG, Burans JP, Ksiazek TG, Del Rosario RA, Miranda ME, Manaloto CR, et al. Outbreak of fatal illness among captive macaques in the Philippines caused by an Ebola-related filovirus. Am J Trop Med Hyg. 1992;46(6):664–71.
102. Barrette RW, Metwally SA, Rowland JM, Xu L, Zaki SR, Nichol ST, et al. Discovery of swine as a host for the Reston ebolavirus. Science. 2009;325(5937):204–6.
103. Nkoghe D, Padilla C, Becquart P, Wauquier N, Moussavou G, Akue JP, et al. Risk factors for Zaire ebolavirus—specific IgG in rural Gabonese populations. J Infect Dis. 2011;204(Suppl 3):S768–75.
104. Muoghalu IS, Moses F, Conteh I, Swaray P, Ajudua A, Nordstrom A. The transmission chain analysis of 2014-2015 Ebola virus disease outbreak in Koinadugu District, Sierra Leone: an observational study. Front Public Health. 2017;5:160.
105. Wendelboe AM, McCumber M, Erb-Alvarez J, Mould N, Childs RW, Regens JL. Managing emerging transnational public health security threats: lessons learned from the 2014 west African Ebola outbreak. Glob Health. 2018;14(1):75.
106. Bausch DG, Schwarz L. Outbreak of ebola virus disease in Guinea: where ecology meets economy. PLoS Negl Trop Dis. 2014;8(7):e3056.
107. Pigott DM, Golding N, Mylne A, Huang Z, Henry AJ, Weiss DJ, et al. Mapping the zoonotic niche of Ebola virus disease in Africa. elife. 2014;3:e04395.
108. Walsh MG, Haseeb M. The landscape configuration of zoonotic transmission of Ebola virus disease in West and Central Africa: interaction between population density and vegetation cover. PeerJ. 2015;3:e735.
109. Ng S, Cowling BJ. Association between temperature, humidity and ebolavirus disease outbreaks in Africa, 1976 to 2014. Euro Surveill. 2014;19(35)
110. Groseth A, Feldmann H, Strong JE. The ecology of Ebola virus. Trends Microbiol. 2007;15(9):408–16.
111. Tambo E, Ugwu EC, Ngogang JY. Need of surveillance response systems to combat Ebola outbreaks and other emerging infectious diseases in African countries. Infect Dis Poverty. 2014;3:29.
112. Varma JK, Prezant DJ, Wilson R, Quinn C, Asaeda G, Cagliuso NV, et al. Preparing the health system to respond to Ebola virus disease in New York City, 2014. Disaster Med Public Health Prep. 2017;11(3):370–4.

113. CDC. Experimental Ebola drug may have helped 2 US patients. [cited Dec 31, 2018]. http://www.cidrap.umn.edu/news-perspective/2014/08/experimental-ebola-drug-may-have-helped-2-us-patients.
114. Dornemann J, Burzio C, Ronsse A, Sprecher A, De Clerck H, Van Herp M, et al. First newborn baby to receive experimental therapies survives Ebola virus disease. J Infect Dis. 2017;215(2):171–4.
115. Henao-Restrepo AM, Longini IM, Egger M, Dean NE, Edmunds WJ, Camacho A, et al. Efficacy and effectiveness of an rVSV-vectored vaccine expressing Ebola surface glycoprotein: interim results from the Guinea ring vaccination cluster-randomised trial. Lancet. 2015;386(9996):857–66.
116. Gsell PS, Camacho A, Kucharski AJ, Watson CH, Bagayoko A, Nadlaou SD, et al. Ring vaccination with rVSV-ZEBOV under expanded access in response to an outbreak of Ebola virus disease in Guinea, 2016: an operational and vaccine safety report. Lancet Infect Dis. 2017;17(12):1276–84.
117. Nkengasong JN, Onyebujoh P. Response to the Ebola virus disease outbreak in the Democratic Republic of the Congo. Lancet. 2018;391(10138):2395–8.
118. Zhang Z, Hou LH. Advances in clinical trials of Ebola vaccine. Infect Dis Inform 2018; 31(05):430–565. (in Chinese).
119. Fischer WA 2nd, Vetter P, Bausch DG, Burgess T, Davey RT Jr, Fowler R, et al. Ebola virus disease: an update on post-exposure prophylaxis. Lancet Infect Dis. 2018;18(6):e183–e92.
120. Shultz JM, Espinel Z, Espinola M, Rechkemmer A. Distinguishing epidemiological features of the 2013–2016 West Africa Ebola virus disease outbreak. Disaster Health. 2016;3(3):78–88.
121. Martinez MJ, Salim AM, Hurtado JC, Kilgore PE. Ebola virus infection: overview and update on prevention and treatment. Infect Dis Ther. 2015;4(4):365–90.
122. Shears P, O'Dempsey TJ. Ebola virus disease in Africa: epidemiology and nosocomial transmission. J Hosp Infect. 2015;90(1):1–9.
123. Bogoch II, Creatore MI, Cetron MS, Brownstein JS, Pesik N, Miniota J, et al. Assessment of the potential for international dissemination of Ebola virus via commercial air travel during the 2014 west African outbreak. Lancet. 2015;385(9962):29–35.
124. WHO, CDC. Infection control for viral haemorrhagic fevers. [cited Dec 31, 2018]. https://www.who.int/csr/resources/publications/ebola/whoem-cesr982sec1-4.pdf.
125. Brolin Ribacke KJ, Saulnier DD, Eriksson A, von Schreeb J. Effects of the West Africa Ebola virus disease on health-care utilization - a systematic review. Front Public Health. 2016;4:222.
126. Liu W, Fang TY, Cao WC. The major progress on the Ebola virus disease study and international Ebola virus testing in Sierra Leone. Chin J Epidemiol. 2015;36(9):1023–5. (in Chinese)
127. Jiang T, Zhao G, Han J, Xin W, Zhuang D, Tan Y, He J, Gao R, Wang H, Chen C, et al. Comparison of international Ebola virus testing laboratories in Ebola virus disease outbreak in Sierra Leone. Chin J Epidemiol. 2015;36(9):1034–7. (in Chinese)

Progress in Dengue Epidemiology

6

Qinlong Jing and Ming Wang

Abstract

Dengue fever is an acute viral infectious disease transmitted by mosquitoes. The increase in incidence rate and mortality rate has brought serious burden to the world. Over the past few decades, significant progress has helped to deepen its epidemiology, including disease burden, distribution, risk factors, control, and prevention measures. Dengue continues to spread to new areas, including high latitudes, and a new serotype (dengue virus serotype 5) has been identified. New progress has been made in vaccine research. The licensed quadrivalent chimeric vaccines of yellow fever and dengue virus are currently undergoing further safety evaluation. In disease surveillance, the detection of dengue virus NS1 antigen has great popularization and application value in grassroots health care institutions because of its simple, rapid, and powerful operation and can be used as an indicator of disease severity. Advances in vector control have promoted new breakthroughs in biotechnology, including *Wolbachia-infected Aedes* and genetically modified *Aedes*. Both *Aedes* mosquito variants are used to block the transmission of dengue virus through population replacement and inhibition. In the future, vector control, together with antiviral drugs and vaccines, should be a key measure to prevent transmission.

Q. Jing · M. Wang (✉)
Guangzhou Center for Disease Control and Prevention,
Guangzhou, Guangdong, People's Republic of China
e-mail: wangming@gzcdc.org.cn

Keywords

Dengue fever · Epidemiology · Disease control and prevention · Progress

6.1 Introduction

Dengue fever is mainly transmitted by female *Aedes aegypti* and *Aedes albopictus*. It is the fastest mosquito-borne virus infection in the world [1]. It occurs suddenly and always leads to large-scale outbreaks, leading to serious public health emergencies, especially in non-epidemic areas. Patients with severe dengue fever have a high probability of death due to bleeding or shock. However, there is no specific antiviral treatment, and licensed vaccines worry about the increased risk of hospitalization due to antibody-dependent effects (ADE) [2, 3]. Although great efforts have been made in research and control practice, rapid spread is still going on, resulting in a huge economic burden. In addition, extensive research over the past few decades has contributed to its epidemiology, including disease burden and distribution, risk factors, and control and prevention measures. Here, we present an updated review that provides a comprehensive overview to raise awareness of the disease.

D.-Q. Ye (ed.), *Progress in China Epidemiology*, https://doi.org/10.1007/978-981-19-2199-5_6

The pathogen of dengue virus (DENV) can lead to a wide spectrum of infection, from inconspicuous subclinical infection to symptomatic infection, from mild and typical dengue fever to severe dengue hemorrhagic fever (DHF) and dengue shock syndrome (DSS), which will increase the risk of death. Among dengue-related infections without clinical symptoms, non-obvious infection accounted for the largest proportion. Obvious infection after 3–15 days incubation period, followed by acute attack. Mild diseases must be distinguished from influenza, colds and other acute febrile diseases. Typical cases of dengue fever usually have a sudden fever (≥38.5 °C), headache, rash, myalgia, joint pain, thrombocytopenia, and leucopenia, with a high medical treatment rate. They are manifested in three natural processes, including fever, crisis, and recovery stages. In the process of defervescence, due to plasma leakage, hypovolemic shock, organ failure, metabolic acidosis, disseminated intravascular coagulation, and severe bleeding, capillary permeability and hematocrit may increase. Severe dengue fever can lead to hepatitis, nervous system diseases, myocarditis, and shock. Without appropriate clinical treatment, the natural mortality can reach 20%, depending on age, virus serotype, and genotype, complications, infection history, and antibodies. However, with appropriate symptoms and supportive treatment, the mortality will be reduced to 1% [1]. In 57% of cases, arthralgia and fatigue occurred within 2 years after onset of the illness [4]. Importantly, dengue fever and malaria, HIV, Chai virus, guinea pig virus and a variety of dengue fever common infections have been reported, which has brought great challenges to diagnosis and treatment.

Because it is difficult to classify and diagnose quickly in clinical practice, especially for severe dengue fever [5], the diagnostic criteria are underestimated and need to be further improved. Classic cases and DHF/DSS were classified in the diagnostic guidelines of the World Health Organization (who) in 1997. Specifically, the diagnosis of DHF requires bleeding tendency and thrombocytopenia (platelet $< 100 \times 10^9$/L) and plasma leakage (increased hematocrit and pleural effusion), although cases without these main features may be under-diagnosed [6]. In the 2009 WHO guidelines, the criteria for severe dengue fever include severe plasma leakage, shock, respiratory distress, severe bleeding and severe organ injury [7]. Compared with the 1997 guidelines, the 2009 guidelines improved the diagnostic sensitivity of severe dengue fever [8–10]. At present, due to the lack of laboratories and health institutions, a new method for early identification of dengue cases is needed. According to the current case definition, some cases of mild diseases are under-diagnosed or unreported [11]. Therefore, prospective multi-center studies need to continue efforts to further improve the classification and diagnostic criteria [7].

6.2 Disease Burden and Epidemiology

According to its morbidity and mortality, dengue fever is the second serious vector-borne disease in the world after malaria [12]. In five American countries such as Brazil, El Salvador, Guatemala, Panama, and Venezuela, and three hyperendemic countries in Southeast Asia such as Cambodia, Malaysia, and Thailand, the economic burden of dengue fever has reached USD 2 billion, exceeding the cost of other viral diseases in addition to media control. In Bhutan, Brunei, Cambodia, Timor-Leste, Indonesia, Myanmar, the Philippines, Singapore, Vietnam, and Taiwan Province of China, the annual burden has reached $ 950 million [13]. The global economic cost of dengue fever in 2011 was estimated to be 3.93 billion dollars [14]. The disease burden of dengue fever is as high as 25.5 disability-adjusted life years per 100,000 population [15]. However, there were no good estimates of the incidence and economic burden of unreported and under-reported infections.

6.2.1 Geographic Distribution

More than 100 countries and regions in tropical and subtropical regions show dengue epidemic, including Southeast Asia, Central and South America, Africa, the Western Pacific, and Eastern

Mediterranean [16]. With regard to WHO estimation, 2.5 billion people live in endemic areas, with 50 million people infected with dengue virus each year, resulting in 25,000 deaths [16]. Notably, the incidence rate has increased 30-fold over the past 50 years and accelerated geographical distribution. It shows that the incidence in the Americas has increased fivefold in the past decade. According to a 2013 study, some 3.6 billion of the world 's population live in areas at risk, with 390 million infections and 96 million symptoms, 500,000 of which develop into DHF or DSS each year [17, 18]. The incidence of dengue fever has increased significantly recently [11], experiencing huge outbreaks in 2014 in South-east countries and China [19, 20]. There are dengue introductions identified in Florida (USA), southeastern France, Madeira Island, Spain, Croatia, and Japan in higher latitude regions [19].

In southern China, the spread frequency and scale of dengue fever have been increasing in the past few decades, and geographical regions, incidence rates, and severe dengue fever rates have been increasing. At present, the epidemic situation of dengue fever is deteriorating [12, 21]. In 1940s, the coastal provinces experienced transmission, reaching Nanchang, Hankou, and other inland areas. Subsequently, after 30 years of silence, Dengue fever reappeared in China with high transmission intensity. It began in Foshan City, Guangdong Province in 1978 and spread to surrounding areas, especially Guangzhou [22]. Subsequently, Hainan, Guangxi, Fujian, Zhejiang, Taiwan, Hong Kong, Macao, and other places experienced local transmission. An outbreak of DHF in Hainan Province from 1985 to 1986 resulted in the death of several hospitalized cases [23].

A total of 10,000 cases were reported in China from 1990 to 2006, including three deaths, with all four serotypes been circulated. As the most important outbreak province, the number of reported cases from Guangdong accounts for 90% of the total number of reported cases in the country [24]. In 2014, the number of cases soared to 450,000. Guangzhou, the capital city of Guangdong Province, reported 380,000 cases, accounting for 84% of Guangdong and 81% of the country. This is 2.4 times the total number of cases (160,000) between 1978 and 2013, including 140,000 hospitalized cases, 308 critically ill cases and five deaths [25]. Since the 2000s, there has been a trend of dengue fever transmission in high latitude areas. For example, dengue fever outbreaks occurred in Henan Province in 2013 and 2014 [20] and outbreaks in Shandong and Zhejiang in 2017, and Jiangxi in 2019.

At present, the origin and prevalence of China are controversial issues in the study. Due to the lack of convincing evidence, especially in non-epidemic and outbreak periods, and the lack of successful virus isolation in local vectors, including larvae and adults, dengue fever in China is mainly considered to be imported, while local transmission is caused by imports and has not been epidemic so far [26]. As strong evidence, Guangzhou reported only two indigenous cases in 2020, thanks to 14 days of strict international quarantine controls at the COVID-19 medical isolation hotel. Due to its geographical location close to the epidemic foci in Southeast Asia, it is suitable for the natural climate and geographical conditions of mosquito growth and reproduction. Once imported cases occur, the probability of local transmission in Guangdong is high. In some studies, there may be local viral cycles, which are endemic in southern China, especially in Yunnan Province.

6.2.2 Temporal Distribution

Periodicity Dengue transmission displays significant periodicity, with variation in different regions. It peaks in 3–5 years in Southeast Asia, while peaks in 4–5 years in Brazil. Before 2010, Guangzhou was the most prevalent region in China and peaked periodicity of 3–5 years [27]. However, the yearly outbreak of Dengue was more frequent in Guangzhou since 2010. With 33, 139, and 1249 cases in 2011, 2012, and 2013, respectively, and with relatively small-scale outbreaks, a record-breaking outbreak occurred in 2014. In 2015, there were only 54 cases. However, the scale continually climbed annually, with 204 cases in 2016, 873 cases in 2017, and exceeding 1000 cases in 2018 and 2019, respectively.

After an outbreak, it may be followed by a growing risk of DHF in the subsequent 3–5 years [19]. For instance, a DHF outbreak occurred in 1981, followed by the 1977 dengue outbreak in Cuba. Similarly, an outbreak of DHF in Hainan province in 1985 was followed by the 1980 dengue outbreak in China. This situation was correlated with ADE, which resulted from the secondary infection with heterogeneous serotypes [28].

The origin of dengue transmission is always under-identification in areas with low population immunity. As such, following the outbreak in Henan province in China in 2013 [29] and Japan in 2014 [30], due to limited systematic surveillance and of non-endemic area, it was difficult to determine the virus origin. Most were ascribed to the introduction of imported cases. The periodicity in endemic areas correlates with the accumulation of epidemic intensity.

Seasonality Dengue circulates year-round in tropical and subtropical areas and is highly correlated with temperature, rainy season, and vector fluctuation with seasonality. With differences in physiographic conditions, the epidemic peak varies. The peak in non-endemic areas is determined by the time of imported cases [31]. However, the peak time in Thailand and Myanmar is from May to October, and June to December in Malaysia and Vietnam. In the Central and South Americas, the peak time was correlated with the rainy season, from February to May in Brazil and July to December in Puerto Rico. In China, the peak season is from June to November in Guangdong province, while July to October in Guangxi, Yunnan, Fujian, and Zhejiang provinces.

6.2.3 Population Distribution

Population of any age can be infected with DENV, of which about 30–60% have symptoms. However, there are differences between epidemic and non-epidemic areas. Infection rates are higher among young adults in non-endemic areas. In the epidemic area, the incidence of children is the highest, accounting for 85% of the total number of cases in Thailand, mainly concentrated in the 8–9 years old. In addition, DHF has become the main cause of hospitalization and death in children. In China, which has the regional characteristics of imported dengue fever, the cases are distributed in all age groups, mainly in young adults, retired, domestic and unemployed people, which is different from the epidemic areas with high incidence of children. There was no difference in infection rate between gender and occupation. The mechanism of age transition to adulthood needs further study [11].

Population infection is directly related to the biting probability of infected *Aedes*. High-risk groups in the population include medical workers. Due to the lack of adequate infection control measures, medical institutions and hospitals are becoming hot spots of outbreaks. Viruses are transmitted to other patients, medical workers and visitors through infected mosquitoes, and the scale of outbreaks is expanded.

6.3 Risk Factors for Transmission

6.3.1 Source of Infection

Humans are the main amplified host of DENV [32]. Cases are the main source of infection, from the day before the onset to the next 5 days for a period of infection, during which *Aedes* bites spread to healthy people [33]. In addition, once infected, the person may enter an unobvious infection at a probability greater than 50%. The ratio of unconspicuous and obvious infections reached 2.2 to 1 [34]. Recessive infections play an important role in transmission [35]. Non-human primates such as chimpanzees, gibbons, and macaques are important natural reservoirs. The source of infection in the jungle epidemic area is concentrated in Southeast Asia [36]. Monkeys, bats, pigs, and chickens are also hosts for storage and spread [37–39]. In the jungle cycle, *Aedes* inhabiting the crown can spread viruses among primates, and then contact with humans to rural and urban areas with high population density, and even to the world through shipping or airlines [40, 41]. In rural and urban circulation, the mode of transmission is *Aedes*-human-*Aedes* [42], which is similar in Guangdong, Hainan, Guangxi, Fujian, and Zhejiang in China. Vertical transmission in vectors of DENV has been demonstrated in the laboratory. However, it is not well demonstrated in the field [1].

6.3.2 Route of Transmission

Aedes is the main vector of DENV, and about 13 subspecies have this ability to spread. *Aedes aegypti*, also known as yellow fever mosquitoes, mainly lives in tropical areas and is the main vector. It often causes harm to human beings before eggs occur and is closely related to human beings. *Aedes albopictus*, named Asian tiger mosquito, exists worldwide compared to *Aedes aegypti*. It is not only seen in Asia and other popular regions but also in Europe and North America. In recent years also caused large-scale outbreaks [25]. However, it is still unclear whether *Culex fatigans* is a DENV reservoir [43]. Dengue is also transmitted through blood products [44] and organ transplantation [45], with an infection rate of 1.6–6% in Singapore [46]. Other means of transmission are rare in humans [47].

In China, *Aedes aegypti* distributes in the south areas of 22°N, including Taiwan, Hainan, west Guangdong, and Beibu Gulf of Guangxi. *Aedes aegypti* was detected in Ruili city in Yunnan in recent years, accounting for 49.56% of the population survey, indicating the latitude as high as 25°N. However, *Aedes albopictus* has a broad distribution covering approximately 75% of China. The north line of distribution from Shenyang city in Liaoning province, to the southwest direction to Xuanhua in Hebei province, Shanxi, Hancheng, Tongchuan, Longxian, and Yangpingguan in Shaanxi province, Yaan, Jiulong, Yanbian in Sichuan province, to Chaou, Motuo of south Tibet, and even to Bhutan and Nepal. South of the line, *Aedes albopictus* profoundly exists, especially with high density in line with 30°N, including Hainan, Taiwan, Guangdong, Guangxi, Fujian, Zhejiang, Jiangxi, Hunan, Guizhou, Chongqing, and Yunnan. Strikingly, No *Aedes aegypti*, while *Aedes albopictus* is widely colonized in Guangzhou, China's important dengue epidemic area [48].

6.3.3 Susceptible Population and Mechanism

In new or imported areas of where DENV is transmitted, populations are all susceptible to DENV infection, and the infection rate is higher in adults [49]. In epidemic areas, most adults carry specific antibodies. At the same time, the incidence of DENV in children is relatively high, which can be explained by the accumulation of immune function in adult populations [50]. After infection, serotype-specific antibodies against the same serotype are produced in the serum for several years or a lifetime. In contrast, heterogeneous serotypes provide immunity for 2 months to 2 years [1]. Surprisingly, secondary infections with heterogeneous serotypes may lead to a higher risk of DHF / DSS, and infants infected with maternal antibodies are more likely to be infected with DHF/DSS than infants not infected with maternal antibodies [51]. The potential mechanism of ADE may be that antibodies are expelled after initial infection to enhance the severity of the disease. The time interval between virus and infection also modulated the outcome of secondary infection. The interval is related to the severity of the disease and the proportion of symptoms [52]. The correlation between atypical antibodies and their impact on population immunity has not been well understood. Studies in Nicaragua and Peru showed that there was reinfection in the same serotype [11]. The people with underlying diseases, such as diabetes, asthma, G6PD deficiency, and sickle-cell anemia, have been recorded with certain risk for severe dengue.

A previous study showed that race, blood type, and human leukocyte antigen (HLA) are related to the susceptibility of DENV [53]. During the outbreak of Cuba in 1981, the DHF/DSS ratio of white, black, and hybrids was 5.5:1:1.8. Chinese people have a higher risk of

DHF than Malaysians. Individuals with AB blood types have a greater risk than those with O, A, and B blood types [54].

The hypothesis of the interaction between HLA and DENV susceptibility to amplify the immune effects of natural immunity and antigen presentation through MHC-I pathway is an important reason for immune pathology. For example, HLA allele polymorphism may be related to T cell morphological diversity in antiviral response [55]. In associations of DF, DHF, and DSS with HLA, the alleles frequencies were significantly different from those in controls matched by age, region and race. Some alleles were associated with specific serotypes of DF and DHF, such as DENV-1 and HLA*0207, DENV-2 and B*52.

6.3.4 Virus and Detection

Dengue virus (DENV) is a icosahedral envelope virus (40–50 nm in diameter) belonging to the genus *Flaviviridae*. Generally, DENV is divided into four serotypes, including DENV-1, DENV-2, DENV-3, and DENV-4 [56–59], and its limited identity is close to 60–70% of its amino acid sequence. The DENV genome is a single positive-strand RNA with a length of 11 kb, containing an open reading frame (ORF), and 96% nucleotides encoding all viral proteins. The genome is divided into two regions. The 5′ side (1/4) encoding three structural proteins (capsid (C), membrane (M), and envelope (E)), and the 3′ side (3/4) encoding seven nonstructural (NS) proteins, including NS1, NS2a, NS2b, NS3, NS4a, NS4b, and NS5 genes (see the Fig. 6.1). In 2013, Malaysia found DENV-5 among a farmer infected in 2007 [60]. It has existed in forest primates for a long time, putting vaccine development in a dilemma.

Phylogenetic analysis shows that the diversity of DENV has existed for a long time, and pedigree change has led to the prosperity and decline of high diversity [62]. Four serotypes that have undergone rapid changes since World War II show new genotypic variations [63]. The difference among nucleotide sequences of serotypes is significant at about 35%, while there are around 3% differences at the amino acid and 6% at the nucleotide level in the same serotype with multiple genotypes [62]. Different serotypes, genotypes and branches lead to changes in clinical manifestations, disease severity, virulence, and epidemic potential [64].

The diagnostic methods for DENV include its genomic sequence, antigen, and serum antibody, depending on the sample time and target, see Fig. 6.2. The virus phase started from 1 day before the onset and 5 days after the onset, overlapping with the infectious phase and the fever phase. In the initial infection, IgG slow growth at low titers, need to detect 8–10 days. In contrast, IgM can be detected within 4 days for 2–3 months. In secondary infections, IgG titers increase rapidly after infection, whereas IgM levels increase transiently after infection [1]. During the fever period, nucleic acid sequence and NS1 were the best targets for the detection of serum by reverse transcription-

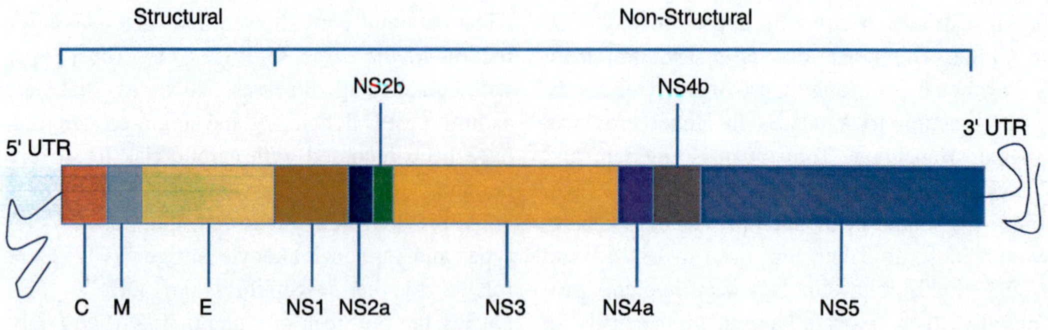

Fig. 6.1 Genome structure of DENV [61]. Note: coding sequence: 5′-I cap-UTR-ACG-C-M-E- NS1-NS2a-NS2b-NS3-NS4a-NS4b-NS5-UTR-3′

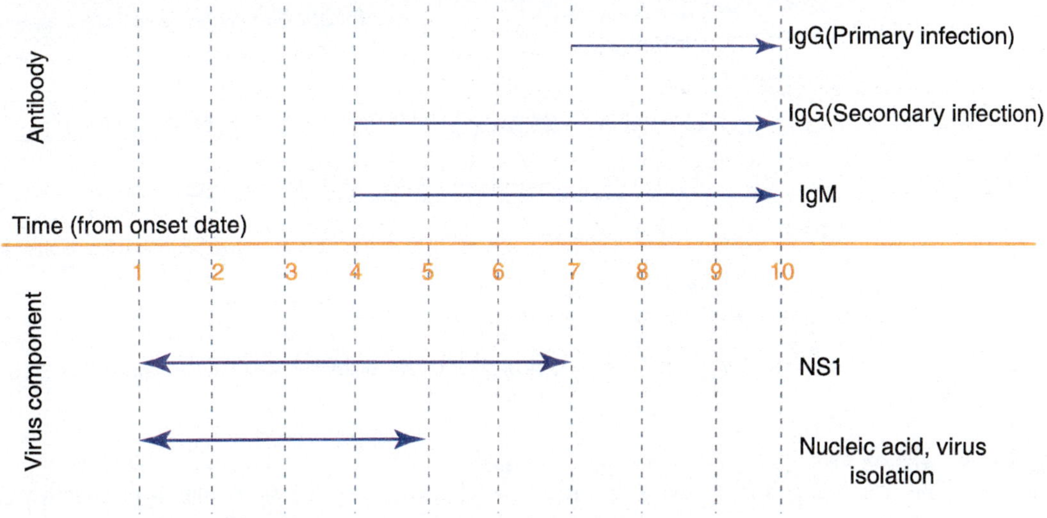

Fig. 6.2 Laboratory test selection for case diagnosis [7]

polymerase chain reaction (RT-PCR) or real-time RT-PCR and enzyme-linked immunosorbent assay (ELISA) to confirm the diagnosis [7]. The rapid lateral flow test of NS1 provides high diagnostic sensitivity, which is widely used in southern China. In primary infection, the sensitivity is as high as 90% and can be detected 9 days after fever [65]. However, the sensitivity was low in 60–80% of secondary infections, which was due to the serological response to previous infections or the memory of other yellow viruses [66]. Confirmatory tests included seroconversion of paired serum IgM and IgG antibodies or a fourfold increase in IgG antibody titers [1]. Single serum IgM positive can be diagnosed in clinical cases, but it cannot be diagnosed because of the cross-reaction between IgG or IgM and other flavivirus pre-infection. IgA and IgE as Candidate Biomarkers for Detection in serum, saliva and urine [67]. Due to the limited accessibility of RT-PCR, IgM or NS1 detection is a practical method for suspected infection in epidemiological surveillance and epidemic investigation of primary medical institutions [68].

Serum is the preferred test sample, followed by plasma, blood and tissues, including liver, spleen, lymph, lung, and brain. Saliva also has test value. Virus isolation is the gold standard for case diagnosis in cell lines, mainly using C6/36. Serotypes were identified using RT-PCR or immunofluorescence of the genome during viremia. Hemagglutination inhibition (HI), ELISA, and IgG neutralization test are the selective methods to detect the specific antibodies after infection. Plaque Reduction Neutralization Test (PRNT) has been used in seroepidemiology and vaccine research, although its repeatability is limited [69]. Microneutralization test (MN), immune spot and flow cytometry can also be used in practice. Recent advances in detection methods include immunomagnetic microspheres, nanodiagnosis, immunosensors, and microarray techniques for screening multiple viruses and biological components [70].

The titer increase of viremia and NS1 are associated with disease severity and can be used as an indicator for early identification and prognosis evaluation for severe dengue [71]. The transfer of DENV-2 can lead to fatal disease, especially in children [72]. Ultrasonography and microarray technology can diagnose severity [73]. HMGB1 (high mobility group box 1 protein) [74] and MCP-1 (monocyte chemotactic protein 1) [75] are two suitable indicators for early diagnosis.

6.3.5 Epidemic Process

DENV circulates between humans and *Aedes*. Once an infected person is bitten by female *Aedes*, the virus enters the mosquito with blood,

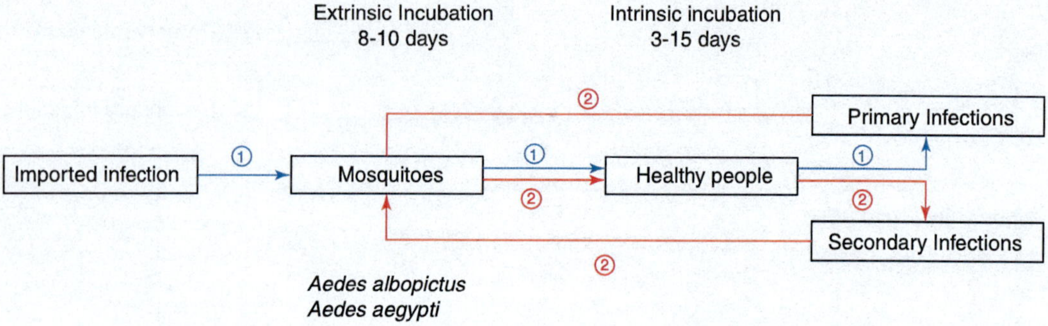

Fig. 6.3 Dengue epidemic process. (1) Blue lines denoting the process of primary infection. (2) Red lines denoting the process of secondary infection

and infectivity is enhanced after 8–10 days of reproduction, which is called the extrinsic incubation period. If another healthy person is bitten three to 15 days after intrinsic incubation period, the virus spreads through the population (see Fig. 6.3). In addition, mechanic transmission through biting can affect the continued transmission of nearby susceptibles. Vertical propagation also exists in the transmission chain.

For emerging DENV cases, control measures should be conducted immediately to prevent spreading by targeting the process of primary infection. However, if secondary cases occur, the number of infections will increase as geometrical progression, and the transmission will spread rapidly.

6.3.6 Impact Factors and Transmission Process

Nature and social factors are two aspects of DENV transmission [76]. In addition to vector factors, climate [77] and geographical factors are two key nature factors. With the increase of precipitation by 1 mm and temperature by 1 °C, the number of local cases in Australia increased by 6% [78]. When the temperature increased by 1 °C per month, the population risk of dengue fever increased by 1.95 times [79].

Social factors include demographic changes [80], urban structure [81], population density, water supply and socioeconomics [82], public health infrastructure, imported cases, geography and ecological environment, human migration [83], trade globalization, sanitary condition, water supply [82], human behaviors (water storage containers, construction sites, park ponding, vacant houses), diagnosis and reporting system (diagnosis criteria, NS1 screening), lack of health knowledge, and emergence response. With the development of global transport, tourism, trade, and population migration, imported dengue cases carrying DENV spread from one region to another is considered to be the main cause of epidemic transmission and increased incidence [84]. The suspected cases of dengue fever should be considered in any patients with fever within 14 days after travelling in the endemic area. Populations in coastal areas and arid areas need water storage containers and aquatic plants in the house, which increases the number of carrier breeding sites. Construction sites with ponds and municipal facilities (sewers, trash cans, artificial mountains with fountains) are high-risk sites in cities. As population density increases, the risk of DENV transmission increases. In the community, home-to-home movement and space-time gathering can exaggerate the spread [64]. Outbreaks can spread freely due to the diversity of clinical symptoms caused by misdiagnosis and missed diagnosis, late reporting, and lack of effective case management and early control measures.

The outbreak of dengue fever is related to the distribution and density of *Aedes*. The cutoff threshold for the Breteau index (BI) is 9.5 [85]. Under the comprehensive factors including temperature, import cases and BI analysis, import cases and BI determine the occurrence of local cases. If the number of import cases exceeds 3.5 within a month, the relative risk value is the highest of 3.00. However, BI and average temperature are two key factors affecting the severity of local propagation. When BI ≥5.29 and average temperature < 27.04 °C, RR of 5.11 is the highest [86].

6.4 Control and Prevention Strategy

The overall goal of dengue fever control is to find dengue cases in time, prevent secondary cases, avoid major epidemic or epidemic, and reduce the harm of dengue fever. At present, although vaccines may play a role in prevention, the main strategy will still rely on vector control to cut off the route of transmission [87]. Further, the most critical measures are environmental control and cleaning up mosquito breeding grounds. Dengue fever is a disease related to environment and community, also known as behavior and ecological decision-making disease. Disease control requires the participation of multiple departments, not just a person, an institution, or a specific government system. In addition, dengue fever cannot be effectively controlled by a single measure [87]. In the WHO strategy, its goal is to reduce mortality and incidence rate by 50% and 25%, respectively in 2020, and adopt four promising measures, such as advanced vector control technology, diagnostic method, classification system, evidence-based clinical intervention and candidate vaccine. In Chinese mainland, the strategy focuses on monitoring, vector density control, prevention of imported cases, improved diagnosis and treatment, and strengthening of multidisciplinary cooperation and population mobilization.

6.4.1 Surveillance and Forecast

6.4.1.1 Epidemic Surveillance

Epidemic situation monitoring is divided into case monitoring and syndrome monitoring. Case identification and epidemic reporting are two methods of case monitoring. Case identification and reporting depend on the hospital, control and quarantine departments to report suspected, clinical or confirmed cases online to specialized agencies within 24 h after diagnosis. The outbreak is defined as three epidemiological related cases occurring in 15 days of population concentration and limited area, such as a community, community, school, village in Chinese mainland. Emergency monitoring is defined as five indigenous cases or more cases in one county or district, or the first indigenous case found in a calendar year. Symptom monitoring includes routine symptom monitoring and emergency response monitoring. Routine monitoring aims to understand the risk of transmission by using designated hospitals to monitor fever with thrombocytopenia and fever with rash [88]. Emergence syndrome aims to find all cases in an epidemic focus in time, conduct door-to-door investigation and screening of fever cases by medical institutions, and take accurate control measures in time. Unknown and underreported infections, including mild or inconspicuous infections, are the key points for assessing the disease burden in the future.

6.4.1.2 Vector Surveillance

The definition of vector surveillance is to estimate the transmission risk and control effect through sampling method and continuous and systematic collection of classification, density, geographical or seasonal variation data of *Aedes*. The target of routine monitoring is the larva or pupa and adult stage. The larva index is BI, house index (HI), container index (CI), route index (RI), dip index (DI), standard space index (SSI), adult density index (bite index), and net capture index. Through human temptation, double-layer net capture, breeding ground capture, and mosquito trap lamp. Ovitrap is a mature oviposition monitoring method.

According to the sample size, accuracy, density, community area, number of houses, and survey resources, a rapid assessment usually requires a survey of 100 houses. The epidemiological significance of the above indicators mainly comes from the experience of yellow fever, such as BI greater than 5 as the alarm threshold. In practice, this change shows volatility due to the classification of ponding and roof drains. In Chinese mainland, larval monitoring is mainly a qualitative investigation of whether there are larvae or pupae in containers. However, quantitative studies on quantity or container size are not well documented, so a large container with 1000 larvae and a small container with 10 larvae have the same weight for the above indicators. Due to environmental and ecological factors such as the size and water quality of containers, the number of containers varies greatly, and the impact on the spread of dengue fever is also different. Recently, scholars have suggested quantitative investigation to accurately control disease vectors.

Adult mosquito monitoring is a key method for measuring density, especially female *Aedes*, to directly measure the risk of dengue transmission. Traditional adult monitoring includes human attraction, breeding ground capture, mosquito trap lamp, net trap, anti-mosquito magnetic method and mosquito ovitrap method. The mosquito ovitrap monitors adults, eggs, larvae, and pupae at all life cycle stages, which shows that it can better reflect seasonal growth and detect the proportion of virus carrying. New advances in adult monitoring include attractors, BG traps [89], mosquito traps for *Aedes* gravidarum [90]. BG trap is a simple attraction and capture tool, which uses upstream air flow and visual temptation to attract *Aedes*, with high capture efficiency. Catching pregnant mosquitoes depends on the habit of pregnant *Aedes* laying eggs on the inner wall of the container. When pregnant mosquitoes lay eggs, the inner wall of the container is covered with a layer of viscose coating to catch them. According to the number of pregnant mosquitoes, the density and number can be calculated. In the field, door-to-door surveys need a larger sample size to avoid researchers' bias, and the trap method can measure short-term changes [87].

6.4.1.3 Forecast, Prediction, and 3S Technology

There is profound temporal and spatial heterogeneity in the transmission of dengue fever, which is related to population distribution, environment and media ecology [91]. 3S technology, including geographic information system (GIS), global positioning system (GPS) and remote sensing system (RS), provides a basic method to reveal this heterogeneity. Using 3S, we can obtain coordinates from GPS, geographic landscape data from RS involving land use, terrain, vegetation, hydrology and climate, and integrate GIS to analyze the relationship between human cases and susceptible population, media and environmental factors.

6.4.2 Control System and Organization

6.4.2.1 Vector Control

Vector control targets larvae and adults to eliminate or mitigate hazards. For larval control, clearing the breeding grounds container management (such as dumping, cleaning, inversion, and covering), social mobilization and education, environmental governance and legislation are important measures. Container operations also include controlled-release preparations (temephos), mosquitoes, copepods and dragonfly larvae. Social mobilization includes education, resource reduction, waste environmental treatment and health management. For adult control, space spraying, indoor residual spraying and personal protection of insecticides are conventional methods, especially relying on ultra-low volume outdoor spraying.

Although there are many vector control methods, the selection and application should be adjusted according to local conditions. Continuous vector management is essential to reduce *Aedes* mosquito density, including chemical control, container management, social mobilization, and legislation. Indoor spraying and residual spraying around lesions have been proved to be a successful method to eliminate *Aedes aegypti* in Tanzania, Greece from 2004 to 2006, and Groote Eylandt in northern Australia from 2006 to 2008 [92]. Source reduction and char spray are also effective in the Americas [93]. Indoor residual spray is neglected in many areas.

However, it can reduce both adult female mosquitoes and the transmission of dengue fever [94]. Indoor ultra-low volume spraying during early outbreak can significantly reduce the incidence rate [95]. In popular areas, because of the reduction in mosquito population and economic costs, it is not recommended to use ultra-low volume space spray installed in air and truck [87]. In addition, the use of DEET, insecticide-treated curtains and mosquito nets and covering water storage containers for personal protection of the public can reduce the number of disease vectors. Vacant sites, houses and dwellings, schools and workplaces are important epidemiological focuses. In addition, the failure of dengue control in some areas is mainly due to the lack of community participation. In addition, for the operational skills of vector control workers, financial investment will also affect the continuous control results.

Although vector control has achieved partial success in reducing the burden of dengue fever, drug resistance remains a prominent problem [96]. The development of pesticides has created efficient, long-lasting, healthy and environmental protection products. Vector control of chemical insecticides mainly depends on pyrethroids and temefos controlled-release preparations, showing shocking drug resistance. In addition, over time, the drug resistance of beta cypermethrin increased 258 times, and the drug resistance of deltamethrin increased 65 times in nine generations [97]. Drug resistance management should strengthen monitoring and classification guidance. Countermeasures include the selection of target insecticides, the application of synergists and mixed insecticides. In addition, the development of new insecticides and molecular insecticides are two ways to deal with this problem.

In recent years, new methods being developed have made progress. *Aedes albopictus* artificially infected with *Wolbachia* and transgenic mosquitoes aimed at reducing population and changing behavior are the most attractive.

The *Aedes albopictus* artificially infected with *Wolbachia* found in the ovary of *Culex* pipiens is a new entomological strategy developed by introducing the intracellular bacterium *Wolbachia* into *Aedes albopictus* [98]. It can spread rapidly into vector population by inducing cytoplasmic incompatibility (CI) [99] and leads to maternal transmission of *Wolbachia*-infected females. Once they mate with infected males, the embryos die. In addition, females infected with *Wolbachia* produce successful offspring, which is not dependent on males [98]. Maternal transmission can rapidly spread *Wolbachia* and make it highly colonized in wild populations. After enough generations, several mosquitoes infected with *Wolbachia* released to a limited area can replace the wild population [100]. *Wolbachia* can inhibit infection and replication in *Aedes albopictus* and human population, so as to control the epidemic of dengue fever [101]. wMelPop-CLA *Wolbachia* provides 65% starting frequency for fixation with minimum apparent adaptation cost and higher maternal genetic induced reproductive phenotype CI [100]. In a field trial in Australia, the *Wolbachia* infection rate remained above 90% 10 weeks after the release of *Aedes aegypti* [99]. Tests in Vietnam and Indonesia also showed satisfactory results. The main method to establish *Wolbachia* strain is microinjection. Adaptive invasion and fixation ability play a key role in successful application [100]. There is no evidence that insects infected with *Wolbachia* are harmful to humans or other vertebrates.

Significant progress has been made in reducing the population of transgenic *Aedes albopictus*, including a field trial. An interesting development is *Aedes aegypti* conditional lethality (RIDL). When transgenic males mate with females, they will lead to sterilization. In addition, only tetracycline was added to the larval feed to improve its productivity. In theory, once transgenic males enter the wild-type population and mate with normal females, almost 100% of their offspring will die in the late larval stage. However, this measure requires a lot of time and sustained release of strains. The experiment was carried out in Malaysia and Brazil. In addition, for this method, the field test must consider the public's response [87]. Another strain OX36404C can cause female death when removing tetracycline (fsRIDL) from larval feed. The reduction of mating competitiveness of transgenic males is the reason for the failure of outdoor field experiment [102]. For the new progress of gene-editing technology, especially CRISPR/cas9, transgenic mosquitoes are promising in vector-borne disease control [103].

Behavior change products that rely mainly on chemicals can prevent mosquitoes from looking for blood from humans, such as space repellents [104]. These active ingredients disrupt the sensation of biting a human host or changing a resting habitat. Metofluthrin has been shown to rapidly reduce mosquito bites and expel them from the home [105].

Among the biological pesticide control measures, environmentally friendly *Acillus thuringiensis* and *Bacillus sphaericus* have the ability to kill rapidly without non-target organisms. At present, they have become a good measure to control larvae.

Aedes aegypti, the main vector of dengue fever, inhabits or near human houses, while *Aedes albopictus* can inhabit areas far away from human houses. The flight distance is relatively short, with a radius of about 100 meters [106–108]. It implements the current basic theory of vector control, and each dengue country mainly focuses on vector control. As the control of mosquito-borne disease malaria has achieved greater results than vector control, dengue fever control benefits from its experience. However, insecticide-treated mosquito nets are not effective in controlling dengue fever. Compared with *Aedes*, *Anopheles* has different living habits. Therefore, Anopheles bites humans mainly at night and outside the urban ecosystem, causing less risk in urban areas [109]. *Aedes* mosquitoes are mainly concentrated in urban areas with high population density, and their biting behavior mainly occurs in the daytime. Since then, major scientific issues, including epidemiological characteristics, risk factors, virus diffusion, epidemic dynamics, human behavior, etc., need in-depth multidisciplinary and cross-regional research on driving factors [83].

6.4.2.2 Case Management

Treatment and isolation are two key case management methods. In public health practice, isolation is an important measure to alleviate transmission through isolation in hospitals or homes with anti-mosquito facilities. At present, this measure has not received enough attention. During the record outbreak of Guangzhou, isolation of infectious hospitals can reduce incidence rate or reduce geographic distribution, especially in the control of new cases [110]. The effect of family isolation control remains to be studied. Good case management of severe dengue fever can reduce mortality [111].

6.4.2.3 Health Education

Health education and protection are the contents of comprehensive prevention and control of dengue fever. Health education popularizes prevention knowledge and skills and guides the public to take appropriate personal behavior, so as to achieve the effect of population control. The control department can provide publicity, communication, electronic media, legislation and publicity days. In order to ensure effectiveness, publicity should be accurate, targeted and rapid for specific groups of people. The effectiveness of advocacy can be assessed through door-to-door surveys and telephone surveys to assess knowledge, attitudes and practices in dengue advocacy and control.

6.4.2.4 Protection of the Susceptible Population

No specific drugs or treatments have been developed. However, vaccine research is a top priority. The vaccine can improve people's immunity and reduce the prevalence of dengue fever. Dengue vaccine has been studied for more than 50 years, but it faces many challenges. The ideal vaccine should provide immunity against all four DENV serotypes, be safe for children and adults, avoid ADE and side effects, and maintain a balance between immunogenicity and reactivity, genetic stability, long-term protection and immunity, and convenient storage and transportation.

There are two factors that hinder the development of vaccines. One is the lack of animal models. The current mouse and monkey models have no or mild symptoms and no DHF/DSS performance. Another limitation is ADE. Specifically, after a serotype infection, secondary different serotypes can increase the risk of severe dengue fever caused by DHF/DSS. Severe dengue fever after secondary infection is associated with baseline antibody concentration, indicating concerns about safe and effective vaccine development [112].

Vaccine types include traditional vaccines, including live attenuated vaccine, inactivated vaccine, subunit vaccine, new tetravalent chimeric dengue fever (CYD) vaccine, DNA vaccine and virus-like particle vaccine. Due to ADE, there is a great risk in developing live attenuated and inactivated vaccines. Subunit vaccines cannot activate the appropriate immunity of dengue vaccine. Until 2015, six candidates participated in the clinical trial, and Sanofi Pasteur's CYD vaccine named Dengvaxia or CYD-TDV completed the phase III clinical trial, showing the protective effect on DENV-1, DENV-3 and DENV-4. However, the efficacy of DENV-2 is low [113]. It is a recombinant attenuated live tetravalent vaccine based on the 17D backbone of yellow fever [114]. In 2015, the vaccine was licensed for public use in the Philippines, Mexico and Brazil and registered in 20 countries until 2020. However, safety issues quickly emerged, increasing the risk of hospitalization for recipients who were not infected with dengue before vaccination [115]. Therefore, WHO recommended pre-vaccination screening should become the preferred strategy, and only seropositive individuals should be vaccinated. Recent advances have proposed two second-generation vaccines. In the experimental study, a candidate TV003/TV005 induced seroconversion of 74–92% of four DENV serotypes and granted near sterilization immunity in the vaccinated population, showing a good prospect [116]. Another candidate virus of Takeda (nct02747927, ClinicalTrials.Gov) contains an attenuated DENV-2 strain and a chimeric virus containing the prM and E genes of DENV-1,3 and 4, which is cloned into the attenuated DENV-2 backbone [117]. Whether the security of the two candidates is still under further study.

6.5 Future Challenge

In fact, dengue fever is a growing problem all over the world [19]. Despite tremendous efforts in the prevention and treatment of dengue fever and various measures taken in practice, the effect of dengue fever prevention is not obvious compared with the high incidence rate of dengue fever and the expanding geographical area, with no exception of developed countries, such as Singapore [118]. Therefore, basic science should focus on prevention, clinical treatment and vector control. Due to the limited use of dengue vaccine, prevention and vector control should be priorities. There is an urgent need to strengthen surveillance, especially population-based active surveillance, in order to accurately and comparably understand the epidemiology of dengue fever and assess the disease burden. In areas where medical infrastructure support is lacking, and dengue fever is neglected, it is important to improve medical awareness of early detection in larger geographical areas and develop and use advanced rapid laboratory testing. It is important to evaluate the effectiveness of the above control measures and make recommendations on best practices [11].

In the past two decades, scientists all over the world have made great progress in basic research. The comprehensive and multivariable control strategy is a consensus, and its core measures are vector control and complementary vaccine development. In the future, nanotechnology and omics will help to deeply understand the interaction between virus host and virus vector, and facilitate the development of diagnostic technology, treatment, prognosis, drugs, pesticides and vaccines. Enhanced surveillance and mathematical modeling contribute to understanding epidemic dynamics, biological behavior, vaccine efficacy, disease burden and cost-effectiveness assessment. In the research design, large-scale prospective cohort research, Internet-based big data technology and new decision support system are important research directions in the future. Improving the understanding of epidemiology will provide scientific and reasonable measures for governments to deal with this global public health challenge.

References

1. WHO. Dengue: guidelines for diagnosis, treatment, prevention and control: New Edition. 2009.
2. Halstead SB. Dengue vaccine development: a 75% solution? Lancet. 2012;380(9853):1535–6.
3. Sabchareon A, Wallace D, Sirivichayakul C, et al. Protective efficacy of the recombinant, live-attenuated, CYD tetravalent dengue vaccine in Thai schoolchildren: a randomised, controlled phase 2b trial. Lancet. 2012;380(9853):1559–67.
4. Kularatne SA. Dengue fever. BMJ. 2015;351:h4661.
5. Rigau-Perez JG. Severe dengue: the need for new case definitions. Lancet Infect Dis. 2006;6(5):297–302.
6. Cucunawangsih NL. Trends of dengue disease epidemiology. Virology (Auckl). 2017;8:1178122X17695836.
7. Simmons CP, Farrar JJ, Nguyen VV, et al. Dengue. N Engl J Med. 2012;366(15):1423–32.
8. Gan VC, Lye DC, Thein TL, et al. Implications of discordance in world health organization 1997 and 2009 dengue classifications in adult dengue. PLoS One. 2013;8(4):e60946.
9. Tsai CY, Lee IK, Lee CH, et al. Comparisons of dengue illness classified based on the 1997 and 2009 World Health Organization dengue classification schemes. J Microbiol Immunol Infect. 2013;46(4):271–81.
10. Narvaez F, Gutierrez G, Perez MA, et al. Evaluation of the traditional and revised WHO classifications of dengue disease severity. PLoS Negl Trop Dis. 2011;5(11):e1397.
11. Sharp TM, Tomashek KM, Read JS, et al. A new look at an old disease: recent insights into the global epidemiology of dengue. Curr Epidemiol Rep. 2017;4(1):11–21.
12. Wu JY, Lun ZR, James AA, et al. Dengue fever in mainland China. Am J Trop Med Hyg. 2010;83(3):664–71.
13. Shepard DS, Undurraga EA, Halasa YA. Economic and disease burden of dengue in Southeast Asia. PLoS Negl Trop Dis. 2013;7(2):e2055.
14. Selck FW, Adalja AA, Boddie CR. An estimate of the global health care and lost productivity costs of dengue. Vector Borne Zoonotic Dis. 2014;14(11):824–6.
15. Shepard DS, Undurraga EA, Betancourt-Cravioto M, et al. Approaches to refining estimates of global burden and economics of dengue. PLoS Negl Trop Dis. 2014;8(11):e3306.
16. Harrington J, Kroeger A, Runge-Ranzinger S, et al. Detecting and responding to a dengue outbreak: evaluation of existing strategies in country outbreak response planning. J Trop Med. 2013;2013:756832.
17. Bhatt S, Gething PW, Brady OJ, et al. The global distribution and burden of dengue. Nature. 2013;496(7446):504–7.
18. Katzelnick LC, Coloma J, Harris E. Dengue: knowledge gaps, unmet needs, and research priorities. Lancet Infect Dis. 2017;17(3):e88–e100.
19. Islam R, Salahuddin M, Ayubi MS, et al. Dengue epidemiology and pathogenesis: images of the future viewed through a mirror of the past. Virol Sin. 2015;30(5):326–43.
20. Lai S, Huang Z, Zhou H, et al. The changing epidemiology of dengue in China, 1990-2014: a descriptive analysis of 25 years of nationwide surveillance data. BMC Med. 2015;13:100.
21. Zhang SX, Wang Y, Yan L, et al. The epidemiological characteristics of dengue fever in China form 2005~2012. Guide China Med. 2013;23(6):401–2.
22. Luo H, Jianfeng HE, Zheng K, et al. Analysis on the epidemiologic features of dengue fever in Guangdong province, 1990–2000. Chin J Epidemiol. 2002;23(6):427–30.
23. Qiu FX, Chen QQ, Ho QY, et al. The first epidemic of dengue hemorrhagic fever in the People's Republic of China. Am J Trop Med Hyg. 1991;44(4):364–70.
24. Liu B. Development on attractant to Aedes alboPictus and Preliminary research on Prewarning indices of dengue. Guangzhou: Southern Medical University; 2010.
25. Luo L, Jiang LY, Xiao XC, et al. The dengue preface to endemic in mainland China: the historical largest outbreak by Aedes albopictus in Guangzhou, 2014. Infect Dis Poverty. 2017;6(1):148.
26. Luo H. Dengue control remains long way to go in China. South China J Prev Med. 2007;33(5):1–3.
27. Luo L, Yang Z, et al. The analysis of the epidemiologic features of dengue fever from 1978 to 2006 in Guangzhou, China. South China J Prev Med. 2008;26(8):490–3.
28. Dejnirattisai W, Jumnainsong A, Onsirisakul N, et al. Cross-reacting antibodies enhance dengue virus infection in humans. Science. 2010;328(5979):745–8.
29. Huang XY, Ma HX, Wang HF, et al. Outbreak of dengue fever in Central China, 2013. Biomed Environ Sci. 2014;27(11):894–7.
30. Kutsuna S, Kato Y, Moi ML, et al. Autochthonous dengue fever, Tokyo, Japan, 2014. Emerg Infect Dis. 2015;21(3):517–20.
31. Jing QL, Cheng Q, Marshall JM, et al. Imported cases and minimum temperature drive dengue transmission in Guangzhou, China: evidence from ARIMAX model. Epidemiol Infect. 2018;146(10):1226–35.
32. Gould EA, Solomon T. Pathogenic flaviviruses. Lancet. 2008;371(9611):500–9.
33. Whitehorn J, Farrar J. Dengue. Br Med Bull. 95:161–73.
34. Wang T, Wang M, Shu B, et al. Evaluation of inapparent dengue infections during an outbreak in southern China. PLoS Negl Trop Dis. 2015;9(3):e0003677.
35. Reiter P. Yellow fever and dengue: a threat to Europe? Euro Surveill. 15(10):19509.
36. Sessions OM, Barrows NJ, Souza-Neto JA, et al. Discovery of insect and human dengue virus host factors. Nature. 2009;458(7241):1047–50.
37. Guirakhoo F, Weltzin R, Chambers TJ, et al. Recombinant chimeric yellow fever-dengue type 2

virus is immunogenic and protective in nonhuman primates. J Virol. 2000;74(12):5477–85.
38. Yong HU, Chen Q, Zhi-Feng LI, et al. The survey of dengue virus and Japanese encephalitis virus in bats in several areas of Guangdong and Guangxi. J Trop Med. 2006;6(6):641–4.
39. Lavergne A, Lacoste V, Germain A, et al. Dengue virus infection in neotropical forest mammals: incidental hosts or potential reservoirs? Med Trop (Mars). 2009;69(4):345–50.
40. Thoisy B, Lacoste V, Germain A. Dengue infection in neotropical forest mammals. Vector-Borne Zoonotic Dis. 2009;9(2):157–70.
41. Maciel-de-Freitas R, Neto RB, Goncalves JM, et al. Movement of dengue vectors between the human modified environment and an urban forest in Rio de Janeiro. J Med Entomol. 2006;43(6):1112–20.
42. Guha-Sapir D, Schimmer B. Dengue fever: new paradigms for a changing epidemiology. Emerg Themes Epidemiol. 2005;2(1):1.
43. Dong Y, Zhao T, Xie C, et al. Study of transmission of dengue virus by Culex pipiens quinquefasciatus in laboratory. Chin J Vector Biol Control. 2000;11(5):363–7.
44. Wilder-Smith A, Chen LH, Massad E, et al. Threat of dengue to blood safety in dengue-endemic countries. Emerg Infect Dis. 2009;15(1):8–11.
45. Stramer SL, Hollinger FB, Katz LM, et al. Emerging infectious disease agents and their potential threat to transfusion safety. Transfusion. 2009;49(Suppl 2):1S–29S.
46. Teo D, Ng LC, Lam S. Is dengue a threat to the blood supply? Transfus Med. 2009;19(2):66–77.
47. Chen LH, Wilson ME. Dengue and chikungunya infections in travelers. Curr Opin Infect Dis. 23(5):438–44.
48. Lu L, Lin H, Tian L, et al. Time series analysis of dengue fever and weather in Guangzhou, China. BMC Public Health. 2009;9:395.
49. Luo L, Liang HY, Hu YS, et al. Epidemiological, virological, and entomological characteristics of dengue from 1978 to 2009 in Guangzhou, China. J Vector Ecol. 2012;37(1):230–40.
50. Ranjit S, Kissoon N. Dengue hemorrhagic fever and shock syndromes. Pediatr Crit Care Med. 12(1):90–100.
51. Kliks SC, Nimmanitya S, Nisalak A, et al. Evidence that maternal dengue antibodies are important in the development of dengue hemorrhagic fever in infants. Am J Trop Med Hyg. 1988;38(2):411–9.
52. Katzelnick LC, Montoya M, Gresh L, et al. Neutralizing antibody titers against dengue virus correlate with protection from symptomatic infection in a longitudinal cohort. Proc Natl Acad Sci U S A. 2016;113(3):728–33.
53. Coffey LL, Mertens E, Brehin AC, et al. Human genetic determinants of dengue virus susceptibility. Microbes Infect. 2009;11(2):143–56.
54. Kalayanarooj S, Gibbons RV, Vaughn D, et al. Blood group AB is associated with increased risk for severe dengue disease in secondary infections. J Infect Dis. 2007;195(7):1014–7.
55. Fink J, Gu F, Vasudevan SG. Role of T cells, cytokines and antibody in dengue fever and dengue haemorrhagic fever. Rev Med Virol. 2006;16(4):263–75.
56. Mason PW, Mcada PC, Mason TL, et al. Sequence of the dengue-1 virus genome in the region encoding the three structural proteins and the major nonstructural protein NS1. Virology. 1987;161(1):262–7.
57. Deubel V, Kinney RM, Trent DW. Nucleotide sequence and deduced amino acid sequence of the nonstructural proteins of dengue type 2 virus, Jamaica genotype: comparative analysis of the full-length genome. Virology. 1988;165(1):234–44.
58. Osatomi K, Sumiyoshi H. Complete nucleotide sequence of dengue type 3 virus genome RNA. Virology. 1990;176(2):643–7.
59. Mackow E, Makino Y, Zhao BT, et al. The nucleotide sequence of dengue type 4 virus: analysis of genes coding for nonstructural proteins. Virology. 1987;159(2):217–28.
60. Mustafa MS, Rasotgi V, Jain S, et al. Discovery of fifth serotype of dengue virus (DENV-5): a new public health dilemma in dengue control. Med J Armed Forces India. 2015;71(1):67–70.
61. Guzman MG, Halstead SB, Artsob H, et al. Dengue: a continuing global threat. Nat Rev Microbiol. 2010;8(12 Suppl):S7–16.
62. Zanotto PM, Gould EA, Gao GF, et al. Population dynamics of flaviviruses revealed by molecular phylogenies. Proc Natl Acad Sci USA. 1996;93(2):548–53.
63. Holmes EC, Twiddy SS. The origin, emergence and evolutionary genetics of dengue virus. Infect Genet Evol. 2003;3(1):19–28.
64. Guzman MG, Harris E. Dengue. Lancet. 2015;385(9966):453–65.
65. Lima Mda R, Nogueira RM, Schatzmayr HG, et al. A new approach to dengue fatal cases diagnosis: NS1 antigen capture in tissues. PLoS Negl Trop Dis. 2011;5(5):e1147.
66. Guzman MG, Jaenisch T, Gaczkowski R, et al. Multi-country evaluation of the sensitivity and specificity of two commercially-available NS1 ELISA assays for dengue diagnosis. PLoS Negl Trop Dis. 2010;4(8):e811.
67. Vazquez S, Cabezas S, Perez AB, et al. Kinetics of antibodies in sera, saliva, and urine samples from adult patients with primary or secondary dengue 3 virus infections. Int J Infect Dis. 2007;11(3):256–62.
68. Fry SR, Meyer M, Semple MG, et al. The diagnostic sensitivity of dengue rapid test assays is significantly enhanced by using a combined antigen and antibody testing approach. PLoS Negl Trop Dis. 2011;5(6):e1199.
69. Rainwater-Lovett K, Rodriguez-Barraquer I, Cummings DA, et al. Variation in dengue virus plaque reduction neutralization testing: systematic review and pooled analysis. BMC Infect Dis. 2012;12:233.

70. Peh AE, Leo YS, Toh CS. Current and nano-diagnostic tools for dengue infection. Front Biosci (Schol Ed). 2011;3:806–21.
71. Vaughn DW, Green S, Kalayanarooj S, et al. Dengue viremia titer, antibody response pattern, and virus serotype correlate with disease severity. J Infect Dis. 2000;181(1):2–9.
72. Lardo S, Utami Y, Yohan B, et al. Concurrent infections of dengue viruses serotype 2 and 3 in patient with severe dengue from Jakarta, Indonesia. Asian Pac J Trop Med. 2016;9(2):134–40.
73. Loke P, Hammond SN, Leung JM, et al. Gene expression patterns of dengue virus-infected children from Nicaragua reveal a distinct signature of increased metabolism. PLoS Negl Trop Dis. 2010;4(6):e710.
74. Allonso D, Vazquez S, Guzman MG, et al. High mobility group box 1 protein as an auxiliary biomarker for dengue diagnosis. Am J Trop Med Hyg. 2013;88(3):506–9.
75. Rathakrishnan A, Wang SM, Hu Y, et al. Cytokine expression profile of dengue patients at different phases of illness. PLoS One. 2012;7(12):e52215.
76. Zhu G, Liu T, Xiao J, et al. Effects of human mobility, temperature and mosquito control on the spatiotemporal transmission of dengue. Sci Total Environ. 2019;651(Pt 1):969–78.
77. Zhang Y, Bi P, Hiller JE. Climate change and the transmission of vector-borne diseases: a review. Asia Pac J Public Health. 2008;20(1):64–76.
78. Hu W, Clements A, Williams G, et al. Spatial patterns and socioecological drivers of dengue fever transmission in Queensland, Australia. Environ Health Perspect. 2012;120(2):260–6.
79. Wu PC, Lay JG, Guo HR, et al. Higher temperature and urbanization affect the spatial patterns of dengue fever transmission in subtropical Taiwan. Sci Total Environ. 2009;407(7):2224–33.
80. Cummings DA, Iamsirithaworn S, Lessler JT, et al. The impact of the demographic transition on dengue in Thailand: insights from a statistical analysis and mathematical modeling. PLoS Med. 2009;6(9):e1000139.
81. Barreto FR, Teixeira MG, Costa MC, et al. Spread pattern of the first dengue epidemic in the city of Salvador, Brazil. BMC Public Health. 2008;8(1):51.
82. Schmidt WP, Suzuki M, Thiem VD, et al. Population density, water supply, and the risk of dengue fever in Vietnam: cohort study and spatial analysis. PLoS Med. 2011;8(8):e1001082.
83. Stoddard ST, Forshey BM, Morrison AC, et al. House-to-house human movement drives dengue virus transmission. Proc Natl Acad Sci USA. 2013;110(3):994–9.
84. Du JW, Pan XH. Prevalent status and features of dengue fever in China. Chin J Epidemiol. 2010;31(12):1429–33.
85. Li X, Luo L, Xiao X, Jing Q, Wei Y, Li Y, et al. Using Breteau index to analyze the nature of sporadic and outbreak cases of dengue fever. Chin J Epidemiol. 2014;35(7):821–4.
86. Jing QL, Luo L, Xiao-Ning LI, et al. Associations of Breteau index, imported cases, and meteorological factors with the risk of local epidemic of dengue fever. South China J Prev Med. 2015;41(5):401–6.
87. Achee NL, Gould F, Perkins TA, et al. A critical assessment of vector control for dengue prevention. PLoS Negl Trop Dis. 2015;9(5):e0003655.
88. Cao Q, Jin QL, Yi-Lan LI, et al. The analysis of dengue antibody in patients with fever and thrombocytopenia in Guangzhou, 2012-2013. J Trop Med. 2015;15(4):552–4.
89. Cui L, Lee YH, Thein TL, et al. Serum metabolomics reveals serotonin as a predictor of severe dengue in the early phase of dengue fever. PLoS Negl Trop Dis. 2016;10(4):e0004607.
90. Gessner BD, Wilder-Smith A. Estimating the public health importance of the CYD-tetravalent dengue vaccine: vaccine preventable disease incidence and numbers needed to vaccinate. Vaccine. 2016;34(20):2397–401.
91. Guo P, Zhang Q, Chen Y, et al. An ensemble forecast model of dengue in Guangzhou, China using climate and social media surveillance data. Sci Total Environ. 2019;647:752–62.
92. Lee C, Jang EJ, Kwon D, et al. Laboratory-acquired dengue virus infection by needlestick injury: a case report, South Korea, 2014. Ann Occup Environ Med. 2016;28:16.
93. Castanha PM, Braga C, Cordeiro MT, et al. Placental transfer of dengue virus (DENV)-specific antibodies and kinetics of DENV infection-enhancing activity in Brazilian infants. J Infect Dis. 2016;214(2):265–72.
94. Vazquez-Prokopec GM, Kitron U, Montgomery B, et al. Quantifying the spatial dimension of dengue virus epidemic spread within a tropical urban environment. PLoS Negl Trop Dis. 2010;4(12):e920.
95. Stoddard ST, Wearing HJ, Reiner RC, et al. Long-term and seasonal dynamics of dengue in Iquitos, Peru. PLoS Negl Trop Dis. 2014;8(7):e3003.
96. Marcombe S, Darriet F, Tolosa M, et al. Pyrethroid resistance reduces the efficacy of space sprays for dengue control on the island of Martinique (Caribbean). PLoS Negl Trop Dis. 2011;5(6):e1202.
97. Guo F. Genetic form and resistance of beta-cypermethrin of Aedes albopictus skuse. Acta Parasitol Med Entomol Sin. 2001;8(2):103–8.
98. Lambrechts L, Ferguson NM, Harris E, et al. Assessing the epidemiological effect of wolbachia for dengue control. Lancet Infect Dis. 2015;15(7):862–6.
99. Hoffmann AA, Montgomery BL, Popovici J, et al. Successful establishment of Wolbachia in Aedes populations to suppress dengue transmission. Nature. 2011;476(7361):454–7.
100. Walker T, Johnson PH, Moreira LA, et al. The wMel Wolbachia strain blocks dengue and invades caged Aedes aegypti populations. Nature. 2011;476(7361):450–3.
101. Moreira LA, Iturbe-Ormaetxe I, Jeffery JA, et al. A Wolbachia symbiont in Aedes aegypti limits infec-

tion with dengue, chikungunya, and plasmodium. Cell. 2009;139(7):1268–78.
102. Tambo E, Chuisseu PD, Ngogang JY, et al. Deciphering emerging Zika and dengue viral epidemics: implications for global maternal-child health burden. J Infect Public Health. 2016;9(3):240–50.
103. Oye KA, Esvelt K, Appleton E, et al. Biotechnology. Regulating gene drives. Science. 2014;345(6197):626–8.
104. Chew CH, Goh PP, Lim TO. Dengue vaccine in regions of endemic disease. N Engl J Med. 2016;374(14):1388.
105. Saville M, L'Azou M, Noriega F. Dengue vaccine in regions of endemic disease. N Engl J Med. 2016;374(14):1388–9.
106. Harrington LC, Scott TW, Lerdthusnee K, et al. Dispersal of the dengue vector Aedes aegypti within and between rural communities. Am J Trop Med Hyg. 2005;72(2):209–20.
107. Maciel-de-Freitas R, Souza-Santos R, Codeco CT, et al. Influence of the spatial distribution of human hosts and large size containers on the dispersal of the mosquito Aedes aegypti within the first gonotrophic cycle. Med Vet Entomol. 2010;24(1):74–82.
108. Reiter P. Oviposition, dispersal, and survival in Aedes aegypti: implications for the efficacy of control strategies. Vector Borne Zoonotic Dis (Larchmont, NY). 2007;7(2):261–73.
109. Hay SI, Guerra CA, Tatem AJ, et al. Urbanization, malaria transmission and disease burden in Africa. Nat Rev Microbiol. 2005;3(1):81–90.
110. Jing QL, Yi-Lan LI, Chen ZQ, et al. Spatial pattern and driving factors of dengue virus-4 epidemics in Guangzhou. J Trop Med. 2016;16(2):244–8.
111. Schwartz LM, Halloran ME, Durbin AP, et al. The dengue vaccine pipeline: implications for the future of dengue control. Vaccine. 2015;33(29):3293–8.
112. Katzelnick LC, Gresh L, Halloran ME, et al. Antibody-dependent enhancement of severe dengue disease in humans. Science. 2017;358(6365):929–32.
113. Guy B, Barrere B, Malinowski C, Saville M, et al. From research to phase III: preclinical, industrial and clinical development of the Sanofi Pasteur tetravalent dengue vaccine. Vaccine. 2011;29(42):7229–41.
114. Wilder-Smith A, Ooi EE, Horstick O, et al. Dengue. Lancet. 2019;393(10169):350–63.
115. Normile D. Safety concerns derail dengue vaccination program. Science. 2017;358(6370):1514–5.
116. Kirkpatrick BD, Whitehead SS, Pierce KK, et al. The live attenuated dengue vaccine TV003 elicits complete protection against dengue in a human challenge model. Sci Transl Med. 2016;8(330):330ra36.
117. Osorio JE, Wallace D, Stinchcomb DT. A recombinant, chimeric tetravalent dengue vaccine candidate based on a dengue virus serotype 2 backbone. Expert Rev Vaccines. 2016;15(4):497–508.
118. Tatem AJ, Hay SI, Rogers DJ. Global traffic and disease vector dispersal. Proc Natl Acad Sci USA. 2006;103(16):6242–7.

Epidemiological Progress of Severe Fever with Thrombocytopenia Syndrome

7

Jiandong Li, Xiaoxia Huang, Fan Ding, Yi Li, Dexin Li, and Qun Li

Abstract

Severe fever with thrombocytopenia syndrome (SFTS) is a truly novel viral infectious disease firstly identified in 2010 in China, characterized by sudden onset of fever, thrombocytopenia, leukopenia, gastrointestinal symptoms, and rapid progression, and with a case fatality of approximately 10%. SFTS is widely distributed in China, and cases acquired through local transmission have also been reported in Japan, South Korea, Vietnam, and Thailand. SFTS virus is mainly transmitted by tick bites and can also cause human-to-human transmission through direct contact with patients and their bloody secretions. In nature, the transmission cycle of the SFTS virus between vertebrates and ticks has been established. The risk of SFTS virus infection among people working and living in epidemic areas cannot be completely avoided. However, if the basic knowledge of disease prevention and control could be widely disseminated in the public, the awareness of early diagnosis and treatment of SFTS could be improved among community or rural medical workers, which can effectively reduce the incidence rate and mortality of this disease. This paper mainly introduces the etiology, epidemiological characteristics, clinical treatment, prevention and control of SFTS, so as to provide a reference for staffs in related fields.

Keywords

Severe fever with thrombocytopenia syndrome virus · SFTS virus · Dabie bandavirus · Tick-borne infectious disease Bunyavirus · Emerging infectious disease

7.1 Introduction

Severe fever with thrombocytopenia syndrome (SFTS) is an acute viral infectious disease caused by severe fever with thrombocytopenia syndrome virus (SFTSV) [1], which is now named as *Dabie bandavirus* classified into a new species in the genus of *Bandavirus Phenuiviridae* family. SFTS was firstly found in Hubei Province in 2009. This disease is characterized by sudden onset of fever, thrombocytopenia, leukopenia, gastrointestinal symptoms, and rapid progression, and approximately 10% of hospitalized patients die from disseminated intravascular coagulation and/or multiple organ failures [2]. In China, the disease occurs mostly in mountainous and hilly areas.

J. Li · X. Huang · D. Li
NHC Key Laboratory of Biosafety, Key Laboratory of Medical and Viral Diseases of the Ministry of Health, National Institute for Viral Disease Control and Prevention, China CDC, Beijing, China

F. Ding · Y. Li · Q. Li (✉)
Public Health Emergency Center, Chinese Center for Disease Control and Prevention, Beijing, China

D.-Q. Ye (ed.), *Progress in China Epidemiology*, https://doi.org/10.1007/978-981-19-2199-5_7

Confirmed cases obtained through local transmission have been reported in South Korea, Japan, Vietnam, and Thailand [3–6].

7.2 Etiology

In 2009, SFTS caused widespread public attention and was called "Tick bite disease" by the public media. After laboratory testing, human granulocytic Anaplasma, leptospirosis, hemorrhagic fever with renal syndrome and Crimean-Congo hemorrhagic fever were excluded from the diagnosis. The former Ministry of Health named it "severe fever with thrombocytopenia syndrome". Subsequently, China CDC and international experts jointly explored the etiology of the disease, in 2010, a novel virus has been successfully isolated from patients' blood at acute stage, and completed the whole genome sequence analysis. Combined with the morphological characteristics of the virus, it was confirmed that the virus belonged to the genus *phlebovirus* of the now-dissolved family *Bunyaviridae*, named as severe fever with thrombocytopenia syndrome virus, SFTSV, and was identified as the cause of the disease [1]. In 2014, SFTSV was classified into a new *phlebovirus* species named SFTS virus by the International Committee on Taxonomy of Viruses (ICTV). Currently, the species was renamed Dabie bandavirus and was moved into a novel genus, *Bandavirus*, in the *Phenuiviridae* Family *Bunyavirales* Order.

7.2.1 Morphology and Structure

SFTSV was spherical or polymorphous under the negative staining electron microscopy, with a diameter of about 80–120 nm, and the surface of virus particles was lipid double-layer coating [1]. Glycoproteins were embedded in the lipid bilayer, and part of them protruded outward, showing a spike appearance. The spike is mainly a heterodimer composed of two viral glycoproteins. Ultrathin sections showed that the virus particles were filamentous or beaded, which might be ribonucleocapsid [1] (Fig. 7.1). X-ray tomographic reconstruction of a single viral particle showed that the internal structure of the virus particle was parallel or rod-shaped, which might be ribonucleoprotein (RNP). Some RNPs were very close to the envelope, suggesting the interaction between RNP and the cytoplasmic tail of glycoprotein [3].

The genome of SFTSV is a single strand of negative RNA, which is composed of three fragments, namely large (L), medium (M), and small (S). The 3′ and 5′ terminus of the genome fragment contain the same complementary nucleotide sequence, and the terminal sequence is highly conserved [1, 7]. The stable stem-loop structure and closed circular RNA can be formed by non-covalently base pairing. Three circular RNAs with different sizes were observed in the RNA extracted from virus particles under an electron microscope. Viral nucleocapsid protein contains a compact C-terminal core domain and an N-terminal extension arm that mediates nucleoprotein polycondensation, forming a hexamer ring structure, which combines with genomic RNA to form L, M, and S nucleocapsids respectively [1]. It is generally believed that these nucleocapsids are helical symmetric structures, but the analysis of RVFV nucleocapsids shows that the nucleocapsids are rope-shaped rather than helical symmetric structures. Under the electron microscope, the nucleocapsid of the virus treated with non-ionic detergent showed a round structure, which indicated that the base pair of the virus genome RNA could still be achieved in the case of binding with protein.

In order to ensure the infectivity, each virus particle should be packaged with at least one copy of L, M, and S nucleocapsid, but mature virus particles do not necessarily contain the same mole ratio of nucleocapsid [8, 9]. The different amounts of ribonucleoprotein in virus particles may be related to the size of virus particles under an electron microscope [10]. The virus particles of RVFV contain three fragments of cRNA, and at least one fragment of cRNA plays a role in the early stage of virus replication. S segment adopts double sense coding strategy. The mRNA

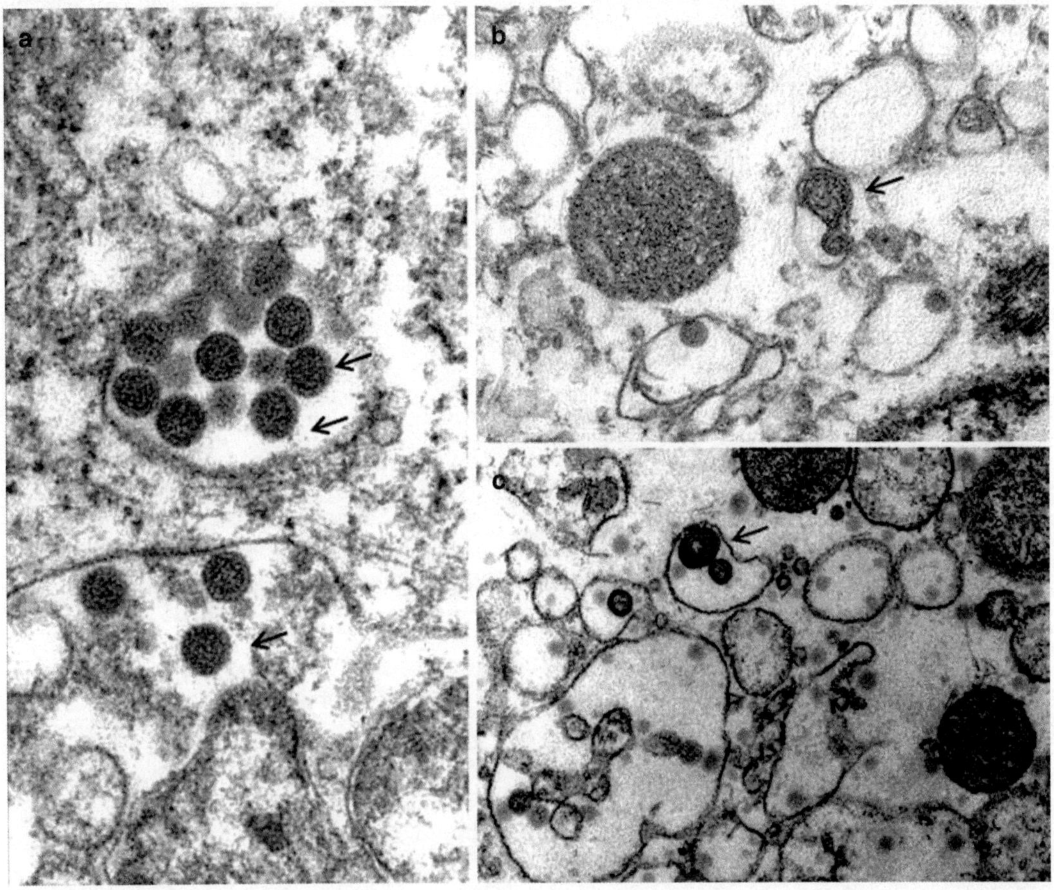

Fig. 7.1 The morphology of SFTS virus (×97,000) observed by transmission electron microscope. As shown by the arrow, the virus can be spherical (**a**) or polytypic (**b**, **c**)

encoding NSs is replicated from cRNA after genome replication. Therefore, NSs protein appears later than N protein after virus infection. However, if the virus particles contain cRNA, NSs and N protein can appear simultaneously after virus infection.

7.2.2 Resistance

SFTSV remained stable at 4 °C for 1 week, the virus titer decreased rapidly at 37 °C. The virus is sensitive to heat and could be inactivated at 60 °C for 30 min. It is sensitive to strong acid, alkali, ultraviolet, organic solvent, and chlorine disinfectant. At pH 3.0, the virus Infectivity was damaged, but the virus could not be completely inactivated.

7.2.3 Infectivity and Virulence

The infectivity and virulence of SFTSV are still not clear. The severity of the disease is related to the immune status, age and underlying medical conditions of the patient. The incubation period of SFTS is generally 5–15 days, and then presents fever, fatigue, and gastrointestinal symptoms. In the experiment, rodents, such as mice and hamsters, can infect SFTSV through muscle, subcutaneous, abdominal cavity, and intracranial injection, which can produce viremia and humoral immune response. The susceptibility to the virus is related to the species of the animals. Infection with c57/BL6 mice can also cause platelet reduction, serum glutathione and glutamine aminotransferase level elevating, and pathological changes in spleen, liver and kidney have been observed, but it cannot cause animal death [11]. Infection of rhesus monkeys only caused slight temperature rise, without obvious gastrointestinal and digestive tract symptoms, bleeding or central nervous symptoms [12].

7.3 Epidemiology

7.3.1 Epidemic Characteristics

1. Geographical distribution

   SFTS is widely distributed in China. Most of the reported cases are distributed in mountainous and hilly areas. The SFTS cases are highly sporadic, but the reported incidence varied significantly among regions, showing a certain regional cluster. Since the discovery of the disease in 2010, suspected or confirmed cases should be reported through the infectious disease reporting system within 24 h. It is similar to the report of category B infectious disease. From 2011 to 2020, 16,257 cases were reported in 26 provinces, and 10,832 laboratory diagnosed cases were reported in 24 provinces in China according to the infectious disease reporting system of China CDC. Among them, 99.25% (16,135 cases) of total reported cases and 99.46% (10,774 cases) of the confirmed cases were reported from 7 provinces, including Henan, Anhui, Hubei, Shandong, Liaoning, Zhejiang, and Jiangsu (Table 7.1). In the past 10 years, a total of 832 death cases were reported, almost all were reported from the above seven high incidence provinces, except for two deaths from Hebei and Jiangxi provinces respectively.

Table 7.1 Incidence and fatality of SFTS in China from 2011 to 2020

	Confirmed cases		Clinical cases		
Province	Cases	Fatality rate (%)	Cases	Fatality rate(%)	Total (case)
Shandong	3663	11.0	979	5.0	4642
Henan	2792	2.0	1812	0.2	4604
Anhui	1558	5.3	1356	2.6	2914
Hubei	1185	5.1	945	2.3	2130
Liaoning	615	4.1	253	0.0	868
Zhejiang	545	11.7	0	–	545
Jiangsu	416	6.3	16	6.3	432
Sichuan	4	0	19	5.3	23
Hunan	17	0	1	0	18
Jiangxi	8	12.5	2	0	10
Guizhou	2	0	6	0	8
Beijing	4	0	3	0	7
Guangxi	1	0	6	0	7
Shaanxi	3	0	3	0	6
Shanxi	1	0	4	0	5
Heilongjiang	3	0	2	0	5
Fujian	4	0	1	0	5
Tianjin	0	–	4	0	4
Hebei	2	50.0	2	0	4
Guangdong	1	0	3	0	4
Gansu	1	0	3	0	4
Jilin	1	0	2	0	3
Shanghai	3	0	0	–	3
Yunnan	2	0	1	0	3
Xinjiang	1	0	1	0	2
Neimenggu	0	–	1	0	1
Total	10,832	6.6	5425	2.1	16,257

In 2012, 4 fatal cases of SFTSV infection were reported in Japan, and 10 fatal cases were reported in South Korea from 2012 to 2013 [13, 14]. After that, there were persistent cases and deaths in both countries. In retrospect, the first two cases of SFTS were described in Japan in 2005 [15]. In addition, confirmed cases have been reported in Vietnam and Thailand [5, 6], and the United States reported similar cases caused by the heartland virus since 2012 [5, 6, 16].

2. Temporal Distribution

   SFTS mainly occurs in spring and summer, with a slight difference in different regions. Every year, cases appear in late March or early April. The number of cases increases gradually in April, reaches the peak from May to July, and then presents a downward trend. However, there will be a small peak again from September to October and decreases rapidly after November. Only a few cases are reported from December to February of the next year. See Fig. 7.2

3. Population distribution

   From 2011 to 2020, a total of 16,257 cases and 832 deaths were reported. Among them, 46.9% were male and 53.1% were female. The ratio of male to female is 1:1.13, but varied in different provinces. Among the seven provinces with high incidence, Henan, Hubei, Anhui, and Zhejiang provinces reported a high proportion of female cases, while Shandong, Liaoning, and Jiangsu provinces reported more male cases than female cases. This may be related to the living and working habits of people in different areas and the chances of contact with ticks. Most of the cases were farmers, mostly engaged in agriculture and forestry production, followed by housework and unemployment. People of all ages can have the disease, mainly in the range of 50–74 years old. The ages of death cases ranged from 37 to 95 years old, and the mortality increased with age. The age and gender distribution of SFTs cases in China from 2011 to 2020 is shown in Fig. 7.3

7.3.2 Host Animals and Vectors

The host animals and vectors of the disease need to be further studied. It has been confirmed that SFTSV could infect non-human primates such as rhesus monkeys, vertebrates such as cattle, sheep, goat dogs, and mice, as well as arthropods such as ticks. The virus did not cause death or serious

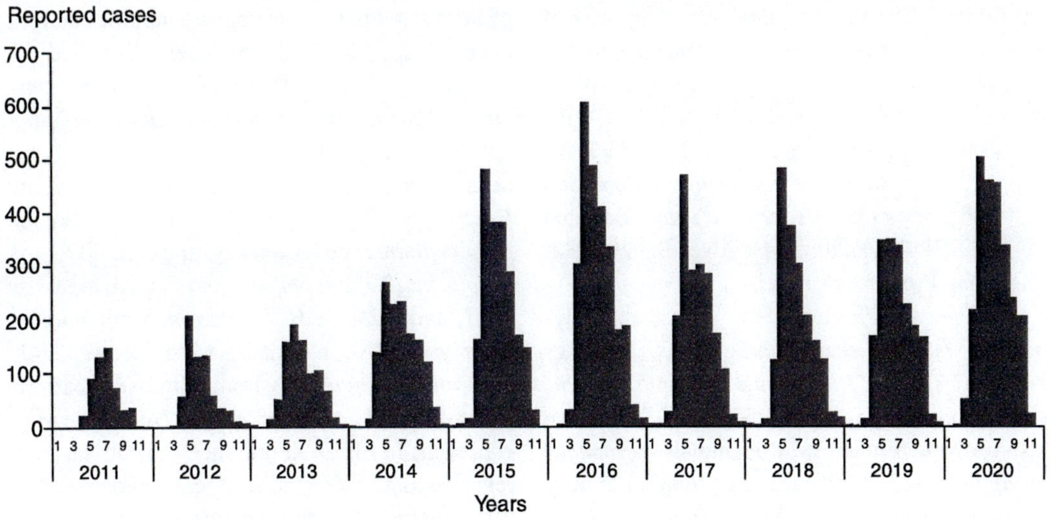

Fig. 7.2 Monthly distribution of SFTS cases in China from 2011 to 2020

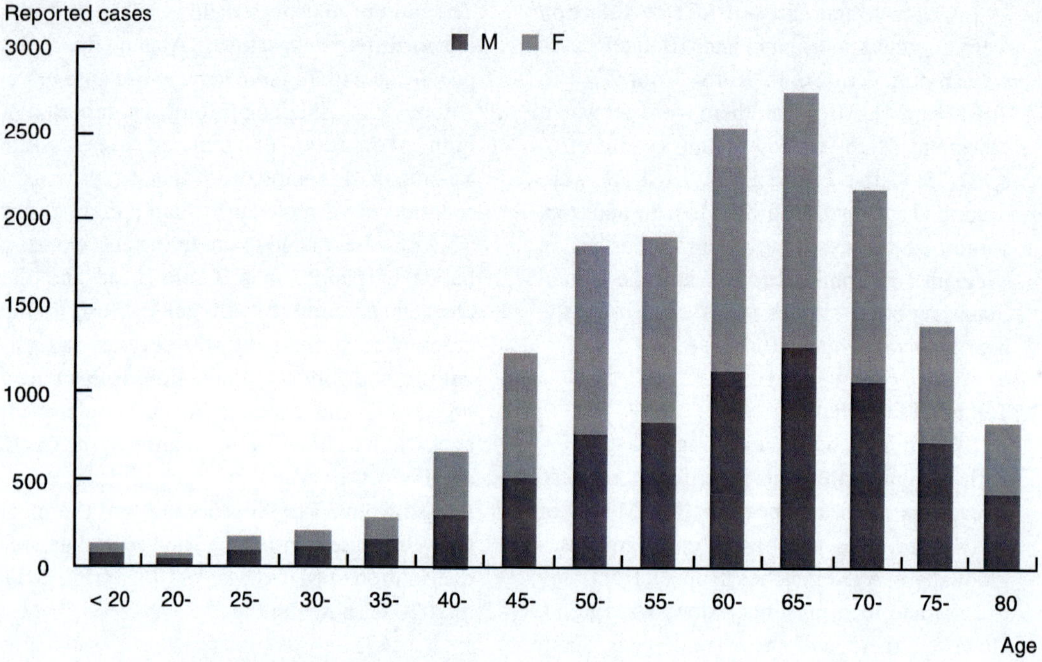

Fig. 7.3 Age and gender distribution of SFTS in China, 2011–2020

symptoms in rhesus monkeys and other vertebrates but could cause fever, thrombocytopenia, leukopenia, elevated transaminase, and myocardial enzymes [11, 12]. Serum prevalence surveys of SFTSV infection among domestic and wild animals revealed a high prevalence rate of virus antibody in the serum of cattle, sheep, goats, and dogs; however, the prevalence varies with different regions. The virus antibody-positive rates of sheep, cattle, dogs, pigs, and chickens in the Yantai area were 70%, 60%, 38%, 3%, and 47%, respectively [17, 18]. And 1.0% /1.1% of mice (*Mus musculus*/*Apodemus agrarius*), 0.9% of rats, 1.2% of hamsters (*Cricetulus tyiton*) and 2.6% of shrews (*Suncus marinus*) were detected to be SFTSV antibody-positive in 2013 at Shandong Province [19].

In Jiangsu Province, the virus antibody-positive rates of sheep, cattle, dogs, and pigs were 57.12%, 31.82%, 5.33%, and 0.98%, respectively [20], and antibodies to SFTSV have also been identified in wild mammals (*Erinaceus europaeus* and *Sorex araneus*) and migratory birds (*Anser cygnoides* and *Streptopelia chinensis*) [21]. Although animal infection rates vary from region to region, it was confirmed that cattle, sheep, dogs, and other vertebrates could be infected with SFTSV and induce antibodies in vivo, suggesting that they might play a role of hosts or intermediate hosts of the virus.

SFTSV is mainly transmitted by tick bites, viral RNA has been detected in ticks at all developmental stages. There are more than 120 species of ticks in China, belonging to 2 families and 11 genera [22]. SFTSV has been identified in *Haemaphysalis longicornis*, *Haemaphysalis concinna*, *Haemaphysalis flava* and *Rhipicephalus microplus*. The infection rate of SFTSV among ticks collected from animals was 4.00% of *Haemaphysalis longicornis* and 4.11% of *Rhipicephalus sanguineus* and 10.00% of *Rhipicephalus boophilus* from Yantai areas in 2011, and 0.2% of *H. longicornis* from Jiaonan County in 2013, in Shandong Province [23, 24]; 3.0% of *H. longicornis* from Jilin, Northeastern China [25]; 21.3% of tick pools (*Haemaphysalis concinna*) in Shaan xi province [26]. It was also reported that SFTSV nucleic acid was detected in *laelapsechidninus* and *Leptotrombidium scutellare* collected from Donghai County in Jiangsu

Province, suggesting that both mites can carry SFTSV [27]. In addition, SFTSV was identified in *Ixodes nipponensis* ticks from lizards and skinks, and in *Amblyomma testudinarium* from snakes in Republic of Korea [28].

7.3.3 Route of Transmission

SFTS is mainly transmitted by tick bites, and can also be transmitted from person to person through direct contact with the blood of infected persons [23, 29].

1. Tick bite

   Related studies suggest that *H. longicornis* is likely to be the main vector of SFTS. Some patients were able to recall history of tick bites within 2 weeks before onset or had definite skin damage before onset. The virus has been isolated from *H. longicornis* in the case finding area, which is highly homologous with the virus isolated from the patient. The viruses have been isolated from ticks collected from patients' body surface and from patients' blood, the genomic sequences of both viruses are identical [23, 30].
2. Human to human

   Human-to-human transmission of SFTS has been reported in China and Korea. People can get infected through direct contact with blood or bloody secretions from patients bearing SFTSV. Possibility of aerosol transmission has been reported [31], but it is very rare.

7.3.4 Susceptible Population

People are generally susceptible to the disease. People engaged in agricultural activities and living in mountainous, hilly and woodland areas, as well as people who go to such areas for tourism and outdoor activities, have a higher risk of infection. The seroepidemiological studies showed that the SFTSV antibodies rate ranged from 0.8% to 10% in general population in endemic areas [32, 33]. 922 healthy people from six districts and counties in Jiangsu Province were investigated, and the positive rate of SFTSV antibody was 0.94%; 237 healthy people from Yiyuan County in Shandong Province were investigated, and the positive rate of SFTSV antibody was 0.8% in 2011 [33]. In one seroprevalence survey in Hubei Province, SFTS antibody was detected in 8.4% of villagers between August 2012 and May 2013 [34]. 2126 healthy people from high incidence areas in Lu'an City in Anhui Province were investigated, and the positive rate of SFTSV antibody was 4.7% in 2014 [35]. In another investigation among a healthy population without previously reported SFTS in a mountainous area of Anhui Province, 6.3% of 270 participants was antibody-positive to SFTSV [36]. These results suggest that SFTS is widely distributed in China and the population is generally susceptible to the virus.

7.4 Clinical Features, Diagnosis, and Treatment

7.4.1 Pathogenesis

The pathogenesis of SFTS has not been fully elucidated. The infection process may be as follows: after the virus enters the human body by tick bite, it enters the local lymph nodes for replication, through the lymphatic system overflow into the blood, and spread to other organs. The virus replicates in lymph nodes, liver, spleen, etc., and then enters the blood again, causing high-level viremia. In the acute stage, the virus can cause disease through a direct cytopathic effect, and in the later stage, it can cause disease through immunopathological damage. The number of T cells in SFTS patients was significantly lower, while the proportion of NK cells increased, especially in the acute stage of severe SFTSV infection. NK cells produce cytokines such as interferon - γ, tumor necrosis factor (TNF) α, IL-10 and granulocyte colony-stimulating factor (G-CSF) to regulate the immune function. Virus infection can induce target cells to release excessive cytokines and form the inflammatory factor "storm," which can lead to pathological damage and play an important role in pathogenesis.

SFTSV can adhere to platelets, which can be recognized and engulfed by splenic macrophages, leading to thrombocytopenia. The virus can replicate in macrophages. In mouse models, macrophages can inhibit the growth of the virus and eventually eliminate it. However, in patients with immunosuppression, the virus can effectively proliferate and lead to multiple organ dysfunction or death.

Virus receptors on the cell surface participate in the process of virus adhesion and infection, which is the first step of virus infection and the decisive factor of virus pathogenesis. Pathogenic and nonpathogenic hantaviruses enter endothelial cells with beta3 and beta1 integrin receptors respectively [37, 38]. The interaction between viruses and integrin receptors interferes with cell-cell adhesion, resulting in the permeability of vascular system and increasing the specific diseases [39]. The replication of sandfly virus in vectors often results in high glycosylation of membrane proteins to high mannose glycoproteins. The dendritic cell surface non-integrin specific intercellular adhesion molecule-3-grabbing non-integral (DC-SIGN) contains carbohydrate recognition domain (CRD) can bind high mannose with high affinity and play an important role in the entry of a variety of sandfly viruses into cells [40, 41]. However, the cells that do not express DC-SIGN can also be infected by the virus. Blocking DC-SIGN can only reduce the level of infection, but can not prevent the virus from entering the cells, indicating that DC-SIGN is not a necessary condition for the virus to enter the cells.

7.4.2 Pathological Features

There are few pathological studies on SFTS patients. The autopsy results of the case died in acute stage due to SFTSV infection show that the liver microtubule system has slight fatty change, mild inflammation around the portal canal, and the renal can see bleeding under epidermis. The main pathological changes appear in lymph nodes, which are lymphocyte depletion, tissue cell infiltration and hemophagocytosis. The phagocytosis was observed in spleen [42]. This phenomenon of infiltration and abnormal enhancement of phagocyte function in peripheral lymphoid organs can also be found in animal infection models [11, 12]. The laboratory infection of C57/BL6 mice and non-human primates rhesus monkeys can cause thrombocytopenia, leucopenia, and viremia. Viral RNA and histopathological changes can be found in spleen, liver, and kidney, but virus replication is only found in spleen. After virus infection, the spleen, liver, and kidney organ of mice showed pathological changes. On the first day after infection, spleen lymphocytes decreased significantly. On the third day, the number of macrophages and platelets increased, and on the 14th day, the liver cells showed degenerative changes and necrosis, glomerular cells increased, marginal thickening, congestion, and lack of inflammatory response [11, 12]. Immunohistochemistry analysis showed that the virus was located in spleen macrophages. Immunofluorescence co-localization studies showed that SFTSV and platelet co-located in the cytoplasm of spleen macrophages, suggesting macrophages phagocytosis virus and platelets, and may also be the target cells for SFTSV infection replication [11, 12].

In vitro studies have found that SFTSV can adhere to human platelets and induce human macrophages to phagocytize platelets, but virus infection has no significant effect on the ability of macrophages to phagocytize platelets, suggesting that clearance of virus adhered platelets by spleen macrophages may play an important role in thrombocytopenia induced by SFTSV infection [11].

7.4.3 Symptoms and Signs

This disease is mostly acute onset. Clinical features mainly manifested as fever, the temperature is usually above 38 °C, and can reach 40 °C or more, and last more than 10 days in some severe cases. Often concomitant with fatigue, general pain, headache, anorexia, nausea, vomiting, and diarrhea. More than half of the patients had unilateral superficial lymph node enlargement with tenderness. Severe cases may have gastrointestinal bleeding, pulmonary hemorrhage, disturbance of consciousness, etc., and may die of shock, disseminated intravascular coagulation (DIC), and multiple organ failure. Patients with chronic underlying diseases have a high risk of severe illness.

The clinical course can be divided into three stages: initial, severe, and recovery stage: the initial stage is generally 1–5 days after the onset. The main clinical manifestations were fever (about 38 °C), fatigue, general soreness and gastrointestinal symptoms. Some patients had unilateral superficial lymph node enlargement with tenderness. At this stage, we can see the decrease of platelet and leucocyte, the increase of LDH, CK, ALT, and AST, and the positive detection of SFTSV RNA. The severe stage is generally 5–14 days after the onset, which is the critical period of clinical outcome. It is characterized by persistent high fever, body temperature up to 39 °C, aggravation of digestive tract symptoms, mental depression, drowsiness, convulsions and disturbance of consciousness in severe cases, skin and mucous membrane hemorrhage in some cases, DIC in severe cases, and interstitial pneumonia in a few cases. At this stage, multiple organ failure may occur, leading to death. Laboratory test showed that platelet and leukocyte decreased significantly, LDH, CK, ALT, AST and other serum enzyme activities increased significantly, and viral RNA test was positive. SFTSV IgM antibody and/or IgG antibody were positive. The recovery period is usually 2 weeks after the onset. The patient's temperature was normal, and the clinical indexes were normal or tended to be normal. The antibody titer of SFTSV increased four times or more.

7.4.4 Laboratory Examination

1. General test

   Blood routine examination, peripheral blood platelets decreased, mostly 30 ~ 60 × 10^9/L, severe cases can be lower than 30 × 10^9/L; white blood cell count decreased, mostly 1.0 ~ 3.0 × 10^9/L, severe cases can be reduced to below 1.0 × 10^9/L; neutrophil ratio, lymphocyte ratio is normal. Urine routine examination showed that more than half of the cases had proteinuria (+ ~ + + +), and a few cases had occult blood or hematuria. Biochemical examination showed that serum enzymes increased in different degrees, especially LDH, CK, ALT, and AST.

2. Specific test

   Detection of viral RNA, antigen or virus in patient's samples can make a diagnosis, which is generally applicable to patients at acute phase. Negative detection can not exclude SFTSV infection. The diagnosis can be made if the antibody titer in sera collected in convalescent phase is four times or higher than that in acute phase. Generally, IgM antibody can be detected 2–3 days after the onset of SFTS. IgM antibody in patients' serum lasts for a long period, and some patients can last more than 1 year. IgG antibody can be detected in most patients 7–10 days after onset, which can last for a long period; in a few severe patients specific antibodies can not be detected in serum from onset to death.

7.4.5 Diagnosis and Differential Diagnosis

The guidelines for the prevention and treatment of fever with thrombocytopenia syndrome (2010 Edition) issued by the National Health Commission of China in 2010 clearly require the diagnosis of the disease [43].

1. Diagnostic criteria

   SFTS can be diagnosed according to the epidemiological history (the history of working, living, or traveling in hills, forest areas, mountains, and other places during the epidemic season, or the history of being bitten by ticks within 2 weeks before the onset), clinical manifestations and laboratory test results. In general, it can be divided into the following two categories:

   ① Suspected cases: Patients with the above epidemiological history, fever, and other clinical manifestations were observed, and peripheral blood platelet and leukocyte decreased.

② Confirmed cases: The suspected cases have one of the following: the nucleic acid test of SFTSV is positive; the IgG antibody titer to SFTSV in the convalescent stage is more than four times higher than that in the acute stage; SFTSV is isolated from the patient.

2. Differential diagnosis

   It should be differentiated from hemorrhagic fever with renal syndrome, dengue fever, sepsis, typhoid fever, thrombocytopenic purpura, and other diseases.

7.4.6 Treatment

There is no specific treatment for SFTS, mainly symptomatic support treatment. Patients should rest in bed, their vital signs and urine volume should be closely monitored.

For the patients who can not feed or who are in critical condition, attention should be paid to supplement nutrition in time and ensure the balance of water, electrolyte, and acid-base, especially for the patients with hyponatremia. For patients with high fever, physical cooling can be used, if necessary, antipyretic drugs can be used. If there is obvious bleeding or platelet reduction (such as less than 30×10^9/L), plasma and platelet can be transfused. In patients with severe neutropenia (less than 1×10^9/L), granulocyte colony-stimulating factor is recommended.

The results of in vitro experiments suggest that ribavirin has an inhibitory effect on the virus and could be used for clinical treatment. Secondary bacterial and fungal infections should be treated with sensitive antibiotics. At the same time, pay attention to the treatment of underlying diseases. There is no evidence to prove the therapeutic effect of glucocorticoid, so it should be used cautiously.

Traditional Chinese medicine believes that this disease belongs to the category of "plague," which should be treated according to different stages of the disease.

7.4.7 Prognosis

More than 80% SFTS cases recovered within 2 weeks. Death in severe cases is usually due to multiple organ failure (MOF). Patients with one of the following situations indicate the patient's condition is critical and the prognosis is poor: chronic underlying diseases in the past; convulsions and disturbance of consciousness; intracavitary hemorrhage; more than one organ failure; laboratory tests show that the viral load continues to increase, platelets and leukocytes significantly decrease, LDH, CK, ALT and AST enzyme activities continue to increase.

7.5 Prevention and Control

1. Case management

   In the process of diagnosis, treatment, and nursing of patients, doctors and nurses should take biosafety and infection control measures. The confirmed cases should be hospitalized, and the severe cases, especially those with bleeding, should be isolated in a separate ward. In the rescue process of severe patients, especially when patients have hemoptysis, hematemesis, and other bleeding phenomena, standard protection and aerosol protection should be taken to avoid direct contact with patients' blood. The patient's blood, secretion, excreta, and the environment and articles polluted by them can be disinfected by spraying or/and soaking with chlorine disinfectant, high temperature and high pressure, etc.

2. Epidemic response capacity

   The awareness of case detection, the ability of diagnosis, report and proper treatment, as well as the ability of field epidemiological investigation, sample collection, laboratory testing and on-site disposal need to be strengthened. It is also necessary to strengthen the education and training of biosafety protection for relevant medical and health workers.

   The relevant government departments should organize and carry out environmental management in time to reduce tick breeding, and take measures such as killing ticks when necessary to reduce the density of ticks in the production and living environment.

3. Health education

   The key knowledge of prevention and control of SFTS should be actively and widely provided to the public through various channels, so that the people can enhance self-protection awareness, take timely and effective preventive measures to prevent the infection, and avoid social panic caused by the epidemic situation.

References

1. Yu XJ, Liang MF, Zhang SY, et al. Fever with thrombocytopenia associated with a novel bunyavirus in China. New Engl J Med. 2011;364:1523–32.
2. Ding F, Guan X-H, Kang K, et al. Risk factors for Bunyavirus-associated severe fever with thrombocytopenia syndrome, China. PLOS Negl Trop Dis. 2014;8(10):e3267.
3. Park S, Han M, Yun S, Park C, Lee W, Ryou J. Severe fever with thrombocytopenia syndrome virus, South Korea, 2013. Emerg Infect Dis. 2014;20(11):1880–2. https://doi.org/10.3201/eid2011.140888.
4. Kobayashi Y, Kato H, Yamagishi T, Shimada T, Matsui T, Yoshikawa T, Kurosu T, Shimojima M, Morikawa S, Hasegawa H, Saijo M, Oishi K, SFTS Epidemiological Research Group Japan. Severe fever with thrombocytopenia syndrome, Japan, 2013–2017. Emerg Infect Dis. 2020 Apr;26(4):692–9.
5. Tran X, Yun Y, Van An L, Kim S, Thao NT, Man PC, et al. Endemic severe fever with thrombocytopenia syndrome, Vietnam. Emerg Infect Dis. 2019;25(5):1029–31. https://doi.org/10.3201/eid2505.181463.
6. Daengnoi C, Ongkittikul S, Watanawong R, Rompho P. Severe fever with thrombocytopenia syndrome virus: the first case report in Thailand. BKK Med J. 2020;16(2):204–6.
7. Elliot RM, Schmaljohn CS. Bunyaviridae. In: Knipe DM, Howley PM, editors. Fields virology. Philadelphia, PA: Lippincott Williams & Wilkins; 2013. p. 1244–77.
8. Bishop D, Shope R. Bunyaviridae. In: Fraenkel-Conrat H, Wagner RR, editors. Comprehensive virology, vol. 14. New York: Plenum Press; 1979. p. 1–156.
9. Hutchinson KL, Peters CJ, Nichol ST. Sin Nombre virus mRNA synthesis. Virology. 1996;224(1):139–49.
10. Talmon Y, Prasad BV, Clerx JP, et al. Electron microscopy of vitrified-hydrated La Crosse virus. J Virol. 1987;61(7):2319–21.
11. Jin C, Liang M, Ning J, et al. Pathogenesis of emerging severe fever with thrombocytopenia syndrome virus in C57/BL6 mouse model. PNAS. 2012;109(25):10053–8.
12. Jin C, Jiang H, Liang M, et al. SFTS virus infection in nonhuman primates. J Infect Dis. 2015 Mar 15;211(6):915–25.
13. Shimojima M, Fukushi S, Tani H, Yoshikawa T, Morikawa S, Saijo M. Severe fever with thrombocytopenia syndrome in Japan. Uirusu. 2013;63(1):7–12.
14. Kim KH, Yi J, Kim G, Choi SJ, Jun KI, Kim NH, Choe PG, Kim NJ, Lee JK, Oh MD. Severe fever with thrombocytopenia syndrome, South Korea, 2012. Emerg Infect Dis. 2013 Nov 19;11:1892–4.
15. Kurihara S, Satoh A, Yu F, Hayasaka D, Shimojima M, Tashiro M, Saijo T, Takazono T, Imamura Y, Miyazaki T, Tsukamoto M, Yanagihara K, Mukae H, Saijo M, Morita K, Kohno S, Izumikawa K. The world first two cases of severe fever with thrombocytopenia syndrome: an epidemiological study in Nagasaki, Japan. J Infect Chemother. 2016 Jul;22(7):461–5.
16. Bosco-Lauth AM, Panella NA, Root JJ, et al. Serological investigation of heartland virus (Bunyaviridae: Phlebovirus) exposure in wild and domestic animals adjacent to human case sites in Missouri 2012–2013. Am J Trop Med Hyg. 2015;92(6):1163–7.
17. Zhao L, Zhai SY, Wen HL, et al. Severe fever with thrombocytopenia syndrome virus, Shandong Province, CHina. Emerg Infect Dis. 2012;18(6):963–5.
18. Cui F, Cao HX, Wang L, et al. Clinical and epidemiological study on severe fever with thrombocytopenia syndrome in Yiyuan County, Shandong Province, China. Am J Trop Med Hyg. 2013;88(3):510–2.
19. Liu JW, Wen HL, Fang LZ, Zhang ZT, He ST, Xue ZF, Ma DQ, Zhang XS, Wang T, Yu H, Zhang Y, Zhao L, Yu XJ. Prevalence of SFTSV among Asian house shrews and rodents, China, January–August 2013. Emerg Infect Dis. 2014 Dec;20(12):2126–8.
20. Wenshuai Z, Xiaoyan Z, Minghao Z, Yongjun J, Tian W, Xiling G, Xian Q, Zhiyang S. Seroepidemiology of severe fever with thrombocytopenia syndrome bunyavirus in Jiangsu Province. Dis Surv. 2011;26(9):676–8.
21. Li Z, Bao C, Hu J, Liu W, Wang X, Zhang L, Ji Z, Feng Z, Li L, Shen A, Liu X, Zhao H, Tan W, Zhou J, Qi X, Zhu Y, Tang F, Cardona CJ, Xing Z. Ecology of the Tick-Borne Phlebovirus causing severe fever with thrombocytopenia syndrome in an endemic area of China. PLoS Negl Trop Dis. 2016 Apr;10(4):e0004574.
22. Chaopin L, editor. Medical arthropodology. Beijing: People's Medical Publishing House; 2009. p. 1702.
23. Wang S, Li J, Niu G, Wang X, Ding S, Jiang X, Li C, Zhang Q, Liang M, Bi Z, Li D. SFTS virus in ticks in an endemic area of China. Am J Trop Med Hyg. 2015 Apr;92(4):684–9.
24. Luo LM, Zhao L, Wen HL, Zhang ZT, Liu JW, Fang LZ, Xue ZF, Ma DQ, Zhang XS, Ding SJ, Lei XY, Yu XJ. Haemaphysalis longicornis ticks as reservoir and vector of severe fever with thrombocytopenia

syndrome Virus in China. Emerg Infect Dis. 2015 Oct;21(10):1770–6.
25. Liu H, Li Z, Wang Z, He B, Wang S, Wei F, Tu C, Liu Q. The first molecular evidence of severe fever with thrombocytopenia syndrome virus in ticks in Jilin, Northeastern China. Ticks Tick Borne Dis. 2016 Oct;7(6):1280–3.
26. Tian H, Yu P, Chowell G, Li S, Wei J, Tian H, Lv W, Han Z, Yang J, Huang S, Zhou S, Brownstein JS, Wang J, Xu B. Severe fever with thrombocytopenia syndrome virus in humans, domesticated animals, ticks, and mosquitoes, Shaanxi Province, China. Am J Trop Med Hyg. 2017 Jun;96(6):1346–9.
27. Qing-Kui W, Heng-Ming G, Zhi-Feng L, Yun-Feng S, Lan C, Yan-Ping W. Vector research of severe fever with thrombocytopenia syndrome virusin gamasid mites and chigger mites. Chin J Vector Biol Control. 2012;23(5):452–4.
28. Suh JH, Kim HC, Yun SM, Lim JW, Kim JH, Chong ST, Kim DH, Kim HT, Kim H, Klein TA, Johnson JL, Lee WJ. Detection of SFTS Virus in Ixodes nipponensis and Amblyomma testudinarium (Ixodida: Ixodidae) collected from reptiles in the Republic of Korea. J Med Entomol. 2016;53(3):584–90.
29. Bao CJ, Guo XL, Qi X, et al. A family cluster of infections by a newly recognized bunyavirus in Eastern China, 2007: further evidence of person-to-person Transmission. Clin Infect Dis. 2011;53:1208–14.
30. Niu G, Li J, Liang M, et al. Severe fever with thrombocytopenia syndrome virus among domesticated animals, China. Emerg Infect Dis. 2013;5:756–63.
31. Gong Z, Gu S, Zhang Y, Sun J, Wu X, Ling F, Shi W, Zhang P, Li D, Mao H, Zhang L, Wen D, Zhou B, Zhang H, Huang Y, Zhang R, Jiang J, Lin J, Xia S, Chen E, Chen Z. Probable aerosol transmission of severe fever with thrombocytopenia syndrome virus in southeastern China. Clin Microbiol Infect. 2015 Dec;21(12):1115–20.
32. Ni H, Yang F, Li Y, Liu W, Jiao S, Li Z, Yi B, Chen Y, Hou X, Hu F, Ding Y, Bian G, Du Y, Xu G, Cao G. Apodemus agrarius is a potential natural host of severe fever with thrombocytopenia syndrome (SFTS)-causing novel bunyavirus. J Clin Virol. 2015 Oct;71:82–8.
33. Zhao L, Zhai S, Wen H, Cui F, Chi Y, Wang L, Xue F, Wang Q, Wang Z, Zhang S, Song Y, Du J, Yu XJ. Severe fever with thrombocytopenia syndrome virus, Shandong Province, China. Emerg Infect Dis. 2012 Jun;18(6):963–5.
34. Xing X, Guan X, Liu L, Zhan J, Jiang H, Liu L, Li G, Xiong J, Tan L, Xu J, Jiang Y, Yao X, Zhan F, Nie S. Natural transmission model for severe fever with thrombocytopenia syndrome bunyavirus in villages of Hubei Province, China. Medicine (Baltimore). 2016 Jan;95(4):e2533.
35. Lyu Y, Ding F, Sun J, Xu PP, Hu JY, Xie SY, Li KC, Chang HW, Qin W, Yu L, Xie H, Li GJ, Yang CW, Huang XX, Wang Q, Zhang XJ. Seroprevalence and risk factors of severe fever with thrombocytopenia syndrome virus infection in endemic areas. Infect Dis (Lond). 2016 Jul;48(7):544–9.
36. Huang X, Zhang Z, Jin G, Wang X, Tan C, Yin H, Wang S. Presence of antibodies against severe fever with thrombocytopenia syndrome virus in non-endemic areas of China. Jpn J Infect Dis. 2017 May 24;70(3):248–51.
37. Schneider-Schaulies J. Cellular receptors for viruses: links to tropism and pathogenesis. J Gen Virol. 2000;81:1413–29.
38. Gavrilovskaya IN, Brown EJ, Ginsberg MH, Mackow ER. Cellular Entry of Hantaviruses which cause hemorrhagic fever with renal syndrome is mediated by beta3 Integrins. J Virol. 1999;73:3951–9.
39. Gavrilovskaya IN, Shaw R, et al. Beta3 integrins mediate the cellular entry of Hantaviruses that cause respiratory failure. Proc Natl Acad Sci USA. 1998;95:7074–9.
40. Gavrilovskaya IN, Peresleni T, Geimonen E, Mackow ER. Pathogenic hantaviruses selectively inhibit beta3 integrin directed endothelial cell migration. Arch Virol. 2002;147:1913–31.
41. Lozach P-Y, Kühbacher A, Meier R, Mancini R, Bitto D, Bouloy M, Helenius A. DC-SIGN as a receptor for phleboviruses. Cell Host Microbes. 2011;10:75–88.
42. Hofmann H, Li X, Zhang X, Liu W, Kühl A, Kaup F, Soldan SS, González-Scarano F, Weber F, He Y, Pöhlmann S. Severe fever with thrombocytopenia virus glycoproteins are targeted by neutralizing antibodies and can use DC-SIGN as a receptor for pH-dependent entry into human and animal cell lines. J Virol. 2013;87(8):4384–94.
43. China National Health and Family Planning Commission. Guideline for prevention and treatment of sever fever with thrombocytopenia syndrome (2010 version). Chin J Clin Infect Dis. 2011;4:193–4.

8 Progress in Epidemiology of Tuberculosis in China

Wei Lu, Limei Zhu, Qiao Liu, Cheng Chen, Peng Lu, Xiaoyan Ding, Yan Shao, and Yan Li

Abstract

9870 thousand people develop tuberculosis (TB) in 2020. Despite being a preventable as well as curable communicable disease, tuberculosis still is the leading communicable disease killer globally. The WHO's End TB Strategy envisions a world free of TB, zero deaths, disease, and suffering due to tuberculosis by 2035. China ranks second for TB cases globally. Over the past 20 years, China has made remarkable achievements in tuberculosis control, with the prevalence and mortality rate of tuberculosis reduced by half compared with 1990. China has achieved the United Nations Millennium Development Goals on tuberculosis control 5 years ahead of schedule. However, in spite of concerted international, regional, and national efforts to address tuberculosis in China, the tuberculosis burden in China is still high. At the same time, China also faces problems such as the high burden of latent TB infection, rifampicin-resistant/multidrug-resistant tuberculosis, and low detection rate of tuberculosis. China needs to further improve the quality of tuberculosis control work to reduce the incidence of tuberculosis and ultimately achieve the goal of ending tuberculosis.

Keywords

Tuberculosis · Epidemiology · Drug resistance · Tuberculosis complications COVID-19

8.1 Introduction

Tuberculosis (TB) is a communicable disease caused by *Mycobacterium tuberculosis*. 9870 thousand people develop tuberculosis (TB) in 2020 with an estimated incidence rate 127/100,000, which has been declining at a slow pace in recent years [1]. The TB incidence rate is falling, but not fast enough to achieve TB elimination [2]. Worldwide, the cumulative reduction from 2015 to 2019 was only 9%, considerably lower than WHO's End TB Strategy first milestone. In China, 833,000 TB cases accounted for 8.4% of all estimated incident cases worldwide. The estimated TB incidence rate in the country in 2019 was 58 cases per 100,000 population.

Globally, in 2019, nearly half a million people have been diagnosed with multidrug-resistant TB (MDR-TB)/rifampicin-resistant TB (RR-TB). The three countries with the largest share of the global MDR-TB burden were India (27%), China (14%), and The Russian Federation (8%). An

W. Lu (✉) · L. Zhu · Q. Liu · C. Chen · P. Lu
X. Ding · Y. Shao · Y. Li
Department of Chronic Communicable Disease, Center for Disease Control and Prevention of Jiangsu Province, Nanjing, Jiangsu Province, People's Republic of China

D.-Q. Ye (ed.), *Progress in China Epidemiology*, https://doi.org/10.1007/978-981-19-2199-5_8

estimated 70,000 new rifampicin-resistant tuberculosis patients occur each year in China, ranking the second highest in the world [1]. There are clear regional differences in the *Mycobacterium tuberculosis* (MTB) infection rate, tuberculosis morbidity, and mortality in China [3]. Tuberculosis rates are substantially higher in rural compared to urban areas and also substantially higher in the west compared to regions in the Central and Eastern regions. Tuberculosis has become among the primary infectious diseases resulting in the return of poverty in rural China. It is a nonnegligible issue in the construction of Healthy China. The government has given importance to the prevention and treatment of tuberculosis and regards tuberculosis as one of the most important diseases in the nation. This chapter summarizes the epidemiology of tuberculosis through discussion of latent tuberculosis infection, active tuberculosis, drug resistance, tuberculosis comorbidities, prevention and control of tuberculosis in key populations, and the impact of the COVID-19 epidemic on tuberculosis control to describe the epidemiology of tuberculosis in China.

8.2 Epidemiology of Latent Tuberculosis Infection

8.2.1 Overview

The "End TB Strategy" aims to reduce TB incidence to fewer than 10 cases per 105 people per year by 2035 [2]. The primary method for achieving this target is to improve efforts to find and treat persons with active TB disease, conduct universal screening of individuals at high risk, and provide preventive therapy for those at risk of progressing to active TB disease [1]. Latent *Mycobacterium tuberculosis* infection (LTBI) is defined by WHO as "a situation of persistent immune response to antigens with no evidence of clinically active tuberculosis disease" [4, 5]. It was estimated that 1.7 billion people have LTBI in the world, and 10% of them are at risk of reactivating into active disease during a lifetime [6]. Around 5% persons infected with TB progress rapidly to active disease, while most of them develop a latent infection and remain at risk for progression to active disease [7]. For persons with latent TB infection, the host maintains a dynamic relationship with *M. tuberculosis* [8].

China has 842,000 tuberculosis patients each year according to WHO report [1]. Even worse, the LTBI persons would contribute to new tuberculosis cases, especially for the rural areas of China as tuberculosis cases from the rural areas accounted for a major proportion of tuberculosis. The results of the fourth Chinese national tuberculosis epidemiological survey in 2000 showed that the average diameter of induration in tuberculin skin test (TST) ≥6 mm for all age groups was 44.5%, ≥10 mm was 28.3%, ≥15 mm was 16.5%, ≥20 mm it was 7.6%. In the TST for children aged 0 to 14 years, the average diameter of induration ≥6 mm is 8.5%, ≥10 mm is 4.5%, and ≥ 15 mm is 2.6% [9]. At the same time, the National Health and Nutrition Survey of the United States from 1999 to 2000 showed that the whole population infection rate of [define the TST induration diameter ≥ 10 mm as positive] was about 4.2% [10], which was extremely lower compared to China.

In the last two decades, great progress has been made in controlling and preventing TB in China. However, the rate of LTBI was not declined as the same speed as the number of TB cases. In 2013, China conducted an epidemiological survey on LTBI with a population of 23,483 participants. The age-standardized and sex-standardized rates of TST positivity (≥10 mm) ranged from 15% to 42%, and the QuantiFERON-TB Gold In-Tube positivity rates ranged from 13% to 20%. This data demonstrated LTBI was still a major issue for TB control in China [11].

8.2.2 Diagnostics of LTBI

Currently, three LTBI tests are recommended by WHO: TST and two interferon-γ release assays (IGRAs), QuantiFERON-TB Gold In-Tube and

T-SPOT TB. Of note, TST and IGRAs cannot differentiate between LTBI and active disease and they should not be used as diagnostic tests for active tuberculosis. Until a decade ago, the only available test for diagnosing LTBI was TST. This involves intradermal injection of MTB antigens and subsequent observation for the induction of cutaneous induration resulted in a delayed-type hypersensitivity response to the antigens [12].

Although TST was inexpensive and simple, there are several limitations associated with the TST. Fundamentally, the test requires a second visit to have the degree of induration assessed. Of particular importance, the test might be affected by prior vaccination with Bacille Calmette–Guérin (BCG) and can produce false positive results in individuals exposed to non-tuberculosis mycobacteria [13]. In China, the prevalence of latent tuberculosis might be overestimated by TST compared to interferon-γ release assays [11]. Furthermore, the TST has lower sensitivity in patients with immunosuppression [14], for example, in young children [13] and individuals with HIV co-infection [15]. These patients represent those most at risk of developing active disease.

IGRAs detect host immune response to MTB antigens in vitro. Commercially, two IGRAs based tests are available and recommended for use in the diagnosis of LTBI. These are branded TSPOT.TB and QuantiFERON Gold In-Tube. Currently, ESAT-6, CFP-10, and TB7.7 were incorporated for IGRAs detection. IGRAs based assays are based on the principle that, upon exposure to MTB antigens in vitro, antigen-specific T cells (both CD4+ and CD8+) present in the blood become activated and secrete IFNγ, a pro-inflammatory cytokine T.

8.2.3 Future Perspectives

A strong public health response will require new diagnostic tools and therapeutic methods along with a better understanding of the microbiological and clinical spectrum of TB infection and the disease. While there are concentrated efforts to develop a new vaccine for TB, but this alone may not be enough to end the TB epidemic [16].

Studies have revealed that age, male gender, smoking, overweight, and close TB contacting might be risk factors for LTBI, while BCG vaccination would be a protective factor for LTBI [17]. Another difficult situation is that the preventive treatment regimens might not be suitable for persons with LTBI who have been exposed to multidrug-resistant tuberculosis or extensively drug-resistant tuberculosis [18]. About one in four individuals is estimated to be infected with *M. tuberculosis*. Whether into active TB depends on several factors, the most important weakened immunological status. There is no gold standard test to diagnose LTBI. The TST and IGRA are currently the most widely used tests for the LTBI.

8.2.4 Recommended Populations for LTBI Testing

The considerations of identifying those are likely to progress to tuberculosis, it is imperative to identify LTBI in high-risk populations, and provide prophylactic treatment of LTBI for the prevention of TB reactivation. The high-risk groups according to the WHO recommendations are as follows:

1. Children aged <5 years old who are household contacts of individuals with bacteriologically confirmed pulmonary TB and who are found not to have active TB.
2. Persons living with HIV (PLWH) or HIV sufferers, or individuals who do not have a positive HIV infection that the clinician considers necessary for treatment who are unlikely to have active TB.
3. Students who are in close contact with confirmed active TB patients and are newly infected with latent infection.
4. Individuals who are initiating anti-TNF treatment, receiving dialysis, preparing for organs or hematological transplant, and who have silicosis.

8.2.5 Preventive Treatment Regimen

The principle of providing preventive treatment regimen for high-risk population is in high priority. Literatures have showed that isoniazid for 6 months and rifampicin for 3–4 months will significantly decrease the risk of developing TB. The recommended preventive treatment for LTBI is shown in Table 8.1.

8.2.5.1 Daily Isoniazid Monotherapy

Daily isoniazid monotherapy is the most recommended treatment therapy in China. The efficacy of daily isoniazid monotherapy (6 months or more) has been confirmed in different individuals and settings in certain systematic reviews. A recent systematic review said that daily isoniazid monotherapy could reduce the overall risk for active TB by 33% (RR 0.67; 95% CI 0.51–0.87), and the preventive efficacy achieved 64% for individuals with a positive TST (RR 0.36; 95% CI 0.22–0.61) [19]. Besides, the efficacy of the 6-month daily isoniazid monotherapy regimen showed no significant difference from that of 12 months (RR 0.58; 95% CI 0.3–1.12) [19]. Furthermore, a recent systematic review also showed a high reduction in TB incidence among participants who have 6-month daily isoniazid monotherapy than in those with placebo (odds ratio, 0.65; 95% CI 0.50–0.83) [20].

8.2.5.2 Weekly Rifapentine Plus Isoniazid

The greatest advantage of weekly rifapentine plus isoniazid is individuals just need to take medicine twice a week, which is easy be accepted. Four reviews have evaluated the efficacy of this regimen [21–24]. Two of the four involved adults with HIV from South Africa showed no statistic difference in the incidence of active TB between two regimen of a 3-month weekly regimen of isoniazid plus rifapentine and 6 or 9 months of isoniazid monotherapy (RR = 0.73, 95% CI, 0.23–2.30). In addition, the risk for hepatotoxicity was much lower in adults with HIV (RR = 0.26, 95% CI 0.12–0.55) and those without HIV (RR = 0.16, 95% CI 0.10–0.27) when compared to isoniazid monotherapy. And the completion rate of rifapentine plus isoniazid is also much high than that of isoniazid monotherapy.

8.2.5.3 Daily Rifampicin plus Isoniazid

Two systematic review conducted for the LTBI guidelines of 2015 and updated in 2017 showed a similar effect for 3–4 months' daily isoniazid plus rifampicin and 6 months of isoniazid [20, 25]. Recent studies also see the same results that fewer participants developed radiographic changes of daily rifampicin plus isoniazid than those being given 9 months of isoniazid (RR = 0.49, 95% CI 0.32–0.76). In addition, the authors also found a higher adherence rate (RR 1.07, 95% CI 1.01–1.14) and a lower risk for

Table 8.1 TB preventive treatment regimen

Treatment regimen	Drugs	Dose				Usage	Treatment course
		Adult (mg/each time)		Children (mg/each time)			
		<50 kg	≥50 kg	mg/kg.	maximum dose (mg/each time)		
Daily isoniazid monotherapy	Isoniazid	300	300	10	300	Once a day	6–9 months
Weekly rifapentine plus isoniazid	Isoniazid	500	600	10 ~ 15	300	Twice a week	3 months
	Rifapentine	450	600	10 (>5 years old)	450 (>5 years old)		
Daily rifampicin plus isoniazid	Isoniazid	300	300	10	300	Once a day	3 months
	Rifampicin	450	600	10	450		
Daily rifampicin monotherapy	Rifampicin	450	600	10	450	Once a day	4 months

adverse events (RR = 0.33, 95% CI 0.20–0.56) among those with 3–4 months' daily rifampicin plus isoniazid [26–28].

8.2.5.4 Daily Rifampicin Monotherapy for 3–4 Months

Two systematic reviews conducted for the LTBI guidelines of 2015 and updated in 2017 showed a similar effect for 3–4 months' daily rifampicin and 6 months of isoniazid (odds ratio = 0.78; 95% CI, 0.41–1.46) [20, 25]. Furthermore, the risk for hepatotoxicity of the daily rifampicin monotherapy for 3–4 months is much lower than that of isoniazid monotherapy (odds ratio, 0.03 = 95% CI 0.00–0.48).

8.2.5.5 Management During the Treatment Course

In the course of treatment, the following management measures should be taken in order to prevent irregular drug use and reduce the occurrence of adverse reactions to anti-TB drugs.

1. Take medicine under the supervision of family members, school doctors, or community health care workers.
2. All patients receiving treatment need to be registered in the Tuberculosis Preventive Treatment Record
3. The monitoring and management of adverse reactions should be strengthened during medication.

8.2.5.6 Withdrawal Criterion

If any of the following conditions occur, the drug should be stopped immediately.

1. Finishing the prescribed course of treatment.
2. Failure to continue to take the medicine due to severe adverse drug reactions during treatment.
3. Not taking medicine regularly for various reasons or failing to complete the entire course of treatment.
4. Active tuberculosis in any part of the body during medication.

8.3 Epidemiology of Active Tuberculosis

8.3.1 The Epidemic of Active TB

Tuberculosis affects all ages and both sexes, and the proportion is highest among adult men. In 2020, 56% of all TB cases were adult men, 33% were adult women, and 11% were children. TB is one of the ten leading causes of death in the world. In 2020, it was estimated that 1.3 million people died from TB in HIV-negative people globally. Additionally, there were 209,000 deaths among people that were living with HIV in 2020 [1].

In 2010, the fifth national tuberculosis prevalence survey showed that the prevalence rate of active pulmonary tuberculosis was 459 per 100,000 population in China, bacteriologically positive rate was 119 per 100,000 population, and smear-positive rate was 66 per 100,000 population. From 2000 to 2010, all pulmonary TB prevalence dropped by 1.5%, the rate of smear-positive TB fell by 61%, and the rate of bacteriologically confirmed TB decreased by 45%. The yearly reduction rate of smear-positive TB, bacteriologically positive TB, and pulmonary TB was 9.0%, 5.8%, and 0.2%, respectively. The prevalence rate of TB enhanced gradually with age. Male was higher than female in all age groups. In rural areas, the prevalence rate of TB was higher than in urbans, also the rates of smear-positive TB and bacteriologically confirmed TB were higher in rural areas [29].

8.3.2 Diagnosis of Active Pulmonary Tuberculosis

In general, the most typical clinical symptoms of pulmonary tuberculosis consist of continuous and productive cough, expectoration, hemoptysis, low-grade fever and weight reduction provides diagnostic basis of the disease. But the most direct and strongest evidence relies on pathogenic examination including sputum smear, culture, and molecular testing.

Through smear staining testing based on acid-fast bacilli or Auramine O procedure under microscope from sputum samples to detect *Mycobacterium tuberculosis* is the standard method in many TB endemic region, especially in low- and middle-income country [30, 31]. Although rapid and inexpensive, the smear microscopy has unsatisfied sensitivity and specificity due to technical factors, especially when non-tuberculosis (NTM) present in the samples [32]. Culturing in liquid or solid media with satisfied efficiency is adopted widely as the gold standard of TB diagnosis now, but it is time-consuming and requires more facilities. Furthermore, biosecurity should been considered seriously through the whole procedure of culture [33, 34]. Nevertheless, the introduction of the nucleic acid amplification test (NAAT) distinctly improved the efficiency of detection and identification of pulmonary tuberculosis [35]. Currently, there are lots of commercial assays based on different molecular mechanisms to amplify and detect *Mycobacterium tuberculosis* recommended by WHO, for instance, Xpert MTB-RIF system, molecular line probe assay, and whole genome sequencing and so on. Owing to fast detection and relative high specificity, molecular tests were wildly applied in clinical diagnosis, but they could not take place of phenotypic methods been used as assistant detection. Besides, the diagnosis of pulmonary TB can also be confirmed by radiological examination, such as chest X-ray or high-resolution computed tomography (HRCT). Alveolar infiltration, lymphadenopathy, pleural effusion, and cavitation are commonly observed through the X-ray from an active pulmonary tuberculosis patient. While centrilobular nodules, patchy, tree-in-bud lesions, or lobular consolidations are the most frequent presentation in HRCT [33, 36].

Like other countries with high pulmonary tuberculosis incidence rate, the standard guidelines of disease diagnosis proposed by national TB control program have been modified from time to time in China. Initially, a diagnosed active TB patient was classified as smear positive and smear negative according to sputum smear testing and chest X-ray examination. Then, culturing mycobacteria was adopted to supply the bacterium pathogenic detection. Since 2018, "Diagnosis for pulmonary tuberculosis" issued by the National Health Commission of the People's Republic of China, molecular biology techniques were added into diagnosis procedure. The principle of diagnosis mainly relied on pathogenic examination, including bacterium and molecular testing, epidemiological background, clinical manifestation, chest radiological examination, other auxiliary inspections such as pathological examination, and differential diagnosis were considered comprehensively for TB identification [37].

8.3.3 Treatment of Tuberculosis

Human beings have been tirelessly engaged in treatment in fighting TB to control and eliminate TB. After nearly a century of trying, tremendous progress had been made in the treatment of TB. For nearly three decades, the anti-TB treatment in China has been developing with the world in step, and has been contributing to the world tuberculosis control.

8.3.3.1 Health Nutrition Therapy

The treatment of tuberculosis began in 1853 by Brehmer. He came up with that TB patients need good rest and adequate nutrition, which gradually developed into the health nutrition therapy. TB patients in European lived in the mountains to have fresh air and nutritious food including cod-liver oil, calcium tablets, and vitamin C. The overall efficiency of the health nutrition therapy was about 25%. Tongren Sanatorium is one of the earliest sanatorium. In China, the work of TB prevention and control led by the public health view began in 1935. A Tuberculosis clinic was established in Dry Lane No. 1 Health Office in Beijing, responsible for health examination, anti-tuberculosis propaganda, and BCG vaccine.

8.3.3.2 The Era of Standard Chemotherapy

Waksman found the streptomycin in 1944, and confirmed it was effective to TB in vitro. Not long after that in 1945, efficacy of the streptomycin has been confirmed by Hinshaw, as the adventure of isoniazid and sodium aminosalicylate, it started the standard chemotherapy of TB, which had brought a revolutionary change to anti-TB treatment.

1. *Isoniazid*

   Meyer and Mally synthesized isoniazid in 1912 in Austria. Domestic isoniazid was synthesized by the Chinese People's Liberation Army Academy of Medical Sciences in 1953. Isoniazid inhibits MTB mycolic acid synthesis through its action on the enoyl-[acyl-carrier-protein] reductase. Isoniazid mainly acts on actively replicating bacilli, which manifest as robust early bactericidal activity (decline in bacillary colony-forming units during the initial few days of therapy), and as a result, isoniazid plays an important role on the initiation of the treatment.
2. *Streptomycin*

   Waksman found the streptomycin in 1944, and confirmed it was effective to TB in vitro. Not long after that in 1945, the efficacy of the streptomycin was been confirmed by Hinshaw. In 1953, Ministry of Health of China had announced streptomycin, sodium p-aminosalicylate, thiourea, and isoniazid could be used to treat blood type disseminated TB, TB meningitis, and invasive lesions, but did not work against fibrous lesions and caseous lesions; however, improper dosage could lead to auditory nerve damage or allergic reaction.
3. *Sodium aminosalicylate*

   In 1946, an effective compound sodium aminosalicylate was found in the derivatives of benzoic acid and salicylic acid. This compound can uniquely inhibit the function of *Mycobacterium* TB. Its important role lies in its use with streptomycin to delay the generation of drug resistance in *Mycobacterium* TB and improve the effect of chemotherapy.
4. *Pyrazinamide*

   Kushner found pyrazinamide has anti-TB effect in 1952. In 1957, pyrazinamide of China was successfully developed and was used in clinics in the 1960s. However, the occurrence of more liver damage had affected its clinical application. In the 1970s, with the advent of rifampin and the re-evaluation of drug modification, the dosage was adjusted from 2.0 g to 1.5 g per day, which is widely used up to now.
5. *Rifampicin*

   In 1959, Lepetit Company isolated an antibiotic from Streptococcus Mediterranean of soil-rifamycins, which had a strong bactericidal effect on Gram-positive bacteria and *Mycobacterium* TB. Its highly effective derivative-rifampicin was discovered in 1965. In 1973, rifampicin was successfully developed by Beijing Tuberculosis Research Institute. Its antimicrobial spectrum, antimicrobial activity, pharmacokinetic parameters, and clinical effects were consistent with those of imported products.
6. *Ethambutol*

   In 1961, Wilkinson had developed ethambutol successfully, and found it had an effect on anti-TB effect. In 1975, ethambutol was successfully developed by Beijing Pharmaceutical Factory. Although the drug only had an inhibitory effect on *Mycobacterium* TB, the drug resistance was delayed when used in combination with rifampicin and biazinamide.

8.3.4 The Era of Standard Chemotherapy for Tuberculosis

As the adventure of isoniazid, the Ministry of Public Health of our country issued the document that recipe of isoniazid treating TB in 1952, indicating that the treatment of TB enters the era of chemotherapy. In 1953, the Ministry of Health has regulated the use of streptomycin, sodium para aminosalicylate, thiourea, and isoniazid, and given the recommended dosage of streptomycin and aminosalicylate. At the national academic conference on TB held in 1963, the main recommended anti-TB treatment regimen was mostly a combination of isoniazid, sodium para aminosalicylate, or streptomycin. In the 1960s, the clinical comparative study of streptomycin, isoniazid, sodium aminohydrochloride and isoniazid alone was carried out, and good curative effect was obtained. In addition to proving the advantages of combined drug use, it was also proved that combined drug use could prevent the occurrence of drug resistance. The standard chemotherapy including streptomycin, isoniazid, sodium aminohydrochloride came out, and the course of treatment was 18–24 months.

8.3.5 The Era of Short-Course Chemotherapy for TB

With the advent of rifampicin, which has a stronger bactericidal effect, anti-TB officially entered the era of short-course chemotherapy. In 1972, W. Fox conducted a study of short-course chemotherapy for TB in East Africa, where a 6–9 month regimen based on elifampicin and biazinamide was designed. The main achievement of the study, which was the result of nine studies over 20 years, was to reduce the conventional 18–24 months of long-term chemotherapy to 6–9 months. In China, the study of short-course chemotherapy began in 1978, and it lasted over 20 years. Finally, the Classic short-course chemotherapy regimen-2HRZE-4HR came out.

8.3.6 Therapeutic Principle

All tuberculosis patients who can be tested for drug sensitivity should be tested drug susceptibility test. In regions where conditions permit, molecular biological drug resistance testing should be carried out, and targeted treatment should be carried out for patients according to drug sensitivity results. The anti-tuberculosis treatment follows the principle of "early, combined, moderate, regular and whole course."

8.3.7 Therapeutic Regimen

At present, patients with rifampicin sensitive TB were treated with first-line anti-tuberculosis agents without special circumstances. First-line anti-TB drugs include Isoniazid (INH or H), Rifampicin (RFP or R), Rifapentine (RFT), Pyrazinamide (PZA or Z), Ethambutol (EMB or E), and Streptomycin (SM or S). Fixed-dose combinations (FDCs) are recommended for anti-tuberculous therapy. Patients with TB who are sensitive to R or whose drug resistance is unknown should be treated with a standardized treatment regimen [38]. Scheme selection requirements are shown in Table 8.2.

8.3.8 Treatment Management of TB Patients

The key to successful treatment is to take medicine regularly during the whole course of TB. During the entire treatment period, all institutions involved in the treatment and management of patients must cooperate closely, strengthen health promotion and communication with patients to ensure patients' treatment compliance.

8.3.9 TB Patients Management

All patients with active pulmonary TB included in the treatment are the target of management, and standardized treatment management should be carried out.

8.3.9.1 Content of Management

1. Urge patients to take anti-TB drugs on time to ensure that patients finish the full course of regular medication.
2. Observe whether patients have adverse reactions after medication, and take measures timely to ensure that patients complete the prescribed course of treatment to the greatest extent.
3. Urge the patient to return to visit regularly, master the change of sputum smear, and make a good record.
4. Health education on tuberculosis prevention knowledge for patients and their family members should be carried out to improve patients'

Table 8.2 Treatment regimens for patients with rifampicin sensitivity (RS) or unknown resistance

Classification of patients		Treatment regimen	Remark
RS	H sensitivity or resistance is unknown	2HRZE/4HR	① Drug sensitivity test should be carried out if the second month of the sputum smear is positive. The regimen of patients with drug resistance is adjusted according to the results of drug sensitivity test, and increase the intense phase for 1 month if RS. However, the treatment plan for the continuation phase remained unchanged, and one more sputum examination was added at the end of the third month. ② Patients with a positive sputum at the fifth month or at the end of the treatment are judged to have treatment failure. ③ Children should be strictly in accordance with the weight of the drug, and use of ethambutol in children under 5 years old should be cautious.
	H resistant	6-9RZELfx	① The regimen of patients with Lfx resistance should be 6-9RZE. ② It is forbidden for pregnant women and can be used in lactating women after stopping breastfeeding. ③ Patients with prolonged Q-T interval were excluded.
Resistance to rifampicin is unknown		2HRZE/4HR	① During the treatment, sputum smear should be tested every month. If sputum smear is positive, drug resistance test should be carried out. The regimen of patients with drug resistance is adjusted according to the results of drug sensitivity test, and increase the intense phase for 1 month if RS. However, the treatment plan for the continuation phase remained unchanged, and one more sputum examination was added at the end of the third month. ② For retreated patients, the intense phase can be extended by 1 month and the continuation phase can be extended by 2–3 months according to the treatment situation and should pay more attention to the resistance test. ③ It is forbidden for pregnant women and can be used in lactating women after stopping breastfeeding. ④ Children should be strictly in accordance with the weight of the drug, and use of ethambutol in children under 5 years old should be cautious.
Tuberculous pleuritis		2HRZE/7HRE	① Critical patients: the continuation phase can be extended by 2–3 months, and the regimen should be 2HRZE/10HRE. ② Once resistance was found during treatment, treatment was carried out according to the resistance protocol
Other tuberculosis or associated diseases		2HRZE/10HRE	① Hematogenous disseminated tuberculosis, tracheobronchial tuberculosis, intrathoracic lymphatic tuberculosis. ② Patients with pulmonary tuberculosis complicated with diabetes and silicosis. ③ Once resistance was found during treatment, treatment was carried out according to the resistance protocol
Tuberculosis with extrapulmonary tuberculosis		Intense phase: 2HRZE continuation phase: HRE; It should be based on the longest treatment course of extrapulmonary tuberculosis.	Once resistance was found during treatment, treatment was carried out according to the resistance protocol

(continued)

Table 9.2 (continued)

Classification of patients		Treatment regimen	Remark
Anti-tuberculosis treatment in HIV infected and AIDS patients		Rifambutin instead of rifampicin and other anti-tuberculosis drugs can be considered as a treatment regimen for anti-tuberculosis treatment; Avoid using rifapentine, which will increase the risk of rifamycin resistance	Once resistance was found during treatment, treatment was carried out according to the resistance protocol

treatment compliance and their family members' sense of responsibility to supervise and take medicine.

8.3.9.2 Medical Staff Management

TB patients take the medicine under the management of medical staff. The medical staff responsible for supervising drug taking are mainly from primary medical and health institutions. Medical staff in designated hospital and Center for Disease Control and Prevention (CDC) can also supervise drug taking.

8.3.9.3 Family Member Management

The spouse, parents, children, and other family members living with the tuberculosis patient can supervise the management of the patient's medication. The requirements for family members to supervise medication include: age above 15, primary school education or above, and with basic medical training they can supervise patients to take medicine, return visit, and fill in relevant records.

8.3.9.4 Volunteer Management

Volunteers (such as teachers, students, cured TB patients, and others) supervise the management of the patient's medication. The requirements for volunteers to supervise medication include: age above 18, junior high school or above education level, and with basic medical training can supervise patients to take medicine, return visit, and fill in relevant records.

8.3.9.5 Intelligent Tools Assist Management

With the help of electronic medicine box, mobile phone, and other intelligent tools, TB patients are supervised to take medicine. Intelligent tools regularly remind people to take medication and record their behavior.

8.4 Epidemiology of Drug Resistance Tuberculosis

8.4.1 Overview

At present, drug-resistant tuberculosis (DR-TB) is increasingly prevalent worldwide, posing a serious threat to global tuberculosis prevention and control. According to WHO estimation, 3.3% of new tuberculosis cases and 20% of previously treated tuberculosis cases worldwide are MDR-TB. About 10% of multidrug-resistant tuberculosis may develop into XDR-TB [39].

According to WHO definition, there are seven major types of DR-TB: ① Mono-drug-resistant tuberculosis (MR-TB): refers to MTB infected by tuberculosis patients confirmed to be resistant to a first-line anti-tuberculosis drug by in vitro drug sensitivity test; ② Poly-drug-resistant tuberculosis

(PR-TB): refers to tuberculosis The patient's infected MTB was confirmed to be resistant to more than one first-line anti-tuberculosis drug through an in vitro drug sensitivity test, but not including isoniazid and rifampicin resistant simultaneously; ③ Rifampicin-resistant tuberculosis (RR-TB): refers to MTB infected by tuberculosis patients confirmed to be resistant to rifampicin by an in vitro drug sensitivity test, regardless of resistance to other anti-tuberculosis drugs; ④ isoniazid-resistant tuberculosis (HR-TB): refers to MTB infected by tuberculosis patients was confirmed to be resistant to isoniazid and susceptible to rifampicin by in vitro drug sensitivity test; ⑤ MDR-TB: refers to tuberculosis patients infected with *MTB* in vitro drug sensitivity test confirmed resistance to at least two first-line anti-tuberculosis drugs including isoniazid and rifampicin simultaneously; ⑥ Pre-extensively-drug resistant (Pre-XDR-TB): TB caused by *MTB* strains that fulfill the definition of multidrug-resistant and rifampicin-resistant TB (MDR/RR-TB) and which are also resistant to any fluoroquinolone; ⑦ Extensively drug-resistant tuberculosis (XDR-TB): TB caused by *MTB (M. tuberculosis)* strains that fulfill the definition of MDR/RR-TB and which are also resistant to any fluoroquinolone and at least one additional Group A drug (Group A anti-TB drugs are the most potent group of drugs in the ranking of second-line medicines for the treatment of drug-resistant TB using a longer treatment regimens and comprise levofloxacin, moxifloxacin, bedaquiline and linezolid).

In 2019, WHO estimates that there are 480,000 new cases of MDR-TB each year, and 190,000 people die from MDR-TB. India, China, and Russia had the highest number of MDR-TB cases, and these three countries accounted for more than 50% of the total number of MDR-TB cases reported globally. Although the global burden of MDR-TB has changed little between 2008 and 2013, in the following countries (for example, China, India, Pakistan, Nigeria, South Africa, Indonesia, Bangladesh, and the Democratic Republic of Congo) the number of rifampin-resistant cases have increased significantly.

The Chinese government has investigated extensive efforts to prevent and control MDR-TB. In 2006, China initiated the fifth round of the Global Fund TB project in Hebei, Jilin, Jiangsu, Yunnan, Guangxi, Sichuan, and Shaanxi Province for MDR-TB. From 2007 to 2008, the Ministry of Health organized a nationwide baseline survey on TB drug resistance [40], and the results indicated that the prevalence of MDR-TB was 8.32% (95%CI, 7.13 to 9.70) with around 120,000 new MDR-TB cases occurring every year, which accounted for about a quarter of the globally total number of new MDR-TB cases in a year. A systematic review and meta-analysis showed that multi-drug resistance among new and retreatment cases was 4.8% (4.0%–5.7%; n/N = 2300/42946) and 26.3% (23.1%–29.7%; n/N = 3125/11589), respectively, from 59 published articles from 2012 to 2015 in China mainland [41].

The fifth national TB epidemiological survey was conducted in 2010, drug-resistant patterns for MTB complex were evaluated as well. Test drugs include isoniazid, rifampicin, streptomycin, ethambutol, p-aminosalicylic acid, kanamycin, amikacin, capreomycin, thiisonicotamine, ofloxacin, and levofloxacin. When the isolated strain is sensitive to the four first-line anti-tuberculosis drugs tested, it is called "sensitive to the first-line drugs." Among the 280 strains of the MTB complex tested in the fifth survey, the prevalence of drug resistance to first-line anti-tuberculosis drugs was 36.8% (95% CI: 31.1–42.7). The prevalence of multi-drug resistance was 6.8% (95% CI: 4.1–10.4%). Compared with the 10.7% multi-drug resistance rate in 2000, it has declined. Drug resistance of second-line anti-tuberculosis drugs was defined when the strains are resistant to any second-line anti-tuberculosis drug, it is called "resistance to second-line drugs. Among the 280 strains of MTB complex, the drug resistance proportion of second-line anti-tuberculosis drugs is 24.6% (95% CI: 19.7–30.1). The extensive drug resistance rate of the isolated strains was 2.1% (95% CI: 0.8–4.6). Among the 280 strains of MTB complex, 162 strains were "susceptible" to the 11 anti-tuberculosis drugs tested, and 118 strains were "drug resistant." The drug resistance rate was 42.1% (95% CI: 36.3–48.2). Among them, the drug resistance rate of newly treated patients was 42.7% (95% CI: 36.4–49.2), of patients who were retreated, the drug resistance rate was 38.5% (95% CI: 23.4–55.4).

8.4.2 Diagnosis

8.4.2.1 Phenotypic Testing on Drug Resistance of *Mycobacterium tuberculosis* Complex

The culture-based phenotypic drug susceptibility test (DST) provides a method for detecting the susceptibility of bacteria to drugs. Conventional DST is usually based on a qualitative method that uses a single critical concentration of the drug to assess bacterial growth. The DST method, used Löwenstein–Jensen slope and proportional method. Count the number of colonies on the drug-containing medium and compare it with the number of colonies on the drug-free medium. If the ratio exceeds the critical ratio of the drug, the strain is classified as drug resistant. DST is also tested in commercial automated cultivation systems such as MGIT 960, and the results can be obtained within 7–12 days [42].

From a clinical perspective, the main disadvantage of DST is the heavy time consumption. At the same time, phenotyping is technically demanding and will be affected by the interaction between the drug and the culture medium and the formation of clumps of hydrophobic MTB.

8.4.2.2 Genotypic Testing on Drug Resistance of *Mycobacterium tuberculosis* Complex

The drug resistance of MTB may result from mutations in the bacterial DNA that make the organism resist to the effects of drugs. The most common cause of resistance is SNPs in genes encoding drug targets or invertases, but large deletions may also lead to resistance [43].

Xpert MTB/RIF is an easy-to-use automated PCR-based test that diagnoses tuberculosis and detects mutations that were predictive of resistance to rifampicin in less than 2 h. The test was endorsed by WHO in 2010 and is recommended as a front-line diagnostic test to assist in the management of MDR tuberculosis. In addition to the GeneXpert technology, WHO has endorsed line probe assay molecular technology for detecting drug susceptibility. Following amplification of the target gene, line probe assay technology reverse-hybridizes samples to a series of oligonucleotide probes immobilized on a membrane.

8.4.3 Treatment [44]

8.4.3.1 The Composition of Longer MDR/RR-TB Regimens

According to the effectiveness and safety, the medicines of longer MDR/RR-TB regimens are divided into three groups (see Table 8.3).

A longer regimen consists of at least four effective anti-TB drugs with a duration of 18–20 months. Principles for making the regimen:

1. The regimen includes all three Group A agents and at least one Group B agent, and contains at least three agents for the remaining course of treatment after stopping bedaquiline. When only one or two drugs can be used in Group A, both drugs in Group B should be selected. Group C drugs can be added when the regimen cannot be developed with drugs from Group A and Group B.
2. The patient's previous medical history and drug sensitivity test results are considered.
3. Oral drugs take precedence over injections.
4. Population resistance levels, drug tolerance, and potential drug interactions should be considered.
5. Monitor and properly manage adverse drug reactions.

Table 8.3 Medicines recommended for use in longer MDR/RR-TB regimens

Groups and steps	Medicine (abbreviation)	Dose (weight-based) <50 kg (mg/day)	≥50 kg (mg/day)	Usual upper daily dose (mg/day)
Group A: Include all three medicines	Levofloxacin (Lfx)/ moxifloxacin (Mfx)	400 ~ 750/400	500 ~ 1000/400	1000/400
	Bedaquiline (Bdq)	400 mg od for first 2 weeks; then 200 mg od Mon/Wed/Fri for 22 weeks		400
	Linezolid (Lzd)	300	300 ~ 600	600
Group B: Add one or both medicines	Clofazimine (Cfz)	100	100	100
	Cycloserine (Cs)	500	750	750
Group C: Add to complete the regimen and when medicines from Groups A and B cannot be used	Ethambutol (E)	750	1000	1500
	Delamanid (Dlm)	100 mg bd		
	Pyrazinamide (Z)	1500	1750	2000
	Imipenem-cilastatin (Ipm-Cln)[a]	1000 mg bd		
	Meropenem (Mpm)[a]	1000 mg bd		
	Amikacin (Am)	400	400 ~ 600	800
	Streptomycin (S)	750	750	750
	Capreomycin (Cm)	750	750	750
	Prothionamide (Pto)	600	600 ~ 800	800
	p-aminosalicylic (PAS)	8000	10,000	12,000

[a]To be used with clavulanic acid

Recommended regimen:

1. Susceptible to fluoroquinolones: 6 Lfx(Mfx) Bdq Lzd(Cs) Cfz /12 Lfx(Mfx)
   Cfz Lzd(Cs). If Bdq and Lzd are not available, the standardized shorter MDR-TB regimen is not preferred and susceptible to second-line injectable agents, following regimen is recommended: 6 Lfx(Mfx) Cfz Cs Am(Cm)Z(E, Pto) /14 Lfx(Mfx) Cfz Cs Z(E, Pto).
2. Resistance to fluoroquinolones: 6 Bdq Lzd Cfz Cs/14 Lzd Cfz Cs

8.4.3.2 The Standardized Shorter MDR/RR-TB Regimen

Regimen: 4–6 Am Mfx Pto Cfz Z Hh E/5 Mfx Cfz Z E.

This regimen consists of an intensive phase and a continuation phase. If sputum culture conversion does not occur after 4 months of treatment, the intensive phase is extended to 6 months. If sputum culture conversion does not occur at the end of 6 months of treatment, a longer MDR/RR-TB regimen should be used.

Inclusion criteria:

RR-TB patients never receive or receive one or more agents included in the shorter RR-TB regimen less than 1 month and susceptible to fluoroquinolones and second-line injections.

Exclusion criteria:

1. Cannot tolerate all drugs in the shorter MDR/RR-TB regimen or risk of drug toxicity;
2. Pregnancy;
3. Hematogenous disseminated TB, meningeal or central nervous system TB;
4. Extrapulmonary TB in people living with HIV;

8.4.4 Management

8.4.4.1 Monitoring

Sputum culture and sputum smear microscopy are recommended for monitoring treatment effect. Sputum culture and sputum smear microscopy to be performed once a month during the intensive phase and to be performed every 2 months during the continuation phase.

Chest radiography to be repeated at 3-months intervals.

8.4.4.2 Treatment Outcomes

1. Cure: Complete the prescribed course of treatment with no evidence of treatment failure and at least three consecutive sputum cultures are negative that taken at a minimum interval of 30 days after the intensive period.
2. Treatment completed: Complete the prescribed course of treatment with no evidence of treatment failure but fail to achieve three consecutive negative sputum cultures that take at a minimum interval of 30 days after the intensive period.
3. Treatment failed: Termination of treatment or change of regimen with at least two anti-TB drugs for: (i) No conversion at the end of the intensive stage; (ii) After conversion to negative bacteriological reversion during the continuation stage; (iii) Resistance to fluoroquinolones or second-line injections; (iv) Adverse drug reactions.
4. Died: During the treatment death from any cause.
5. Lost to follow-up: Treatment interruption for 2 months or more.
6. Not evaluated: Treatment outcome is not registered.
7. Successfully treated: Cured and treatment completed are included.

8.4.4.3 Care and Support for Patients with MDR/RR-TB

The key point to successful treatment is regular medication for a full course. Management of patients' treatment should be provided throughout the treatment period. We should take patient-centered care to ensure adherence [45]. Health education on the knowledge of TB prevention and treatment for patients and their families should be provided to improve compliance. In addition we can offer a treatment compliance interventions to patients on TB treatment which include psychological support, social support, and tracers.

The treatment administration options include: directly observed treatment (DOT) and video-observed treatment (VOT). If we can use video communication technology, DOT may be replaced by VOT.

8.4.4.4 Health Care Service and Funding Mechanisms of MDR/RR-TB

The prevention and control of drug-resistant TB has been an important part of China's national TB control program [46]. China has established a cooperation model between designated hospitals and TB dispensaries. Hospitals are responsible for diagnosis, treatment, and management of adverse reaction for MDR/RR-TB patients. TB dispensaries are responsible for tracking patients' management and supervision. China has taken a series of measures for MDR/RR-TB control such as: build a new funding model, designate hospitals at the prefecture level for diagnosis and treatment of MDR/RR-TB, increase human resources, and optimize an appropriate patient discovery strategy. China has introduced policies to cover MDR/RR-TB care into health insurance, with 70% reimbursement, 30% self-payment. If the patients meet the eligibility criteria for civil assistance, they will get an additional 20% subsidy.

Although China has aimed to develop an appropriate service system for MDR/RR-TB control, implementation varies in different parts of China. In some areas the self-payment for MDR/RR-TB services is high and catastrophic health expenditure in MDR/RR-TB treatment has happened from time to time [47].

8.5 Epidemiology of Tuberculosis Comorbidity

8.5.1 HIV/TB Co-infection

8.5.1.1 Overview

Acquired immune deficiency syndrome (AIDS), namely acquired immunodeficiency syndrome, is a chronic infectious disease caused by HIV. HIV is a kind of lentivirus within the family Retroviridae. It mainly invades and destroys human helper lymphocyte T through sexual, blood, and mother-to-infant transmission, resulting in cellular immune deficiency. Since the first case of AIDS was reported in 1981, it has spread rapidly around the world. According to WHO, in 2020, there were totally 37.7 million people living with HIV/AIDS (PLWHA) in the world, of which 1.5 million people newly infected with HIV and 680,000 people died from HIV-related causes [48]. In 2018, there were 850,000 PLWHA and 18,780 deaths have been reported in China [49]. At present, the AIDS epidemic in China is on the rise and spread a wide range. Low prevalence in the general population and high prevalence coexists in local areas and the specific population, meanwhile, the epidemic spreads from high-risk groups to the general population [50].

8.5.1.2 The Relationship Between Tuberculosis and HIV/AIDS

Human beings are generally susceptible to HIV and MTB pathogens, which can be infected successively or at the same time, resulting in co-infection of HIV and MTB [51]. HIV and MTB co-infection is not a simple superposition of two diseases, but a process of mutual influence and mutual promotion.

In the areas with high burden of tuberculosis, HIV infection accelerates the process of tuberculosis infection to active tuberculosis. HIV infection destroys the immune system of patients, increases the susceptibility to infection and the risk of tuberculosis recurrence [52]. It is mainly caused by the damage to the cellular immune function when infected with HIV. HIV infection will change the clinical manifestations of tuberculosis. There are increasing sputum smear-negative tuberculosis patients and extrapulmonary tuberculosis patients among PLWH. The decline of patients' immune function makes anti-tuberculosis treatment more complex and weakens the effect of anti-tuberculosis treatment [53, 54]. Furthermore, the susceptibility of MTB is related to the cytokines of T lymphocytes. T1 lymphocytes can release interferon (INF) and defense center of bacteria; T2 lymphocytes can release interleukin-4 (IL-4) and interleukin-10 (IL-10). The production of INF decreases in HIV-positive patients when exposed to MTB, indicating that the decreased response of T1 lymphocytes. Besides, HIV can destroy the balance of Th1/Th2, thus weakening the body's control of MTB [55–57].

Tuberculosis is the most common related infectious disease and the cause of death in patients with HIV/AIDS [58–60]. Tuberculosis infection can promote HIV invasion, accelerate HIV replication, and shorten the time from asymptomatic infection to AIDS. Compared with HIV/AIDS patients without tuberculosis, HIV/AIDS patients with tuberculosis are several times more likely to develop other opportunistic infections and death [61]. The mechanism is mainly manifested in the following aspects [62, 63]: Frist, the secretion level of inflammatory cytokines decreases and cannot prevent HIV from invading the target cells. Second, T lymphocytes are activated in vivo, and the cytokines released by them can significantly increase the transcription of HIV provirus, accelerate virus replication, and promote the deterioration of the disease. Third, the production of Th2 cells inhibits the body's ability to resist intracellular infection, which is not conducive to the elimination of latent HIV in cells. Last, MTB infection also increases the number of CXC chemokine receptor 4 receptors on the surface of dendritic cells, which promotes the infection process of HIV in dendritic cells.

8.5.1.3 HIV/TB Co-infection Clinical Features

The most common symptoms of PLWHA complicated with tuberculosis are fever, fatigue, poor appetite, cough, and weight loss [64]. Compared with HIV-negative tuberculosis patients, systemic poisoning symptoms are more common in PLWHA with tuberculosis, and superficial lymphadenopathy occurs in more than 1/3 of patients [65]. In the early stage of HIV/TB co-infection, the clinical manifestations of tuberculosis patients were similar to those without co-infection patients. However, when entering AIDS phase, symptoms and signs of AIDS and tuberculosis are superimposed on each other, and the symptoms of tuberculosis lose the diagnostic specificity. Studies have shown that the sensitivity of comprehensive clinical symptoms to diagnose TB in HIV/TB co-infection patients was 79%, whereas the specificity is only 50% [66, 67]. It have been reported that the most common symptom of HIV-negative tuberculosis patients is cough, accounting for 81%, while the most common symptoms of HIV/TB co-infection patients are fever, fatigue, poor appetite, cough, and weight loss, accounting for 85.6%, 68.4%, 65.6%, 52.6%, and 50.2%, respectively [68].

The X-ray manifestations of pulmonary tuberculosis are atypical in patients with AIDS combined with pulmonary tuberculosis. Compared with TB patients without HIV infection, patients with HIV/TB co-infection have more extrapulmonary tuberculosis and disseminated tuberculosis. In the early stage of HIV infection, the immune level of the body is not been significantly suppressed. The pathological changes of tuberculosis are similar to those of HIV-negative tuberculosis patients. The lesions are mostly located in the apical and posterior segments of the upper lobe and the back of the lower lobe, and there may be cavities. When the immune function impaired, it reduces the inflammatory response and the formation of lung injury cavity. So cavities in the lungs are rare in HIV/TB co-infection patients [69].

Extrapulmonary tuberculosis is more common, mostly without pulmonary manifestations [70]. The most common type of extrapulmonary tuberculosis is lymph node tuberculosis, including superficial lymph node tuberculosis (neck lymph node, axillary lymph node, inguinal lymph node tuberculosis), and deep lymph node tuberculosis (mediastinal lymph node, lung). Hilar lymph nodes, retroperitoneal lymph nodes; followed by tuberculous pleurisy [68].

The positive rate of TST is much lower. Due to immunosuppression, the TST positive rate of HIV/TB co-infection is only 15%–40% [71]. Previous studies have shown that the positive rate of TST in HIV/TB co-infection patients is half of that in patients without HIV/TB co-infection. Due to the immunodeficiency, the false negative rate of TST is higher in PLWHA, so TST negative results cannot exclude the diagnosis of LTBI [72]. It has been reported in related literature that when CD4+ lymphocytes are less than 100×10^6/L, TST is of little significance in the diagnosis of HIV with LTBI [73].

8.5.1.4 The Prevalence of HIV/TB Co-infection

Meta-analysis showed that the global TB/HIV co-infection rate ranged from 2.93% to 72.34%, while the co-infection rate in Africa was 31.25% (95%CI: 19.30–43.17), and the rate in Asian countries, European countries, Latin American countries, and America was 17.21% (95%CI: 9.97–24.46), 20.11% (95%CI: 13.82–26.39), 25.06% (95%CI: 19.28–30.84), and 14.84% (95%CI: 10.44–19.24), respectively [74]. In 2014, the co-infection rate of HIV/TB was 5.2%, 3%, and 4% in Vietnam, Cambodia, and India, respectively. The HIV/TB co-infection rate in Asian countries with high burden of TB was 16% in Indonesia, 13% in Thailand, and 11% in Myanmar [75].

Tuberculosis is the most common opportunistic infection of AIDS patients in developing countries. There was 25%–65% HIV/AIDS population infected with TB in developing countries, while the co-infection rate was relatively low in developed countries [76]. Compared with the incidence of tuberculosis about 5% in general population, half of PLWHA with LTBI develop tuberculosis within 60 days [77]. In Guinea, HIV/TB co-infection accounted for 20.27% of the PLWH from 1991 to 1992 [78]. Zhao et al. also reported that in Vietnam, 31.6% of 1206 new PLWHA were HIV/TB co-infection. Thailand began to screen for HIV in tuberculosis patients in 1989, HIV/TB co-infection accounted for 10% of all newly registered tuberculosis patients by 1994. Babajide et al. covered that 31% of new tuberculosis cases in Sub-Saharan Africa were HIV/TB co-infection [79].

Gao et al. [80]. conducted a meta-analysis of 29 literatures on HIV/TB two-way screening, showing that the proportion of PLWH among tuberculosis patients in mainland China was 0.9% (0.6%–1.4%) and the prevalence of tuberculosis in PLWHA was 7.2% (4.2%–12.3%).

The proportion of tuberculosis in AIDS patients was 22.8%. The data from 1032 TB patients in areas with severe HIV infection showed that the HIV/TB co-infection proportion was 3.3% [81]. A study of 2300 tuberculosis patients in Guangxi showed HIV/TB co-infection proportion was 0.5% (12/2300) [82]. From 1994 to 1999, 309 cases of PLWH were found in Taiwan province, of which 77 cases were combined with tuberculosis and the co-infection accounted for 24.9% of all PLWH. From 1984 to 2000, 1542 cases of HIV-infected people were found in Hong Kong and 109 cases were complicated with tuberculosis, accounting for 21.8% of the HIV infection.

8.5.1.5 HIV/TB Co-infection Control Strategy

In 2010, the former Ministry of Health issued *the National Implementation Plan for the Prevention and Control of Tuberculosis/HIV Dual Infection (Trial)*, which requires strengthening leadership, establishing a cooperative mechanism between TB and HIV/AIDS prevention, and implementing a two-way screening strategy [83]. That is, providing tuberculosis examination for all newly registered and followed-up HIV/AIDS, and providing HIV testing for tuberculosis patients in areas with a high and moderate prevalence of HIV/AIDS. Mobilize tuberculosis patients with high-risk behaviors of AIDS in low prevalence areas to receive HIV test, and provide corresponding treatment and follow-up management services for confirmed HIV/TB co-infection patients. *National Tuberculosis Prevention and Control Plan (2011–2015)* required that the HIV screening rate in tuberculosis patients in HIV/AIDS epidemic key counties (cities) should reach 70%. *China's 12th Five-Year Plan of Action for Containment and Prevention of AIDS* required that more than 90% of PLWHA receive tuberculosis examination at least once a year, and the proportion of anti-tuberculosis and anti-virus treatment for co-infection patients reaches more than 80%.

The prevention and control mechanism between HIV/AIDS and tuberculosis is well-developed, and two-way screening was carried out in many areas. In 2013, the proportion of X-ray or sputum smear examination among HIV/AIDS people reached 84.9%, and the proportion of HIV detection among tuberculosis patients in 294 key counties reached 88.8%. The proportion of people with co-infection receiving anti-tuberculosis and AIDS treatment increased from 35.6% in 2011 to 57.2% in 2013.

8.5.1.6 Problems and Challenges

HIV/TB dual infection has become a prominent problem in the prevention and treatment of HIV/AIDS and tuberculosis. Although some progresses have been made in the diagnosis and treatment of HIV/TB in recent years, there are still many problems to be solved. HIV screening coverage and antiviral treatment coverage are not high. The early diagnosis of tuberculosis needs to be strengthened. The symptoms of HIV/TB patients are atypical and the number of non-tuberculosis mycobacterial diseases is increasing year by year. It brings great challenges in the diagnosis and distinguish of HIV/TB dual infection. Tuberculosis and AIDS prevention and control work is still relatively independent, and there is no cooperation mechanism between tuberculosis and HIV/AIDS prevention and control in some areas. The interaction between anti-tuberculosis drugs and antiviral drugs has many side effects and affects the treatment outcomes. There is low LTBI preventive therapy in HIV/AIDS patients and lack of funds for the prevention and treatment of HIV/TB co-infection.

The prevalence of AIDS and tuberculosis has fallen into a vicious circle of mutual promotion. How to prevent, diagnose, treat, and manage HIV/TB co-infection has become a very serious problem. It is still the focus of future work that we should strengthen cooperation, carry out two-way screening, participate in the diagnosis, treatment, and management of HIV/TB double infection patients, strengthen joint work supervision, information communication and exchange, and strengthen epidemic information monitoring.

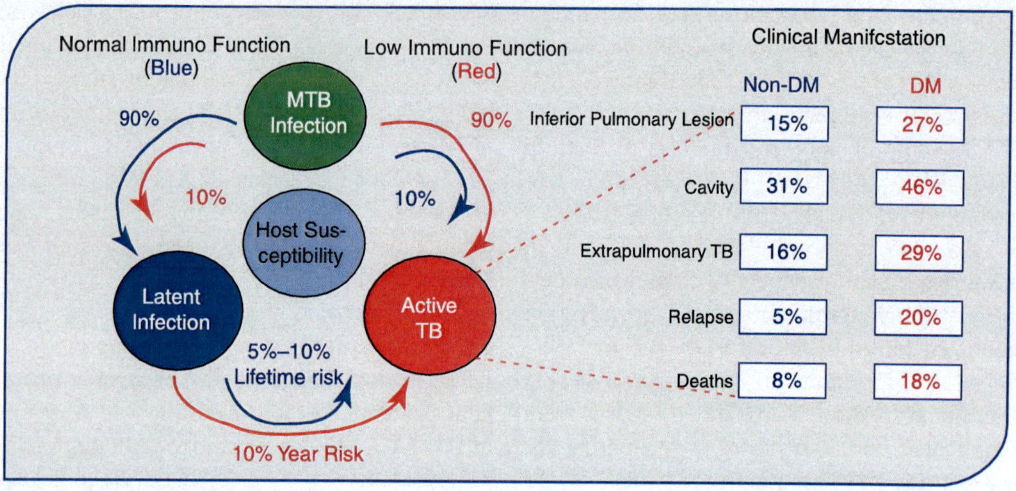

Fig. 8.1 The impact of diabetes on the clinical manifestations and treatment outcomes of tuberculosis

8.5.2 Epidemiology of DM in PTB

8.5.2.1 Mutual Effect of PTB-DM

With the increase in the global incidence of diabetes and its potential effect on tuberculosis control, the co-epidemic of tuberculosis and diabetes has drawn public attention again. Since 1980, the global prevalence of diabetes has almost doubled, from 4.7% to 8.8% in the adult population. The prevalence of diabetes in low- and middle-income countries rose faster than that in high-income countries [84], especially in low- and middle-income countries where the burden of tuberculosis was the heaviest, the prevalence of diabetes has increased significantly [85, 86]. According to the data from the International Diabetes Federation (IDF) [84], the prevalence of diabetes in mainland China was 10.9% in 2017, with approximately 114 million diabetic patients, accounting for 26.8% of global cases, which ranked first in the world [84]. It is estimated that 15% of tuberculosis incidence and 11% of tuberculosis deaths attributed to diabetes worldwide [87]. In 2014, WHO proposed the End TB Strategy, which aimed to achieve a TB-free world [2]. However, based on the current epidemic trend of diabetes and its effect on tuberculosis, the goal of ending TB by 2035 will be difficult to achieve [88], and diabetes has become the main obstacle to achieving it.

Diabetes has a negative influence on the incidence and prognosis of tuberculosis (Fig. 8.1). It is estimated that the risk for diabetes patients to develop TB was 2 to 3 times that for the general population. Moreover, suffering from diabetes can change the clinical manifestations of tuberculosis, increase the scope of lung lesions [89], and result in the increased risk of treatment failure [89, 90], death [91, 92], relapse and drug resistance [89, 93]. Although increasing evidence have shown that diabetes increased the risk of tuberculosis, treatment outcomes and effect mechanisms [94, 95], the research on the effect of tuberculosis on blood glucose metabolism was still in its infancy, and studies have revealed that tuberculosis can cause hyperglycemia [96]. As an infectious disease, tuberculosis can affect the blood glucose changes of patients through oxidative stress and other pathways, which causes insulin resistance in vivo, resulting in transient hyperglycemia [97, 98] and blood glucose variation, and even developing diabetes in the acute phase of active tuberculosis [98, 99] (Fig. 8.2).

8.5.2.2 The Prevalence of PTB-DM

In recent years, the co-epidemic of tuberculosis and diabetes has attracted worldwide attention. The results of five national epidemiologic sampling surveys for tuberculosis in China [100]

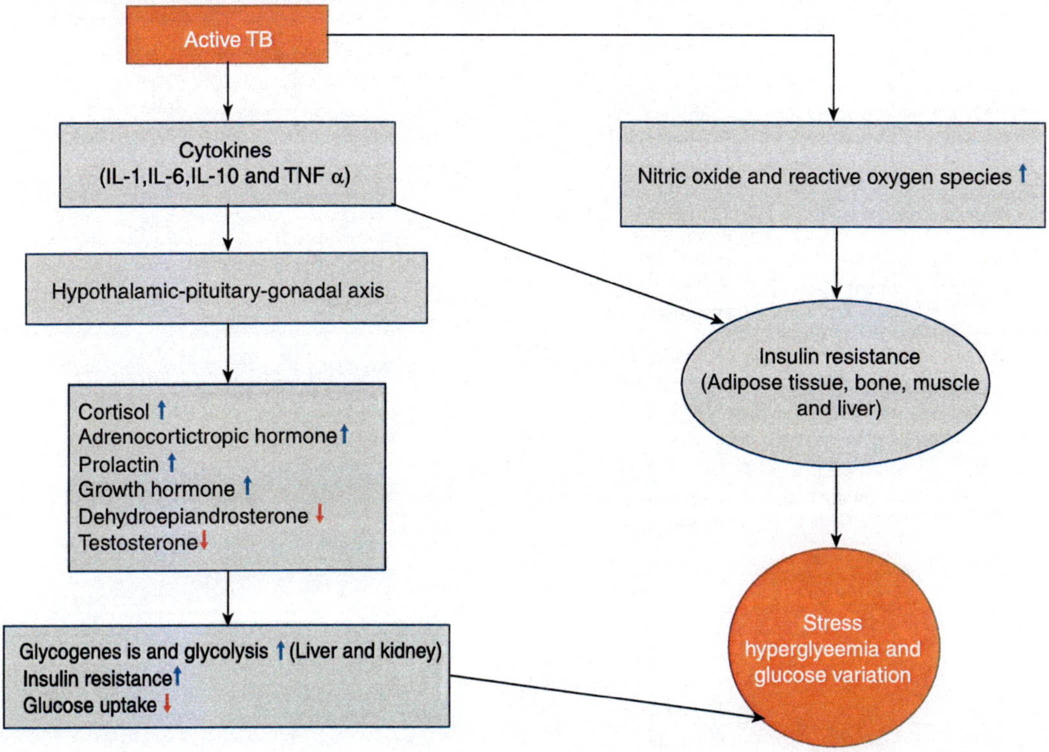

Fig. 8.2 Tuberculosis causes metabolic and endocrine changes leading to stress hyperglycemia. Tuberculosis stimulates the release of pro-inflammatory and anti-inflammatory cytokines and the production of cortisol. Prolactin growth hormorne increases gluconeogenesis amd glycolysis is in the liver and kidney, increases insulin resistance, reduces glucose intake, and leads to elevated blood sugar. Increased nitric oxide and reactive oxygen species can also increase insulin resistance

showed that the prevalence of tuberculosis was 717/100,000, 5.5/100,000, 523/100,000, 367/100,000, and 495/100,000 respectively, indicating a general downward trend. However, the control of tuberculosis in rural areas and Western China was unsatisfactory. Despite the global prevalence of tuberculosis is on the decline, the prevalence of diabetes increases year by year, so the situation of diabetes combined with tuberculosis is more serious.

A systematic review conducted by Harvard School of Public Health [101] showed that the risk of suffering from TB in diabetic patients was 3.1 times that of non-diabetic population. A study [102] found that the percentages of population attributable risk for tuberculosis attributed to diabetes and human immunodeficiency virus infection were 25% and 5%, respectively. Poor glycemic control is also associated with the risk of tuberculosis. Hong Zhu et al. [21] found that the risk of developing tuberculosis in patients with poor glycemic control was 8.7 times that of those with good glycemic control. The above results suggest that the level of glycemic control and the severity of the disease in diabetic patients are closely related to the risk of tuberculosis.

The results of tuberculosis screening among 15,342 diabetic patients in 5 provinces and regions in China [103] showed that 0.6% (92 cases) of the subjects were screened for sputum positive tuberculosis patients, which was higher than the prevalence of healthy control population, of which 48 patients were newly diagnosed with tuberculosis. In 2003, the new registration rate of tuberculosis patients with diabetes in Haikou city was 0.6/100,000 [104], which increased to 1.8/100,000 in 2008, with an annual increase rate of 24.6%. According to the data from Chengdu

Table 8.4 The prevalence of DM-TB in China

Authors	Region	Sample source	Year	Number of patients with TB	Number of patients with TB-DM	The comorbidity rate
Liang et al.	Beijing	Community	2001	1061	87	8.2
Zhu et al.	Jiangsu	Community	2002	2238	88	3.93
Zhang et al.	Zhejiang	Community	2002	2737	231	8.44
Li et al.	Xinjiang	Community	2003	1073	35	3.26
Liu et al.	Henan	Hospital	2003	1256	158	12.58
Zheng et al.	Shanghai	Community	2006	4573	335	7.33
Yue et al.	Sichuan	Community	2006	5049	105	2.08
Chen et al.	Zhejiang	Community	2006	526	28	5.32
Yang et al.	Chongqing	Community	2007	3884	285	7.34
Chen et al.	Hainan	Community	2009	4453	126	2.83
Wang et al.	Hebei	Community	2009	669	64	9.57
Yuan et al.	Hunan	Community	2009	1833	110	6
Yang et al.	Zhejiang	Community	2009	946	52	5.5
Kuang et al.	Guangdong	Community	2010	16,899	1047	6.2
Cao et al.	Beijing	Community	2010	1085	110	10.14
Huang et al.	Jiangsu	Community	2011	578	34	5.88
Lin et al.	Zhejiang	Community	2011	1569	59	3.76
Li et al.	Guangxi	Hospital	2011	833	75	9
Xi et al.	Shanghai	Hospital	2012	725	75	10.34
Cai et al.	Tianjin	Hospital	2012	2612	227	8.69
Sun et al.	Gansu	Community	2012	1080	90	8.33
Gu et al.	Beijing	Community	2013	1126	182	16.16

Tuberculosis Control Institute [105], the proportion of inpatients with tuberculosis complicated with diabetes increased from 3.35% in 2001 to 6.71% in 2004. In 2014, the proportion of tuberculosis patients with diabetes in Tianjin was 10.36% [103]. The age distribution of patients with tuberculosis complicated with diabetes has certain characteristics, most of which are elderly patients, and the incidence increases significantly after 40 years old, which overlaps with the age of onset of diabetes. Xuejun Gu et al. [106] found that middle-aged and elderly people in China were the population with a high risk of tuberculosis combined with type 2 diabetes, which may be related to the poor nutritional status of the elderly, low cellular immune function, and decreased ability of the body to defend against infection (Table 8.4).

8.5.2.3 Risk Factors for PTB-DM

Sociodemographic characteristics and economic factors: Relevant studies [107] have found that males were at a higher risk of developing TB combined with diabetes, and males are a risk factor for TB with diabetes. The elderly population is a risk factor for TB complicated with diabetes, and the reason may be related to the decreased immune status and more likely to develop TB and diabetes. It has also been reported that urban residence was a risk factor for the formation of TB with diabetes [108]. In addition, place of birth, ethnicity, high-income, and occupational class were also risk factors [109].

Behavioral factors: Illicit drug use and a sedentary lifestyle have been reported to be risk factors for TB with diabetes [110]. Behavioral characteristics such as smoking and alcohol consumption, as risk factors, have been associated with TB with diabetes [111]. Smoking causes inflammation and oxidative stress increases the risk of diabetes [112]. Conversely, regular outdoor activity is a protective factor for TB with diabetes [113], which may be related to the increased peripheral insulin sensitivity after the increase of physical activity, resulting in more glucose uptake of body muscles.

Clinical factors: Long duration of diabetes, poor glycemic control, liver cirrhosis, and the history of hypertension are all risk factors for TB with diabetes [114]. Poor glycemic control is usually associated with diabetes duration, which can impair both the innate and adaptive immune responses necessary to combat the spread of tuberculosis. Family history of diabetes, history of tuberculosis, TB treatment, more side effects, and long duration of anti-TB treatment are risk factors for TB with diabetes [114]. Receiving TB treatment after abandoning has also been identified as a low-risk factor for TB with diabetes [115].

Other factors: It has been reported [116] that contacting confirmed TB patients was a risk factor for TB development in diabetic patients. Frequent exposure can lead to the transmission of tuberculosis. Patients with a history of incarceration have been associated with the occurrence of TB with diabetes, indicating a high incidence of these two diseases during incarceration in view of overcrowding and stressful living conditions [111]. Kept in certain institutions (prison, hospices, orphanages, psychiatric hospitals, etc.) was a risk factor for TB with diabetes.

8.5.2.4 The Mechanism of PTB-DM

The mechanisms underlying the high incidence of diabetes in patients with tuberculosis have not been expounded very well. When the observational population epidemiological study found that the two diseases were concurrent [117], it was difficult to predict the order of their onset, which added difficulties to the study of related mechanisms. Studies have pointed out that among patients with active tuberculosis, almost all of the screened diabetic patients had been diagnosed as diabetes before the diagnosis of tuberculosis, which may be caused by the effect of diabetes on the body's anti-tuberculosis immunity. At present, it is believed that the effect mechanism of diabetes on tuberculosis may be caused by the direct effects of hyperglycemia and cellular insulin deficiency [118], as well as the indirect effects of macrophages and lymphocytes functions. The most important effector cells which limit the development of tuberculosis are phagocytes and lymphocytes. Chronic hyperglycemia would cause damage to the immune system and affect the chemotaxis, phagocytosis, activation, and antigen presentation of phagocytes in response to tuberculosis, which promotes the occurrence of active tuberculosis. Animal experiments [119] have shown that diabetic mice had a delayed adaptive immune response in the initial stage of tuberculosis infection, which promoted the spread of bacteria from the lungs to the lymph nodes and the accumulation of lymphocytes at the infected site. In the initial stage of lymphocytes activation, phagocytes acted as antigen-presenting cells, and the conjugated antigen was then processed and presented through the Fc receptor. Once the cells were activated, interleukin (IL) can be produced to enhance T cell proliferation. When lacking insulin, it would cause damage to the Fc receptor binding element, thus affecting cell activation. Some studies [120] have speculated that the increased susceptibility of diabetic patients to tuberculosis is caused by Th1 (T helper cell 1, Th1) cytokines deficiency in T helper cells (Th). Macrophages recognize MTB to trigger cell activation and cytokines production and further promote self-activation as well as cytokines production. This cascade of cytokines is critical in the immune response and the control of tuberculosis infection outcome.

Diabetic patients generally have abnormal liver function, which leads to a lack of vitamin A in vivo, reduces the resistance of the respiratory mucosa, and reduces the ability to eliminate MTB [121]. T-lymphocyte-mediated cellular immunity is the most important immune response of anti-tuberculosis immunity. The cellular immunity of patients with diabetes combined with tuberculosis reduces significantly than patients with simple tuberculosis. The main manifestations are the reduction of CD3+ and CD4+T lymphocytes, leading to the inability to kill MTB. The relative increase in CD8+T lymphocytes and the enhanced effect of lyzing macrophages cause the release and spread of MTB, and the number of helper T cells is significantly reduced, cellular immunity is suppressed, thereby reducing the successful cure rate of diabetes and tuberculosis patients. Recent studies [114] have shown that patients with active tuberculosis (with or without diabetes) had lower levels of interferon-γ (IFN-γ), while other pro-inflammatory factors and interleukin-4 (IL-4) levels were higher. In addition, gluconic acid, triglycerides, and ketone bodies in diabetic patients accumulate in the blood and tissues, which can provide sufficient nutrients and a good acidic environment for the reproduction and growth of MTB; at the same time, diabetic microangiopathy lesions could involve the lungs providing a suitable place for the invasion and reproduction of MTB. Relevant studies [122] have shown that changes in glucose and lipid metabolism led to a change from an anti-inflammatory environment to a pro-inflammatory environment, making diabetic patients more susceptible to bacterial infections. Due to the decrease of reduced glutathione, diabetic patients have poor ability to regulate the level of active oxygen in the body, and the increase of reduced nicotinamide adenine dinucleotide phosphate reduces the regeneration ability of reduced glutathione, thereby intensifying the reduction of reduced glutathione.

8.5.2.5 PTB-DM Treatment Outcome

After tuberculosis patients co-infect with diabetes, due to the mutual influence of the two diseases, it develops more rapidly. It has the characteristics of rapid lesions, wide range and easy formation of pulmonary cavities, which leads to changes in the clinical manifestations of tuberculosis and poor prognosis of treatment [123], such as increased bacterial load in sputum, increased numeration of leukocyte, acute phase reactions, and fever. The incidence of clinical symptoms in patients with diabetes combined with tuberculosis is significantly higher than that in patients with simple tuberculosis, and the lesions are mostly distributed in the lower lobes of the lung, commonly with pulmonary consolidation, multiple cavities, and tree bud-shaped bronchial foci. In a number of prospective studies and retrospective studies [124], the effect of anti-tuberculosis treatment in patients with hyperglycemia or diabetes was poor. Therefore, the WHO recommends screening for diabetes in all tuberculosis patients and optimizing blood glucose control during anti-tuberculosis treatment, thereby improving tuberculosis treatment outcomes.

Diabetes affects the treatment of tuberculosis patients, which is mostly manifested in the rate of sputum negative conversion, drug resistance, relapse, and mortality in tuberculosis patients. Patients with tuberculosis combined with diabetes have a higher positive rate of sputum test than patients with simple tuberculosis, a longer time for sputum negative conversion, and a lower rate of sputum negative conversion. At the same time, diabetes increases the risk of drug-resistant tuberculosis. Studies [125] have found that after taking rifampicin 6 h, the maximum blood concentration of patients co-infected with diabetes and tuberculosis was only half that of non-diabetes TB patients. Due to the low blood concentration, MTB was more resistant to drugs. These differences in pharmacokinetics may be an important mechanism for drug resistance of MTB. Other studies have found that patients co-infected with tuberculosis and diabetes had increased bacterial load, longer treatment time, and higher treatment failure rate than those with simple tuberculosis, and were more likely to transform into multi-drug-resistant tuberculosis.

Therefore, for patients co-infected with tuberculosis and diabetes, health education should be strengthened to improve treatment compliance. When standard treatment plans are adopted, the course of treatment ought to be appropriately extended according to the actual conditions of the patients to reduce the recurrence rate and the production of drug-resistant tuberculosis. Good blood glucose control is of great significance for improving the effect of anti-tuberculosis treatment in patients with tuberculosis.

8.5.2.6 Prevention and Control Strategy of PTB-DM

In conjunction with the work of basic public health service projects, active screening for tuberculosis should be performed in diabetic patients managed within the jurisdiction. When basic medical and health institutions conduct quarterly follow-ups of diabetic patients, they must screen for suspected tuberculosis symptoms and provide health education. For people with suspected tuberculosis symptoms, qualified primary medical and health institutions should perform imaging screening of those with suspicious symptoms at first. If the chest X-ray is abnormal, then refer them to designated tuberculosis medical institutions at the county (district) level; unconditional primary medical and health institutions will directly refer people with suspicious symptoms to designated tuberculosis medical institutions at county (district) level for tuberculosis examinations.

In addition to the quarterly symptom screening, qualified primary medical and health institutions can also perform chest imaging examinations once a year for diabetic patients with high-risk factors (such as previous tuberculosis patients, underweight malnutrition, poor blood sugar control, etc.). If abnormal chest X-rays are found, they should be referred to designated tuberculosis medical institutions at county (district) level for tuberculosis examination.

8.5.3 Rare Complications of Tuberculosis

In addition to the most common diabetes and HIV infection, clinical tuberculosis is also prone to other diseases, including silicosis, chronic obstructive pneumonia, lung cancer, acute respiratory distress syndrome, and so on. Although the incidence of these comorbidities is relatively low, they have a significant impact on the treatment outcome of tuberculosis. Therefore, attention should be paid to the diagnosis and treatment of tuberculosis. In a retrospective study from 2011 to 2017 in Suzhou, Jiangsu Province, it has been reported that 72.70% of inpatient pulmonary tuberculosis had complications, of which extrapulmonary tuberculosis, diabetes, hemoptysis, drug resistance, and adverse drug reactions were the most common types [126]. The Beijing Chest Hospital analyzed the complications of inpatient pulmonary tuberculosis from 2012 to 2016. Among them, 8 types of pulmonary tuberculosis complications accounted for the main clinical types, including malnutrition, type 2 diabetes, anemia, leukopenia, and viral hepatitis. And respiratory system-related lung cancer, chronic obstructive pulmonary disease, and silicosis were all associated with the patient's age and gender. Male patients older than 60 had a significantly higher probability of comorbidities than other groups [127]. Elderly pulmonary tuberculosis patients combined with other diseases have more complicated clinical symptoms, and their anti-tuberculosis treatment outcomes are often unsatisfactory. Comprehensive treatment methods should be applied to improve the treatment effect. Taking elderly pulmonary tuberculosis with chronic obstructive pneumonia as an example, studies have shown that such patients often have no characteristic clinical manifestations and atypical imaging features. They are prone to complicated bacterial infections and mixed bacterial infections, and there are mostly moderate to severe changes in their lung function. Moreover, systemic adverse reactions and body immunity are affected to varying degrees. Therefore, under the principle of anti-tuberculosis treatment, it is necessary to select antibiotics according to pathogenic bacteria and drug sensitivity and give reasonable individualized treatment to achieve a better outcome [128]. Low immunity combined with hypoproteinemia caused by long-term use of glucocorticoids can easily induce acute respiratory distress syndrome in patients with tuberculosis, and the mortality rate is high. So, effective mechanical ventilation is required as soon as possible [129]. In conclusion, as for rare complications of tuberculosis more detailed and comprehensive diagnosis and differential diagnosis are required and the therapeutic schedule should be individually designed to ensure the treatment effect.

8.6 Prevention and Control of Tuberculosis in Key Populations

Strengthening detecting TB patients in key places and key populations and carrying out standardized treatment management can effectively reduce the spread of TB and accelerate the decline of TB epidemic.

8.6.1 Students

Although the TB incidence numbers have been decreasing in recent years, the number of new TB patients is still large every year due to the large population and high population infection rate. Due to the heavy study burden, the developing immune system, and the limited protective effect of BCG vaccine, students are prone to active TB after being infected with tuberculosis bacteria. The campus is crowded, and it is liable to cause TB outbreak once there is an index patient. In China, TB outbreaks often occur in school settings like kindergartens, primary schools, high school, and colleges [130, 131]. Compared to other school settings, boarding schools have a higher risk of TB outbreaks, where adolescents often flock together under relatively overcrowded conditions [132, 133]. Therefore, students are one of the key populations of tuberculosis.

8.6.1.1 Characteristics of the Epidemic

The reported incidence of TB among students is about one-fifth of that among the whole population, and the overall trend is decreasing. From the perspective of population classification, the reported incidence of TB in students accounted for about 4%–6% of the total reported incidence of TB in population, second only to the number of patients in farmers, workers, and retirees. In terms of reporting age, the 15–24 years old age group accounts for about 85% of the total number of reported cases of students, that is, students in high school, undergraduate and junior college students, especially the age group around 18 years old has the highest proportion.

8.6.1.2 Characteristics of Public Health Emergencies of TB in Schools

In recent years, China has reported many public health emergencies of tuberculosis in schools, showing the following characteristics:

First, being focused on boarding schools; Second, high school is the majority; Third, the proportion of TB patients with positive bacteria is low; Fourth, emergencies in low-epidemic areas occur more often in schools with more students from high-epidemic areas. In addition, there have been outbreaks of MDR-TB transmission within schools.

8.6.1.3 School Routine Preventive Control Measures

1. *Physical examination*

   Physical examination is an important tool for early detection of TB patients. Schools should carry out TB-related examinations in the *Physical examination* at the entrance for freshmen and regular physical examinations for faculty and staff, and incorporate the results of the physical examinations into the health files of students and staffs.

2. *Entrance examination*

   (a) *New students enrolled in kindergarten, primary school, and non-boarding secondary school*

   Inquire about the patient's close contact history and suspicious symptoms of tuberculosis. For students with a history of close contact with tuberculosis patients or suspicious symptoms, they will receive TST. The students with suspected pulmonary TB symptoms or strong positive TST results (mean induration of diameter ≥ 15 mm or local double circles, blisters, necrosis, and lymphangitis) should be examined by chest X-ray.

   (b) *New students entering high school and boarding junior high school*

   Questionnaire for suspicious symptoms of tuberculosis and TST. The students with suspected pulmonary TB symptoms or strong positive TST results should be examined by chest X-ray.

   (c) *College freshmen*

   Questionnaire for suspicious symptoms of tuberculosis and chest X-ray.

   (d) *Physical examination of staff*

   Questionnaire for suspicious symptoms of tuberculosis and chest X-ray.

3. *Health education*

   School tuberculosis health education refers to carrying out health education of the knowledge and skills in TB prevention and treatment to make them develop good habits of study, hygiene and living, prevent the transition of tuberculosis, eliminate concealment reporting of TB from teachers and students, and reduce the risk of TB spreading on campus.

4. *Environmental health of school*

   Schools, in accordance with the relevant regulations and standards of school hygiene, guarantee the per capita use area for students to study and live, and strengthen the ventilation of classrooms, dormitories, libraries, and other crowd gathering places, do a good job in cleaning the campus environment.

5. *Illness absence monitoring and cause tracking of students*

   (a) *Morning check*

   It applies to nursery institutions and primary and secondary schools. It can also be carried out in colleges and universities where conditions permit. The class monitor is assigned by the head teacher or the designated student, who is responsible for the morning check and record work. The school doctor trained the monitors in each class, and the monitors were responsible for the morning examination every day to know whether each student had cough, phlegm, fever, night sweats, and other symptoms. If students have cough, expectoration, or other suspicious symptoms, the monitor should report them to the school clinic (health room/health room) in time. The school designates personnel or notifies parents to accompany students with suspicious symptoms to the local tuberculosis designated medical institutions for examination.

   (b) *Cause tracking and registration of absence due to illness*

   Attention should be paid to the tracking and management of students/staff who ask for leave due to illness. And this work falls on head teacher (counselor), class cadre, dormitory leader, school hospital and clinic (health care room/clinic) should be established. Students who are absent from school should be confirmed whether they are absent due to illness, especially those who have chronic cough, expectoration, and other suspicious symptoms of TB. The school designates personnel or notifies parents to accompany students with suspicious symptoms to the local tuberculosis designated medical institutions for examination.

   (c) *Standard of suspension*

   Students who meet one of the following conditions for tuberculosis shall be suspended from school.

   ① TB patients with positive bacteria;
   ② Chest radiographs show extensive lung lesions and/or cavitation in TB patients with negative bacteria.
   ③ Patients with obvious symptoms of TB, such as cough, expectoration, hemoptysis, etc.
   ④ Other conditions, according to the actual situation of the patient.

   (d) *Standard of resumption of schooling*

   Bacteria-positive pulmonary TB patients and severe bacteria-negative pulmonary TB patients (including cavity/large caseous necrosis lesions/miliary pulmonary TB, etc.) have completed the full course of treatment after standard treatment, reaching the standard of cure or completion of treatment.

   Other bacteria-negative pulmonary TB patients: After 2 months of standard treatment, the symptoms were relieved or disappeared, and the lesion on chest X-ray was obviously absorbed. Have at least two sputum smear tests and one *Mycobacterium* TB culture test (at least 1 month between each test) after the end of 3 months of treatment.

6. *Management process of school TB outbreak*

   (a) *Definition*

   Sporadic outbreaks of tuberculosis in schools: a case of TB is found in a school but has not yet up to a public health emergency.

   Public health emergencies of TB in schools: the occurrence of 10 or more epidemiologically linked TB cases or deaths from TB in the same term in a school.

Close contacts: ① Students and teachers who study in the same classroom and live in the same dormitory with the TB patient. ② Family members who have contacted with the TB patient in the same residence for up to 7 days between 3 months before diagnosis and 14 days after treatment begins. ③ Other patients with bacteria-positive/severe bacteria-negative/obvious-symptom bacteria-negative patients who have been in direct contact for 8 h or more or cumulatively up to 40 h in a closed space from 3 months before diagnosis to 14 days after starting treatment, or with other bacteria-negative patients who have accumulated 40 h of exposure in the 1 month before diagnosis.

If the patient has more than 3 months from the onset of symptoms to a clear diagnosis, the above definition of close contacts should be updated from the onset of symptoms to 14 days after the start of treatment.

General contacts: those who study and live together in the same teaching floor or dormitory floor as the indicative case.

Occasional contacts: Those who study and live together on the same teaching building or dormitory building but not on the same floor as the indicative case, or who have occasional contact with teachers and students.

(b) *The screening process*

After finding the active TB of students, the CDC staff immediately conducted field epidemiological investigations. At first, perform TST and chest X-ray among close contacts. If new TB cases are found in the first screening, or the strong positive rate of TST detection in close contacts is significantly higher than that in the same age group in the area, the scope of contact screening should be expanded to all general contacts. It also needs to screen all close contacts of newly detected cases. Then if new TB cases are found in the expanded screening, or the strong positive rate of TST detection in close contacts is significantly higher than that in the same age group in the area, the scope of contact screening should be expanded to all occasional contacts. It also needs to screen all close contacts of newly detected cases.

(c) *Dispose after screening*

Active TB: Standardized anti-TB treatment and supervised medication management should be started as soon as possible, and management of suspension and resumption of schooling should be carried out in accordance with relevant regulations.

Suspected pulmonary TB patient: Should be segregated first, and wait for diagnosis or exclude from pulmonary TB, then undertake follow-up processing according to relevant requirements.

For individuals with strong TST (PPD $\geq$ 15 mm) or IGRA test, preventive treatment should be provided under the principle of informed consent. For those who did not receive preventive treatment, health education and health monitoring should be strengthened. If suspicious symptoms of TB occur, they should go to designated medical hospitals for TB treatment in time. Chest X-ray examination should be conducted at the end of third month, the end of sixth month, and the end of twelfth month after the first screening, respectively. Prophylaxis is strongly recommended when detecting three or more cases of TB. For individuals with PPD < 15 mm and > 5 mm, health education should been developed and strengthen health monitoring should be strengthened. When appearing TB suspicious symptom, go to designate medical hospitals in time. When detecting three or more cases of TB, it is recommended that those who are with PPD < 15 mm and > 5 mm should be re-examined by chest X-ray after 3 months. Should develop health education and strengthen health monitoring among individuals with negative TST (PPD < 15 mm) or IGRA test. When appearing

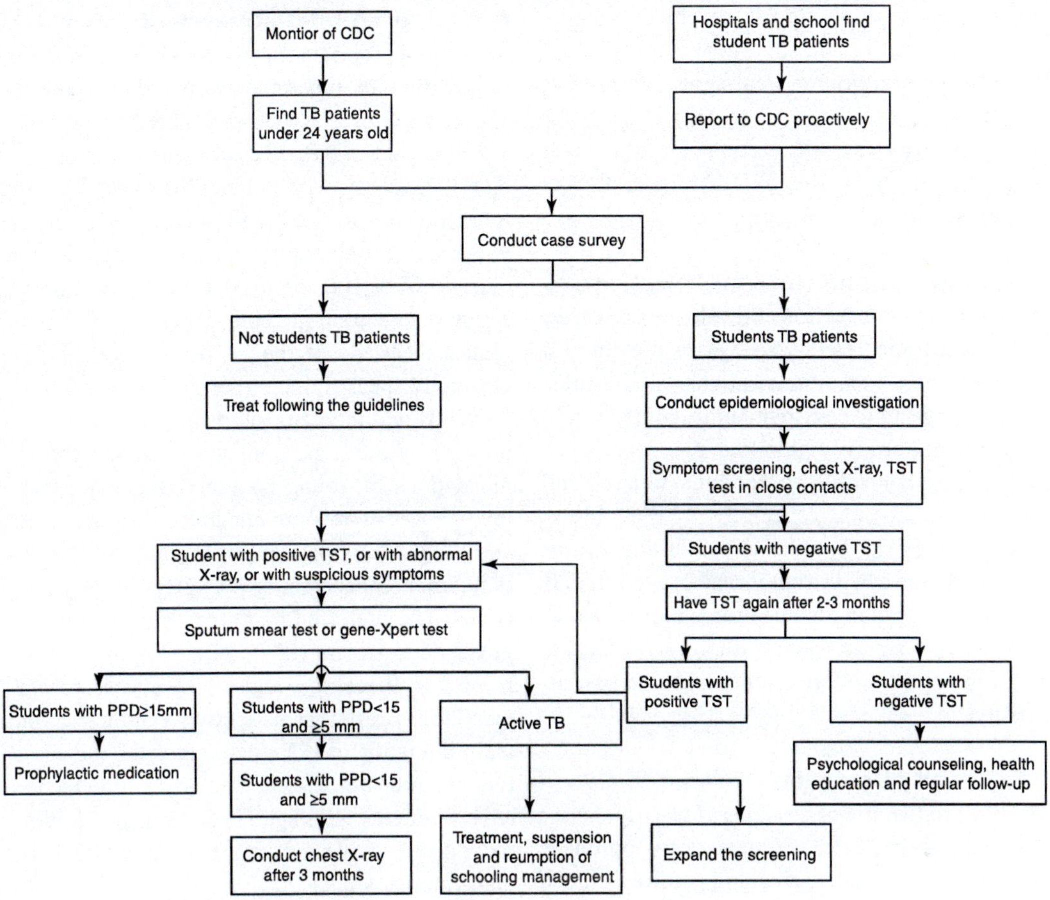

Fig. 8.3 Flowchart of TB outbreak dispose

TB suspicious symptom, go to designate medical hospitals in time. When appearing a public health emergency of TB in schools, TST or IGRA tests should be performed again after 3 months, and chest X-rays should be performed on individuals with positive conversion of TST and IGRA (Fig. 8.3).

8.6.2 The Elderly

With declining fertility rates and longer life expectancy, the pace of aging population is getting faster and faster all over the world. It was estimated that the global population over 60 will exceed 2 billion by 2050. The impacts TB epidemiology have on aging population are rather complicated, and vary among countries and regions [39]. Studies confirmed that TB incidence and mortality are higher in the vulnerable elderly population both in developing and developed countries with higher TB burden, such as India, Indonesia, and China. It was reported, that the notification rates of TB in people over the age of 65 were significantly higher than that of any other 10-year interval group. Tuberculosis is rapidly becoming a major public health challenge for the elderly all over the world. With the increase of age, the risk of TB infection in elderly cohorts is higher, as well as the possibility of remaining latent before reactivation. These are the main obstacles to the elimination of tuberculosis. The control and prevention strategies of tuberculosis in the elderly were divided into four categories, such as preventive transmission, program management, appropriate treatment, and early detection [134]. The aim of the intervention was to identify cases as early as possible so as to avoid delays in the treatment and further transmission.

8.6.2.1 Preventing Transmission

It is known that infection control was one of the most direct and effective ways to prevent TB transmission. Administrative measures, engineering and environmental control, and personal protective equipment play an important role in controlling infectious sources and vulnerable persons, especially in the elderly institutions [134]. In elderly institutions, symptomatic patients with radiographic signs of TB should be placed in the airborne infection isolation room, a single room with surgical masks, or transferred to an appropriate isolation facility.

8.6.2.2 Early Detection

There were two major strategies for early detection of tuberculosis: Strategies to optimize actions and systematic screening pathway (direct observation and short-course treatment) along the pathways initiated by patients.

The system screening pathway plays important role in the early detection of tuberculosis patients, especially in the elderly population, including:

1. Symptom screening: Observe and ask whether there are suspicious symptoms of pulmonary tuberculosis.
2. Chest imaging examination: Chest X-ray examination is the first choice for screening.
3. Pathogen-detecting: Smear microscopy or mycobacterium culture examination should be performed for suspected pulmonary tuberculosis patients.
4. Nucleic acid detection of MTB should be carried out in areas where conditions permit.
5. Immunological examination: TST, γ-IFN test were used as auxiliary examination methods.

8.6.2.3 Appropriate Treatment

Without appropriate interventions to prevent the progression of tuberculosis in elderly patients with tuberculosis, as well as to prevent new transmission and adverse treatment outcomes in elderly patients with tuberculosis, early latent tuberculosis infection and tuberculosis testing will become useless. Preventive treatment for the elderly cohort is recognized as the most effective single intervention method, which could directly reduce the scale of the latent reservoirs [135]. Generally speaking, treatment recommendations for LTBI and tuberculosis in the elderly are not necessarily different from the treatment recommendations of young people. Generally speaking, treatment recommendations for the LTBI and tuberculosis patients in the elderly population are not necessarily different from young adults. The preferred treatment is isoniazid prophylactic treatment (IPT), with a regime ranging from 6 to 9 months, and 12 months is recommended for different patients. Nevertheless, the main limitation of IPT treatment is the increased risk of hepatotoxicity and drug interaction adverse effects with age [136, 137]. In addition, older people may need longer duration of therapy than younger adults.

8.6.2.4 Programmatic Management

The aim of programmatic management was to effectively promote the strategic plan by improving the following key methods. In the designated national surveillance system, all of the elderly TB patients should be identified and reported promptly both in active and passive case-finding strategies. Health education on tuberculosis related knowledge should be provided to medical staff, patients, family members, visitors, and staff so that they can understand and participate in TB control programs. Health education of tuberculosis related knowledge should be provided to patients, medical staff, family members, and visitors so that they can understand and participate in TB control programs. A continuous assessment is required to evaluate and monitor activities consistent with TB control programs and responsibilities [138].

8.6.3 The Migration

Although there is no consistency in definition for migrant population, period of residence and spatial span are accepted as major elements. Therefore, the migrant population is the population who moves to a new living place without changed registered permanent residence except schooling, traveling, or enrollment of military and so on. Due to economic integration, migration is a global issue resulting in many hygiene problems, especially infectious diseases. In China, internal migration which means population moved among different provinces and migrant population commonly flowed into east coastal areas from relatively under-developed middle-west areas for better job, business, and health service. According to a study conducted between 2005 and 2015, the Eastern regions of China accounted for the highest levels of internal immigrants including Beijing (31.15%), Tianjin (19.6%), Shanghai (34.86%), Zhejiang (18.51%), and Guangdong (20.19%) provinces. Meanwhile, the TB clusters were mainly located in Central-Southern China which was emigrants clustered area [139].

Previous studies indicated that the migrating population is one of the vulnerable groups. Usually, they are engaged in work with high-risk but low socioeconomic status, such as architecture, manufacture, express delivery industry, and retail industry.

Therefore, migrant population is more likely to encounter diagnosis delay and unfavorable treatment. Compared to urban population, the incidence of TB was relatively higher among migrant population [140]. Researchers found that 75% of culture-positive tuberculosis occurred among migrants in Shanghai [141]. Meanwhile, another spatial and temporal analysis in Zhejiang Province revealed similar findings. Because of massive migrants, Wenzhou county which is one of the wealthiest regions had a significant higher risk of TB infection compared with other counties in the province [142]. Although the migrant population has been specialized as target population in national policy of TB control, the free treatment of TB could relieve the financial burden on TB immigration faintly. Due to different medical insurance systems, internal migrants who are from countryside are usually covered by the new rural cooperative medical system which only could been demonstrated in their local place. It is reasonable that once a migrant got TB, he would like to return to his hometown for anti-TB treatment under the health insurance. Furthermore, the high-speed railway also makes it convenient for people to move between provinces within a few hours. Nowadays, the available strategies for free diagnosis and treatment of TB achieved landmark decline in TB incidence, but the barrier to accessing TB care for immigrants in China remains a problem [143].

Besides, treatment defaults among urban migrants who move between cities and provinces were another major risk factor for TB control. The strengthened TB control program applied in the Eastern area of China improved the urban migrants' received medical service but the treatment success rate was still below the target set by the WHO. Furthermore, many urban migrant TB patients transferred during their treatment period could not been followed up again [144].

In conclusion, comprehensive health insurance coverage providing the thorough free detection and treatment of TB is a valuable policy for migrant TB control. Migrant TB patient should be diagnosed timely and treated as local resident completely without transfer frequently. There was a good model conducted in Shenzhen achieved distinct success. In the past 20 years, through establishing a specialized comprehensive TB management system for the internal migrating population, a population-wide TB control strategy was implemented in Shenzhen. As a result, the prevalence of SS+ TB among migrants has dropped by 54.2% and treatment success rate increased to 90.3% [145].

8.6.4 Prisoner

As a risk factor, prisoner is a vulnerable group of TB infection worldwide. Due to overcrowding, limited health services, poor ventilation, and lacked infection control, prisoners are more likely to develop active TB and disease transmission [146]. In South Africa, 3.5% of prisoners not taking tuberculosis treatment were detected as culture positive for MTB [147]. Meanwhile, a high prevalence of latent TB was declared in Spanish prisons which was related to age, sex, and nationality origin [148]. In China, the epidemic of tuberculosis in prison also was severer. A study choosing two prisons in Central China to screen TB patients. The active TB prevalence (1156/100000) was significantly higher than that of the province and China's general population ($P < 0.01$) [149]. Besides exaggerated TB prevalence in prison, the treatment success rate of TB patient in prison was lower than the target according to WHO [150]. Therefore, many studies concerned the specific control strategy to improve the obstacle. Considering the characteristics of TB epidemic in prison, male prisoners is needed to be paid more attention and screening of latent TB in the prison unit, especially among high-risk groups should be emphasized. Furthermore, it is also necessary to establish a consummate and effective management system to enhance the treatment outcome.

8.7 Conclusion and Future Trends

Currently, tuberculosis is a major cause of ill health, ranked in the top 10 causes of death worldwide, and becomes the leading cause of death from a single infectious agent. In 2015, WHO has launched the stopping and ending the global TB epidemic as an aspiration for the next 20 years of tuberculosis control, with the targets of 90% reduction in tuberculosis incidence, 95% reduction in tuberculosis deaths, and an end to catastrophic personal costs to individuals and families affected by tuberculosis. Current rates of decline in tuberculosis incidence are between 1% and 2% per year, but achieving the 90% target requires >15% reductions annually for the next 20 years. Accelerating the implementation of currently available tools would increase the rate of decline according to the mathematical calculation, but we would still fall short.

At the end of 2019, most WHO regions and many high TB burden countries were not on track to reach the 2020 milestones of the End TB Strategy. Even though the global TB incidence rate is falling, it was not fast enough to reach the 2020 milestone of a 20% reduction between 2015 and 2020. Meanwhile, the annual number of TB deaths is falling globally, but not fast enough to reach the 2020 milestone of a 35% reduction between 2015 and 2020. Since 2015, a total of 17 countries have completed a national survey of costs faced by TB patients and their households. However, on average 49% of people with TB and their households faced catastrophic costs.

The COVID-19 pandemic threatens to reverse recent progress in reducing the global burden of TB disease. Negative impacts on many essential TB services include the reallocation of human, financial, and other resources from TB to the COVID-19 control. Two modeling analyses have reached similar conclusions about the potential impact of the COVID-19 pandemic on global TB deaths. They suggested that the annual number of TB could rise to the levels seen in 2015 or even 2012. Overall, it is crucial to maintain and strengthen TB services as an essential component of overall progress toward universal health coverage, and to ensure synergies in the control of both TB and COVID-19.

To end the global TB epidemic, the world needs to expand affordable and accessible rapid point-of-care tests for diagnosing TB infection and TB disease, and for detecting drug resistance; shorter, safer, and more effective regimens for treating TB infection, drug-susceptible and drug-resistant TB; a TB vaccine that is effective before and after exposure, as well as across a range of age groups and geographical settings; and innovative strategies to address broader determinants of TB, such as poverty, undernutrition, HIV infection, smoking, and diabetes.

References

1. WHO. Global tuberculosis report 2021. Geneva: World Health Organization; 2021.
2. Uplekar M, Weil D, Lonnroth K, Jaramillo E, Lienhardt C, Dias HM, Falzon D, Floyd K, Gargioni G, Getahun H. WHO's new end TB strategy. Lancet. 2015;385:1799–801.

3. Wang Y. Compilation of the fifth national tuberculosis epidemiological sample survey. Beijing: Military Medical Science Press; 2011.
4. Getahun H, Matteelli A, Chaisson RE, Raviglione M. Latent Mycobacterium tuberculosis infection. New Engl J Med. 2015;372:2127.
5. Jagger A, Reiter-Karam S, Hamada Y, Getahun H. National policies on the management of latent tuberculosis infection: review of 98 countries. Bull World Health Organ. 2018;96:173–184F.
6. Lu P, Cheng J, Lu X, Liu E, Zhou L, Lu W. Scientific preventive treatment to accelerate the process of tuberculosis control (in Chinese). Chin J Antituberc. 2020;42:316–21.
7. Cadena AM, Fortune SM, Flynn JL. Heterogeneity in tuberculosis. Nat Rev Immunol. 2017;17:691–702.
8. Barry CE, Boshoff HI, Dartois V, Dick T, Ehrt S, Flynn J, Schnappinger D, Wilkinson RJ, Young D. The spectrum of latent tuberculosis: rethinking the biology and intervention strategies. Nat Rev Microbiol. 2009;7:845–55.
9. Duanmu H. Report on fourth national epidemiological sampling survey of tuberculosis (in Chinese). Chin J Tuberc Respir Dis. 2002;25:3–7.
10. Bennett DE, Courval JM, Onorato I, Agerton T, Gibson JD, Lambert L, McQuillan GM, Lewis B, Navin TR, Castro KG. Prevalence of tuberculosis infection in the United States population: the national health and nutrition examination survey, 1999–2000. Am J Respir Crit Care Med. 2008;177:348–55.
11. Gao L, Lu W, Bai L, Wang X, Xu J, Catanzaro A, Cárdenas V, Li X, Yang Y, Du J. Latent tuberculosis infection in rural China: baseline results of a population-based, multicentre, prospective cohort study. Lancet Infect Dis. 2015;15(3):310–9.
12. Vukmanovic-Stejic M, Reed JR, Lacy KE, Rustin MH, Akbar AN. Mantoux test as a model for a secondary immune response in humans. Immunol Lett. 2006;107:93–101.
13. Bakir M, Dosanjh DP, Deeks JJ, Soysal A, Millington KA, Efe S, Aslan Y, Polat D, Kodalli N, Yagci A. Use of T cell-based diagnosis of tuberculosis infection to optimize interpretation of tuberculin skin testing for child tuberculosis contacts. Clin Infect Dis. 2009;48:302–12.
14. Kim S-H, Song K-H, Choi S-J, Kim H-B, Kim N-J, Oh M-d, Choe K-W. Diagnostic usefulness of a T-cell-based assay for extrapulmonary tuberculosis in immunocompromised patients. Am J Med. 2009;122:189–95.
15. Cobelens FG, Egwaga SM, Ginkel Van T, Muwinge H, Matee MI, Borgdorff MW. Tuberculin skin testing in patients with HIV infection: limited benefit of reduced cutoff values. Clin Infect Dis. 2006;43:634–9.
16. Pai M, Nicol MP, Boehme CC. Tuberculosis diagnostics: state of the art and future directions. Microbiol Spectr. 2016;4:16.
17. Chen C, Zhu T, Wang Z, Peng H, Kong W, Zhou Y, Shao Y, Zhu L, Lu W. High latent TB infection rate and associated risk factors in the Eastern China of low TB incidence. PLoS One. 2015;10:e0141511.
18. Van der Werf MJ, Langendam MW, Huitric E, Manissero D. Multidrug resistance after inappropriate tuberculosis treatment: a meta-analysis. Eur Respir J. 2012;39:1511–9.
19. Lewinsohn DA, Zalwango S, Stein CM, Mayanja-Kizza H, Okwera A, Boom WH, Mugerwa RD, Whalen CC. Whole blood interferon-gamma responses to Mycobacterium tuberculosis antigens in young household contacts of persons with tuberculosis in Uganda. PLoS One. 2008;3:e3407.
20. Rangaka MX, Wilkinson RJ, Boulle A, Glynn JR, Fielding K, Van Cutsem G, Wilkinson KA, Goliath R, Mathee S, Goemaere E. Isoniazid plus antiretroviral therapy to prevent tuberculosis: a randomised double-blind, placebo-controlled trial. Lancet. 2014;384:682–90.
21. Martinson NA, Barnes GL, Moulton LH, Msandiwa R, Hausler H, Ram M, McIntyre JA, Gray GE, Chaisson RE. New regimens to prevent tuberculosis in adults with HIV infection. N Engl J Med. 2011;365:11–20.
22. Sterling TR, Scott NA, Miro JM, Calvet G, La Rosa A, Infante R, Chen MP, Benator DA, Gordin F, Benson CA, Chaisson RE, Villarino ME. Three months of weekly rifapentine and isoniazid for treatment of Mycobacterium tuberculosis infection in HIV-coinfected persons. AIDS. 2016;30:1607–15.
23. Sterling TR, Villarino ME, Borisov AS, Shang N, Gordin F, Bliven-Sizemore E, Hackman J, Hamilton CD, Menzies D, Kerrigan A, Weis SE, Weiner M, Wing D, Conde MB, Bozeman L, Horsburgh CR Jr, Chaisson RE. Three months of rifapentine and isoniazid for latent tuberculosis infection. N Engl J Med. 2011;365:2155–66.
24. Villarino ME, Scott NA, Weis SE, Weiner M, Conde MB, Jones B, Nachman S, Oliveira R, Moro RN, Shang N, Goldberg SV, Sterling TR. Treatment for preventing tuberculosis in children and adolescents: a randomized clinical trial of a 3-month, 12-dose regimen of a combination of rifapentine and isoniazid. JAMA Pediatr. 2015;169:247–55.
25. Sharma SK, Vashishtha R, Chauhan LS, Sreenivas V, Seth D. Comparison of TST and IGRA in diagnosis of latent tuberculosis infection in a high TB-burden setting. PLoS One. 2017;12:e0169539.
26. Spyridis NP, Spyridis PG, Gelesme A, Sypsa V, Valianatou M, Metsou F, Gourgiotis D, Tsolia MN. The effectiveness of a 9-month regimen of isoniazid alone versus 3- and 4-month regimens of isoniazid plus rifampin for treatment of latent tuberculosis infection in children: results of an 11-year randomized study. Clin Infect Dis. 2007;45:715–22.
27. Galli L, Lancella L, Tersigni C, Venturini E, Chiappini E, Bergamini BM, Codifava M, Venturelli C, Tosetti G, Marabotto C, Cursi L, Boccuzzi E, Garazzino S, Tovo PA, Pinon M, Le Serre D, Castiglioni L, Lo Vecchio A, Guarino A, Bruzzese E, Losurdo G, Castagnola E, Bossi G, Marseglia GL,

Esposito S, Bosis S, Grandolfo R, Fiorito V, Valentini P, Buonsenso D, Domenici R, Montesanti M, Salvini FM, Riva E, Dodi I, Maschio F, Abbagnato L, Fiumana E, Fornabaio C, Ballista P, Portelli V, Bottone G, Palladino N, Valenzise M, Vecchi B, Di Gangi M, Lupi C, Villani A, de Martino M. Pediatric tuberculosis in Italian children: epidemiological and clinical data from the Italian Register of Pediatric Tuberculosis. Int J Mol Sci. 2016;17:960.

28. Van Zyl S, Marais BJ, Hesseling AC, Gie RP, Beyers N, Schaaf HS. Adherence to anti-tuberculosis chemoprophylaxis and treatment in children. Int J Tuberc Lung Dis. 2006;10:13–8.
29. Wang L, Zhang H, Ruan Y, Chin DP, Xia Y, Cheng S, Chen M, Zhao Y, Jiang S, Du X, He G, Li J, Wang S, Chen W, Xu C, Huang F, Liu X, Wang Y. Tuberculosis prevalence in China, 1990–2010; a longitudinal analysis of national survey data. Lancet. 2014;383:2057–64.
30. Kwon YS, Koh W-J. Diagnosis of pulmonary tuberculosis and nontuberculous mycobacterial lung disease in Korea. Tuberc Respir Dis. 2014;77:1.
31. Saini V, Garg K. Case finding strategies under National Tuberculosis Elimination Programme (NTEP). Indian J Tuberc. 2020;67:S101–6.
32. Aber VR, Allen BW, Mitchison DA, Ayuma P, Edwards EA, Keyes AB. Quality control in tuberculosis bacteriology. 1. Laboratory studies on isolated positive cultures and the efficiency of direct smear examination. Tubercle. 1980;61:123–33.
33. Lewinsohn DM, Leonard MK, LoBue PA, Cohn DL, Daley CL, Desmond E, Keane J, Lewinsohn DA, Loeffler AM, Mazurek GH, O'Brien RJ, Pai M, Richeldi L, Salfinger M, Shinnick TM, Sterling TR, Warshauer DM, Woods GL. Official American Thoracic Society/Infectious Diseases Society of America/Centers for Disease Control and Prevention Clinical practice guidelines: diagnosis of tuberculosis in adults and children. Clin Infect Dis. 2017;64:111–5.
34. WHO. Laboratory services in tuberculosis control: culture part III. Geneva: World Health Organization; 1998.
35. Machado D, Couto I, Viveiros M. Advances in the molecular diagnosis of tuberculosis: from probes to genomes. Infect Genet Evol. 2019;72:93–112.
36. Jeong YJ, Lee KS. Pulmonary tuberculosis: up-to-date imaging and management. AJR Am J Roentgenol. 2008;191:834–44.
37. China NHCoTPsRo. Diagnosis for pulmonary tuberculosis (in Chinese). 2017.
38. Dai Z, Xiao D, Wan L. The history of Chinese anti-tuberculosis (in Chinese). 2013.
39. WHO. Global tuberculosis report 2020. 2020.
40. Zhao Y, Xu S, Wang L, Chin DP, Wang S, Jiang G, Xia H, Zhou Y, Li Q, Ou X, Pang Y, Song Y, Zhao B, Zhang H, He G, Guo J, Wang Y. National survey of drug-resistant tuberculosis in China. N Engl J Med. 2012;366:2161–70.
41. Duan Q, Chen Z, Chen C, Zhang Z, Lu Z, Yang Y, Zhang L. the prevalence of drug-resistant tuberculosis in Mainland China: an updated systematic review and meta-analysis. PLoS One. 2016;11:e0148041.
42. Martin A, Portaels F, Palomino JC. Colorimetric redox-indicator methods for the rapid detection of multidrug resistance in Mycobacterium tuberculosis: a systematic review and Meta-analysis. J Antimicrob Chemother. 2007;59:175–83.
43. Coll F, McNerney R, Preston MD, Guerra-Assuncao JA, Warry A, Hill-Cawthorne G, Mallard K, Nair M, Miranda A, Alves A, Perdigao J, Viveiros M, Portugal I, Hasan Z, Hasan R, Glynn JR, Martin N, Pain A, Clark TG. Rapid determination of anti-tuberculosis drug resistance from whole-genome sequences. Genome Med. 2015;7:51.
44. WHO. WHO consolidated guidelines on tuberculosis: module 4: treatment: drug-resistant tuberculosis treatment. Geneva: World Health Organization; 2020.
45. Long Q, Qu Y, Lucas H. Drug-resistant tuberculosis control in China: progress and challenges. Infect Dis Poverty. 2016;5:9.
46. Steve Olson RAE, Claiborne AB. The global crisis of drug-resistant tuberculosis and leadership of China and the BRICS: challenges and opportunities: summary of a joint workshop. Washington, DC: The National Academies Press; 2014.
47. Tang S, Wang L, Wang H, Chin DP. Access to and affordability of healthcare for TB patients in China: issues and challenges. Infect Dis Poverty. 2016;5:10.
48. UNAIDS. Global AIDS update 2020. Geneva: UNAIDS; 2020.
49. Lyu P, Chen F. National HIV/AIDS epidemic estimation and interpretation in China. Zhonghua Liu Xing Bing Xue Za Zhi. 2019;40:1191–6.
50. Health Mo. HIV/AIDS prevention and control regulations (in Chinese). 2006.
51. Shen J, Lu H. Diagnosis, treatment, and control of HIV and TB co-infection: the works in progress. Chin J AIDS STD. 2015;2015:543–6.
52. Corbett EL, Watt CJ, Walker N, Maher D, Williams BG, Raviglione MC, Dye C. The growing burden of tuberculosis: global trends and interactions with the HIV epidemic. Arch Intern Med. 2003;163:1009–21.
53. Apers L, Wijarajah C, Mutsvangwa J, Chigara N, Mason P, Van der Stuyft P. Accuracy of routine diagnosis of pulmonary tuberculosis in an area of high HIV prevalence. Int J Tuberc Lung Dis. 1947;2004(8):945–51.
54. Mtei L, Matee M, Herfort O, Bakari M, Horsburgh CR, Waddell R, Cole BF, Vuola JM, Tvaroha S, Kreiswirth B. High rates of clinical and subclinical tuberculosis among HIV-infected ambulatory subjects in Tanzania. Clin Infect Dis. 2005;40:1500–7.
55. Mcshane H. Co-infection with HIV and TB: double trouble. Int J STD AIDS. 2005;16:95–101.

56. Kwan CK, Ernst JD. HIV and tuberculosis: a deadly human syndemic. Clin Microbiol Rev. 2011;24:351–76.
57. Toossi Z, Hirsch C, Wu M, Mayanja-Kizza H, Baseke J, Thiel B. Distinct cytokine and regulatory T cell profile at pleural sites of dual HIV/tuberculosis infection compared to that in the systemic circulation. Clin Exp Immunol. 2011;163:333–8.
58. Harries AD. Deaths from tuberculosis in Sub-Saharan African countries with a high prevalence of HIV-1. Lancet. 2001;357:1519–23.
59. Mukadi YD, Maher D, Harries A. Tuberculosis case fatality rates in high HIV prevalence populations in Sub-Saharan Africa. AIDS. 2001;15:143–52.
60. Meintjes G. Why are people still dying of HIV in Africa. Int J Infect Dis. 2014;21:12–3.
61. WHO. WHO policy on collaborative TB/HIV activities: guidelines for national programmes and other stakeholders. Review. 2012;160:1–6.
62. Toossi Z, Funderburg N, Sirdeshmuk S, Whalen C, Nanteza M, Johnson D, Mayanjakizza H, Hirsch C. Systemic immune activation and microbial translocation in dual HIV/tuberculosis-infected subjects. J Infect Dis. 2013;207:1841–9.
63. Sullivan Z, Wong E, Ndungu T, Kasprowicz V, Bishai W. Latent and active tuberculosis infection increase immune activation in individuals co-infected with HIV. EBioMedicine. 2015;2(4):334–40.
64. Kalichman SC, Rompa D, Cage M. Distinguishing between overlapping somatic symptoms of depression and HIV disease in people living with HIV-AIDS. J Nerv Ment Dis. 2000;188:662–70.
65. Eramova I, Matic S. 2 management of opportunistic infections and general symptoms of HIV/AIDS. Clinical Protocol for the WHO European Region. 2006.
66. Getahun H, Kittikraisak W, Heilig CM, Corbett EL, Ayles H, Cain KP, Grant AD, Churchyard GJ, Kimerling M, Shah S, Lawn SD, Wood R, Maartens G, Granich R, Date AA, Varma JK. Development of a standardized screening rule for tuberculosis in people living with HIV in resource-constrained settings: individual participant data meta-analysis of observational studies. PLoS Med. 2011;8:e1000391.
67. Padmapriyadarsini C, Narendran G, Swaminathan S. Diagnosis and treatment of tuberculosis in HIV co-infected patients. Indian J Med Res. 2011;134:850.
68. Mo Z. The epidemiological investigation of HIV and TB co-infection. Wuhan: Wuhan University; 2014.
69. Burman WJ, Jones BE. Clinical and radiographic features of HIV-related tuberculosis. Semin Respir Infect. 2003;2013:263–71.
70. Korzeniewska-Kosela M. Spectrum of tuberculosis in patients with HIV infection in British Columbia: report of 40 cases. Can Med Assoc J. 1992;146:1927–34.
71. Zhang D. Modern phthisiology (in Chinese). Beijing: People's Military Medical Publishing House; 2000.
72. Chen Y. Clinical features analysis of 53 cases about AIDS complicated with pulmonary tuberculosis (in Chinese). Med Recapitulate. 2009;15:3663–5.
73. Zhang K, Ma D, Lv F, Zhao D, Wu H, Xu L. Clinical diagnosis and treatment of acquired immunodeficiency syndrome complicated by tuberculosis (in Chinese). Chin J Tuberc Respir Dis. 2001;24:682–4.
74. Junling G, Pinpin Z, Hua F. Prevalence of TB/HIV co-infection in countries except China: a systematic review and meta-analysis. PLoS One. 2013;8:e64915.
75. Trinh QMNH, Do TN, Nhung NV, Hoa NB, Nguyen TV, Sintchenko V, Marais BJ. Tuberculosis and HIV co-infection in Vietnam. Int J Infect Dis. 2016;44:64–5.
76. Sharma SK, Mohan A, Kadhiravan T. HIV-TB co-infection: epidemiology, diagnosis & management. Indian J Med Res. 2005;121:550–67.
77. Pathni AK, Ls C. HIV/TB in India: a public health challenge. J Indian Med Assoc. 2003;101(3):148–9.
78. Sabbatani S, Ferro A, Gomez V, Rezza G. AIDS–TB complex in Guinea Bissau: an epidemiological updating. Le infezioni in Medicina. 1996;4:146–8.
79. Keshinro B, Diul MY. HIV-TB: epidemiology, clinical features and diagnosis of smear-negative TB. Trop Doct. 2006;36:68–71.
80. Gao L, Zhou F, Li XW, Jin Q. HIV/TB co-infection in Mainland China: a meta-analysis. PLoS One. 2010;5:e10736.
81. Xu J, Tang W, Cheng S, Mahapatra T, Zhou L, Lai Y, Jiang Y, Liu F, Zhen X, He J. Prevalence and predictors of HIV among Chinese tuberculosis patients by provider-initiated HIV testing and counselling (PITC): a multisite study in South Central of China. PLoS One. 2014;9:e89723.
82. Wang LLW, Wang L, et al. HIV prevalence among pulmonary tuberculosis patients in Guangxi, China. J Acquir Immune Defic Syndr. 2010;53(suppl 1):S61.
83. Council GOotS. National tuberculosis control program (2011–2015) (In Chinese). 2011.
84. International Diabetes Federation. IDF Diabetes Atlas. 8th ed. Brussels, Belgium: International Diabetes Federation; 2017.
85. Guariguata L, Whiting DR, Hambleton I, Beagley J, Linnenkamp U, Shaw JE. Global estimates of diabetes prevalence for 2013 and projections for 2035. Diabetes Res Clin Pract. 2014;103:137–49.
86. International Diabetes Federation. IDF Diabetes Atlas. 7th ed. Brussels, Belgium: International Diabetes Federation; 2015.
87. Kyu HH, Maddison ER, Henry NJ, Mumford JE, Murray CJ. The global burden of tuberculosis: results from the Global Burden of Disease Study 2015. Lancet Infect Dis. 2018;18:261–84.
88. Pan S-C, Ku C-C, Kao D, Ezzati M, Fang C-T, Lin H-H. Effect of diabetes on tuberculosis control in 13 countries with high tuberculosis: a modelling study. Lancet Diabetes Endocrinol. 2015;3:323–30.

89. Jiménez-Corona ME, Cruz-Hervert LP, García-García L, Ferreyra-Reyes L, Delgado-Sánchez G, Bobadilla-del-Valle M, Canizales-Quintero S, Ferreira-Guerrero E, Báez-Saldaña R, Téllez-Vázquez N. Association of diabetes and tuberculosis: impact on treatment and post-treatment outcomes. Thorax. 2013;68:214–20.
90. Viswanathan V, Vigneswari A, Selvan K, Satyavani K, Rajeswari R, Kapur A. Effect of diabetes on treatment outcome of smear-positive pulmonary tuberculosis—a report from South India. J Diabetes Complicat. 2014;28:162–5.
91. Faurholt-Jepsen D, Range N, Praygod G, Jeremiah K, Friis H. Diabetes is a strong predictor of mortality during tuberculosis treatment: a prospective cohort study among tuberculosis patients from Mwanza, Tanzania. Trop Med Int Health. 2013;18:822–9.
92. Baker MA, Harries AD, Jeon CY, Hart JE, Kapur A, Lonnroth K, Ottmani S-E, Goonesekera SD, Murray MB. The impact of diabetes on tuberculosis treatment outcomes: a systematic review. BMC Med. 2011;9:81.
93. Lee P-H, Fu H, Lai T-C, Chiang C-Y, Chan C-C, Lin H-H. Glycemic control and the risk of tuberculosis: a cohort study. PLoS Med. 2016;13:e1002072.
94. Critchley JA, Restrepo BI, Ronacher K, Kapur A, Bremer AA, Schlesinger LS, Basaraba R, Kornfeld H, Van Crevel R. Defining a research agenda to address the converging epidemics of tuberculosis and diabetes. Part 1: epidemiology and clinical management. Chest. 2017;152(1):174–80.
95. Ronacher K, Van Crevel R, Critchley J, Bremer AA, Schlesinger LS, Kapur A, Basaraba R, Kornfeld H, Restrepo BI. Defining a research agenda to address the converging epidemics of tuberculosis and diabetes. Part 2: underlying biological mechanisms. Chest. 2017;152(1):174–80.
96. Dooley KE, Tang T, Golub JE, Dorman SE, Cronin W. Impact of diabetes mellitus on treatment outcomes of patients with active tuberculosis. Am J Trop Med Hyg. 2009;80:634–9.
97. McGuinness OP. Defective glucose homeostasis during infection. Annu Rev Nutr. 2005;25:9–35.
98. Dungan KM, Braithwaite PSS, Preiser JC. Stress hyperglycaemia. Lancet. 2009;373:1798–807.
99. Odegaard AO, Jacobs DR Jr, Sanchez OA, Goff DC Jr, Reiner AP, Gross MD. Oxidative stress, inflammation, endothelial dysfunction and incidence of type 2 diabetes. Cardiovasc Diabetol. 2016;15:51.
100. Wang L, Cheng S, Chen M, Zhao Y, Zhang H, Jiang S, He G, Lv Q, Du X, Chen W, Liu X, Ruan Y, Wang S, Xia Y, Yu L, Li J, Li X. The fifth national tuberculosis epidemiological survey in 2010 (in Chinese). Chin J Antituberc. 2012;34:485–508.
101. Jeon CY, Murray MB. Diabetes mellitus increases the risk of active tuberculosis: a systematic review of 13 observational studies. PLoS Med. 2008;5:e152.
102. Restrepo BI, Fau CAJ, Rahbar MH, Fau RMH, Wang W, Fau WW, Restrepo MA, Fau RM, Zarate I, Fau ZI, Mora-Guzmán F, Fau M-GF, Crespo-Solis JG, Fau C-SJG, Briggs J, Fau BJ, JB MC, Fau MCJB, Fisher-Hoch SP, Fisher-Hoch SP. Cross-sectional assessment reveals high diabetes prevalence among newly-diagnosed tuberculosis cases. Bull World Health Organ. 2011;89:352–9.
103. Lin Y, Fau LL, Mi F, Fau MF, Du J, Fau DJ, Dong Y, Fau DY, Li Z, Fau LZ, Qi W, Fau QW, Zhao X, Fau ZX, Cui Y, Fau CY, Hou F, Fau HF, Zachariah R, Fau ZR, Kapur A, Fau KA, Lönnroth K, Fau LK, Harries AD, Harries AD. Screening patients with diabetes mellitus for tuberculosis in China. Trop Med Int Health. 2012;17:1302–8.
104. Xia Z, Yang S. Epidemiological analysis of type 2 diabetes mellitus among residents in Meilan District of Haikou City in 2011. Pract Prev Med. 2012;19:1081–3.
105. Wu G, Zhou X, Luo T, Mao Y, Ma Y, Huang X, Yue J. Analysis of the anti-tuberculosis drugs resistance of Mycobacterium tuberculosis in Chengdu area (in Chinese). Mod Prev Med. 2010;37:1753–4.
106. Gu X. Analysis of clinical features of diabetes mellitus combined with tuberculosis. Med Philos. 2008;2018:80.
107. Balakrishnan S, Fau VS, Nair S, Fau NS, Subramoniapillai J, Fau SJ, Mrithyunjayan S, Fau MS, Wilson N, Fau WN, Satyanarayana S, Fau SS, Dewan PK, Fau DPK, AMV K, Fau KA, Karthickeyan D, Fau KD, Willis M, Fau WM, Harries AD, Fau HA, Nair SA, Nair SA. High diabetes prevalence among tuberculosis cases in Kerala, India. PLoS One. 2012;7:e46502.
108. Amare H, Fau GA, Anagaw B, Fau AB, Gelaw B, Gelaw B. Smear positive pulmonary tuberculosis among diabetic patients at the Dessie referral hospital, Northeast Ethiopia. Infect Dis Poverty. 2013;2:1–8.
109. Suwanpimolkul G, Grinsdale JA, Jarlsberg LG, Higashi J, Osmond DH, Hopewell PC, Kato-Maeda M. Association between diabetes mellitus and tuberculosis in United States-born and foreign-born populations in San Francisco. PLoS One. 2014;9:e114442.
110. Baldé NM, Fau CA, Camara LM, Fau CL, Diallo MM, Fau DM, Kaké A, Fau KA, Bah-Sow OY, Bah-Sow OY. Associated tuberculosis and diabetes in Conakry, Guinea: prevalence and clinical characteristics. Int J Tuberc Lung Dis. 2006;10:1036–40.
111. Alladin B, Fau MS, Singh A, Fau SA, Singh C, Fau SC, Smith B, Fau SB, Cummings E, Fau CE, Hershfield E, Fau HE, Mohanlall J, Fau MJ, Ramotar K, Fau RK, La Fleur C, La Fleur C. Tuberculosis and diabetes in Guyana. Int J Infect Dis. 2011;15:e818–21.
112. Ping PA, Zakaria R, Islam MA, Yaacob LH, Muhamad R, Wan Mohamad WMZ, Yusoff HM. Prevalence and risk factors of latent tuberculosis infection (LTBI) in patients with type 2 diabetes mellitus (T2DM). Int J Environ Res Public Health. 2021;18:305.

113. Wang Q, Ma A, Han X, Zhao S, Cai J, Ma Y, Zhao J, Wang Y, Dong H, Zhao Z, Wei L, Yu T, Chen P, Schouten EG, Kok FJ, Kapur A. Prevalence of type 2 diabetes among newly detected pulmonary tuberculosis patients in China: a community based cohort study. PLoS One. 2013;8:e82660.
114. Webb EA, Fau HAC, Schaaf HS, Fau SHS, Gie RP, Fau GRP, Lombard CJ, Fau LCJ, Spitaels A, Fau SA, Delport S, Fau DS, Marais BJ, Fau MBJ, Donald K, Fau DK, Hindmarsh P, Fau HP, Beyers N, Beyers N. High prevalence of Mycobacterium tuberculosis infection and disease in children and adolescents with type 1 diabetes mellitus. Int J Tuberc Lung Dis. 2009;13:868–74.
115. Kibirige D, Fau SR, Mutebi E, Fau ME, Worodria W, Worodria W. Overt diabetes mellitus among newly diagnosed Ugandan tuberculosis patients: a cross sectional study. BMC Infect Dis. 2013;13:122.
116. Lönnroth K, Fau WBG, Cegielski P, Fau CP, Dye C, Dye C. A consistent log-linear relationship between tuberculosis incidence and body mass index. Int J Epidemiol. 2010;39:149–55.
117. Dobler CC, Fau FJ, Marks GB, Marks GB. Risk of tuberculosis among people with diabetes mellitus: an Australian nationwide cohort study. BMJ Open. 2012;2:e000666.
118. Shimizu H, Shimomura Y, Fau HR, Fau HR, Ohtani K, Fau OK, Sato N, Fau SN, Futawatari T, Fau FT, Mori M, Mori M. Serum leptin concentration is associated with total body fat mass, but not abdominal fat distribution. Int J Obes Relat Metab Disord. 1997;21:536–41.
119. Nissapatorn V, Fau KI, Jamaiah I, Fau JI, Fong MY, Fau FM, Rohela M, Fau RM, Anuar AK, Anuar AK. Tuberculosis in diabetic patients: a clinical perspective. Southeast Asian J Trop Med Public Health. 2005;36:213–20.
120. Singla R, Fau KN, Al-Sharif N, Fau A-SN, Ai-Sayegh MO, Fau A-SM, Shaikh MA, Fau SM, Osman MM, Osman MM. Influence of diabetes on manifestations and treatment outcome of pulmonary TB patients. Int J Tuberc Lung Dis. 2006;10:74–9.
121. Yu Pang JA, Shu W, Huo F, Chu N, Gao M, Qin S, Huang H, Chen X, Xu S. Epidemiology of extrapulmonary tuberculosis among inpatients, China, 2008–2017. Emerg Infect Dis. 2019;25:457–64.
122. Baker MA, Fau LH, Chang H-Y, Fau CH, Murray MB, Murray MB. The risk of tuberculosis disease among persons with diabetes mellitus: a prospective cohort study. Clin Infect Dis. 2012;54:818–25.
123. Yoon YS, Jung JW, Jeon EJ, Seo H, Ryu YJ, Yim JJ, Kim YH, Lee BH, Park YB, Lee BJ, Kang H, Choi JC. The effect of diabetes control status on treatment response in pulmonary tuberculosis: a prospective study. Thorax. 2017;72:263–70.
124. Nandakumar KV, Duraisamy K, Balakrishnan S, Sunilkumar M, Jaya Sankar S, Sagili KD, Satyanarayana S, Ajay Kumar MV, Enarson DA. Outcome of tuberculosis treatment in patients with diabetes mellitus treated in the revised national tuberculosis control programme in Malappuram District, Kerala, India. PLoS One. 2013;8:e76275.
125. Delgado-Sánchez G, García-García L, Castellanos-Joya M, Cruz-Hervert P, Ferreyra-Reyes L, Ferreira-Guerrero E, Hernández A, Ortega-Baeza VM, Montero-Campos R, Sulca JA, Martínez-Olivares Mde L, Mongua-Rodríguez N, Baez-Saldaña R, González-Roldán JF, López-Gatell H, Ponce-de-León A, Sifuentes-Osornio J, Jiménez-Corona ME. Association of pulmonary tuberculosis and diabetes in Mexico: analysis of the National Tuberculosis Registry 2000–2012. PLoS One. 2015;10:e0129312.
126. Yao L, Xia-Fang W, Xing-Hua S, Jian-Ping Z, Zi-Wei B, Shi C-LSY-J, Pei-Jun T, Mei-Ying W. Cause analysis and distribution trend of 9528 cases of tuberculosis complications in Suzhou area from 2011 to 2017 (in Chinese). Anti Infect Pharm. 2019;16:258–61.
127. Yang Xinting JJ, Jun A, Jimin G, Li. Weimin retrospective analysis of patients with tuberculosis complications in Beijing Chest Hospital in 2012–2016 (in Chinese). Dis Surv. 2018;33:320–3.
128. Ying Liu XL, Liu R. Investigation and analysis of 50 cases of chronic obstructive pulmonary disease complicated with pulmonary tuberculosis in elderly (in Chinese). Contemp Med. 2012;18:39–40.
129. Wu Wenjuan TC, Birong X. Clinical analysis of pulmonary tuberculosis complicated with acute respiratory distress syndrome (in Chinese). J Clin Pulm Med. 2011;16:217–8.
130. Ma MJ, Yang Y, Wang HB, Zhu YF, Fang LQ, An XP, Wan KL, Whalen CC, Yang XX, Lauzardo M, Zhang ZY, Cao JF, Tong YG, Dai EH, Cao WC. Transmissibility of tuberculosis among school contacts: an outbreak investigation in a boarding middle school, China. Infect Genet Evol. 2015;32:148–55.
131. Abubakar I, Matthews T, Harmer D, Okereke E, Crawford K, Hall T, Collyns T, Smith G, Barrett A, Baugh S. Assessing an outbreak of tuberculosis in an English college population. Eur Respir J. 2011;38:976–8.
132. Kaiser C, Cole B, Saruwatari K, Leon R. Rapid large-scale deployment of tuberculosis testing in a high school - Riverside County, California, 2013–2014. MMWR Morb Mortal Wkly Rep. 2015;64:574–7.
133. Huang Y, Zhong J, Wu Q, Liu Z, Pan A, Zhu L, Wang X. Investigation of a large school-based outbreak of tuberculosis infection in Eastern China. Pediatr Pol. 2016;91:541–6.
134. Organization WH. WHO consolidated guidelines on tuberculosis: module 1: prevention: tuberculosis preventive treatment. Geneva: World Health Organization; 2020.
135. Mori T, Leung CC. Tuberculosis in the global aging population. Infect Dis Clin N Am. 2010;24:751–68.
136. Campbell JR, Sasitharan T, Marra F. A systematic review of studies evaluating the cost utility of screening high-risk populations for latent tuber-

culosis infection. Appl Health Econ Health Policy. 2015;13:325–40.
137. Walsh K. Guidelines for the prevention and control of tuberculosis in the elderly. Nurs Pract. 1994;19:79–84.
138. WHO. WHO consolidated guidelines on tuberculosis: tuberculosis preventive treatment. Geneva: WHO; 2020.
139. Liao W-B, Ju K, Gao Y-M, Pan J. The association between internal migration and pulmonary tuberculosis in China, 2005–2015: a spatial analysis. Infect Dis Poverty. 2020;9:5.
140. Liu LWJ, Zhao XQ. The impact of migrant workers on the tuberculosis transmission: General models and a case study for China. Math Biosci Eng. 2012;9:785–807.
141. Yang C, Lu L, Warren JL, Wu J, Jiang Q, Zuo T, Gan M, Liu M, Liu Q, DeRiemer K, Hong J, Shen X, Colijn C, Guo X, Gao Q, Cohen T. Internal migration and transmission dynamics of tuberculosis in Shanghai, China: an epidemiological, spatial, genomic analysis. Lancet Infect Dis. 2018;18:788–95.
142. Ge E, Zhang X, Wang X, Wei X. Spatial and temporal analysis of tuberculosis in Zhejiang Province, China, 2009–2012. Infect Dis Poverty. 2016;5:11.
143. Zhou C, Chu J, Geng H, Wang X, Xu L. Pulmonary tuberculosis among migrants in Shandong, China: factors associated with treatment delay. BMJ Open. 2014;4:e005805.
144. Neyrolles O, Chen J, Qi L, Xia Z, Shen M, Shen X, Mei J, DeRiemer K, Zheng'an Y. Which Urban Migrants Default from Tuberculosis Treatment in Shanghai, China? PLoS One. 2013;8:e81351.
145. Tan Weiguo GH, Wu Q, Lu P, Chuangyue H, Peixuan L, Mingzhen L, Chen RYW. The implement effects and innovative strategies for tuberculosis controlling among migrants. Electron J Emerg Infect Dis. 2020;5:145–9.
146. Owokuhaisa J. Prevalence of pulmonary tuberculosis among prison inmates at Mbarara Central Prison, South Western Uganda. Adv Res. 2014;2:618–25.
147. Wilkinson RJ, Telisinghe L, Fielding KL, Malden JL, Hanifa Y, Churchyard GJ, Grant AD, Charalambous S. High tuberculosis prevalence in a South African prison: the need for routine tuberculosis screening. PLoS One. 2014;9:e87262.
148. de Goicoechea Saiz ML, Sternberg F, Portilla-Sogorb J. Prevalence and associated risk factors of latent tuberculosis infection in a Spanish prison. Rev Esp Sanid Penit. 2018;20:4.
149. Tong Y, Jiang S, Guan X, Hou S, Cai K, Tong Y, Cai L, Liu J, Lu Q. Epidemic situation of tuberculosis in prisons in the Central Region of China. Am J Trop Med Hyg. 2019;101:510–2.
150. Berihun YA, Nguse TM, Gebretekle GB. Prevalence of tuberculosis and treatment outcomes of patients with tuberculosis among inmates in Debrebirhan Prison, North Shoa Ethiopia. Ethiop J Health Sci. 2018;28:347.
151. Lu R, Zhao X, Li J, Niu P, Yang B, Wu H, Wang W, Song H, Huang B, Zhu N. Genomic characterisation and epidemiology of 2019 novel coronavirus: implications for virus origins and receptor binding. Lancet. 2020;395:565–74.
152. Hoehl S, Rabenau H, Berger A, Kortenbusch M, Cinatl J, Bojkova D, Behrens P, Böddinghaus B, Götsch U, Naujoks F. Evidence of SARS-CoV-2 infection in returning travelers from Wuhan, China. New Engl J Med. 2020;382:1278–80.
153. Ye Q, Wang B, Mao J, Fu J, Shang S, Shu Q, Zhang T. Epidemiological analysis of COVID-19 and practical experience from China. J Med Virol. 2020;92:755–69.
154. Yang Y, Lu Q, Liu M, Wang Y, Zhang A, Jalali N, Dean N, Longini I, Halloran ME, Xu B. Epidemiological and clinical features of the 2019 novel coronavirus outbreak in China. MedRxiv. 2020.
155. Guan W-j, Ni Z-y, Hu Y, Liang W-H, Ou C-Q, He J-X, Liu L, Shan H, Lei C-L, Hui DS. Clinical characteristics of 2019 novel coronavirus infection in China. MedRxiv. 2020.
156. Ichikawa M, Nakahara S, Wakai S, Hong-Jen C, Huang N. Lowered tuberculosis notifications and deterred health care seeking during the SARS epidemic in Hong Kong/Chang and Huang respond. Am J Public Health. 2005;95:933.
157. WHO. Global tuberculosis report 2019. Geneva, Switzerland: WHO; 2019.
158. Fei H, Yinyin X, Hui C, Ni W, Xin D, Wei C, Tao L, Shitong H, Miaomiao S, Mingting C. The impact of the COVID-19 epidemic on tuberculosis control in China. Lancet Reg Health West Pac. 2020;3:100032.
159. Cilloni L, Fu H, Vesga J. The potential impact of the COVID-19 pandemic on tuberculosis: a modelling analysis. medRxiv. 2020;28:100603.
160. Ragonnet R, Trauer JM, Geard N, Scott N, McBryde ES. Profiling Mycobacterium tuberculosis transmission and the resulting disease burden in the five highest tuberculosis burden countries. BMC Med. 2019;17:1–12.
161. McCreesh N, White RG. An explanation for the low proportion of tuberculosis that results from transmission between household and known social contacts. Sci Rep. 2018;8:1–9.
162. Alene KA, Wangdi K, Clements AC. Impact of the COVID-19 pandemic on tuberculosis control: an overview. Trop Med Infect Dis. 2020;5:123.

9 Recent Advances in Genetic Epidemiology of Colorectal Cancer in Chinese Population

Jianbo Tian, Xiaoping Miao, and Dongxin Lin

Abstract

Colorectal cancer is the most common malignant tumor in digestive system, ranks third in the incidence of cancers, but second in terms of cancer mortality all around the world. With the development of socioeconomic, the burden of colorectal cancer incidence and mortality is also rapidly growing in China. Moreover, the average age of patients developing colorectal cancer continues to decline, making it an urgent public health problem to be solved. Primary prevention remains the key strategy to reduce the increasing global burden of colorectal cancer. Tumorigenesis is a multistage and multistep process involving multiple factors, and the occurrence of colorectal cancer is closely related to gene–environment interactions. Environmental factors, such as diet patterns, physical activity, smoking, alcohol intake, overweight, occupational hazards, etc., could initiate the development of colorectal cancer. Additionally, genetic factors determine the individual susceptibility to cancer. Genome-wide association studies (GWASs) have identified about one hundred single nucleotide polymorphisms (SNPs) associated with colorectal cancer. Post-GWAS strategies integrate molecular, metabolic, computational together with statistical approaches to explain the underlying mechanism of association. These identified genetic susceptibility variants are of great importance in risk prediction, precision medicine, and drug development. Despite genetic epidemiology obtained notable successes, a substantial portion of colorectal cancer heritability remains unexplained. Besides, these statistical associations lack thorough investigation to clarify their mechanisms. Transforming research results to application in disease early screening, clinical diagnosis, and individualized treatment remains primary issue in future. Here, in addition to introducing the epidemiology and risk factors of colorectal cancer, we also summarized study strategies, potential benefits and challenges of genetic epidemiology to systematically characterize genetic epidemiology of colorectal cancer in Chinese population.

Keywords

Colorectal cancer · Epidemiology · Risk factors · GWAS · SNP · Precision prevention

J. Tian · X. Miao (✉)
Department of Epidemiology and Biostatistics, School of Public Health, Wuhan University, Wuhan, China
e-mail: xpmiao@whu.edu.cn

D. Lin
Department of Etiology and Carcinogenesis, National Cancer Center/Cancer Hospital, Chinese Academy of Medical Sciences and Peking Union Medical College, Beijing, China

D.-Q. Ye (ed.), *Progress in China Epidemiology*, https://doi.org/10.1007/978-981-19-2199-5_9

9.1 Epidemiology of Colorectal Cancer

According to the estimates from the International Agency for Research on Cancer (IARC) in 2020 [1], the incidence of colorectal cancer (CRC) worldwide is predicted to increase to 1.9 million new cases, accounting for 10% of total new cancer cases, and ranks third in the incidence of cancers. CRC is the second most common cancer diagnosed in women and the third most in men. 935,173 cases are predicted to die of CRC, accounting for 9.4% of total cancer deaths in the world, and ranks second in the mortality of cancers. With continuing progress in China, the estimated number of new cases of CRC is about 555,477 in 2020, and the population standard incidence is 23.9 per 100,000, ranking third in the incidence of cancers; while the estimated deaths of CRC are about 286,162 cases, and the population standard mortality rate is 12.0 per 100,000, ranking fifth in the mortality of cancers.

9.1.1 Temporal Trend

9.1.1.1 Temporal Trend of CRC Prevalence Worldwide

The incidence and mortality of CRC among most countries and regions are on the rise worldwide. According to the data from GLOBOCAN, the incidence of CRC increased from 1.4 million to 1.8 million new cases from 2012 to 2018, and the mortality also raised from about 700,000 deaths in 2012 to 881,000 deaths in 2018. Assessing the incidence and mortality trends, there are three distinct global temporal patterns related to level of development [2, 3]: (1) increasing incidence and mortality in the last decade (e.g., Baltic States, Russia, China, and Brazil); (2) increasing incidence and decreasing mortality (Canada, United Kingdom, Denmark, Singapore), the incidence of CRC in the United Kingdom has increased slightly, but the mortality rate has declined since 1971; and (3) both decreasing incidence and decreasing mortality (the United States, Japan, and France), those countries where organized screening and early detection programs have been established since the 1990s, for example, incidence rates (33.36% off) and mortality rates (28.4% off) had decreased in the United States since 1990 until 2006. Generally, the incidence and mortality rates of CRC are still rising rapidly in many low-income and middle-income countries; a stable or declining trends to be observed in highly developed countries, where mortality rates remain among the highest in the world. As a matter of fact, CRC has become the second most common cancer while replaced the infection-related cancers in several middle-income countries, particularly among women; underscores the significant challenge of CRC control in countries, which are undergoing major socioeconomic transition, and the importance of continued efforts to monitor trends in CRC incidence, mortality, and survival worldwide.

9.1.1.2 Temporal Trend of CRC Prevalence in China

Refer to the data from National Cancer Center in 2015 [4], CRC ranked third in most commonly diagnosed malignancy. The population standard incidence is 18.02 per 100,000 in 2015, and the incidence rate was higher in males than in females. And the population standard incidence is 8.21 per 100,000, which was also higher in males. According to the estimates from IARC in 2020, the population standard incidence of CRC is predicted to increase to 23.9 per 100,000, and the population standard mortality rate is 12.0 per 100,000. Compared to historical data, the burden of cancer continuing to rise, which may suggest adapting nationwide screening programs and uptake of colonoscopy in general.

9.1.2 Regional Distribution

9.1.2.1 Distribution of CRC Worldwide

According to the estimates from IARC in 2020, the highest incidence rates of colon cancer are found in parts of Europe (e.g., Hungary, Slovenia, Slovakia, The Netherlands, and Croatia), Australia/New Zealand, Northern America, and Eastern Asia (Japan, Singapore, and the Republic of Korea), with Hungary and Norway topping the list for males and females, respectively (Fig. 9.1). Rectal cancer incidence rates have a similar regional distribution, although the highest rates are seen in Portugal among males and in Brunei Darussalam among females.

In 2020, CRC incidence varies considerably by region, with the incidence of colon and rectal cancer being eight-fold and six-fold variations, respectively. Disease can be considered a marker of socioeconomic development, and for example, in countries undergoing major development transition, their incidence rates tend to rise uniformly with increasing human development index (HDI) [3]. It is noteworthy that more than two-thirds of all cases and about 60% of all deaths occur in countries with a high or very high HDI. Temporal patterns of CRC incidence rates and mortality also vary globally.

9.1.2.2 Distribution of CRC in China

Cancers are complex diseases caused by a combination of social environmental and genetic factors. China is a vast country with significant regional differences, which is characterized by ethnic cultural diversity and changeable geographical environment, resulting in differences in the lifestyle and living environment of people in different regions. Therefore, the burden of cancer in different regions also has regional characteristics. According to statistics in 2015, the east Coast of China presented a higher mortality rate than Central and Western China. Additionally, China had a higher case-fatality ratio and mortality/incidence ratio than other developed countries [5].

Considering great differences in economic level, living conditions, and health resources between urban and rural areas in China, the incidence rate of CRC was higher in urban areas than in rural areas in 2015, which could be observed both among males and females. Whereas, the mortality of CRC showed an adverse trend when comparing urban and rural areas.

9.1.3 Population Distribution

9.1.3.1 Age

Cancers may occur at all ages, but in general, the incidence of cancers before age of 40 is at a relatively low level. After 40, the incidence increases rapidly with the increase of age and reaches a peak at the age of 80–85. Similarly, the incidence rates and mortality rates of CRC increase with age. According to statistics estimated by IARC in

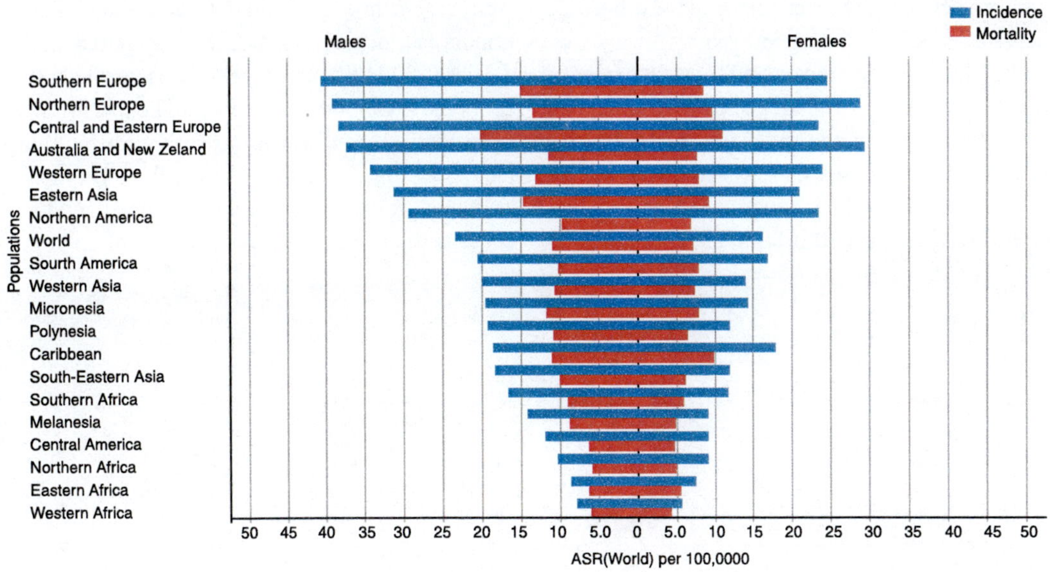

Fig. 9.1 Estimated incidence and mortality rates of CRC in different regions. (Data from: WHO IARC 2020)

2020, the rates increase rapidly after age 50 years, with an estimated 90% of global cases and deaths occurring after this age, and the rates are higher in males than in females at any age. Moreover, the age-standardized morbidity and mortality of CRC are extremely low under the age of 25, rising slowly from 25 to 55, and increasing rapidly after the age of 55 (Fig. 9.2a).

In China, according to the estimates of IARC on the number of new cases and deaths, morbidity and mortality of CRC increase with age, and the older the age, the faster the increase. The most common group to develop CRC are those over 50 years old, which accounts for 91.05% new cases or 94.34% death cases. CRC patients with age older than 70 years attributed to the highest rate of CRC, followed by the 60–69 years old group and 50–59 years old group (see Fig. 9.2b).

9.1.3.2 Gender

The incidence and mortality of CRC are generally higher in males than in females all around the world. According to the estimates of IARC, the age-adjusted rates are higher in males than in females in 2020, yielding an approximately 1.44-fold and 1.53-fold difference for incidence (23.4 versus 16.2 cases per 100,000 persons per year) and death (11.0 versus 7.2 deaths per 100,000 persons per year), respectively, and the difference becomes evident after age 50 years.

In China, the incidence and mortality rates of CRC in males and females show a similar pattern. According to the estimates of IARC, the number of new cases of CRC in 2020 will be 319,486 and 235,991 among males and females, respectively, ranking third in most common cancer diagnosed both in males and females. According to statistics, among the male cancer deaths in China, there are 164,959 CRC, ranking the fifth; and among the 1.18 million female cancer deaths in China, there will be 121,203 cases of CRC ranked second. As for the age-adjusted rates, they are also higher in males than in females in 2020, yielding an approximately 1.47-fold and 1.57-fold difference for incidence (28.6 versus 19.5 cases per 100,000 persons per year) and death (14.8 versus 9.4 deaths per 100,000 persons per year), respectively.

9.1.3.3 Race

As an example of racial or ethnic disparity, according to the statistics from the United States in 2015, it suggest that the distribution of age-standardized rates for the USA population in 2000 was highest in black population, while those of Asian or Pacific Islander background was lowest, in terms of incidence (43.2 and 28.8 cases per 100,000 persons per year) and deaths (18.6 and 9.9 deaths per 100,000 persons per year). Genetic factors may play a role in this racial disparity [6].

9.2 Risk Factors of CRC

Apart from about 5% of CRCs are hereditary tumors [7], most cases of CRC are sporadic and develop slowly over several years through the adenoma–carcinoma sequence. The occurrence of cancer is a multistage process with multiple factors acting, and risk factors will vary by cancer types. It has been widely acknowledged that CRC as the result of the cooperation of environ-

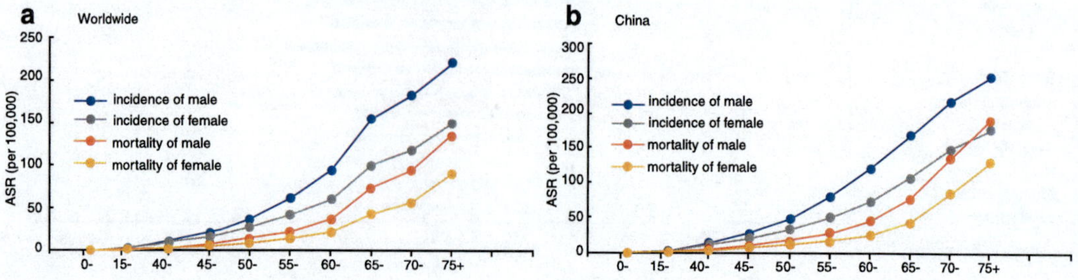

Fig. 9.2 Age-standardized incidence and mortality rates of CRC in the world or China. (Data from WHO IARC 2020)

mental factors and genetic factors progresses from adenoma in to adenocarcinoma. These risk factors could be divided into modifiable factors (e.g., smoking and drinking) and non-modifiable factors, like a person's age and family history. The accumulation and superposition of these risk factors will increase the risk of colorectal polyps or CRC, but this does not mean that having more risk factors will definitely get cancer. At present, several risk factors that might increase the risk of developing colorectal polyps or CRC have be identified.

9.2.1 Modifiable Risk Factors

9.2.1.1 Overweight or Obesity

The WHO definition for overweight is a body mass index (BMI, weight/(height in m)^2) $\geq$ 25 kg/m^2 and for obesity BMI $\geq$ 30 kg/m^2. The relationship between body weight and different cancers is now well recognized [8, 9]. For colon cancer, the relative risk attributable to obesity is 1.24 for men; it ranges between 1.04 and 1.13 depending on the country [9]. Additionally, epidemiology studies have provided evidence for an association between obesity-related metabolic or inflammatory factors and CRC risk, including changes in insulin-like growth factor 1 signaling, adipokines, sex hormones, and systemic inflammation. Obesity-associated changes in the intestinal microbes and their metabolites may also contribute to carcinogenesis [10].

9.2.1.2 Physically Active and Sedentary Behavior

Regular physical exercise can reduce the risk of CRC, and individuals with the highest level of physical activity have a 19% lower risk of colon cancer than individuals with the lowest level, but physical activity has not been associated with rectal cancer. On the contrary, prolonged sedentary behavior can increase the risk of advanced colon adenoma, which indicates that sedentary behavior is an early factor contributing to cancer [11]. The effects of physical activity or sedentary behavior, or both, on the immune system, epigenetics, protein translation, and microbiome, including in relation to cancer development, are under active study [12, 13].

9.2.1.3 Dietary Patterns

Red and Processed Meats High intake of red meats (such as beef, pork, lamb, or liver) and processed meats (e.g., hot dogs and some luncheon meats) increases the risk of CRC [14]. Recently, a meta-analysis indicated an approximately 20% higher risk of CRC per 100 g/day increase in red meat and 50 g/day increase in processed meat [15]. The risk increases linearly with increasing intake of red and processed meats up to approximately 140 g/day; beyond this level, the risk increase is less pronounced. It may be related components other than fat and protein in red and processed meat, which contribute to the carcinogenic effects. Thus, based on current evidence it would be reasonable to recommend substitution of poultry or fish for red and processed meat as a strategy for CRC prevention [15].

Vegetables and Fruits There is a statistically significant nonlinear inverse association between fruit and vegetable intake and CRC incidence [16], with the greatest risk reduction associated with increasing fruit intake up to about 100 g/day and vegetable intake to about 100–200 g/day, with little evidence for further reduction with higher intake [15]. Fruit and vegetables are good sources of fiber that can prevent CRC by increasing stool bulk, decreasing transit time in the colon, and diluting potential carcinogens [17].

Whole Grains In contrast with refined grains that retain only the endosperm, whole grains contain germ and bran, which are rich sources of various substances with anticancer properties, including fiber, antioxidants, and phytochemicals. High intake of whole grain has been related to lower CRC risk [18]. Given the well-established role of insulin in promoting colonic growth, whole grain may exert its beneficial effect on colorectal carcinogenesis by lowering insulin [15].

Dairy Products Milk intake is associated with a reduction in CRC risk, which represents that no substantial change in CRC incidence below ~200 g/day and the greatest reduction over consumption of 500–800 g/day [19]. Dairy products may protect against colorectal neoplasia because of their high content of calcium, other micronutrients, and bioactive constituents. Fermented dairy products, such as yogurt, also could reduce the risk of CRC. The lactic acid bacteria of fermented milk products may alter the composition or function of a host's endogenous gut microbiota, reduce absorption of mutagens from cooked foods, inactivate intestinal carcinogens, and dampen intestinal inflammation [15].

Tree Nuts Nut consumption is inversely associated with the risk of cancer incidence and mortality. A higher consumption of nuts is not only significantly associated with a lower cancer risk [20], but also reduces the incidence of cancer recurrence and death in patients with stage III colon cancer [21]. Nuts inhibit cancer progression by altering lipid metabolism, reducing endothelial dysfunction, lipid peroxidation, and insulin resistance [20].

Vitamin D, C and Others Vitamin D deficiency increases the risk of developing cancer, so avoiding deficiency and adding vitamin D supplements might be an economical and safe way to reduce cancer incidence and improve cancer prognosis and outcome [22]. It would be reasonable to ensure that patients obtain a sufficient level of vitamin D to maintain a plasma level of 25(OH)D greater than at least 36 ng/ml [15].

Recommending adequate folate intake may abrogate the increased risk of CRC consistently observed with folate deficiency. Antioxidants or reactive oxygen species scavengers, including carotenoids (e.g., beta carotene, vitamin A precursor, and lycopene), vitamin C, and vitamin E, protect cells from oxidative stress that can initiate and promote carcinogenesis by inducing gene mutations, DNA damage, genome instability, cell proliferation, and inflammation [15].

9.2.1.4 Smoking

Smoking is a well-known cause of lung cancer, and it is linked to a lot of other cancers as well. Compared to non-smokers, people who have smoked tobacco for a long time are more likely to develop and die of CRC. Twenty-six studies provided adjusted risk estimates for ever smokers vs never smokers, leading to a pooled relative risk of 1.18 (95% confidence interval [CI], 1.11–1.25). Smoking was associated with an absolute risk increase of 10.8 cases per 100,000 person-years (95% CI, 7.9–13.6) [23]. This may involve a variety of biological mechanisms, including changes in the intestinal microbiota caused by smoking [23], molecular mechanisms [24], etc.

9.2.1.5 Alcohol Intake

CRC has been linked to the moderate to heavy alcohol use. Even light-to-moderate alcohol intake has been associated with certain risks. After ruling out the influence of race/ethnicity, lifestyle factors, alcoholic beverage type, and anatomical subsite of tumors, beer and wine, but not liquor, consumption was positively related to CRC risk. The association was stronger for rectum and left-colon tumors than for right-colon tumors [25].

9.2.1.6 Occupational Hazards

Work Stress Epidemiological studies in different regions and countries of the world show that there is a positive correlation between work stress and the risk of CRC, which indicates that work pressure is an important risk factor for CRC. However, this relationship may be caused by differences in cancer incidence among different genders or geographic regions. Therefore, prospective studies with larger sample sizes are still needed to seek further verification [26].

Night Shift Work Risk for rectal cancer significantly increased with shift work duration, suggesting that long-term circadian disruption may play a role in rectal cancer development [27].

Asbestos Exposure The risk of CRC mortality increases as the level of asbestos exposure rises. Although the effect size is small and the heterogeneity among studies is large, these findings indicate that occupational exposure to asbestos is a risk factor for CRC [28].

9.2.2 Non-modifiable Risk Factors

9.2.2.1 Hereditary Factors

Genetic Predisposition CRC has a substantial heritable component. According to a large twin study, 35% of CRC risk might be attributable to heritable factors [29]. Hereditary CRC accounts for 3%–5% of all cases of CRC, which can be subdivided as non-polyposis (Lynch syndrome and familial CRC) and polyposis syndromes. Lynch syndrome is caused by a dysfunction of the DNA mismatch repair system, characterized by expansion or contraction of microsatellite regions in the tumor compared with healthy tissue, called microsatellite instability (MSI), and found at molecular analysis.

Apart from above hereditary forms, which are determined by well-known genetic aberrations, but account for less than 5% of all CRC, genetic factors that determine the risk of disease are still incompletely understood. Genome-wide association studies have identified an increasing number of single nucleotide polymorphisms (SNPs) showing statistically significant, but it can only explain about 7%-8% heritability [30].

Family History Positive family history has a part in approximately 10–20% of all patients with CRC [31]. Individual with a history of CRC in a first-degree relative (parent, sibling, or child) are at increased risk. The risk is even higher if that relative was diagnosed with cancer when they were younger than 50, or if more than one first-degree relative is affected. Additionally, having family members who have had adenomatous polyps is also linked to a higher risk of colon cancer.

9.2.2.2 Other Risk Factors

Age and Male Gender The risk of CRC is low at ages younger than 50 years, but strongly increases with age. Median age at diagnosis is about 70 years in developed countries. Besides, incidence is higher in men than women [7].

Ethnicity Mediation analyses suggested that stage at diagnosis had the greatest influence on overall racial/ethnic survival disparities accounting for 24% of disparities in breast cancer, 24% in prostate cancer, and 16% to 30% in CRC [32].

Inflammatory Bowel Disease Patients of ulcerative colitis (UC) or Crohn's colitis have a higher risk rate of CRC which can account up to 10% of all deaths in patients of inflammatory bowel disease (IBD). The risk depends on disease duration, extent of inflammation, presence of primary sclerosing cholangitis, and backwash ileitis [33].

Aspirin or NSAID Use A recent pooled analysis of 10 cohort and case–control studies demonstrated that aspirin use was associated with a 29% reduction in the incidence of CRC (OR = 0.71, 95% CI = 0.66–0.77) [34]. Use of anti-inflammatory drugs (NSAIDs) is also associated with lower risk of CRC. However, the timing of and the subtype of CRC that would benefit the most from using aspirin and other nonsteroidal in relation to survival are unclear.

9.3 Strategy for Genetic Epidemiological Study in CRC

Most cases of CRC are sporadic, in which low-penetrance genetic polymorphism plays an important role. As the most common type of human genetic variation, SNPs appear in the genome at a frequency of approximately one in 1000 base pairs (bp). SNPs may exert their effects via influencing promoter activity (gene expression), messenger RNA (mRNA) conformation (stability), translational efficiency, and function of gene product protein. Therefore, systematical identification of dozens of variations in genome and exploration of their function may lead to a better understanding of their impact on gene function and health of an individual [35]. Here, we systematically summarized common approaches used in genetic epidemiological study in CRC (Fig. 9.3).

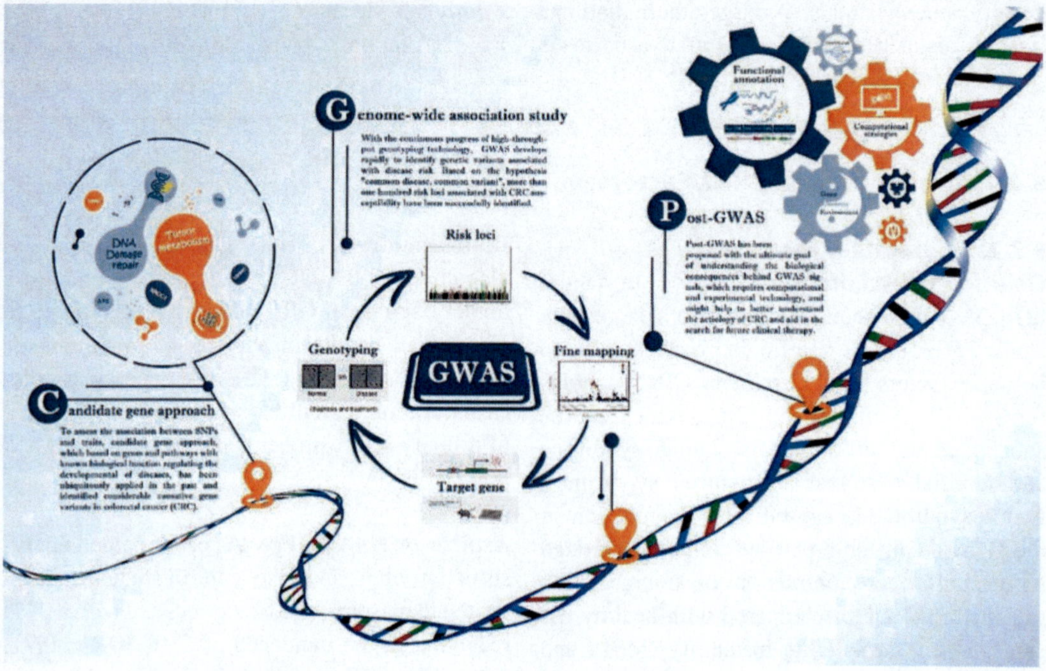

Fig. 9.3 Key advances in the strategies for genetic epidemiological study in CRC

9.3.1 Association Analysis Based on Candidate Gene Approach

Candidate genes are generally the genes with known biological function regulating the developmental processes of the investigated traits directly or indirectly. SNPs located in the coding or regulatory regions of those genes are selected for association analysis, to evaluate their effects on disease susceptibility. The candidate gene approach has been extensively applied for gene–disease research and genetic association studies, identifying considerable causative gene variants [36].

Researches on the genetic susceptibility of CRC mainly focused on *APC* and DNA damage repair genes, carcinogen metabolism genes, cell cycle and apoptosis pathway genes, etc. [37]. Folate is an essential nutrient for the human body; their deficiency can cause alterations in DNA methylation, disruption of DNA synthesis and repair, thereby increasing the incidence of cancer. Miao et al. investigated the association between genetic variations in methylenetetrahydrofolate reductase (MTHFR) and the risk of CRC in 198 CRC cases and 420 controls, finding that *MTHFR* 677TT genotypes had a 67% increased risk of CRCs than 677CC genotype [38].

Apart from these candidate genes, some pathways also play a pivotal role in tumor initiation and progression, such as the FAS and FASL system could regulate apoptotic cell death, and corruption of this signaling pathway has been shown to participate in tumorigenesis. Yang et al. found FAS-1377G/A and FASL-844 T/C polymorphisms may be genetic susceptibility factors for CRC among the Chinese population, by applying PCR-RFLP method to determine the genotypes in 382 CRC patients and 648 controls [39]. Gong et al. also identified that SNPs in genes of TGF-β signaling pathway could affect the miRNA/mRNA bindings and eventually contributed to CRC susceptibility [40].

The candidate gene approach has proven to be effective and economical for direct gene discovery. Nevertheless, the dependence on existing knowledge about the known or assumed biology of the phenotype under investigation is the biggest limitation of the practicability of traditional candidate gene approach, but unfortunately the underlying molecular mechanism of most biological traits remains unknown. To develop new strategies for breaking the restriction of information bottleneck is quite necessary.

9.3.2 Genome-Wide Association Study

With the more comprehensive understanding of the human genome, the increasing automation degree of DNA sequencing technology, and the continuous progress of high-throughput genotyping technology, the candidate gene approach is gradually replaced by genome-wide association study (GWAS) in recent years.

"Common disease, common variant" hypothesis is the underlying principle for GWAS, indicating that common diseases are attributable in part to allelic variants present in more than 1–5% of the population [41]. Through an agnostic genome-based approach, GWAS compares the frequency of common variants in members of unrelated patients with those in matched healthy population to identify genetic variants correlated with disease risk [42]. Based on the staged strategy, GWAS could refrain from high cost of commercial SNP arrays but retain statistical power. In a two-stage design, all tag SNPs are genotyped with high-throughput SNP chips covering the whole genome during the first stage on a small subset of cases and controls. During the second stage, significant SNPs (such as $P < 10^{-8}$), comprising approximately 10% of the SNPs tested, are screened for validation on all remaining samples [43]. Since the reduction of cost of arrays and the formation of international consortia, many analyses are entirely based on the meta-analysis of genome-wide SNP data.

Owing to technological and methodological advances, GWAS has successfully identified risk loci in complex diseases such as tumors, cardiovascular diseases, and rheumatism, as well as complex traits including blood lipid levels, and height. In recent years, there have been over fifty GWAS studies of CRC that were conducted worldwide, and brought the number of independent signals to about one hundred [44]. However, many variants revealed by European population GWASs show only weak or no effects among Asians, suggesting the occurrence of genetic heterogeneity between European and Asian ethnicities [45, 46]. Zeng et al. conducted a two-phase case–control study in the East-Asian population and found 4 loci correlated with CRC risk, revealing that the susceptibility of CRC might be connected with protein synthesis and degradation, steroid hormone, and autophagy pathways and providing additional insight into the mechanism of CRC pathogenesis [47]. These loci identified account for only ~7.7% of the genetic risk of CRC among East Asians, additional susceptibility regions for CRC remain to be further explored in Asians. Wang et al. conducted a GWAS in 1023 cases and 1306 controls, followed by the replicate stage in seven independent samples from China, which was comprised of 5317 cases and 6887 controls. The variant at 12p13.2 was found to be associated with CRC risk (rs2238126 in *ETV6*, $P = 2.67 \times 10^{-10}$), with G allele of rs2238126 confers earlier age at onset of CRC ($P = 1.98 \times 10^{-6}$), and reduce the binding affinity of transcriptional enhancer MAX [48]. The difference between Asian and European individuals in MAFs may exert an effect on patterns of linkage disequilibrium (LD) for index SNPs and causal SNPs. Therefore, further studies among different ethnic groups are warranted.

GWAS method represents an important advance than candidate gene studies in identifying novel variant–trait associations and novel biological mechanisms. However, it still has some limitations. First, GWAS explains only a modest fraction of the missing heritability. The over-rigorous statistical screening criteria of GWAS ($P < 5 \times 10^{-8}$) may leave out some SNPs that do not meet the statistical criteria but have biological functions. Based on the hypothesis of "common disease, common variant," some low-frequency genetic variants but with high penetrance may not be systematically identified. Second, GWAS do not inevitably pinpoint causal variants and genes. Because of LD, it is challenging to identify a single causal variant among multiple correlated variant. Moreover, gene–gene and gene–environment interactions are disregarded. Genetic susceptibility to disease should be studied under the consideration of environmental risk factors [49, 50].

To address these limitations, researchers are beginning to dig deeper into existing GWAS data, applying novel and accurate analytical methods, and combining functional genomics to explore the biological implications of GWAS results. These heralds the arrival of the post-GWAS era.

9.3.3 Post Genome-Wide Association Study

GWAS genotyping arrays typically contain 300,000–5,000,000 SNPs [51], which do not necessarily pinpoint causal variants. To identify the truly functional variants underlying observed GWAS signals, the information about all possible causal variants is required [52]. Post-GWAS focuses on illuminating the functional mechanisms of GWAS-identified genetic risk loci by applying novel and precise analytical methods.

9.3.3.1 Using Computational Strategy

Computational strategies could link signals to effector genes; the availability of increasingly large sample sizes, deeply sequenced reference panels, and ethnically diverse populations that allow variants not captured by genotype arrays to be imputed and allow genetic association signals to be refined to smaller regions.

Genotype Imputation With a high density of genotyped SNPs, such as the HapMap, genotype imputation allows the estimation of genotypes in a target data set by seeking common haplotypes between an individual's genome and a reference panel [53], 1000 Genomes projects [54]. The imputation of sporadic missing genotypes could increase power to detect genetic association, and guide fine-mapping. Moreover, imputation of SNPs can harmonize data from different GWAS genotyping arrays to conduct a pooled or meta-analysis, since the combination of data from different arrays can raise issues generated by different quality of genotyping among array technologies as well as the density of SNP genotypes.

Methodological Developments After imputation, the conduction of conditional association analysis to search independent signals within regions is crucial for downstream fine-mapping, since these multiple independent signals can interfere with each other in the statistical analyses.

By shrinking small effect estimates toward zero, penalized regression models perform estimation of SNP effect sizes and SNP selection into a model at the same time. Tuning parameters, estimated by cross-validation to choose a model with minimum prediction error, are used to select SNPs into a model and remove SNPs with small effect sizes. Penalized models tend to perform better than forwarding selection when using a very stringent *P*-value threshold to select SNPs, since a liberal threshold increases the chance of incorrect selection of SNPs [55]. Popular penalized models are lasso, minimax concave penalty, and a normal-exponential-γ shrinkage prior [55, 56].

Bayesian approaches assign posterior probabilities of causality to each variant, resulting in a "credible set" of candidate causal variants. In contrast with approaches based on *P*-values, Bayesian posteriors can be applied to compare variants directly, either within the same study or across different studies, which can be critical for large international collaborations in complex disease genetics. Additionally, by incorporating prior knowledge of functional annotation or consequence, Bayesian analysis could weigh evidence for a given variant more straightforwardly [52]. Recently, Li et al. constructed an integrative risk gene selector (iRIGS), a Bayesian framework which integrates multi-omics data and gene networks to predict functional genes in GWAS loci, contributing to the translation of GWAS to biology and therapeutic targets for multiple complex diseases [57].

Quantitative Trait Locus Analysis The vast majority of variants identified by GWAS reside in non-coding regions, the target genes of them might not be the nearest. Quantitative trait locus (QTL) analysis is an effective approach to evaluate the effects of genetic variants on intermediate molecular phenotype and discern the causal variant located in GWAS loci [58].

Expression quantitative trait locus (eQTL) analysis links gene expression to specific genomic regions [59–61]. Multiple studies have provided sufficient evidence that GWAS signals are enriched with eQTL in a tissue-specific manner, stressing their utility in illuminating the mechanisms underlying GWAS signals [51]. Zou et al. integrated genome-wide data with eQTL data to identify causal trait-relevant SNPs, demonstrating that rs27437 disrupts the TF-binding site within upstream of *SLC22A5* to decrease gene expression and subsequently lead to higher CRC risk in the Chinese population (OR = 1.31, 95% CI = 1.17–1.47) [62].

Previous eQTL analyses were mainly based on data derived from mRNA expression, ignoring the non-coding RNA expression which could also carry out diverse functions in cancer. By combining a large-scale population study with a comprehensive eQTL analysis, which tests the determinants of germline variants in established GWAS risk loci on mRNA and long non-coding RNA (lncRNA) expression in CRC tissues, Tian et al. prioritized a potential causal candidate variant. rs174575 could act as an allele-specific enhancer to distally regulate expression of both *FADS2* and lncRNA *AP002754.2* via long-range enhancer–promoter interaction loops, and *AP002754.2* further activated a transcriptional activator to upregulate *FADS2* expression that eventually facilitated CRC development (OR = 1.26; 95% CI = 1.17–1.36, Fig. 9.4) [63]. Moreover, several databases have provided eQTLs of mRNA [64] and non-coding RNA [65],

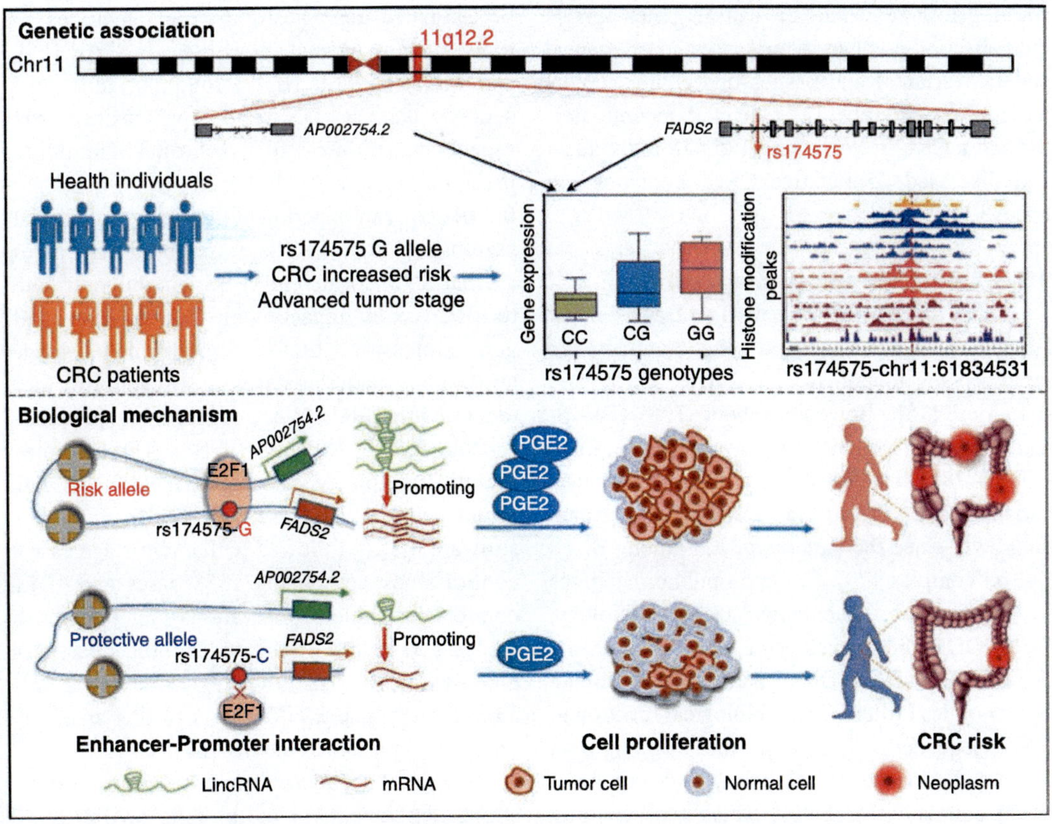

Fig. 9.4 SNP rs174575 acts as an allele-specific long-range enhancer of *FADS2* and lncRNA *AP002754.2* expression by mediation of E2F1 transcription factor (Cancer Res. 2020 May 1;80 (9):1804–1818)

contributing to the fine-mapping of post-GWAS and identification of therapeutic biomarkers for cancer.

In addition, the effect of variants on gene expression levels through post-transcriptional processes such as mRNA splicing [66] and stability [67] has also been evaluated. Other studies have associated genetic variants with altered levels of DNA methylation [68], immune cells infiltration [69] and protein expression [70], and some of these reports show significant overlap of these variants with disease-associated variants as well.

Transcriptome-Wide Association Studies With the wide application of transcriptome sequencing (RNA-seq) in specific tissues, transcriptome-wide association studies (TWAS) integrating GWAS and gene expression datasets to identify gene–trait associations have been conducted for many traits and tissues [71, 72]. TWAS could prioritize candidate causal genes (genes mediating the phenotypic effects of causal genetic variants) and tissues underlying GWAS loci more accurately [73]. Guo et al. recently performed a CRC TWAS using 125,478 individuals and disclosed 25 putative CRC predisposition genes [74].

9.3.3.2 Fine-Mapping: Integrating Functional Annotation Data

Disease- and trait-associated genetic variants are rapidly being identified with GWAS and related strategies [75]. To date, about 100 GWAS-identified risk loci of CRC have been identified [44, 76–78]. However, the vast majority of causal variants that drive the associations remain unknown, since the patterns of LD among SNPs can be complex [79]. Common public databases for annotation, including Gene Ontology, GENCODE, the Encyclopedia of DNA Elements (ENCODE), FANTOM, and the Roadmap Epigenomics Project, assign biological function to DNA sequences. Therefore, fine-mapping can select and prioritize causal variants based on functional annotation of SNPs, which are generally categorized on the basis of whether they occur in non-coding regions versus coding regions.

Non-coding Regions Annotation More than 90% of GWAS-identified SNPs are in non-coding regions [75]. It is believed that SNPs located in various regulatory element sequences are more likely to be causal SNPs, which may alter the regulatory mechanism of these regulatory elements through their allelic changes and affect the expression level of related genes, thereby exerting influence on the risk of disease [80]. Common non-coding annotation are promoters, enhancers, long non-coding RNA (lncRNA) loci, transcription start sites, transcription factor binding sites (TFBS), regulatory sequences, features of chromatin accessibility and histone modification patterns, and DNase I hypersensitive sites [81]. Annotation databases, such as GWAS4D [82] and RegulomeDB [83], provide regulatory impact scores for non-coding SNPs by aggregating multiple evidence sources of functional importance.

Variant impacts on putative TFBS motifs can be estimated upon position weight matrices by tools, such as AnimalTFDB [84], JASPAR [85], and MATCH [86]. High-throughput functional assays such as DNase I-hypersensitive site sequencing (DNase-seq) and chromatin immunoprecipitation assays followed by sequencing (ChIP-seq) can experimentally detect functional regions including TFBSs. Based on the hypothesis that SNPs located at TFBSs might contribute to CRC risk by impacting on TF regulations and gene expressions, Lou et al. performed systematic bioinformatics analyses on susceptibility loci identified by CRC GWASs to screen out potential functional SNPs located at TFBSs. Through integrating multiple types of data from ENCODE project, dbSNP database, and TFBS prediction software Match, followed with a two-stage case–control study comprising 1353 cases and 1448 controls in Chinese populations and functional analyses, rs6695837 exhibited significant associations with CRC risk (OR = 1.31, 95% CI = 1.06–1.63) by acting as a TFBS and exerting an effect on *LAMC1* promoter activity [87].

A class of regulatory regions with unusually strong enrichment for the binding of transcriptional coactivators has been found and termed as super-enhancers (SEs) [88]. Compared to typical enhancers, SEs are larger in size, bind with higher density of TFs, and possess greater capacity to activate gene transcription. Ke et al. performed systematical bioinformatics analysis on multi-omics data to screen potential SNPs in cancer-specific SEs, and then evaluated their contributions to CRC risk in a two-stage case–control study consisted of 4929 cases and 7083 controls from the Chinese population. Further functional assays elucidated that protective rs11064124-G disrupts the binding affinity with vitamin D receptor (VDR) and increases enhancer activity and interactions with promoters of two target genes *CD9* and *PLEKHG6*, coactivating the transcription of these two putative tumor suppressor genes for CRC [89].

LncRNA as a diverse class of transcript which could not serve as templates for proteins, has been massively authenticated with the advances in deep sequencing [90]. Increasing evidence shows that up to 90% of the non-coding transcripts in the human genome have important and different biological roles [91]. Recent researches have demonstrated that many lncRNAs are abnormally expressed in cancers, with potentially carcinogenic or tumor suppressor roles [92, 93]. Among the lncRNAs, a subset of the lncRNAs can function as a miRNA decoy or sponge by interacting with miRNAs by complementary sequence, which indirectly affect the miRNA regulation of other protein-coding genes. Gong et al. first comprehensively screened functional SNPs that could influence lncRNA:miRNA binding in CRC GWAS loci, revealing that rs2147578(G) allele within in lnc-LAMC2-1:1 may augment the risk of CRC (OR = 1.29, 95% CI = 1.11–1.51) in Chinese populations by losing the binding of miR-128-3p [94]. Moreover, they constructed the lncRNASNP database to profile comprehensive information about lncRNA related SNPs in human and mouse by characterizing all SNPs in lncRNA exon sequences and predicting their effects on lncRNA secondary structure and lncRNA–miRNA interaction, which could contribute to the exploration of their potential functions [95].

Coding Regions Annotation Although less than 10% of the SNPs are located in the coding region of the human genome, these SNPs may cause amino acid changes, which further change the stability, structural or biochemical properties of the protein, and post-translational modification (PTM). Examples of annotation include whether a SNP occurs in an intron, an exon, or a splice site or whether it is involved in alternative splicing [81]. A large number of bioinformatics annotation methods, such as CADD [96] and REVEL [97] methods, are available to functionally profile coding SNPs and provide impact scores to predict their deleterious effect. Our research team has also developed a database that integrates SNPs and multiple PTM information, providing clues for researchers to study the function of genetic variation in coding regions [98].

9.3.3.3 Deep Sequencing and Exon Array Research

Based on the hypothesis of "common diseases-common mutations," GWAS can only identify the common variants (minor allele frequency, MAF > 5%) associated with diseases and miss the association between low-frequency genetic variants (1% < MAF ≤ 5%) or rare variants (MAF ≤ 1%) and common disease [99]. Moreover, these common variants only explain a small proportion of the genetic risk. For instance, a study including 8025 cases and 10,814 controls of CRC GWAS reported the heritability explained by all common SNPs was merely 7.42%, indicating the impact of common variants on disease is limited [30].

With the progress of deep sequencing technology, technical barriers to detection of low-frequency variants and rare variants have been eliminated. Deep sequencing can not only accurately identify existing common variants, but also effectively discover new low-frequency and rare variants in complex diseases. Latest research performed whole-genome sequencing of 1439 cases and 720 controls and identified 40 new independent signals, including a strongly protective 0.3% frequency variant signal at *CHD1*. Their result suggests that CRC risk is highly polygenic, larger and more comprehensive studies will enable rare variant identification, thus improve understanding of functional effects of this risk, determine personalized screening strategies, and facilitate drug development [44].

Although the current sequencing technology advances, sequencing the whole genome still requires a high cost, and whole-exome sequencing is a relatively cost-effective method. Based on the hypothesis that genetic variants in genes involved in telomere maintenance could predispose individuals to CRC, Li et al. captured germline variations in 192 patients with CRC by sequencing the coding regions of 13 core components participant in telomere biology. Combing with a two-stage case–control study and functional exploration, a rare variant P507L in *TPP1* was identified to confer higher risk of CRC through disrupting TPP1-TIN2 interaction, damaging telomerase processivity, and shrinking telomere length. This approach highlights the role of rare variants in cancer development and provides new insights into the prevention of CRC [100].

Subsequently, Chang et al. performed an exome-wide association analysis to systematically investigate the low-frequency or rare coding risk variants in patients with CRC from Chinese populations. Two variants were identified to be significantly associated with CRC risk: a novel rare missense variant in *TCF7L2* (rs138649767, OR = 2.08, 95% CI: 1.69–2.57, $P = 5.66 \times 10^{-12}$) and a previous identified 3'-UTR variant within *ATF1* from European GWAS (rs11169571, OR = 1.18, 95% CI: 1.13–1.24, $P = 1.65 \times 10^{-12}$), the rare missense variant exhibits higher effect size than most GWAS-identified common susceptible variants (Fig. 9.5) [101]. In the post-GWAS era, deep sequencing of exomes and candidate regions, identified by previous GWAS, can complement with traditional GWAS strategies, providing unprecedented opportunities for comprehensively revealing the genetic mechanisms of CRC.

9.3.3.4 Experimental Post-GWAS

As associations detected by GWAS do not yield casual variants or genes, computational strategies are first level of assessment of candidate SNPs, and functional annotations further refine genetic association signals to smaller regions. Whereas,

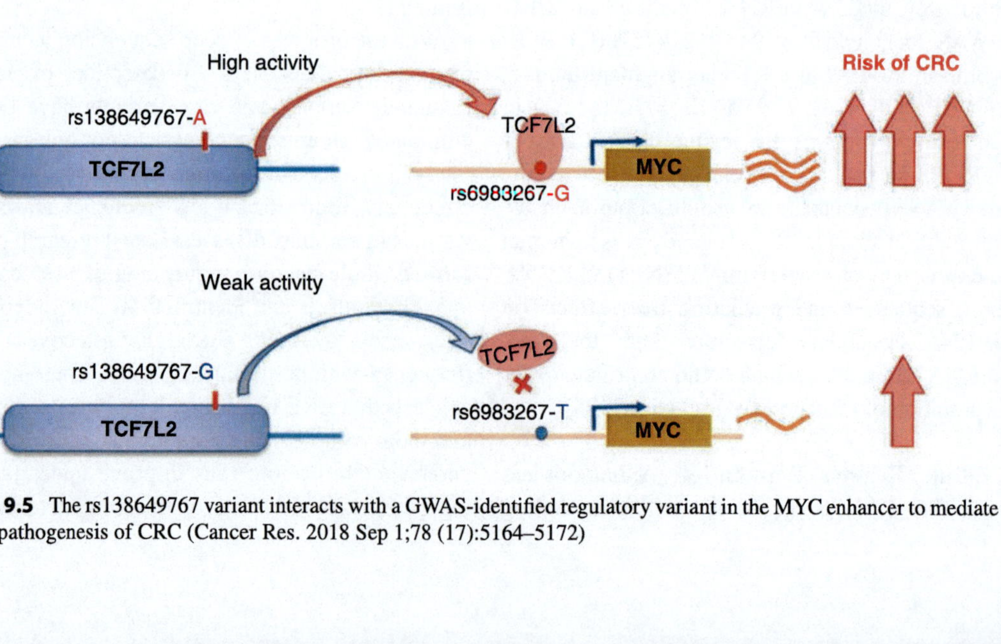

Fig. 9.5 The rs138649767 variant interacts with a GWAS-identified regulatory variant in the MYC enhancer to mediate the pathogenesis of CRC (Cancer Res. 2018 Sep 1;78 (17):5164–5172)

these strategies usually only provide indirect evidence of an association, and experimental approaches are necessary for confirming its functional relevance. To date, relatively few risk loci have been systematically studied. Insights into the genetic and biological basis of cancer susceptibility mediated through common variation are emerging [42].

Methods for Functional Validation of Coding Variants Protein-coding variants are easiest to build a case for prioritization and to design experiments to assay functional effects, mainly focusing on the functional interpretation of the non-synonymous genetic variation. Non-synonymous mutations can result in amino acid substitutions, which might modify protein stability, structure or biochemical properties, subcellular localization, and modification status [102]. Real-time PCR (RT-qPCR) is universally applied to detect effect of those variants on mRNA expression levels. Methods to evaluate different SNP genotypes on protein expression level are mainly based on antigen antibody response, such as western blotting (WB), enzyme linked immunosorbent assay (ELISA), and immunofluorescence. Mass spectrometry (MS)-based proteomics has been developed extensively in the past decade and is becoming the standard approach for comprehensively characterizing different post-translational modifications (PTMs) on a global scale, including phosphorylation, SUMOylation, and glycosylation. In addition, recent researches have also discovered that germline variants or mutations located in the coding region may change the status of gene RNA m^6A modification (N^6-Methyladenosine), which affects the occurrence, development, and prognosis of diseases through different functional mechanisms [103–106]. Using exome-wide association data, Tian et.al first systematically explored the association of m^6A modification related variants with CRC risk in 1062 CRC cases and 2184 controls and followed by two replication sets including 7341 CRC cases and 7902 controls. The A allele of missense variant rs8100241 located in *ANKLE1* was associated with the decreased risk of CRC (OR = 0.88, 95% CI = 0.84–0.92). Using a specific antibody against m^6A, RNA immunoprecipitation (RIP) assay followed by a real-time qPCR elucidated that rs8100241[a] allele increased *ANKLE1* m^6A modification level, and Western blotting detected the ANKLE1 protein expression. Mechanistically, the germline missense variant linked to CRC risk by increasing *ANKLE1* mRNA m^6A level and thus facilitating ANKLE1 protein expression, which can function as potential tumor suppressor [107].

In addition to disrupting protein function, coding variants could have more subtle effects including tag functional non-coding variants [108]. Chang et al. identified a significant interaction between the *TCF7L2* missense variant rs138649767 and a previous GWAS-identified regulatory variant rs6983267 in the *MYC* enhancer. Considering previous studies that the binding affinity of *TCF7L2* to *MYC* enhancer region in 8q24 could be affected by a GWAS-identified rs6983267 variant, they transfected the pGL3-basic vector which contained the *MYC* promoter and enhancer with different rs6983267 alleles into LoVo and SW480 cells, followed by overexpressing different *TCF7L2* rs138649767 variants to perform reporter assay. Compared to transfection of TCF7L2[G], transfection of TCF7L2[A] significantly activates the *MYC* enhancer, especially for enhancer with rs6983267[G]. This functional interaction result validated the population analysis, highlighting an important role of rare missense variant in the development of CRC (see Fig. 9.5) [101].

Methods for Functional Validation of Non-coding Variants Most disease-associated variants identified from GWAS do not alter protein-coding sequences but rather reside in non-coding regions. Differing from the accurate prediction and identification of biological mechanisms involved in coding region variants, non-coding variants may result in enhancer–promoter contact inhibition, transcription factor binding disturbances, and chromatin openness.

Transcriptional regulatory activity of genetic variants can be assayed using reporter genes in vitro [109] and/or in vivo [110]. Protein binding can be assessed by in vitro assays such as electrophoretic mobility shift assays (EMSAs), for which knowledge of the bound proteins is not required. To further test which proteins mediate allele-specific binding, antibodies against TFs of interest are used in supershift EMSA experiments [51]. Besides, ChIP-Seq methodologies are currently applied to identify histone modifications and transcription-factor-occupied regions, yielding signals of less than 1 kb DNA stretches for detailed analyses [111]. In order to further investigate the long-range regulation of remote target genes by regulatory elements, chromosome conformation capture (3C) and its derivatives (4C, 5C, Hi-C, ChIA-PET, and Capture-HiC) and other three-dimensional topological association domain methods have been widely applied [112, 113]. CRISPR/Cas gene editing has transformed functional genomics, enabling researchers to potentially edit any desired region of the genome [114].

The methods described above are mainly focusing on the function identification of individual candidate variants. Whereas, computational studies have suggested that many disease risk loci are driven by multiple variants, emphasizing the importance of experimentally testing all candidate causal variants at a given locus. High-throughput sequencing-based assays enable genome-wide loss-of-function screening. Analysis of functional importance of noncoding variants in promoters and enhancers can be achieved in a high-throughput manner using a modification of cis-regulatory element analysis by sequencing (CRE-seq) [115]. Self-transcribing active regulatory region sequencing (STARR-seq) is an alternative method for characterizing enhancer variants, in which enhancer libraries are flanked by synthetic adaptor DNA sequences and cloned downstream of a transcription reporter construct [116]. Recently, Arensbergen et al. developed a higher throughput method, a survey of regulatory elements reporter technology (SuRE), which could survey the effect of 5.9 million SNPs on enhancer and promoter activity [117].

Knockout, knockdown, and activation screens are complementary methods that together will contribute to a more complete understanding of biological systems. Functional genomic screening based on a high-throughput RNA interference (RNAi) [118] or CRISPR-Cas9 [119] interrogation has been proved to be a powerful tool for unraveling disease-related genes and gene interaction networks. Through this high-throughput RNAi functional screen, Tian explored genes associated with proliferation in the CRC risk loci of Asian populations, *ATF1* which located in the 12q13.12 region was identified to have most significant effect on the identified genes and promotes CRC xenograft growth by affecting cell apoptosis. Further fine-mapping analysis followed by a two-stage affected control study consisting of 6213 affected individuals and 10,388 controls, and multipronged experiments. Two risk variants rs61926301 and rs7959129, located in the *ATF1* promoter and first intron, respectively, could facilitate a promoter–enhancer interaction, though the synergy of SP1 and GATA3 to upregulate *ATF1* expression, thus synergistically predisposing to CRC risk (OR = 1.77, 95% CI = 1.42–2.21, $P = 3.16 \times 10^{-7}$; $P_{\text{multiplicative-interaction}} = 1.20 \times 10^{-22}$; $P_{\text{additive-interaction}} = 6.50 \times 10^{-3}$). These findings revealed the clinical potential of *ATF1* in CRC development and illuminated a promoter–enhancer interaction module between the *ATF1* regulatory elements, and bring a closer understanding to the molecular drivers of cancer (Fig. 9.6) [120].

In general, these approaches will might be especially suitable for loci harboring multiple functional variants that all contribute to disease risk.

9.3.3.5 Gene–Gene and Gene–Environment Interaction Studies

In contrast to simple Mendelian disorders, common complex traits are caused by a combination of multiple genetic and environmental risk factors, pointing that genetic susceptibility to disease should be investigated under the context of environmental risk factors. Gene–gene and gene–environment (GxE) interactions are expected to explain part of the missing heritability [121]. This might be especially important for diseases, including CRC, which susceptibility is inextricably linked with the environment.

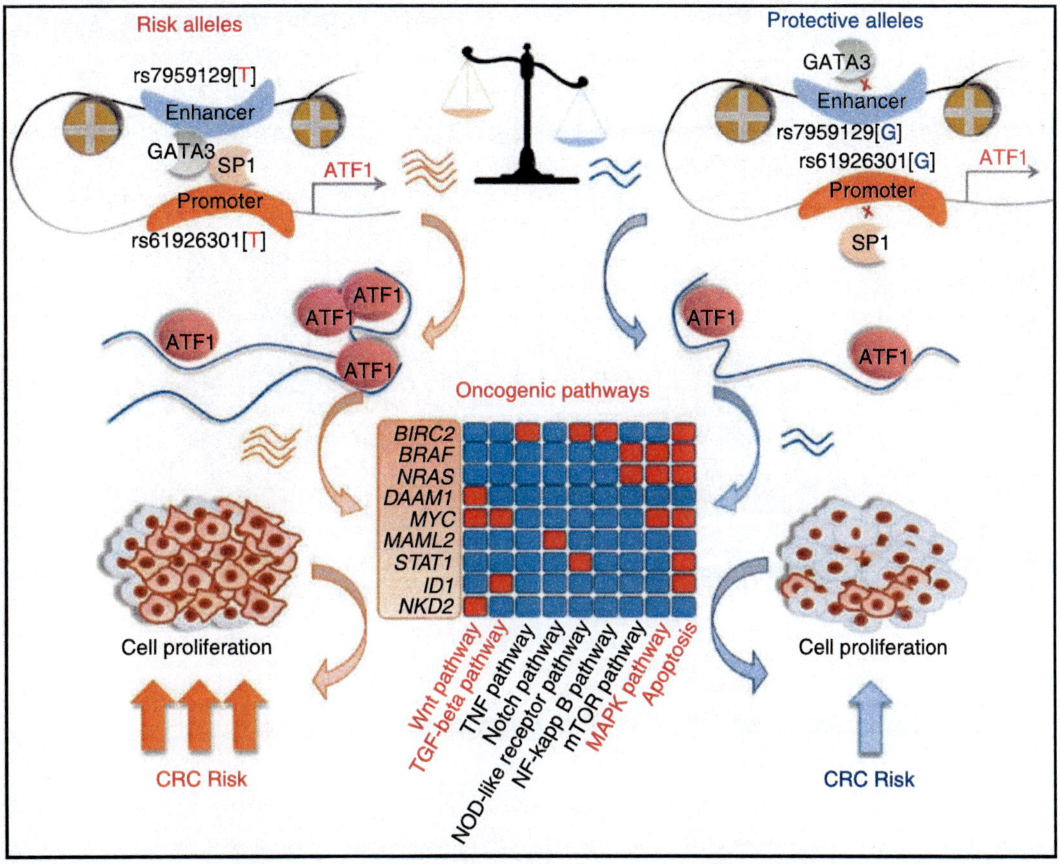

Fig. 9.6 rs61926301 and rs7959129 facilitate a promoter–enhancer interaction that regulates *ATF1* expression and thus synergistically predisposing to CRC risk (Am J Hum Genet. 2019 Jul 3;105 (1):29–47)

Many disease risk loci are driven by multiple variants spanning multiple enhancers that target the same gene [122]. Considering the interaction between genetic variants would increase the risk of CRC, Gong et al. systematically integrated ChIP-Seq, DNase-Seq, and transcription factor motif data to screen variants with potential ability to affect the MYC binding affinity (Fig. 9.7a). Based on a two-stage case–control study (Fig. 9.7b) in the Chinese population to identify risk polymorphisms and interactions between genetic variants, a novel polymorphism rs11777210 in *KBTBD11* was validated to harbor significantly interaction with *MYC* nearby rs6983267. Subjects carrying rs6983267 GG and rs11777210 CC genotypes exhibited higher susceptibility to CRC (2.83-fold) than those carrying rs6983267 TT and rs11777210 TT genotypes. Further functional analysis demonstrated that rs6983267 T > G increased *MYC* expression, and MYC bound to and negatively regulated *KBTBD11* expression only when the rs11777210 C risk allele occurred (Fig. 9.7c). This study highlights the identification of interaction between the genetic variants [123].

After identifying a novel missense variant by exome chip described above, Chang et al. further performed functional analysis, a missense variant rs138649767 lies in *TCF7L2* gene was identified to significantly interact with a previous GWAS-identified regulatory variant rs6983267 located in the *MYC* enhancer ($P_{\text{interaction}} = 0.0002$, see Fig. 9.5). These results illuminate the functional importance of genetic risk loci in the molecular pathogenesis of CRC and provide insight into pathways that might be targeted to prevent CRC [101].

Diet, lifestyle, and other environmental factors are thought to have a strong impact on CRC

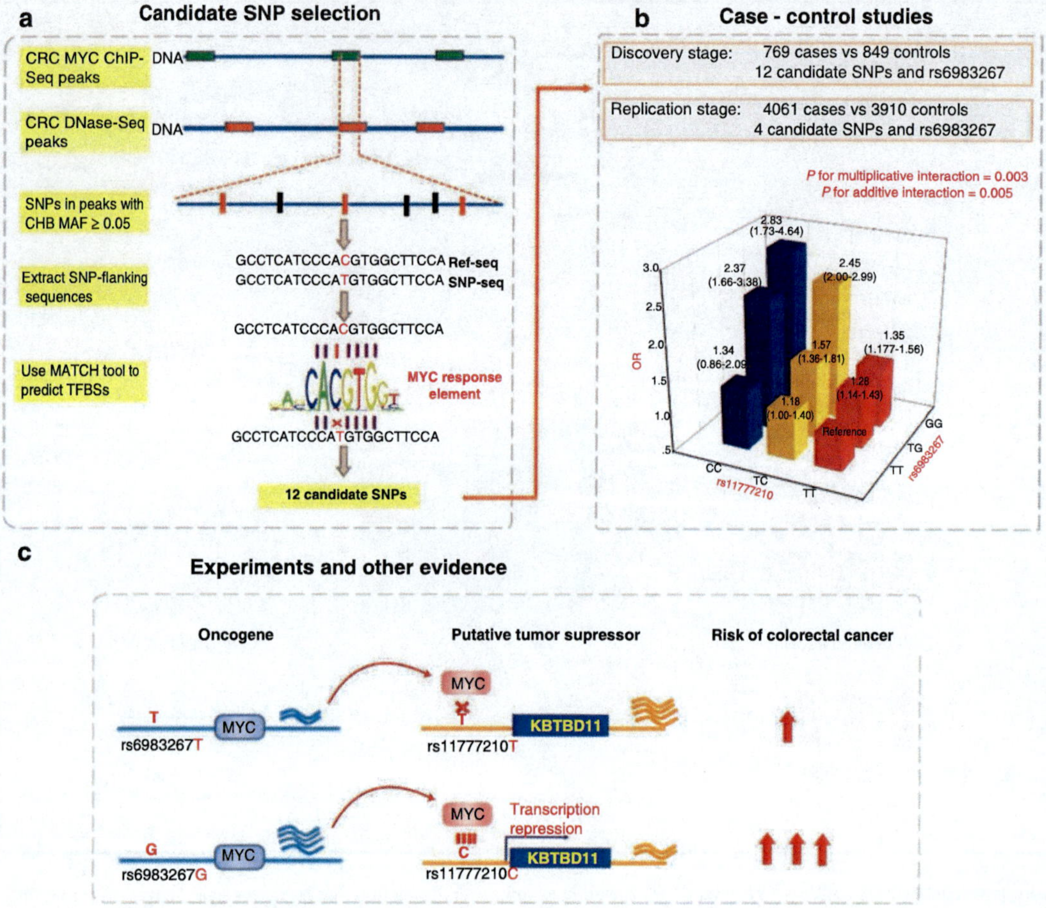

Fig. 9.7 Integrative multistage methodology to illuminate the effects of variants in *MYC* response elements on CRC risk (Ann Oncol. 2018 Mar 1;29 (3):632–639)

risk, underlying the important role of the environment in CRC etiology. The interaction between environmental factors and genes is an area of growing interest. Individual components of the TGF-β signaling pathway interact with each other to form a complex network, which triggered speculation that expression of TGF-β components might be affected by the potential synergy of multiple common genetic variations and environmental exposures, and eventually lead to enhanced tumor growth and metastatic potential. Based on a two-staged case–control study among Chinese population, Zhong et al. comprehensively explored associations of common genetic variations in the TGF-β signaling pathway and environmental factors with CRC risk. Combining random forest and multilocus genotype patterns could capture the complex interaction effects among high-dimensional data, through this approach, potential interactions between *SMAD7* rs11874392, *TGFBR1* rs10988706, rs6478972 and smoking were found to enhance the risk of CRC at both stages [124]. This study emphasized the substantial role of the TGF-β signaling pathway and their interaction with smoking in CRC development.

Gene–environment studies could be used to identify novel environmental and genetic risk factors and enable people to understand the etiologic role of those factors in disease. However, GxE studies still have many challenges, among which the most important is the quantification of environmental exposure, such as exposure dose, exposure time, and exposure range.

9.3.3.6 Population Validation in a Prospective Cohort Study

GWASs mainly apply case–control studies to find disease-associated SNPs, which need to be validated by prospective cohorts. The ideal prospective cohort has following the advantages: a) is longitudinal, with data collected annually before, during, and after the disease, b) includes participants without other diseases that confuse the associated outcome, c) collects information more comprehensively and accurately, including phenotypes of endogenous, exogenous, environmental, and molecular factors. Population validation based on prospective cohort could facilitate the identification of factors that determine outcomes and assessment of the interactions between gene and environment.

Although current cohorts are expensive to build and maintain, some longitudinal cohorts are long running and population based. Research institutes and government agencies around the world have their own longitudinal cohort of people, such as China Kadoorie Biobank (CKB) and Dongfeng Tongji Cohort in China [125]; the Twins UK Registry [126], UK Biobank [127], and 1958 Birth Cohort in UK [128]; Study of Health in Pomerania (SHIP) in Germany [129]; the Nurses' Health Study in the United States [130]; the Northern Finland Birth Cohort (NFBC) [131], and Lifelines in Finland [132], as well as the Human Genome Project created 500FG Cohort [133]. These projects focused on the investigation of environmental and genetic risk factors for cardiovascular disease, metabolic disease, cancer, and aging, while collecting a wide range of phenotypic characteristics of an individual, each contributing significantly to various aspects of population health. In particular, the large-scale CRC cohort in American, Prostate, Lung, Colorectal and Ovarian Cancer Screening Trial (PLCO) provides GWAS datasets for confirmation [134].

9.4 The Potential Benefits and Challenges of Genetics Epidemiology for CRC

It is preferred to understand the determinants of CRC in an age of growing healthcare costs and burgeoning burden of cancer. Genetic epidemiology emerged in the 1960s through the integration between genetics and epidemiology, which studies the role of inherited factors, along with the environmental contributors in disease etiology. Benefits of genetic epidemiology in CRC are numerous, including an improved understanding of its biological mechanisms, effective clinical treatments, and dosage regimens for pharmaceuticals. In order to fully appreciate the contributions of genetic epidemiology research to CRC, it is helpful to be familiar with the applications and the current challenges researchers face.

9.4.1 The Potential Benefits of Genetics Epidemiology for CRC

9.4.1.1 Polygenic Risk Score (PRS) in CRC Risk

A polygenic score (PGS) or PRS is a single value estimate of an individual's genetic liability to a phenotype, calculated according to their genotype profile derived from GWAS summary statistic data. These scores were employed for the first time to identify individuals at high risk for disease in the late 2000s [135]. This was first successfully applied in empirical research in 2009 by researchers who organized a GWAS of schizophrenia to construct scores of risk propensity. As GWAS sample sizes increase and PRSs become more powerful, PRSs analyses become an integral part of research and stratified medicine.

As CRC has a sizable heritable fraction (heritability estimates ranging from 12 to 35%) [29] and is polygenic in nature with probably thousands of genetic variants contributing to its development [136], utilizing genome-wide data to predict risk holds promise for risk stratification for primary and secondary prevention. The developed PRS offers a way to improve CRC risk prediction and translate to optimize clinical decision-making.

Li et al. initially conducted a case–control study in a Chinese Han population to assess the association between 21 discovered SNPs and CRC risk in multiple models combining genetic and non-genetic factors. This study found that multiple genetic GWAS loci jointly influenced the CRC risk. The combination of genetic factors and conventional non-genetic factors improved the performance of risk predictive model for CRC [137].

The AUC can be further improved perhaps by combining the PRS with other predictive factors, such as rare variants, colorectal tissue-specific functional data, or environmental/lifestyle risk factors which will further substantially improve risk prediction. The modifiable risk factors for the CRC are an important component of risk prediction because the best approach to primary prevention is avoidance or elimination of these risk factors. For secondary prevention, both genetics and modifiable risk factors would contribute to determining optimal CRC screening timing and frequency. At this point in time, the accuracy of PRSs may only be well-characterized for European ancestry populations. More research is needed to derive the data for making PRSs useful for other populations.

PRSs are not yet routinely used by health professionals because there are no practical guidelines and researchers are still refining how these scores are generated. PRSs will always be probabilities, not certainties. However, some healthcare and companies have already begun generating PRSs for their consumers and they may 1 day serve as an complementary tool to guide healthcare decisions.

9.4.1.2 Precision Medicine in CRC Treatment

Unlike traditional medicine, precision medicine (PM) is referred to as a model of medicine that proposes the customization of healthcare, where medical decisions, treatments, practices, or products are tailored to a group of patients, rather than a one-drug-fits-all model [138]. The idea of PM is not new, but recent advances in science and technology have helped accelerate the pace of research in this area.

It is common that patients with CRC were treated with one-size-fits-all drugs and provided with consistent guideline care in the past few decades. In addition to the standard colorectal surgery, recommendations for drug therapy, radiation, and combination procedures based on the tumor staging have been successful in improving overall survival in patients and stopping cancer from recurring [139]. However, due to tumor heterogeneity, it is too simple to rely solely on CRC staging to determine treatment options. This has likely led to many cases of treatment failure, adverse drug reactions, and multiple side effects.

Information on an individual's genetic makeup is key to estimating their likelihood of developing disease and creating personalized drugs that work better. Since the U.S. Food and Drug Administration approved next generation sequencing (NGS) devices for clinical diagnosis in 2013 [140], the application of NGS technology has skyrocketed and is becoming a mainstream option for diseases investigation. NGS can be applied to noninvasively detect circulating tumor DNA (ctDNA) in CRC patients for monitoring the disease in real time, facilitating sensitive, specific, and cost-efficient detection of cancer progression [141]. For instance, KRAS mutant alleles detected in plasma has become crucial for clinical decision-making in CRC treatments before cancer progression [142].

In summary, the purpose of PM is to develop a tailor-made treatment for each individual and his or her unique condition to maximize benefit and minimize potential harms. The stratification of patients through the use of biomarkers is thus key. As the use of newer therapeutic agents connected with specific genetic sup-type(s) will increase, ultimately increasing patients' quality of life and life expectancy.

9.4.1.3 Integrating Genetics into the Drug Development

Compared to established (non-genomic) approaches to drug discovery and development, it has long been expected that genetic approach would provide a systematic and reliable way to explain inter-individual variability in drug response. Conventional small molecule drugs and biotherapeutics act by directly perturbing the function of proteins. Drug development is therefore predicated on identifying those proteins that both play a causal role in a disease and are also "druggable" [143]. Genomics now provides a tool to accurately identify proteins that both play a controlling role in a disease and which are amenable to targeting by drugs. In many (but perhaps not all) cases, the rediscovery by GWAS of over 70 drug targets suggests that genes influencing disease onset can provide useful insight on targetable pathways for the prevention of progression or recurrence of common conditions.

In contrast to established non-genomic approaches to preclinical drug development, GWAS fueled the rapid development and evaluation of colorectum-specific drug for clinical use. Human genetic will soon be universally regarded as a mechanism to prioritize molecular targets early in drug development stage toward potentially more efficacious models. By improving the reliability and efficiency of target identification, GWAS and other genetic study designs offer the potential to overturn the currently poor odds of success currently beleaguering drug development.

In the context of drug development, GWAS are yet to be optimally designed or sufficiently widely deployed to maximize their potential impact on target discovery. Over 90% of GWAS associated variations do not reside in genes encoding druggable targets but in non-coding regions. The range of diseases studied has also been limited. Sample sizes in most GWAS may not have been enough to detect all responsible genes and all relevant drug targets.

At present, revolutionary steps in drug development through human genomics could have the consequence of reducing wasted investment, increasing value for investors and, eventually, reducing the inflationary pressure on drug prices for healthcare providers. The drug development through human genomics might provide the sorely needed stimulus for true drug development innovation, to the benefit of patients, health systems, business, and society.

9.4.2 Challenges in Post-GWAS Analysis for CRC

Despite remarkable successes, genetic epidemiology has yet to fully elucidate the genetic basis of disease. Generally, the post-GWAS field lacks well-established strategies to implement comprehensive criteria to elucidate the causal variants and their mechanisms. Indeed, as we develop better techniques enforcing rigorous experimental criteria and considering the genomic 3D architecture and interaction with the tumor microenvironment, we get closer to clearly defining the causal variants and confidently declaring a gene or genes as implicated in the impact of those causal variants in CRC oncogenesis. Nevertheless, additional challenges encountered during analysis of the valuable GWAS data that need to be surmounted in order to maximize the accuracy and precision of post-GWAS analyses are noted below.

9.4.2.1 Genetic Association of Causal SNPs Could be Missed by Current GWAS

Decade years ago, it was widely expected that the genetic basis of common disease would be resolved by GWAS. However, the bulk of heritable variance remains unexplained. The low resolution of GWAS does not allow for full coverage of the SNP density present in the human genome and thus candidate causal loci [144]. Particularly, some variants in the lower frequency and larger effects domains might be missed in GWAS, fine-mapping, and imputation statistical procedures [145]. It is postulated that much of the missing heritability of CRC is enshrined in high-impact rare alleles, which are mechanistically and clinically important [146]. Thus, it is crucial to include them in the subsequent post-GWAS analysis. To detect structural variants in CRC, many high-throughput sequencing-based GWAS have gained attention as methods to detect them. However, it is technically challenging owing to the low-resolution maps of current sequencing technologies. Imputation methods also have their own limitations that can be minimized by expanding reference panels of genomic variation. Information emerging from projects such as the Haplotype Reference Consortium will facilitate the investigation of the lower frequency spectrum without the need for de novo sequencing. Because the reference panels are limited to European ancestry population and given the genetic heterogeneity among various populations, more diverse reference panels including sets of worldwide populations are needed to increase the yield of intriguing rare variants.

9.4.2.2 Target Genes of Regulatory SNPs Are Not Always the Nearest or Embedded Genes

One default approach has been to assign the top associated SNP to the nearest gene at each locus. Unfortunately, relying on physical proximity alone has not yet been tested empirically since SNPs can influence gene expression over long gnomic ranges, with studies based on eQTL data suggesting that two-thirds of the causal genes at GWAS loci are distinct from the nearest genes. A typical example of how misleading the traditional approach could be is the regulatory variant SNP rs9930506, which led to the initiation of drug design and preclinical studies in adiposity. Initially, the fat mass and obesity-associated (FTO) gene was considered the target gene of this SNP, which is located within the intronic region of FTO. However, further studies demonstrated that this variant is functionally connected to the gene Iroquois homeobox 3 (IRX3) via a long-range interaction [147]. EQTL analysis has been commonly used for the discovery of allele-specific regulatory elements and target gene(s). However, eQTL mapping hinges on statistical association, which may fail to detect the direct target. Additionally, functional study of risk loci should include different modulators to result in genuine causality discoveries. The protein QTL, methylation QTL or metabolites QTL, and splice QTL studies together with eQTLs may be useful to examine correlations between proteomics, epigenomics, and transcriptomic data along with genomics data.

9.4.2.3 Overlooking Tumor Microenvironment and Tissue Specificity

CRC is a complex and molecularly heterogeneous disease, characterized by different genomic, pigenomic, transcriptomic, and immune landscapes [148]. Limited tissue-specific expression resources could be a hurdle to discovering functional SNPs. This is of high importance in the case of regulatory variants owing to a strong degree of tissue specificity in crucial interactions of regulatory machinery. Moreover, studies in animal models and human samples have regarded the concept of the tumor microenvironments as a functional component central to tumorigenesis and tumor progression. Aside from the original disease-relevant tissue, disease-related cell types can harbor functional variants that are involved in CRC manifestations. For example, cells from the immune system and other cells in the tumor microenvironment play an important role in CRC development and progression along with cancer cells [149]. The recent development of in vitro 3D organoid models has opened new avenues for recapitulating the in vivo complexity of tumorigenesis. Integration of data from all available resources for specific cancer cell types and/or tissue might be helpful to overcome this challenge. Understanding the transcriptome at the single-cell level by identifying single-cell QTLs will enable us to dissect heterogeneity in cell populations hidden in bulk analysis and explore rare cell types associated with tumorigenesis and metastasis.

9.4.2.4 Consideration of Genetic, Epigenetic, and Environmental Factors

The phenotypic heterogeneity in patients with CRC depends on specific combinations of genome composition, epigenetic components, and environmental inputs. For example, CRC is characterized by diverse genetic alterations in both germline and somatic variants that disrupt normal biology and provide selective advantage to cells during tumorigenesis, suggesting that germline variants may cooperate with somatic mutations as "co-oncogenes" or "co-tumor suppressors." Recent efforts investigating SNP–SNP interactions try to expand association studies to a higher level of cross-associations of risk loci. Moreover, various epigenetic profile analyses comparing healthy and cancer cells indicate that epimutations have been proposed as driver mutation in CRC initiation and progression together with genetic lesions [150]. Environmental factors, particularly diet and lifestyle, can affect the overall impact of functional loci on the cell phenotype at various levels and make the interpretation of consequences even more complex. Studies of non-genetic factors such as smoking, body fatness, and alcohol drinks [10, 151]try to understand the evidence of gene–environment interaction beyond genetics factors to affect CRC incidence. The Mendelian randomization approach can be used to investigate causality of other risk factors (adiposity, hyperlipidemia and fatty acid profile, and so on) in CRC [152, 153]. Methods such as summary-data-based Mendelian randomization (MR), which was created based on Mendelian randomization using GWAS and gene expression data, are helpful to explore the potential causal association between an exposure and CRC. MR can be performed using only GWAS summary statistics, making it potentially an extremely cost-effective technique with wide applicability. It is valuable in the development of new therapeutic strategies.

References

1. Rimbert H, Darrier B, Navarro J, et al. High throughput SNP discovery and genotyping in hexaploid wheat. PLoS One. 2018;13:e0186329.
2. Arnold M, Sierra MS, Laversanne M, et al. Global patterns and trends in colorectal cancer incidence and mortality. Gut. 2017;66:683–91.
3. Fidler MM, Soerjomataram I, Bray F. A global view on cancer incidence and national levels of the human development index. Int J Cancer. 2016;139:2436–46.
4. Zheng RS, Sun KX, Zhang SW, et al. Report of cancer epidemiology in China, 2015. Zhonghua Zhong Liu Za Zhi. 2019;41:19–28.
5. Sun KXZRS, Zhang SW, et al. Report of cancer incidence and mortality in different areas of China. China Cancer. 2015;28:1–11.
6. Keum N, Giovannucci E. Global burden of colorectal cancer: emerging trends, risk factors and prevention strategies. Nat Rev Gastroenterol Hepatol. 2019;16:713–32.
7. Brenner H, Kloor M, Pox CP. Colorectal cancer. Lancet. 2014;383:1490–502.
8. Bardou M, Barkun AN, Martel M. Obesity and colorectal cancer. Gut. 2013;62:933–47.
9. Renehan AG, Tyson M, Egger M, et al. Body-mass index and incidence of cancer: a systematic review and meta-analysis of prospective observational studies. Lancet. 2008;371:569–78.
10. Song M, Chan AT, Sun J. Influence of the gut microbiome, diet, and environment on risk of colorectal cancer. Gastroenterology. 2020;158:322–40.
11. Kerr J, Anderson C, Lippman SM. Physical activity, sedentary behaviour, diet, and cancer: an update and emerging new evidence. Lancet Oncol. 2017;18:e457–e71.
12. Hibler E. Epigenetics and colorectal neoplasia: the evidence for physical activity and sedentary behavior. Curr Colorectal Cancer Rep. 2015;11:388–96.
13. Robinson MM, Dasari S, Konopka AR, et al. Enhanced protein translation underlies improved metabolic and physical adaptations to different exercise training modes in young and old humans. Cell Metab. 2017;25:581–92.
14. Vieira AR, Abar L, Chan DSM, et al. Foods and beverages and colorectal cancer risk: a systematic review and meta-analysis of cohort studies, an update of the evidence of the WCRF-AICR continuous update project. Ann Oncol. 2017;28:1788–802.
15. Song M, Garrett WS, Chan AT. Nutrients, foods, and colorectal cancer prevention. Gastroenterology. 2015;148:1244–60.e16.
16. Aune D, Lau R, Chan DS, et al. Nonlinear reduction in risk for colorectal cancer by fruit and vegetable intake based on meta-analysis of prospective studies. Gastroenterology. 2011;141:106–18.
17. Wiseman M. The second World Cancer Research Fund/American Institute for Cancer Research expert report. Food, nutrition, physical activity, and the prevention of cancer: a global perspective. Proc Nutr Soc. 2008;67:253–6.
18. Pollak M. The insulin and insulin-like growth factor receptor family in neoplasia: an update. Nat Rev Cancer. 2012;12:159–69.
19. Aune D, Lau R, Chan DSM, et al. Dairy products and colorectal cancer risk: a systematic review and meta-analysis of cohort studies. Ann Oncol. 2012;23:37–45.
20. Zhang D, Dai C, Zhou L, et al. Meta-analysis of the association between nut consumption and the risks of cancer incidence and cancer-specific mortality. Aging (Albany NY). 2020;12:10772–94.

21. Fadelu T, Zhang S, Niedzwiecki D, et al. Nut consumption and survival in patients with stage III colon cancer: results from CALGB 89803 (Alliance). J Clin Oncol. 2018;36:1112–20.
22. Feldman D, Krishnan AV, Swami S, et al. The role of vitamin D in reducing cancer risk and progression. Nat Rev Cancer. 2014;14:342–57.
23. Botteri E, Iodice S, Bagnardi V, et al. Smoking and colorectal cancer: a meta-analysis. JAMA. 2008;300:2765–78.
24. Lei Z, Xiaomin Y, He H, et al. Nicotine downregulates microRNA-200c to promote metastasis and the epithelial-mesenchymal transition in human colorectal cancer cells. J Cell Physiol. 2019;234:1369–79.
25. Park SY, Wilkens LR, Setiawan VW, et al. Alcohol intake and colorectal cancer risk in the multiethnic cohort study. Am J Epidemiol. 2019;188:67–76.
26. Yang T, Qiao Y, Xiang S, et al. Work stress and the risk of cancer: a meta-analysis of observational studies. Int J Cancer. 2019;144:2390–400.
27. Papantoniou K, Devore EE, Massa J, et al. Rotating night shift work and colorectal cancer risk in the nurses' health studies. Int J Cancer. 2018;143:2709–17.
28. Kwak K, Paek D, Zoh KE. Exposure to asbestos and the risk of colorectal cancer mortality: a systematic review and meta-analysis. Occup Environ Med. 2019;76:861–71.
29. Lichtenstein P, Holm NV, Verkasalo PK, et al. Environmental and heritable factors in the causation of cancer: analyses of cohorts of twins from Sweden, Denmark, and Finland. N Engl J Med. 2000;343:78–85.
30. Jiao S, Peters U, Berndt S, et al. Estimating the heritability of colorectal cancer. Hum Mol Genet. 2014;23:3898–905.
31. Dekker E, Tanis PJ, Vleugels JLA, et al. Colorectal cancer. Lancet. 2019;394:1467–80.
32. Ellis L, Canchola AJ, Spiegel D, et al. Racial and ethnic disparities in cancer survival: the contribution of tumor, sociodemographic, institutional, and neighborhood characteristics. J Clin Oncol. 2018;36:25–33.
33. Nadeem MS, Kumar V, Al-Abbasi FA, et al. Risk of colorectal cancer in inflammatory bowel diseases. Semin Cancer Biol. 2020;64:51–60.
34. Nan H, Hutter CM, Lin Y, et al. Association of aspirin and NSAID use with risk of colorectal cancer according to genetic variants. JAMA. 2015;313:1133–42.
35. Shastry BS. SNPs: impact on gene function and phenotype. Methods Mol Biol. 2009;578:3–22.
36. Zhu M, Zhao S. Candidate gene identification approach: progress and challenges. Int J Biol Sci. 2007;3:420–7.
37. Te Paske I, Ligtenberg MJL, Hoogerbrugge N, et al. Candidate gene discovery in hereditary colorectal cancer and polyposis syndromes-considerations for future studies. Int J Mol Sci. 2020;21:8757.
38. Miao XP, Yang S, Tan W, et al. Association between genetic variations in methylenetetrahydrofolate reductase and risk of colorectal cancer in a Chinese population. Zhonghua Yu Fang Yi Xue Za Zhi. 2005;39:409–11.
39. Yang S, Miao XP, Zhang XM, et al. Genetic polymorphisms of apoptosis-associated genes FAS and FASL and risk of colorectal cancer. Zhonghua Yi Xue Za Zhi. 2005;85:2132–5.
40. Gong J, Shen N, Zhang HM, et al. A genetic variant in microRNA target site of TGF-beta signaling pathway increases the risk of colorectal cancer in a Chinese population. Tumour Biol. 2014;35:4301–6.
41. Manolio TA, Collins FS, Cox NJ, et al. Finding the missing heritability of complex diseases. Nature. 2009;461:747–53.
42. Sud A, Kinnersley B, Houlston RS. Genome-wide association studies of cancer: current insights and future perspectives. Nat Rev Cancer. 2017;17:692–704.
43. Stadler ZK, Gallagher DJ, Thom P, et al. Genome-wide association studies of cancer: principles and potential utility. Oncology (Williston Park). 2010;24:629–37.
44. Huyghe JR, Bien SA, Harrison TA, et al. Discovery of common and rare genetic risk variants for colorectal cancer. Nat Genet. 2019;51:76–87.
45. Ho JW, Choi SC, Lee YF, et al. Replication study of SNP associations for colorectal cancer in Hong Kong Chinese. Br J Cancer. 2011;104:369–75.
46. Xiong F, Wu C, Bi X, et al. Risk of genome-wide association study-identified genetic variants for colorectal cancer in a Chinese population. Cancer Epidemiol Biomarkers Prev. 2010;19:1855–61.
47. Zeng C, Matsuda K, Jia WH, et al. Identification of susceptibility loci and genes for colorectal cancer risk. Gastroenterology. 2016;150:1633–45.
48. Wang M, Gu D, Du M, et al. Common genetic variation in ETV6 is associated with colorectal cancer susceptibility. Nat Commun. 2016;7:11478.
49. Tam V, Patel N, Turcotte M, et al. Benefits and limitations of genome-wide association studies. Nat Rev Genet. 2019;20:467–84.
50. Hirschhorn JN, Lohmueller K, Byrne E, et al. A comprehensive review of genetic association studies. Genet Med. 2002;4:45–61.
51. Edwards SL, Beesley J, French JD, et al. Beyond GWASs: illuminating the dark road from association to function. Am J Hum Genet. 2013;93:779–97.
52. Spain SL, Barrett JC. Strategies for fine-mapping complex traits. Hum Mol Genet. 2015;24:R111–9.
53. Altshuler DM, Gibbs RA, Peltonen L, et al. Integrating common and rare genetic variation in diverse human populations. Nature. 2010;467:52–8.
54. Abecasis GR, Auton A, Brooks LD, et al. An integrated map of genetic variation from 1,092 human genomes. Nature. 2012;491:56–65.
55. Ayers KL, Cordell HJ. SNP selection in genome-wide and candidate gene studies via penalized logistic regression. Genet Epidemiol. 2010;34:879–91.
56. Breheny P, Huang J. Penalized methods for bi-level variable selection. Stat Interface. 2009;2:369–80.

57. Wang Q, Chen R, Cheng F, et al. A Bayesian framework that integrates multi-omics data and gene networks predicts risk genes from schizophrenia GWAS data. Nat Neurosci. 2019;22:691–9.
58. Vandiedonck C. Genetic association of molecular traits: a help to identify causative variants in complex diseases. Clin Genet. 2018;93:520–32.
59. Westra HJ, Peters MJ, Esko T, et al. Systematic identification of trans eQTLs as putative drivers of known disease associations. Nat Genet. 2013;45:1238–43.
60. Zhu Z, Zhang F, Hu H, et al. Integration of summary data from GWAS and eQTL studies predicts complex trait gene targets. Nat Genet. 2016;48:481–7.
61. Nica AC, Montgomery SB, Dimas AS, et al. Candidate causal regulatory effects by integration of expression QTLs with complex trait genetic associations. PLoS Genet. 2010;6:e1000895.
62. Zou D, Lou J, Ke J, et al. Integrative expression quantitative trait locus-based analysis of colorectal cancer identified a functional polymorphism regulating SLC22A5 expression. Eur J Cancer. 2018;93:1–9.
63. Tian J, Lou J, Cai Y, et al. Risk SNP-mediated enhancer-promoter interaction drives colorectal cancer through both FADS2 and AP002754.2. Cancer Res. 2020;80:1804–18.
64. Gong J, Mei S, Liu C, et al. PancanQTL: systematic identification of cis-eQTLs and trans-eQTLs in 33 cancer types. Nucleic Acids Res. 2018;46:D971–d6.
65. Li J, Xue Y, Amin MT, et al. ncRNA-eQTL: a database to systematically evaluate the effects of SNPs on non-coding RNA expression across cancer types. Nucleic Acids Res. 2020;48:D956–D63.
66. Tian J, Wang Z, Mei S, et al. CancerSplicingQTL: a database for genome-wide identification of splicing QTLs in human cancer. Nucleic Acids Res. 2019;47:D909–D16.
67. Yang Y, Zhang Q, Miao YR, et al. SNP2APA: a database for evaluating effects of genetic variants on alternative polyadenylation in human cancers. Nucleic Acids Res. 2020;48:D226–d32.
68. Gong J, Wan H, Mei S, et al. Pancan-meQTL: a database to systematically evaluate the effects of genetic variants on methylation in human cancer. Nucleic Acids Res. 2019;47:D1066–D72.
69. Tian J, Cai Y, Li Y, et al. CancerImmunityQTL: a database to systematically evaluate the impact of genetic variants on immune infiltration in human cancer. Nucleic Acids Res. 2021;49:D1065–d73.
70. Pai AA, Cain CE, Mizrahi-Man O, et al. The contribution of RNA decay quantitative trait loci to inter-individual variation in steady-state gene expression levels. PLoS Genet. 2012;8:e1003000.
71. Mancuso N, Shi H, Goddard P, et al. Integrating gene expression with summary association statistics to identify genes associated with 30 complex traits. Am J Hum Genet. 2017;100:473–87.
72. Gusev A, Mancuso N, Won H, et al. Transcriptome-wide association study of schizophrenia and chromatin activity yields mechanistic disease insights. Nat Genet. 2018;50:538–48.
73. Wainberg M, Sinnott-Armstrong N, Mancuso N, et al. Opportunities and challenges for transcriptome-wide association studies. Nat Genet. 2019;51:592–9.
74. Guo X, Lin W, Wen W, et al. Identifying novel susceptibility genes for colorectal cancer risk from a transcriptome-wide association study of 125,478 subjects. Gastroenterology. 2020.
75. Maurano MT, Humbert R, Rynes E, et al. Systematic localization of common disease-associated variation in regulatory DNA. Science. 2012;337:1190–5.
76. Broderick P, Carvajal-Carmona L, Pittman AM, et al. A genome-wide association study shows that common alleles of SMAD7 influence colorectal cancer risk. Nat Genet. 2007;39:1315–7.
77. Jia WH, Zhang B, Matsuo K, et al. Genome-wide association analyses in East Asians identify new susceptibility loci for colorectal cancer. Nat Genet. 2013;45:191–6.
78. Lu Y. et al. Large-scale genome-wide association study of east asians identifies loci associated with risk for colorectal cancer. Gastroenterology. 2019;156:1455–66. https://doi.org/10.1053/j.gastro.2018.11.066.
79. Tehranchi A, Hie B, Dacre M, et al. Fine-mapping cis-regulatory variants in diverse human populations. Elife. 2019;8:e39595.
80. Gao L, Uzun Y, Gao P, et al. Identifying noncoding risk variants using disease-relevant gene regulatory networks. Nat Commun. 2018;9:702.
81. Schaid DJ, Chen W, Larson NB. From genome-wide associations to candidate causal variants by statistical fine-mapping. Nat Rev Genet. 2018;19:491–504.
82. Huang D, Yi X, Zhang S, et al. GWAS4D: multidimensional analysis of context-specific regulatory variant for human complex diseases and traits. Nucleic Acids Res. 2018;46:W114–W20.
83. Boyle AP, Hong EL, Hariharan M, et al. Annotation of functional variation in personal genomes using RegulomeDB. Genome Res. 2012;22:1790–7.
84. Hu H, Miao YR, Jia LH, et al. AnimalTFDB 3.0: a comprehensive resource for annotation and prediction of animal transcription factors. Nucleic Acids Res. 2019;47:D33–D8.
85. Mathelier A, Zhao X, Zhang AW, et al. JASPAR 2014: an extensively expanded and updated open-access database of transcription factor binding profiles. Nucleic Acids Res. 2014;42:D142–7.
86. Kel AE, Gossling E, Reuter I, et al. MATCH: a tool for searching transcription factor binding sites in DNA sequences. Nucleic Acids Res. 2003;31:3576–9.
87. Lou J, Gong J, Ke J, et al. A functional polymorphism located at transcription factor binding sites, rs6695837 near LAMC1 gene, confers risk of colorectal cancer in Chinese populations. Carcinogenesis. 2017;38:177–83.
88. Hnisz D, Abraham BJ, Lee TI, et al. Super-enhancers in the control of cell identity and disease. Cell. 2013;155:934–47.

89. Ke J, Tian J, Mei S, et al. Genetic predisposition to colon and rectal adenocarcinoma is mediated by a super-enhancer polymorphism coactivating CD9 and PLEKHG6. Cancer Epidemiol Biomarkers Prev. 2020;29:850–9.
90. Rinn JL, Chang HY. Genome regulation by long noncoding RNAs. Annu Rev Biochem. 2012;81:145–66.
91. Geisler S, Coller J. RNA in unexpected places: long non-coding RNA functions in diverse cellular contexts. Nat Rev Mol Cell Biol. 2013;14:699–712.
92. Sun QL, Zhao CP, Wang TY, et al. Expression profile analysis of long non-coding RNA associated with vincristine resistance in colon cancer cells by next-generation sequencing. Gene. 2015;572:79–86.
93. Yang X, Song JH, Cheng Y, et al. Long non-coding RNA HNF1A-AS1 regulates proliferation and migration in oesophageal adenocarcinoma cells. Gut. 2014;63:881–90.
94. Gong J, Tian J, Lou J, et al. A functional polymorphism in lnc-LAMC2–1:1 confers risk of colorectal cancer by affecting miRNA binding. Carcinogenesis. 2016;37:443–51.
95. Gong J, Liu W, Zhang J, et al. lncRNASNP: a database of SNPs in lncRNAs and their potential functions in human and mouse. Nucleic Acids Res. 2015;43:D181–6.
96. Kircher M, Witten DM, Jain P, et al. A general framework for estimating the relative pathogenicity of human genetic variants. Nat Genet. 2014;46:310–5.
97. Ioannidis NM, Rothstein JH, Pejaver V, et al. REVEL: an ensemble method for predicting the pathogenicity of rare missense variants. Am J Hum Genet. 2016;99:877–85.
98. Yang Y, Peng X, Ying P, et al. AWESOME: a database of SNPs that affect protein post-translational modifications. Nucleic Acids Res 2019;47:D874–D80.
99. Cirulli ET, Goldstein DB. Uncovering the roles of rare variants in common disease through whole-genome sequencing. Nat Rev Genet. 2010;11:415–25.
100. Li J, Chang J, Tian J, et al. A rare variant P507L in TPP1 interrupts TPP1-TIN2 interaction, influences telomere length, and confers colorectal cancer risk in Chinese population. Cancer Epidemiol Biomarkers Prev. 2018;27:1029–35.
101. Chang J, Tian J, Yang Y, et al. A rare missense variant in TCF7L2 associates with colorectal cancer risk by interacting with a GWAS-identified regulatory variant in the MYC enhancer. Cancer Res. 2018;78:5164–72.
102. Farashi S, Kryza T, Clements J, et al. Post-GWAS in prostate cancer: from genetic association to biological contribution. Nat Rev Cancer. 2019;19:46–59.
103. Chen M, Wei L, Law CT, et al. RNA N6-methyladenosine methyltransferase-like 3 promotes liver cancer progression through YTHDF2-dependent posttranscriptional silencing of SOCS2. Hepatology. 2018;67:2254–70.
104. Meyer KD, Saletore Y, Zumbo P, et al. Comprehensive analysis of mRNA methylation reveals enrichment in 3' UTRs and near stop codons. Cell. 2012;149:1635–46.
105. Wang X, Zhao BS, Roundtree IA, et al. N(6)-methyladenosine modulates messenger RNA translation efficiency. Cell. 2015;161:1388–99.
106. Zhang S, Zhao BS, Zhou A, et al. m(6)A demethylase ALKBH5 maintains tumorigenicity of glioblastoma stem-like cells by sustaining FOXM1 expression and cell proliferation program. Cancer Cell. 2017;31(591–606):e6.
107. Tian J, Ying P, Ke J, et al. ANKLE1 N(6)-methyladenosine-related variant is associated with colorectal cancer risk by maintaining the genomic stability. Int J Cancer. 2020;146:3281–93.
108. Mercer TR, Edwards SL, Clark MB, et al. DNase I-hypersensitive exons colocalize with promoters and distal regulatory elements. Nat Genet. 2013;45:852–9.
109. Jia L, Landan G, Pomerantz M, et al. Functional enhancers at the gene-poor 8q24 cancer-linked locus. PLoS Genet. 2009;5:e1000597.
110. Visel A, Blow MJ, Li Z, et al. ChIP-seq accurately predicts tissue-specific activity of enhancers. Nature. 2009;457:854–8.
111. Freedman ML, Monteiro AN, Gayther SA, et al. Principles for the post-GWAS functional characterization of cancer risk loci. Nat Genet. 2011;43:513–8.
112. Corradin O, Scacheri PC. Enhancer variants: evaluating functions in common disease. Genome Med. 2014;6:85.
113. Kempfer R, Pombo A. Methods for mapping 3D chromosome architecture. Nat Rev Genet. 2020;21:207–26.
114. Bonjoch L, Franch-Exposito S, Garre P, et al. Germline mutations in FAF1 are associated with hereditary colorectal cancer. Gastroenterology. 2020;159(227–40):e7.
115. Mogno I, Kwasnieski JC, Cohen BA. Massively parallel synthetic promoter assays reveal the in vivo effects of binding site variants. Genome Res. 2013;23:1908–15.
116. Arnold CD, Gerlach D, Stelzer C, et al. Genome-wide quantitative enhancer activity maps identified by STARR-seq. Science. 2013;339:1074–7.
117. Van Arensbergen J, Pagie L, FitzPatrick VD, et al. High-throughput identification of human SNPs affecting regulatory element activity. Nat Genet. 2019;51:1160–9.
118. McDonald ER 3rd, de Weck A, Schlabach MR, et al. Project DRIVE: a compendium of cancer dependencies and synthetic lethal relationships uncovered by large-scale, deep RNAi screening. Cell. 2017;170(577–92):e10.
119. Fulco CP, Munschauer M, Anyoha R, et al. Systematic mapping of functional enhancer-promoter connections with CRISPR interference. Science. 2016;354:769–73.

120. Tian J, Chang J, Gong J, et al. Systematic functional interrogation of genes in GWAS loci identified ATF1 as a key driver in colorectal cancer modulated by a promoter-enhancer interaction. Am J Hum Genet. 2019;105:29–47.
121. Aschard H, Chen J, Cornelis MC, et al. Inclusion of gene-gene and gene-environment interactions unlikely to dramatically improve risk prediction for complex diseases. Am J Hum Genet. 2012;90:962–72.
122. Corradin O, Saiakhova A, Akhtar-Zaidi B, et al. Combinatorial effects of multiple enhancer variants in linkage disequilibrium dictate levels of gene expression to confer susceptibility to common traits. Genome Res. 2014;24:1–13.
123. Gong J, Tian J, Lou J, et al. A polymorphic MYC response element in KBTBD11 influences colorectal cancer risk, especially in interaction with an MYC-regulated SNP rs6983267. Ann Oncol. 2018;29:632–9.
124. Zhong R, Liu L, Zou L, et al. Genetic variations in the TGFbeta signaling pathway, smoking and risk of colorectal cancer in a Chinese population. Carcinogenesis. 2013;34:936–42.
125. Wang F, Zhu J, Yao P, et al. Cohort profile: the Dongfeng-Tongji cohort study of retired workers. Int J Epidemiol. 2013;42:731–40.
126. Moayyeri A, Hammond CJ, Hart DJ, et al. The UK adult twin registry (TwinsUK resource). Twin Res Hum Genet. 2013;16:144–9.
127. Bycroft C, Freeman C, Petkova D, et al. The UK Biobank resource with deep phenotyping and genomic data. Nature. 2018;562:203–9.
128. Power C, Elliott J. Cohort profile: 1958 British birth cohort (National Child Development Study). Int J Epidemiol. 2006;35:34–41.
129. Volzke H, Alte D, Schmidt CO, et al. Cohort profile: the study of health in Pomerania. Int J Epidemiol. 2011;40:294–307.
130. Colditz GA, Philpott SE, Hankinson SE. The impact of the nurses' health study on population health: prevention, translation, and control. Am J Public Health. 2016;106:1540–5.
131. Sabatti C, Service SK, Hartikainen AL, et al. Genome-wide association analysis of metabolic traits in a birth cohort from a founder population. Nat Genet. 2009;41:35–46.
132. Scholtens S, Smidt N, Swertz MA, et al. Cohort profile: LifeLines, a three-generation cohort study and biobank. Int J Epidemiol. 2015;44:1172–80.
133. Tigchelaar EF, Zhernakova A, Dekens JA, et al. Cohort profile: LifeLines DEEP, a prospective, general population cohort study in the Northern Netherlands: study design and baseline characteristics. BMJ Open. 2015;5:e006772.
134. Prorok PC, Andriole GL, Bresalier RS, et al. Design of the prostate, lung, colorectal and ovarian (PLCO) cancer screening trial. Control Clin Trials. 2000;21:273S–309S.
135. Wray NR, Goddard ME, Visscher PM. Prediction of individual genetic risk to disease from genome-wide association studies. Genome Res. 2007;17:1520–8.
136. Zhang YD, Hurson AN, Zhang H, et al. Assessment of polygenic architecture and risk prediction based on common variants across fourteen cancers. Nat Commun. 2020;11:3353.
137. Li J, Chang J, Zhu Y, et al. Risk prediction of colorectal cancer with common genetic variants and conventional non-genetic factors in a Chinese Han population. Zhonghua Liu Xing Bing Xue Za Zhi. 2015;36:1053–7.
138. Yau TO. Precision treatment in colorectal cancer: now and the future. JGH Open. 2019;3:361–9.
139. Wilkinson NW, Yothers G, Lopa S, et al. Long-term survival results of surgery alone versus surgery plus 5-fluorouracil and leucovorin for stage II and stage III colon cancer: pooled analysis of NSABP C-01 through C-05. A baseline from which to compare modern adjuvant trials. Ann Surg Oncol. 2010;17:959–66.
140. Sheridan C. Milestone approval lifts illumina's NGS from research into clinic. Nat Biotechnol. 2014;32:111–2.
141. Diaz LA Jr, Bardelli A. Liquid biopsies: genotyping circulating tumor DNA. J Clin Oncol. 2014;32:579–86.
142. Misale S, Yaeger R, Hobor S, et al. Emergence of KRAS mutations and acquired resistance to anti-EGFR therapy in colorectal cancer. Nature. 2012;486:532–6.
143. Hingorani AD, Kuan V, Finan C, et al. Improving the odds of drug development success through human genomics: modelling study. Sci Rep. 2019;9:18911.
144. Sham PC, Purcell SM. Statistical power and significance testing in large-scale genetic studies. Nat Rev Genet. 2014;15:335–46.
145. McCarthy MI, Abecasis GR, Cardon LR, et al. Genome-wide association studies for complex traits: consensus, uncertainty and challenges. Nat Rev Genet. 2008;9:356–69.
146. Chubb D, Broderick P, Dobbins SE, et al. Rare disruptive mutations and their contribution to the heritable risk of colorectal cancer. Nat Commun. 2016;7:11883.
147. Livingstone KM, Celis-Morales C, Papandonatos GD, et al. FTO genotype and weight loss: systematic review and meta-analysis of 9563 individual participant data from eight randomised controlled trials. BMJ. 2016;354:i4707.
148. Dienstmann R, Vermeulen L, Guinney J, et al. Consensus molecular subtypes and the evolution of precision medicine in colorectal cancer. Nat Rev Cancer. 2017;17:268.
149. Angelova M, Mlecnik B, Vasaturo A, et al. Evolution of metastases in space and time under immune selection. Cell. 2018;175:751–65.

150. Fearon ER. Molecular genetics of colorectal cancer. Annu Rev Pathol. 2011;6:479–507.
151. Ocvirk S, O'Keefe SJD. Dietary fat, bile acid metabolism and colorectal cancer. Semin Cancer Biol. 2020.
152. Murphy N, Carreras-Torres R, Song M, et al. Circulating levels of insulin-like growth factor 1 and insulin-like growth factor binding protein 3 associate with risk of colorectal cancer based on serologic and Mendelian randomization analyses. Gastroenterology. 2020;158(1300–12):e20.
153. Thrift AP, Gong J, Peters U, et al. Mendelian randomization study of height and risk of colorectal cancer. Int J Epidemiol. 2015;44:662–72.

10 Research Progress in Infectious Agents of Malignant Tumors

Xiaoming Shi and Ni Li

Abstract

Malignant tumors are one of the primary diseases influencing human health and remain a leading cause of death worldwide. Infectious agents are among a few known causes of cancer and contribute to malignancies in different pathogeneses. This chapter focuses on several infectious agents, including human papillomavirus (HPV), hepatitis B (HBV) and C viruses (HCV), *Helicobacter pylori* (*H. pylori*), Epstein-Barr virus (EBV), human herpesvirus 8 (HHV-8), and human immunodeficiency virus (HIV), which play critical roles in developing different cancers. We introduce the biology of the abovementioned agents, describe the epidemic trends worldwide and in China, and summarize the association of the risks of cervical cancer, anal cancer, gastric cancer, liver cancer, nasopharyngeal cancer, Burkitt lymphoma, non-Hodgkin's lymphoma, Kaposi's Sarcoma, and other related tumors. We also depict perspectives of future research on cancer prevention and control. Early diagnosis and treatment of the infectious agents could be beneficial to preventing cancer development and optimizing cancer control strategies. Persistent efforts should be devoted to tailoring optimal cancer screening strategies which are suitable for china's national conditions and contributing to the Healthy China Blueprint. It is also a pressing issue to understand the interaction between infectious agents and cancers. A growing number of cost-effective vaccines against infection-related malignant tumors need to be developed.

Keywords

Infectious agents · Malignant tumors · Biology · Epidemiology · Cancer prevention

10.1 Introduction

Malignant tumors are one of the primary diseases influencing human health and remain the world's second leading cause of death in 2018. In recent decades, the disease burden of malignant tumors has continued to increase. Infectious agents are among the few known causes of cancer and contribute to different malignancies. According to the International Agency for Research on Cancer (IARC), 15–20% of new cancer cases worldwide were associated with infections. The

X. Shi (✉)
China CDC Key Laboratory of Environment and Population Health, National Institute of Environmental Health, Chinese Center for Disease Control and Prevention, Beijing, China
e-mail: shixm@chinacdc.cn

N. Li
National Cancer Center/National Clinical Research Center for Cancer/Cancer Hospital, Chinese Academy of Medical Sciences and Peking Union Medical College, Beijing, China

D.-Q. Ye (ed.), *Progress in China Epidemiology*, https://doi.org/10.1007/978-981-19-2199-5_10

percentage of infection-related cases in developing countries (23%) was much higher than in developed countries (7%), partially because certain infectious agents were more prevalent in developing areas.

Infections may increase the risk of cancer development in various pathogeneses. A few viruses can insert their genes into the cell, disrupt biochemical signaling, and cause out-of-control cell growth and proliferation. Some infections may weaken a person's innate immune system and make their body more vulnerable to cancer. Some viral and bacterial infections are related to chronic inflammation and eventually lead to cancers. Infectious agents, including human papillomavirus (HPV), hepatitis B (HBV) and C viruses (HCV), *Helicobacter pylori* (*H. pylori*), Epstein-Barr virus (EBV), human herpesvirus 8 (HHV-8), and human immunodeficiency virus (HIV), play essential roles in developing different cancers.

Some high-risk strains of HPVs, including HPV 16, 18, and a few others, have been tied to the leading causes of cervical cancer. In 2020, an estimated 604,127 women were diagnosed with cervical cancer worldwide, and over 340,000 women died from this disease. In China, cervical cancer was the sixth most common cancer and ranked as the eighth leading cause of cancer death in women in 2015. The number of new cases in China accounted for 18% of all new cervical cancer cases globally among females in 2020. The incidence and mortality of cervical cancer in China have increased over the past 20 years. Close attention should be paid to the morbidity and mortality of cervical cancer among younger females.

Liver and gastric cancers are common malignant tumors of the digestive system and are responsible for an estimated 2 million new cases in 2020 globally, especially in developing and underdeveloped areas. Liver and gastric cancers both remained in China's top five cancer incidences and mortality in 2015. *H. pylori* was identified as a Group 1 (definite) carcinogen in 1994 because long-term infection with *H. pylori* may lead to gastric carcinoma over time. *H. pylori* colonizes about 50% of the world's population. The infection rates are much higher in developing nations and older age groups. Hepatocellular carcinoma (HCC) is the most common type of liver cancer, in which most cases are related to cirrhosis associated with chronic HBV/HCV infections. HBV and HCV have been classified as Group 1 carcinogens with sufficient evidence for causing HCC in humans by the IARC in 2011.

Nasopharyngeal carcinoma (NPC) originates in the nasopharynx, rare in most other areas worldwide. Its occurrence in Southeast Asia is considerably high. This tumor is prevalent and the sixth most common cancer among males in South Asia. NPC was once endemic in Southern China in the early twentieth century, including Guangdong and Hong Kong. However, the incidence has been decreasing after that. According to the World Health Organization (WHO), cases in China account for 80% of all NPC cases worldwide. NPC poses a severe threat to the health of the population in China. EBV infection is the most studied etiological agent engaged in the pathogenesis of NPC. EBV was classified as a Group 1 carcinogen by the IARC based on its association with epithelial and lymphoid malignancies. The attendance of EBV in several stages of B-cell development and its ability to infect epithelial cells may contribute to carcinoma and lymphoma.

Kaposi's sarcoma develops when infected cells form in the lining of lymph or blood vessels. HHV-8 and HIV are undoubtedly associated with Kaposi's sarcoma. Among the healthy population, HHV-8 infection usually appears asymptomatically because the immune system prevents it from developing lesions. However, HHV-8 may trigger Kaposi's sarcoma when the immune system of the human body is damaged. Kaposi's sarcoma remains a common and widely recognized cancer among people living with HIV.

This chapter introduces infectious agents' characteristics associated with malignant tumors, describes its epidemiology, and reviews the latest research progress to summarize shreds of scientific evidence for the control and prevention of infectious agent-related tumors.

10.2 HPV Infection and Cervical Cancer, Anal Cancer, and Other Cancers

10.2.1 Introduction to the Biology of HPV

HPV belongs to the *Papillomaviridae* family as a spherical double-stranded DNA circular virus without enveloping. It has an obvious host and tissue specificity and human is its only host. The molecular length of HPV DNA is about 7.8–8.0 kb. According to the function, the gene structure can be divided into three functional regions including early region (E), late region (L), and long control region (LCR). The early region contains 8 open reading frames (ORFs) including E1, E2, E3, E4, E5, E6, and E7, which encode E1–E8 early proteins and relate to DNA replication, transcription, translation, regulation, and cellular transformation of viruses. The late region contains two ORFs, called L1 and L2. Given the L1 ORF is relatively conserved, it is used for HPV classification, which encodes major capsid proteins. L2 is variable, reflecting polymorphism of HPV antigen and encoding minor capsid protein. The HPV genome is coated with these two structural proteins. The long control region is a noncoding region, consisting of about 1000 bp, containing multiple binding sites and a series of regulatory factors, which regulate early and late gene transcription and viral replication. Unlike other viruses, HPV has a life cycle that requires basal cells that have the potential to proliferate. Amplification of the HPV gene requires the expression of all the early gene products of the virus. And after the invasion of the upper basal cells, the late genes (L) express. Therefore, most early ORFs express in the whole viral life circle, but only late ORFs that encode capsid proteins and E4 gene express in infected terminally differentiated reproductive tract epithelial cells. The expression of late proteins contributes to the assembly of viral particles in the upper epithelial cells, the shedding of apoptotic keratinocytes (the natural process of the cell cycle), and the release of HPV particles to infect other cells or spread to other individuals.

10.2.2 The Global and China Epidemic Trend of HPV and the Burden of Relevant Cancers

As a common sexually transmitted pathogen, HPV infection is very common. Worldwide, the majority of women have had HPV infection during their lifetime and the rate of infection is closely related to age and sexual behavior. Young and sexually active women have higher rates of HPV infection, which peaks in their mid-20s. And with increasing age, the new cervical HPV infection rate showed a significant downward trend. However, compared with young women, older people are more likely to suffer from persistent HPV infection, which may be related to the decline in the ability of individuals to self-clear HPV caused by the decline of immune function with age. Some studies have revealed that the second peak of HPV infection occurs in the perimenopausal period of women aged 45–50 years, which is partly attributed to physiological factors causing hormonal changes in the body. And most studies confirm that it is the infection caused by the contact between themselves or their spouses with new sexual partners.

The overall infection rate of high-risk HPVs among women in mainland China was 19.0% (95% confidence interval [CI], 17.1–20.9%), and the top 5 HPV subtypes with the highest infection rates included 16, 52, 58, 53, and 18. The total infection rates among cervical intraepithelial neoplasia I (CINI), CINII+, and cervical cancer patients were 59.6% (95% CI, 52.7–66.4%), 84.8% (95% CI, 81.2–88.5%), and 89.9% (95% CI, 86.6–93.1%), respectively. The high-risk HPV infection rates and common subtypes in women of various age groups in various regions were different, and the high-risk HPVs and subtypes among cervical cancer patients in various regions were also different [1, 2].

The most common subtype of infection is HPV16 worldwide, existing in about 70% of cervical cancer samples, followed by HPV18 (about 15%). A meta-analysis of cancer patients in China showed an overall HPV detection rate of 83.87%. The first four subtypes of infection were

HPV16, 18, 58, and 52, accounting for 58.7%, 11.0%, 7.2%, and 3.6% of the total infection, respectively.

So far, more than 200 types of HPV DNA have been clearly identified. HPV is a kind of DNA virus with a strict host range and tissue specificity. According to the difference in tissue affinity, it can be divided into skin type and mucosal type. Most HPVs are skin type, which infect squamous epithelium of skin surface. Others are mucosal type (around 60 types), which infect squamous epithelium of mucosa including the genital tract and oral cavity. Based on the level of tumorigenicity, mucosal HPV could be divided into low-risk type and high-risk type. Low-risk HPV usually causes benign hyperplastic lesions of skin and mucosa, such as genital papilloma, exophytic condyloma lesions, and low-grade cervical intraepithelial neoplasia, but it hardly causes cancer. Low-risk virus subtypes mainly include HPV6, 11, 30, 40, 42, 43, 44, 54, 61, 70, 72, and 81. High-risk HPV can cause not only genital warts but also genital cancer, cervical cancer, and high-grade cervical intraepithelial neoplasm. High-risk virus subtypes contain HPV16, 18, 31, 33, 35, 39, 45, 51, 52, 56, 58, 59, 68, 73, 82, etc.

HPV causes most cervical cancers and is the cause of a substantial fraction of other anogenital and oropharyngeal cancers. Understanding the HPV-attributable cancer burden can enhance HPV vaccination and HPV-based cervical screening programs.

Worldwide, 4.5% of all cancers (630,000 new cancer cases per year) are due to HPV: 8.6% in women and 0.8% in men. AF (attributable fraction) in women varies from lower than 3% in Australia/New Zealand and The United States of America to more than 20% in India and Sub-Saharan Africa. Cervical cancer accounts for 83% of HPV-attributable cancers, two-thirds of which take place in less developed countries. Other HPV-attributable anogenital cancers include 8500 vulvar, 12,000 vaginal, 35,000 anal (half occurring in men), and 13,000 penile. As for head and neck, HPV-attributable cancers reach the number of 38,000 cases, of which 21,000 are oropharyngeal cancers in more developed countries. The relative contribution of HPV16/18 is 73% and the corresponding figure of HPV6/11/31/33/45/52/58 is 17%. Universal access to vaccination is the key to preventing most cases of HPV-attributable cancer. The regnant burden of HPV16/18 and the possibility of cross-protection underline the importance of the introduction of more affordable vaccines in less developed countries [3].

In China, a total of 110,650 new cancer cases and 36,714 cancer deaths attributable to HPV infection were estimated to have occurred in 2015, of which cervical cancer occupied 85.6% and 78.1%, respectively. The age-standardized incidence rate (ASIR) of HPV-attributable cancers was 5.63 per 100,000 person-years and the age-standardized mortality rate (ASMR) was 1.81 per 100,000 person-years. Both the ASIR and ASMR varied by anatomic site, with the highest rates known for cervical cancer at 4.83 and 1.42 per 100,000 person-years, respectively. And the ASMR for anal cancer was 0.13. Between 2005 and 2015, ASIR and ASMR of all cancers attributed to HPV almost tripled. Cervical cancer ASIR and ASMR increased more than threefold.

Between 2005 and 2015, cervical cancer made up the vast majority of HPV-attributable cancers and its incidence and mortality both increased rapidly in China. The comprehensive prevention of cervical cancer is still the most important target in the prevention of HPV-attributable cancers [4].

10.2.3 The Association Between HPV and the Risk of Cervical Cancer, Anal Cancer, and Other Tumors

In 1976, Dr. Zur Hausen first proposed the hypothesis that HPV infection can induce cervical cancer. After Laverty observed the presence of HPV particles in cervical biopsy tissue under electron microscope, scientists from all over the world successively joined in the research on the relationship between HPV and cervical cancer. In 1995, the IARC workshop concluded that HPV infection is the major cause of cervical cancer. Later, epidemiologists and biologists have done a lot of research on the relationship between HPV and cervical cancer. The IARC, respectively in 2007 and 2012, summarized the new study evidence and further confirmed that HPV was a pathogenic factor of cervical cancer, and that high-risk type HPV infection can cause almost all cervical cancer. The odds ratio of correlation strength between high-risk type HPV infection and CIN3 or cervical cancer can be as high as 50, and the OR value is higher, particularly among persistent high-risk type HPV infections. Cohort studies have found that the risk of cervical cancer in the following 10 years is lower in the patients with negative results of high-risk type detected by the second-generation hybrid capture (HC) technology. At present, researchers have reached a consensus on the relationship between HPV and cervical cancer, that is, HPV infection, especially the high-risk type of HPV infection is a requirement for the occurrence of cervical cancer.

The most common high-risk subtypes were HPV16 and 18. Global data showed that the rates of HPV16/18 infection in women with normal cytology, low-grade lesions, and high-grade lesions were 3.9%, 25.5%, and 51.5%, respectively. Among cervical cancer patients, the infection rate of HPV16/18 was the highest (about 70%). Notably, the IARC's summary report on HPV suggests that the current data is likely to underestimate the rate of HPV infection among cervical cancer patients because of limitations in testing methods.

Only infection of HPV that belongs to the α genus has been clearly linked to all or almost all squamous intraepithelial lesions and cancers of the cervix and anus. The HPV genus is also related to a subset of penile, vulvar, and vaginal cancers. Among the 14 most common oncogenic HPV types associated with these three cancers, HPV 16 is the most common and associated one with the highest risk of progression to cancer. Exactly the same α HPV genotypes (or "types") that cause cervical cancer also cause most cases of anal cancer and a considerable proportion of oropharyngeal cancer in men and women, a fair proportion of vulvar and vaginal cancer, and a significant proportion of penile cancer. For example, a meta-analysis of anogenital cancers in Europe, North America, Asia, and South America revealed that HPV 16 type was discovered in 75% of HPV-positive non-cervical anogenital cancers.

An increasing body of evidence manifests a relationship between HPV infection, especially with HPV 16 type, and squamous cell carcinoma of the oral cavity, particularly in people under 50-years of age [5].

10.2.4 Future Perspectives

At present, the most effective measures to prevent cervical cancer include primary prevention and secondary prevention. Cervical cancer screening for women of appropriate age, early diagnosis and treatment of cervical cancer and precancerous lesions, and reducing potential exposure to cervical cancer risk factors, all can effectively reduce the incident rate and mortality rate of cervical cancer. The discovery of HPV and its association with cervical cancer has greatly promoted the primary and secondary prevention of cervical cancer. Not only has it promoted the development of cervical cancer screening technology, making the detection of HPV infection a screening measure for cervical cancer, but also it has promoted the birth of a vaccine to prevent HPV infection, which makes it possible for cervical cancer to be the first malignant tumor prevented by vaccines. At home and abroad plenty of effective evaluation research of cervical cancer screening have confirmed that the mature HPV DNA detection methods as early cervical cancer screening method, has high sensitivity (higher than 90%) and is objective, reliable, repeatable, and convenient. It can greatly reduce the workload of cytology reading and increase screening efficiency.

The prevention and control of cervical cancer in China have achieved distinguished results. Three kinds of preventive HPV vaccines marketed in other areas of the world have also got approval to be marketed in China, and the preventive bivalent HPV vaccine which is independently developed by China is also about to be marketed. Plenty of existing cervical cancer screening technologies are ready to be clinically validated, which will provide evidence for the development of screening programs suitable for regions with disparate economic conditions. At the same time, Chinese experience in cervical cancer prevention and control will provide precious experience and models for other developing countries and enhance international radiation-driven capacity. In addition, WHO has initiated a call for action on the elimination of cervical cancer worldwide. As such, China has made active responses and helped build the health silk road, which can help the world recognize the importance of China's role in the global elimination of cervical cancer.

However, cervical cancer prevention and control in China still has a long way to go. In the future, researches need to be carried out in monitoring cervical cancer and HPV trend, increasing prophylactic HPV vaccination rates, improving screened people coverage, applying and promoting product of artificial intelligence in cervical cancer prevention and control of practice. A system of comprehensive prevention and control system needs to be constructed, which will make scientific advances applied to the practice of prevention and cure of cancer as soon as possible.

10.3 HBV and HCV Infection and Liver Cancer

10.3.1 Introduction to the Biology of HBV and/or HCV

There are three types of particles in the serum of hepatitis B virus (HBV) infected persons: Dane particles with a diameter of 42 nm are composed of an envelope and a core. The core contains circular double-stranded DNA, DNA polymerase, and core antigen, which is the main body of virus replication; small spherical particles; filamentous or nuclear particles with a diameter of 22 nm. Small spherical particles and filamentous and nuclear particles are composed of hepatitis B surface antigen (HBsAg), are hollow pericardium, contain no nucleic acid, and are not infectious [6, 7]. In general, HBV-infected patients have the smallest spherical particles in the serum, and Dane particles the least. The double-stranded circular DNA in the core of the Dane particle is the HBV genome. It is composed of a positive strand and a negative strand. The positive strand is shorter, and the total length is 50–75% of the negative strand. The positive strand is a semi-closed circular DNA. It has no transcription and translation functions. The negative strand is a long chain, which is a closed circular DNA, which combines with the positive strand in a base-pairing manner to form double-stranded DNA, which has the function of transcribing and translating proteins [8]. There are 4 open reading frame regions in the HBV genome, namely the S, C, P, and X gene regions. The S region is involved in encoding the outer capsid protein of HBV, which are namely HBsAg, preS1 antigen, and preS2 antigen; C region encodes hepatitis B core antigen (HBcAg) and hepatitis B e antigen (HBeAg); P region is the longest and encodes DNA polymerase; X region encodes hepatitis B x Antigen (HBxAg). Epidemiological investigations and clinics often use the detection of serum HBsAg and anti-HBs, HBeAg, anti-HBe, and anti-HBc as a means of confirming HBV infection [9]. If any of HBsAg, HBeAg, anti-HBe, and anti-HBc is positive, it is HBV infection. HBV is very resistant to the outside world, and has strong resistance to heat, low temperature, dryness, ultraviolet rays, and general concentrations of disinfectants. It can survive for 7 days at 37 °C, at least 6 months at 30 ~ 32 °C, and 15 years at −20 °C. High-pressure steam sterilization at 121 °C for 20 min, boiling at 100 °C for 2 min, and 65 °C for 10 h. 0.2% benzalkonium bromide, 0.5% peracetic acid, 3% bleaching powder, 5% sodium hypochlorite, and ethylene oxide can inactivate HBV [8].

Hepatitis C virus (HCV) is a spherical particle with a diameter of 40–60 nm. It is composed of an envelope, a nucleocapsid, and a virus core. The virus core contains viral nucleic acid. The HCV genome is a single-stranded positive-stranded RNA with a total length of about 9.6 KB. The two sides of the genome are noncoding regions with a single open reading frame in the middle. The coding region includes structural region and nonstructural region: the structure is divided into core region and envelope region, which respectively encode structural proteins such as the core protein and envelope protein of the virus; the nonstructural region encodes 7 nonstructural proteins that replicate in the HCV genome play an important role in the process [10]. HCV has strong resistance to the external environment and heat resistance. It can inactivate the virus for 5 minutes at 100 °C and 10 hours at 60 °C. HCV is sensitive to general chemical disinfectants. 10%–20% chloroform and 1:1000 formaldehyde can kill HCV [9, 11, 12].

10.3.2 The Global and China Epidemic Trend of HBV and/or HCV and the Burden of Liver Cancer

Due to differences in economic and health levels in different regions, the intensity of HBV infection varies greatly. According to the severity of the epidemic, it can be divided into three types of epidemic areas: high, medium, and low. The HBsAg carrier rate in highly endemic areas is 8–20%. Adults and children have more chances of infection. HBV infection is widespread from the start of newborns, represented by tropical Africa, Southeast Asia, and China; HBsAg carrier rate in moderately endemic areas 2–7%, mainly adult infections, but newborns and children also have infections, represented by Eastern Europe, the Mediterranean, Japan, and Russia; the HBsAg carrier rate in low endemic areas is 0.2–0.5%, and childhood infections are rare. The 20 to 29 years age group is the peak incidence, represented by North America, Western Europe, and Australia [13]. Epidemiological data in 2006 showed that the total infection rate of hepatitis B in China was 7.18%, and the infection rate of children under 5 years was about 0.96%. It was higher in rural areas than in cities, higher in the west than in the east, and higher in the South than in the North [14]. Jiang et al. found that the incidence of hepatitis B in China from 2004 to 2012 was highest in Qinghai, Gansu, and Xinjiang, and the lowest in Shanghai, Beijing, Jiangsu, and Tibet, with more men than women. Farmers have the largest occupational composition, followed by workers and students [15]. China included hepatitis B vaccine in its childhood immunization program in 1992. In recent years, the HBsAg-positive rate in the general population has dropped significantly, from 9.75% to 7.18% [14].

The prevalence of HCV infection varies greatly in different regions and countries. In most developed countries, the infection rate is less than 1%, some countries in Africa and most parts of South America are between 2.5% and 9.9%, and some countries in Southeast Asia, Mongolia, and most parts of Africa exceed 10%. HCV infection can occur at all ages, but the infection is concentrated in the age of 15 years and older, and the incidence is high among young adults. In China in 2006, the Chinese Center for Disease Control and Prevention conducted an investigation using the sera retained in the "2006 China Hepatitis B Seroepidemiological Survey." The survey data shows that the anti-HCV-positive rate among people aged 1–60 years is 0.43%. The prevalence of anti-HCV among the population in Central China (0.54%) is slightly higher than that in the Eastern and Western regions (0.27% and 0.40%), and the prevalence of anti-HCV in the Northern population (0.53%) is significantly higher than that in the Southern region. The prominent feature of the HCV epidemic in China is the low prevalence rate in general areas, and the high prevalence rate in some areas, which are scattered and unevenly distributed [16].

The epidemic of HBV and HCV has caused the disease burden of liver cancer. A study on the burden of liver cancer disease in the Chinese population indicated that the total number of liver cancer deaths in the Chinese population in 2013 was about 358,100, and the mortality rate was 258.5 per 100,000. Among them, about 163,600 (45.69%) died of liver cancer secondary to hepatitis B and about 134,200 (37.48%) died of liver cancer secondary to hepatitis C. The disability-adjusted life-year (DALY) caused by liver cancer is 40,804 million person-years. According to the DALY ranking, the first is still the liver cancer secondary to hepatitis B (4.65 million person-years), and the second is the liver cancer secondary to hepatitis C (200,000 person-years). The DALY of liver cancer secondary to liver disease in men is significantly higher than that in women.

Compared with the data in 1990, the standardized mortality rate of liver cancer dropped 25.0%, the absolute value of DALY of liver cancer rose 16.95%, while the age-standardized DALY rate of liver cancer dropped 33.47%; among them, the burden of liver cancer which secondary to hepatitis C has become increasingly worsening. The standardized mortality rate has increased by 106.18% and the standardized DALY rate has increased by 91.68% in the past 23 years. Overall, in recent years, the burden of liver cancer which secondary to hepatitis B has dropped, but the burden of liver cancer which secondary to hepatitis C has risen significantly. The burden of liver cancer in men is significantly higher than that of women, and targeted prevention and control measures are imminent [17, 18].

10.3.3 The Association Between HBV and/or HCV and the Risk of Liver Cancer and Other Tumors

In 1981, Beasley et al. published the world's first prospective research report on the relationship between HBV and liver cancer [19]. Since then, research on the relationship between HBV infection and liver cancer has attracted widespread attention. A 12-year cohort study conducted by China in Haimen, Jiangsu Province in 1992 indicated that HBsAg positive is the most important risk factor for male and female primary liver cancer in this cohort (male: hazard ratio [HR] = 15.97, 95% CI: 14.29–17.85; female: HR = 21.63, 95% CI: 16.16–28.96) [20]. A prospective cohort study conducted in Qidong, Jiangsu Province in 1997 also showed that the risk of liver cancer in HBsAg-positive people was 13.51 times that of negative people [21]. Further research found that when the HBV DNA load is less than 106 cps/ml, the risk of liver cancer increases with the increase of the viral load, suggesting that HBV infection is related to the incidence of liver cancer [22]. In 2008, a nested case-control study in Shanghai showed that the relative risk ratio of male HBsAg-positive liver cancer was 24.00, while the relative risk ratio of female HBsAg-positive liver cancer was 6.30, indicating that HBV infection will significantly increase the risk of liver cancer [23]. In 2016, a South Korean cohort data suggested that the incidence of liver cancer in the population of HBV-positive people over 40 years old after standardized antiviral treatment will drop by 58.8% after 5 years, which also suggests that HBV infection may be related to the incidence of liver cancer [24]. In the same year, a large prospective cohort study in Taiwan found that HBeAg seropositivity and elevated serum ALT, AFP, and HBsAg levels at the time of diagnosis of liver cirrhosis are risk predictors of hepatocellular carcinoma in patients with chronic hepatitis B in liver cirrhosis [25].

Studies have shown that the HCV infection rate in patients with liver cancer is as high as 6–70%, suggesting that the incidence of liver cancer may be related to HCV infection [26]. In the 1970s, a case-control study conducted in Greece showed that the risk of liver cancer in HCV-positive people was 6.3 times that of negative people [27]. Further studies found that in the HBsAg-positive population, the risk of liver cancer in the HCV-positive patients was 20.0 times higher than that in the negative people, suggesting that HCV infection was a risk factor for liver cancer, and there may be a synergistic effect of HBV/HCV dual infection on the occurrence of liver cancer [28]. Beginning in 1995, a 17-year cohort study conducted in Taiwan, China showed that the risk of liver cancer among HCV-positive people is about 25.10 times that of negative people [29]. At the same time, a cohort study conducted in Southern Italy showed that HCV infection increased the risk of liver cancer by 61.0 times, suggesting an association between HCV infection and liver cancer [30]. A large cohort study in Asia found that among patients with cirrhosis, HCV genotype 6 was significantly associated with HCC compared to patients with non-6 genotypes, with the adjusted HR = 2.12 (1.33–3.39), $P < 0.05$ [31]. While another 18-year cohort study found that the cumulative lifetime (30–80 years) risk of liver cancer for patients infected with non-1b and 1b HCV was 19.2 and 29.7%, respectively ($P < 0.001$) [32]. Therefore, we suggest that in patients with HCV subtype 1b and HCV genotype 6, antiviral therapy should be given high priority to reduce the risk of HCC and vigilantly follow HCC surveillance.

Meta-analysis studies showed that the risk of hepatocellular carcinoma (HCC) and intrahepatic cholangiocarcinoma (ICC) in HBV-infected persons is relatively high, HCC: odds ratio [OR] = 14.1(95% CI: 10.6–18.8), ICC: OR = 5.54(95% CI: 3.19–9.63); while the risk of HCC and ICC in infected persons is relatively low, HCC: OR = 4.6 (95% CI: 3.6–5.9), ICC: OR = 3.38 (95% CI: 2.72–4.21) [33–35]. Another meta-analysis in 2016 showed that the risk of developing liver cancer in HBV-positive people was 58 times that of negative people, and the risk of developing liver cancer in HCV-positive people was 2.34 times that of negative people, while the risk of developing liver cancer in patients with HBV and HCV infection increased 11.39 times, further confirming that HBV and/or HCV infection increased the risk of developing liver cancer [36]. The risk ratio of HCC development in subjects coinfected with HBV and HCV was evaluated in a prospective community cohort in Asia. They found that the HRs of HBV and HCV single infection and HBV/HCV coinfection were 17.1 (CI: 8.4–34.8), 10.4 (CI: 4.9–22.1), and 115.0 (CI: 32.5–407.3), respectively. HBV/HCV combined infection also has a proliferative synergistic effect on the risk of HCC (synergistic index: 4.5, CI: 1.3–15.5) [37].

In addition to liver cancer, HBV and HCV also suggest that they are related to the occurrence of other tumors. In 2008, Hassan et al. reported for the first time that there may be a link between the incidence of pancreatic cancer and HBV infection [38]. The study suggests that patients who have developed antibodies after recovery from previous HBV infections and patients with latent HBV infection are at increased risk of developing pancreatic cancer. At the same time, a number of retrospective or prospective cohort studies also discussed this issue. A cohort study from Taiwan, China, found that HbsAg positive increased the risk of pancreatic cancer, and patients with HbeAg positive or HBV-DNA test >300 cps/ml have a further increase in pancreatic cancer risk [39]. In addition to chronic liver disease and liver cancer, the main diseases caused by HCV infection include acute kidney injury (AKI) and chronic kidney disease (CKD). HCV is known to affect kidney health. In patients with HCV-infected CKD and AKI, the clinical outcome is poor. The prevalence of HCV infection is abnormally high in dialysis and kidney transplant patients worldwide. According to various parts of the world, it is estimated that 5–25% or more of patients who rely on dialysis will be affected by chronic HCV. Nearly half of all deaths in CKD patients, including those with HCV infection, are due to cardiovascular disease, and HCV-infected patients have a higher mortality rate [40]. Currently, there are relatively few studies on HCV infection and other tumors. Some studies suggest that HCV infection may be positively associated with gastric cancer and bowel cancer [41, 42]. A meta-analysis suggests that HBV infection is related to some B-cell Non-Hodgkin-Lymphoma types, increasing the risk of intrahepatic cholangiocarcinoma, and is also related to pancreatic cancer [43]. However, further research and exploration are needed.

HBV and/or HCV infection is currently recognized as an important cause of liver cancer. Some studies have found that HBV and/or HCV infection is related to other non-liver cancer tumors. With the continuous deepening of current epidemiological research, people's understanding of HBV and/or HCV is gradually deepening, and antiviral therapy related research will still be an important research field in the future.

10.3.4 Preventive Effect of Hepatitis B Vaccine on Liver Cancer

Hepatitis B is a globally widespread infectious disease caused by hepatitis B virus, and it is the clearest risk factor for liver cancer. The risk of liver cancer in patients with hepatitis B cirrhosis is tens to hundreds of times higher than that of healthy people [44], and about 80% of liver cancer patients are positive for hepatitis B surface antigen [45]. Vaccination of hepatitis B vaccine cannot only prevent hepatitis B virus infection, but also reduce the risk of liver cancer. It is one of the most economical and effective measures to prevent hepatitis B and liver cancer. In 1997, "The New England Journal of Medicine" confirmed that the hepatitis B vaccine was a cancer vaccine that reduced the incidence of liver cancer by 75% [46]. According to statistics, the protection rate of mother-to-child transmission of hepatitis B vaccine is 87.8%, which can protect more than 95% of the population from the threat of hepatitis B virus [47]. In 1992, national health commission of the People's Republic of China included hepatitis B vaccine in the management of childhood immunization; In 2002, general office of the state council of the People's Republic of China approved the inclusion of hepatitis B vaccine in children's planned immunization. In 2005, national health commission of the People's Republic of China made hepatitis B a key infectious disease to control and proposed a strategy to strengthen hepatitis B vaccination for people other than newborns. Therefore, the prevention of liver cancer should be vaccinated in time, and after the hepatitis B vaccine, check whether the hepatitis B surface antibody is produced to determine the effect of the vaccination. If the antibody titer is not enough, the injection should be strengthened. At the same time, cancer screening can be used for early detection, early diagnosis, and early treatment to improve the survival rate of patients and reduce the mortality rate.

10.3.5 Future Perspectives

Studying the relationship between HBV/HCV and liver cancer is of vital importance to tumor prevention and control. Currently, the most effective measures to prevent liver cancer include primary prevention and secondary prevention. HBV/HCV is an important pathogenic factor in causing primary liver cancer. In the process of liver cancer prevention, hepatitis B vaccine immunization should be actively implemented to implement effective primary prevention [48]; strengthen viral hepatitis-related publicity work, so that the masses understand the relevant knowledge and skills of prevention and control, increase their attention to the prevention and control of viral hepatitis, understand the dangers of this type of disease, and carry out scientific health education [49]. We also need to conduct secondary prevention through HBsAg screening of blood donors, and those who are positive are not allowed to participate in blood donation. Take Jiangsu Qidong as an example. Since the 1970s, Qidong has been the first to carry out hepatitis B vaccination in China. According to the data on the prevention and treatment of hepatitis B in the past 40 years, the standardized rate of local liver cancer incidence in China has dropped from 49.95 per 100,000 in 1972 to 25.75 per 100,000 in 2011, a decrease of 44.35% in 40 years. In terms of Qidong liver cancer mortality, the standardization rate of China's population dropped from 45.11 per 100,000 in 1972 to 24.12 per 100,000 in 2011, a decrease of 44.20% from 1972 [50]. The "Guidelines for the Prevention and Treatment of Chronic Hepatitis B" (2019 Edition) [51] and the "Guidelines for the Diagnosis and Treatment of Primary Liver Cancer" (2019 Edition) [52] issued by China in recent years emphasize the importance of antiviral treatment for patients with liver cancer. The "Guidelines for Prevention and Treatment of Hepatitis C" (2019 Edition) [53] also mentioned that antiviral therapy can delay the occurrence of liver cancer. The expert group of the Liver Disease Branch of the Chinese Medical Association gave recommendations to select treatment options for patients with chronic HBV or HCV infection in accordance with the "Guidelines for Prevention and Treatment of Chronic Hepatitis B" (2019 Edition) or "Guidelines for Prevention and Treatment of Hepatitis C" (2019 Edition). This is an important secondary prevention measure to prevent HBV/HCV-related liver cancer. With the continuous deepening of current epidemiological research, people's understanding of HBV/HCV is gradually deepening, and antiviral therapy-related research will still be an important research field in the future.

10.4 *Helicobacter pylori* and Gastric Cancer

10.4.1 Introduction to the Biology of *Helicobacter pylori*

Helicobacter pylori (*H. pylori*), discovered by Australian scholars Marshall and Warren in 1983 [54], is a Gram-negative, microaerophilic, flagellated, and spiral-shaped bacterium. It can colonize the gastric mucosa by flagella and its own production of urea enzyme. The complete sequencing of *H. pylori*'s genome was completed in 1997, containing about 1.6 million bases and 1500 open reading frames. And there is 20–30% variation between different types of *H. pylori*'s genomes, which is generally believed to be due to its high spontaneous mutation rate and recombination frequency. Areas of high variation include the "plasticity zone" and "cytotoxin-associated gene pathogenicity islands" (Cag-PAI), and the multiple structural proteins encoded by Cag-PAI play a key role in *H. pylori* colonization of gastric epithelial cells [55]. *H. pylori* is one of the main causes of gastric cancer, peptic ulcers, and gastritis. Cytotoxin associated gene A (CagA), vacuolating cytotoxin A, blood group antigen-binding adhesin and Gamma-glutamyl transpeptidase, etc. are major virulence factors of *H. pylori*, some of them are the predictors of severe poor prognosis [56]. *H. pylori* is estimated to colonize the human stomach of approximately 50% of the world's human population, and usually does not cause symptoms. Especially, more than 80% of the population may harbor the bacterium in many developing countries. Individuals are primarily infected by *H. pylori* during childhood, and it usually stays with the host's whole life when left untreated. *H. pylori* can spread through fecal–oral, oral–oral, and iatrogenic routes [57, 58].

10.4.2 Trends in the Prevalence of *Helicobacter pylori* Infection in China and Worldwide

H. pylori infection is a well-known main risk factor for gastric cancer, and it remains to be a major public health issue over the world.

A meta-analysis of global prevalence of *H. pylori* infection published in 2017 indicates that more than 50% population worldwide are infected by *H. pylori*, and there is extreme variation in prevalence among different regions [59]. This analysis pools the prevalence estimate data of *H. pylori* infection from 184 articles of 62 countries which were published from January 1970 through January 2016. Based on the 2015 world population and regional prevalence of *H. pylori*, there are about 4.4 billion people estimated to be infected by *H. pylori* globally in 2015. Among 62 countries included in this study, Nigeria has the highest prevalence (87.7%; 95% confidence interval [CI], 83.1%–92.2%), while Switzerland has the lowest pooled prevalence of *H. pylori* infection (18.9%; 95% CI, 13.1%–24.7%). Nevertheless, even in Switzerland, there are still about 1.6 million infected individuals. The prevalence in China is 55.8% (95% CI, 51.8–59.9%) and the estimation of *H. pylori*-positive population is 768,110,552 based on the data of 21 reports with a total of 103,128 participants. This meta-analysis also analyzes the *H. pylori* prevalence of two time periods (1970–1999 and 2000–2016) in different regions to estimate the trend of *H. pylori* prevalence along with time. Compared to 1970–1999, *H. pylori* prevalence during 2000–2016 is lower in Northern America (42.7–26.6%), Europe (48.8–39.8%), and Oceania (26.6–18.7%). However, the prevalence of *H. pylori* infection during the 4 decades is almost unchanged in Asia (53.6%–54.3%) and Latin America and the Caribbean (62.8%–60.2%). In China, it is estimated that the prevalence of *H. pylori* infection in 2000–2016 is 52.2% (95% CI, 48.1–56.4%), which is lower than that in 1970–1999 (60.5%; 95% CI, 53.0–68.0%).

It has been mentioned in the Chinese consensus that the infection rate of *H. pylori* in China is 40–60% [60]. In the light of a meta-analysis of 66 epidemiological investigations published from 1990 to 2002 in China, the average infection rate of *H. pylori* is 58.07% which is similar to the result in 1970–1999 of the above meta-analysis, and there are regional differences and familial aggregation. The average infection rate is 64.4% in rural areas and 48.7% in urban areas, indicating a large difference between urban and rural areas.

In the family of *H. pylori*-positive patients, the infection rate of other members is 62.96%. And remarkably, the average infection rate of children aged 1–10 years is 38.28% [61]. Another survey between 2005 and 2011 involving 51,025 people from 24 regions in China reveals the *H. pylori* infection rate is 49.5%, and the infection rate still reaches 37.1% in people aged below 20 years [62]. And according to a meta-analysis based on the data from 34 articles covering 18 regions of total 149,391 individuals during 2009–2013, the *H. pylori* infection rate is 42.06% [63].

In summary, *H. pylori* infections remain a significant public health burden around the world. And there is a huge differential gap in prevalence between different regions which is generally due to different levels of socioeconomic and hygiene status. In most developing countries, the prevalence of *H. pylori* plateaued at a high level whereas in developed countries the prevalence has been declining. The prevalence of *H. pylori* has declined in China over the 40 years, but it remains high now. It has been mentioned that approximately 89% of all gastric cancers can be attributed to *H. pylori* infection [64]. The global burden of gastric cancer caused by *H. pylori* infection is considerable, which deserves further attention.

10.4.3 The Association Between *Helicobacter pylori* and the Risk of Gastric Cancer

In 1994, International Agency for Research on Cancer defined *H. pylori* as a Group I carcinogen. Numerous studies have shown that *H. pylori* is one of the major risk factors for gastric diseases such as gastric cancer and makes a vast difference in the occurrence and development of peptic ulcer disease and chronic gastritis, etc.

Early in the 1990s, some results of studies about the relation between *H. pylori* infection and gastric carcinoma had been published. A global multicenter epidemiological study finds that gastric cancer incidence cumulative rates (0–74 years) are associated with the prevalence of *H. pylori* infection (regression coefficients = 2.68, P = 0.001) [65]. A prospective cohort study of 5908 Japanese American men indicates that men with a positive test for *H. pylori* antibodies have an elevated risk of gastric cancer (OR = 6.0; 95% CI, 2.1–17.3), and there is excessive risk of gastric cancer with the level of titers rising (P for trend = 0.0009) [66]. In a cohort study in British, the estimated OR for the risk of gastric cancer in participants infected by *H. pylori* is 2.77 (95% CI, 1.04–7.97) [67]. In another nested case-control study in British, the OR for *H. pylori* infection is 3.6 (95% CI, 1.8–7.3) [68]. A study in Norway suggests that cardia cancer is negatively associated with *H. pylori* infection (OR = 0.27, 95% CI, 0.12–0.59) and *H. pylori* infection is related to an augmented risk of non-cardia cancer (OR = 4.75, 95% CI, 2.56–8.81) [69]. In Germany, a large prospective cohort study that includes 9949 participants with an average 13.8-year follow-up shows that infection of *H. pylori* without expression of CagA is associated with an increase in non-cardia gastric cancer incidence (HR = 5.2; 95% CI, 1.00–27.1). And an 18.2-fold (95% CI, 4.3–77.4) increased risk of non-cardia gastric cancer is also observed in infection with expression of CagA [70].

Especially in East Asian countries, gastric cancer is recognized as a substantial public health issue, and more and more attention are paid to its high incidence rates. A number of studies related to gastric cancer and *H. pylori* have been conducted in Japan. A total of 19,028 individuals were followed-up from 1993 to 2009 to assess the impact of the risk factors associated with gastric cancer by using a parametric survival model. According to research findings, one of the most vital risk factors is *H. pylori* infection (HR = 7.58; 95% CI, 4.16–13.79) [71]. In another cohort of 4655 middle-aged (40–59 years old) male healthy asymptomatic subjects with 16-year follow-up, Yoshida et al. found that significant cancer risk elevations are seen in chronic atrophic gastritis (CAG)-negative subjects who are infected by *H. pylori* (HR = 8.9; 95% CI, 2.7–54.7) [72]. Now some researchers have speculated that the population with high-negative anti-*H. pylori* IgG antibody titers (3- < 10 U/mL) have a higher risk of gastric cancer. And a large-scale cohort study including 19,106 Japanese who were followed up from 1993 to 2013 found that the elevated risk of gastric cancer among participants with a high-negative titer is statistically significant (HR = 2.81; 95% CI, 1.62–4.89) when compared with those with a low-negative anti-*H. pylori* IgG titer (≤3 U/mL) [73].

Some systematic reviews and meta-analyses show similar results. A meta-analysis published in 1998 indicates that the pooled OR for the risk of gastric cancer in *H. pylori*-infected patients is 1.92 (95% CI, 1.32–2.78) in all 19 qualified studies worldwide including cohort studies and case-control studies with a total of 2491 patients and 3959 controls [74]. In 1999, another meta-analysis of 8 cohort studies and 34 case-control studies shows that *H. pylori* infection is in relation to a 2.04-fold increased risk of gastric cancer (95% CI, 1.69–2.45). However, as the progression of gastric cancer is relatively long and the patients are older at the time of diagnosis, *H. pylori* infection in the stomach might not be easily detected [75]. A meta-analysis, based on 16 qualified studies with a total of 2284 cases and 2770 controls, indicates that compared to *H. pylori* infection alone, participants infected by CagA-positive strains of *H. pylori* have more risks for gastric cancer. *H. pylori* infection significantly adds to the risk for gastric cancer by 2.28-fold and people with CagA seropositivity have a 2.87-fold increased risk. And CagA-positive strains' infection increases the risk of gastric cancer (pooled OR = 1.64; 95% CI, 1.21–2.24) among *H. pylori*-infected populations, and increases the risk of non-cardia gastric cancer by 2.01-fold (95% CI, 1.21–3.32) overall [76]. A meta-analysis of the relation between *H. pylori* infection and early gastric cancer (EGC) based on the articles published up to June 2006 founds that compared to non-neoplasm controls or advanced gastric cancer (AGC) controls, *H. pylori* infection is significantly correlated with EGC. And the OR for EGC in relation to *H. pylori* infection is 3.38 (95% CI, 2.15–5.33) compared with non-neoplasm controls. The prevalence of *H. pylori* infection in participants with EGC is higher than that in AGC patients (OR = 2.13; 95% CI, 1.75–2.59) [77].

In China, You et al. built the gastric cancer research site at Linqu County, Shandong Province, one of the areas with the highest incidence of gastric cancer in China. Many epidemiological investigations have been conducted to explore risk factors and prevention of gastric cancer since 1983. Based on the baseline data of 1989–1990 and follow-up data in 1994, participants who had been infected by *H. pylori* at baseline are more likely with progression to gastric cancer or dysplasia during the 4.5-year follow-up (OR = 1.8; 95% CI, 1.2–2.6) [78]. During the 10-year follow-up, incidence rate of gastric cancer in *H. pylori*-positive population is higher than in negative population (OR = 1.87; 95% CI, 1.01–3.46), which is similar to the result of 4.5-year follow-up. And the gastric cancer incidence rate in *H. pylori*-positive population of baseline chronic gastritis group is significantly higher than in *H. pylori*-negative [79]. In 1984, the Cancer Institute of China Medical University established the gastric cancer research center in Zhuanghe, Liaoning Province. And the survey of high-risk population in 1998 shows that the positive rate of *H. pylori* infection in residents of the Zhuanghe area is as high as 60.7%, much higher than that in the Shenyang area (12.6%), and *H. pylori* infection is positively correlated with gastric cancer or precancerous lesions, indicating that *H. pylori* infection may be one of the reasons for the high incidence of gastric cancer in Zhuanghe [80]. A retrospective cohort study conducted in Shandong, Zhejiang, and Jiangsu shows a heightened risk of mortality due to gastric cancer in the *H. pylori* infected population compared with H. pylori negative population (rate ratio [RR] = 1.99; 95% CI, 1.00–3.93), and the result of the nested case-control shows that H. pylori infection is strongly related to the increase of gastric cancer risk (OR = 4.47; 95% CI, 1.16–17.19) [81]. And a prospective dynamic cohort study conducted in Shanghai in 1986 found that the average risk of gastric cancer in *H. pylori*-positive patients is 1.8 times of the negative group during 12 years of follow-up, and further analysis found that the OR is 3.7 in those who are followed for more than 5 years [82]. Also started in the 1980s, a cohort study in Lin County founds that the OR of *H. pylori* infection in cardia cancer patients to non-cancer control group is 1.87, and that in non-cardia cancer patients is 2.29, and the pooled OR of the two is 2.04, suggesting that *H. pylori* infection may have different risks for gastric cancer at different sites [83]. According to the finding of study in an area with relatively low risk of gastric cancer suggests that *H. pylori* infection is also a risk factor and makes a difference in the progression of precancerous gastric lesions (OR = 4.2; 95% CI, 1.7–10.0) [84]. In 2019, a multicenter cross-sectional study with subjects aged 40–80 years indicates that there is a higher risk of gastric cancer in people of anti-*H. pylori* IgG antibody positive compared with those of anti-*H. pylori* IgG antibody negative (Adjusted OR = 1.26; 95% CI, 1.12–1.62) [85]. A new prospective study cohort of natural population in areas with high risk of gastric cancer has been conducted in Gansu Province of China from 2013, namely Wuwei Gastric Cancer Cohort (WGCC). The cross-sectional baseline data from March 2013 to April 2016 suggests that the risk of precancerous lesion of gastric cancer in *H. pylori*-infected patients is 1.53 times (95% CI, 1.38–1.70) to uninfected patients [86]. And the result of a nationwide multicenter cross-sectional study published in 2019 shows that *H. pylori* infection is weakly correlated with gastric cancer (Adjusted OR = 1.26; 95% CI, 1.12–1.62) [85].

In 2001, a meta-analysis of 21 papers in China suggests that pooled OR for gastric cancer related to *H. pylori* infection is 3.00 (95% CI, 2.42–3.72) [87]. And another meta-analysis of 66 epidemiological studies in China from 1990 to 2002 covering 52 regions in 21 provinces demonstrates the pooled OR is 1.92 (95% CI, 1.26–4.48) of the association between *H. pylori* infection and gastric cancer. And the case-control studies of *H. pylori* are analyzed especially in the meta-analysis, and the result shows that compared with cardia cancer (OR = 1.41; 95% CI, 1.05–3.34) and diffuse gastric cancer (OR = 1.70; 95% CI, 0.79–3.56), the pooled OR of *H. pylori* infection is especially higher in non-cardiac carcinoma (OR = 3.95; 95% CI, 1.83–8.54) and intestinal gastric carcinoma (OR = 3.38; 95% CI, 2.42–7.23). And it also shows that there is no significant correlation between intermediate and advanced gastric cancer and *H. pylori* infection (OR = 1.12; 95% CI, 0.71–3.13) which indicates the progression of gastric cancer after the occurrence has little relationship with *H. pylori* infection [61]. In 2010, a meta-analysis pooling 34 studies on cardiac cancer and non-cardiac cancer shows that *H. pylori* infection results in a greater risk of non-cardiac gastric cancer than that of cardiac cancer, and the results are similar to the study of Lin County in China and the above meta-analysis.

Many systematic reviews and meta-analyses indicate that eradication therapy for *H. pylori* has been related to a decline in gastric cancer incidence. In a meta-analysis, after adjusting for the baseline incidence of gastric cancer, it seems that patients after eradication of *H. pylori* have a lower risk of gastric cancer than those without eradication treatment (pooled incidence rate ratio [RR] =0.53; 95% CI, 0.44–0.64) [88]. A randomized intervention trial in Linqu County, China which started in 1995 and were followed up through 2017 shows that *H. pylori* treatment has a protective effect on gastric cancer incidence and the protective effect persists 22 years post-intervention (OR = 0.48, 95% CI, 0.32–0.71) [89]. Many studies indicate eradication of *H. pylori* can slow the occurrence and development of gastric cancer in healthy asymptomatic *H. pylori*-infected individuals [90]. These results provide additional evidence for the association between *H. pylori* and gastric cancer.

These studies suggest that the relationship between *H. pylori* and gastric cancer is closer than previously thought. And series of epidemiological studies continue to be carried out worldwide, which may shift toward a greater focus on genetic polymorphism and interaction with other factors. People's understanding of *H. pylori* gradually deepens.

10.4.4 Future Perspectives

Gastric cancer remains one of the most common forms of cancer worldwide, with more than 50% of cases in the world coming from China and other East Asian countries. And the prognosis is very poor, a five-year survival rate of less than 30% after diagnosis [91]. Therefore, the prevention and control of gastric cancer are particularly important [92]. A large number of epidemiological and basic medical studies have proved that *H. pylori* infection is a key pathogenic factor in causing gastric cancer.

Early detection and eradication of *H. pylori* are essential parts of secondary prevention. A variety of tests to diagnose *H. pylori* infection are now available. One is invasive testing, which requires endoscopy to obtain gastric tissue and then conducts microculture, histopathological examination, rapid urease testing, DNA probes, PCR analysis, gene diagnosis, and other experiments. The other is noninvasive testing that does not require endoscopy including stool antigen test, urea breath test, and gastric juice PCR [93]. A recently published meta-analysis in 2020 suggests that in East Asian countries the incidence of gastric cancer declines after *H. pylori* eradication therapy in both healthy populations (Relative Risk [RR] = 0.54; 95% CI, 0.40–0.72) and patients with gastric neoplasia (RR = 0.49; 95% CI, 0.34–0.70), and the therapy also reduces the mortality from gastric cancer in healthy individuals (RR = 0.61; 95% CI, 0.40–0.92) [94]. In China, a study has shown that screening and eradication of *H. pylori* in young adults are estimated to help prevent about 16.7–25.0% of gastric cancer cases [95]; and the result of an evaluation of the epidemiologic efficacy demonstrates that after eradication therapy of *H. pylori*, the relative risk reduction is about 77% on the development of non-cardiac gastric cancer [96]. In 2019, a newly published result of a randomized intervention trial of *H. pylori* treatment in a high-risk region for gastric cancer in Shandong shows the protective effect on gastric cancer incidence lasted 22 years after *H. pylori* treatment intervention (OR = 0.48; 95% CI, 0.32–0.71) [89]. And a long-term cohort study of mass eradication of *H. pylori* in Taiwan suggests that after six rounds of screening and eradication the effectiveness in reducing incidence and mortality of gastric cancer is 53% (95% CI, 30–69%) and 25% (95% CI, 14–51%) compared with the period before 2004 [97]. Now, the Taipei global consensus supports that all individuals infected with *H. pylori* should receive eradication therapy [98].

At present, many researchers have paid attention to the development of *H. pylori* vaccine, which provides the possibility for the primary prevention of *H. pylori* infection. We have to further understand the pathogenesis of gastric cancer induced by *H. pylori*, which might help with vaccine development. Although the prevalence of *H. pylori* infection is comparatively low in developed countries, the absolute number of infected people is still significant. Therefore, *H. pylori* vaccination has still been shown to be cost-effective for preventing gastric cancer in developed countries not only in developing countries [99]. Now, some progress has been made in vaccine development. In China, a phase 3 trial of an oral recombinant vaccine has shown that after vaccination there is a strongly reduced risk of *H. pylori* infection among young people [100].

In the future, we will be committed in developing new strategies of prevention and treatment to identify high-risk groups, and to stratify individuals' risk of gastric cancer and thus to guide targeted screening and precision prevention. In addition, *H. pylori* recurrence remains a problem, especially in developing countries [101], and we also need to focus more on the problem of a growing prevalence of antimicrobial resistance in *H. pylori* for preventing for reversing the good trend of reducing prevalence in the last few decades around the world [102].

10.5 Epstein-Barr Virus and Nasopharyngeal Carcinoma, Burkitt Lymphoma, Non-Hodgkin's Lymphoma

10.5.1 Introduction to the Biology of Epstein-Barr Virus

10.5.1.1 Biological Characteristics of Epstein-Barr Virus

Epstein-Barr virus (EBV), a γ herpesvirus known as human herpesvirus 4 or HHV-4, is discovered from a line of Burkitt Lymphoma cells in 1964. EBV transmission generally begins with contact with respiratory secretions. After pharyngeal infection, the virus spreads throughout the body. B lymphocytes are the primary target. As a DNA virus with about 184 kb pairs, EBV can encode 100 proteins. EVB is composed of an envelope, spikes, core, capsid, and tegument [103]. In terms of appearance and structure, the capsid of EBV particles is icosahedral when immature, with a diameter of about 75 nm, and spherical when mature, with a diameter of about 180 nm. All these structures help make the virus successful in the infection process and avoid detection from the human immune system.

10.5.1.2 EBV Tumorigenic Mechanism

EBV is related to the development of about 1.5% of cancers in the world, however, most people in the world are infected with EBV without any disease. EBV-associated cancers are mainly B cell-derived lymphomas and epithelial cell cancers [104].

People usually contact with EBV in childhood, and infection lasts for life. The life cycle of EBV is usually divided into latent and lytic periods. The virus suspends lytic replication until the infectious agent senses a more favorable environment during the latent period [105], which would be closely related to the occurrence of tumors once activated.

According to which latent genes are being expressed, latency can be divided into 3 different stages. In latency I, there is only EBNA1 expressed, while in latency II, in addition to EBNA1, other intermediate levels of EBNAs and LMP proteins are also expressed together. Latency II can be subdivided into IIa and IIb defined by EBNA2 and LMP1 expression status, in IIa, only EBNA2 but not LMP1 is expressed, and the expression is just the opposite in IIb. In latency III, the complete latent viral proteome is expressed [106]. Several non-coding RNAs and micro-RNAs are also produced during latency. The expression of protein during latency causes DNA damage and inhibits repair, inactivates the starting point of the cell cycle, and causes the instability of cell genes, which in turn causes cancer.

10.5.2 Epidemiological Characteristics of Epstein-Barr Virus in China and Worldwide

EBV, infecting approximately 90% of the worldwide population, is a ubiquitous virus. EBV is transmitted orally and infects the epithelial cells of the oropharynx. Exposure typically occurs early in life, and most children in developing countries are seropositive by 5 years old. Although the onset of infection is delayed in areas with rapid socio-economic development, almost all adults are positive. Symptoms of EBV infection include pharyngitis, fever, fatigue, swollen lymph nodes in the neck, enlarged spleen, liver swelling, and skin rash. Patients with different ages and immune statuses show different symptoms of EBV infection. Prevalence rates of EBV vary between different countries. In England, the prevalence of EBV among children aged 11–24 years is 74.6%. The prevalence is low for 11–14 years of age, and 93% of young people aged 22 to 24 years [107]. There is a study from Tehran, Iran found that EBV IgG antibody seropositivity rate of the study population is 81.4% [108].

In China, a study found the prevalence of Chinese children at the age of 3 years was over 50%, and over 90% at the age of 8 to 9 years in 2014. The EBV infection rate of children in rural areas in China is higher than that in urban children, and the age of onset is also later. Meanwhile, another retrospective cohort study shows that approximately 98% of Chinese patients with EBV infection appear before the age of 30 and the highest rate of acute EBV infection occurs in patients under 5 years old [109].

One study found that between June and August, the EBV infection rates tend to increase, which suggests that EBV infection may be seasonal.

10.5.3 The Association Between Epstein-Barr Virus and Nasopharyngeal Carcinoma, Burkitt Lymphoma, and Non-Hodgkin's Lymphoma

10.5.3.1 The Association Between Epstein-Barr Virus and Nasopharyngeal Carcinoma

Undifferentiated nasopharyngeal carcinoma (NPC) is found to have the closest association with EBV infection. NPC shows a distinctive geographical and ethnic distribution on a global scale. Although NPC rarely occurs in most parts of the world, it is very common in Southern China, where the risk may be 50-fold higher than in non-endemic areas [110]. Cloning is the origin of EBV infection in NPC. Lytic replication is the default procedure for EBV infection of epithelial cells. However, EBV infection in NPC is mainly in the form of latent infection. One of the early stages of NPC pathogenesis has been identified as a latent EBV infection in the nasopharyngeal epithelial cells before infiltration [111].

A large number of studies have shown that there are distinctive anti-EBV antibody profiles for NPC patients and individuals at high-risk of developing into NPC, who have IgA antibodies against specific EBV antigens, such as VCA-IgA, EA-IgA, Zta-IgA, and EBNA1-IgA. Previous cohort studies conducted in NPC endemic areas in South China and Taiwan found that there are several serological biomarkers in high-risk groups that can be used for screening and early diagnosis. Compared with seronegative people, individuals with higher antibody levels may increase the risk of NPC by 20-fold [112, 113]. These cohort studies reported that antibody levels were elevated, and the serological window could be detected before the onset of NPC, indicating that EBV serum reaction may be causally related to the occurrence of NPC. Meanwhile, Jia et al. found that there are significant differences in the EBV load of people in high- and low-incidence areas of NPC [114]. The median amount of virus carried in the oral cavity of healthy people in Guangdong high-incidence areas is several folds that of the Northern population, suggesting that EBV may be associated with the incidence of NPC.

10.5.3.2 The Association Between Epstein-Barr Virus and Burkitt Lymphoma

Based on clinical features and disease epidemiology, Burkitt lymphoma (BL), a highly aggressive non-Hodgkin B-cell tumor, can be divided into three variants, Endemic BL (EBL), Sporadic BL (SBL), and AIDS-related BL. EBL infections mainly occur in young children in equatorial Africa and Papua New Guinea, accounting for about 50% of all pediatric cancers. Jaw tumors is a common manifestation of the high-incidence form of this disease, which is EBV positive in almost every case. SBL, with a much lower incidence, could be found all over the world and affects older children. In the northeastern part of Brazil where the incidence of BL appears to be high, the EBV rate may exceed 80%. AIDS-related BL affects HIV-infected individuals. There is study found compared with sporadic cases, the incidence of BL in HIV-infected patients is more than 100-folds higher, and about 30–40% of tumors are EBV positive [115]. In China, there are relatively few studies on the association between BL and EBV.

10.5.3.3 The Association Between Epstein-Barr Virus and Non-Hodgkin's Lymphoma

The role of EBV in other non-Hodgkin's lymphomas (NHLs) is still unclear, but a mild decrease in immune function may lead to EBV activation and subsequent NHL.

Some researchers combined their own case-control studies with 8 previous case-control studies and nested case-control studies for meta-analysis. Early antigen (EA) and viral capsid antigen (VCA) were selected as indicators, and the results showed both EA (OR = 1.52) and VCA (OR = 1.20) were positively associated with NHL risk [116]. These results indicate that

EBV may be associated with a wider range of NHL subtypes, but further research is needed to confirm and fully understand these associations.

10.5.4 Future Perspectives

10.5.4.1 The Role of EBV Vaccine in the Prevention and Control of Nasopharyngeal Carcinoma, Burkitt's Lymphoma, and Non-Hodgkin's Lymphoma

In China, NPC has become the main cancer type and mortality factor of malignant tumors of otolaryngology. Although the incidence of BL and NHLs in China is not high, it still necessary to prevent and control the diseases for it is harmful. As mentioned above, EBV infection is a key risk factor for the onset of these malignant tumors.

Some researchers have carried out vaccine research and development. Three preventive EBV vaccine candidates have been tested in humans. Two of them are based on gp350, which allows the virus to attach to the CD21 receptor of human B lymphocytes and subsequently infect them. Although it is shown in the Phase 2 trial that monomeric EBV gp350 cannot reduce the incidence of EBV infection, the newer gp350 preparations may be more effective. Vaccines that also contain other viral glycoproteins, cleavage proteins, or incubation period proteins may also increase the effectiveness of the EBV gp350 vaccine [117].

10.5.4.2 The Role of EBV Detection in the Prevention and Control of Nasopharyngeal Carcinoma, Burkitt Lymphoma, and Non-Hodgkin's Lymphoma

EBV detection will play an important role in prevention and control of these diseases. There are many detection methods for EBV, and serological testing is mostly used in the field of screening. Deng Hong, Zeng Yi, et al. used immune-enzymatic method to detect EB virus VCA-IgA and EA-IgA antibodies in 413,164 natural populations in Guangdong, Guangxi, and Hainan, China for NPC, the early diagnosis rate of which was 86.78% [118]. Zeng et al. used the EBV synthetic peptide chain as the capture antigen and saliva as the specimen to diagnose nasopharyngeal carcinoma by ELISA. The positive coincidence rate was 72.6–77.3% [119].

In recent years, some researchers have performed early tumor diagnosis by detecting EBV DNA in plasma, which seems to be much more specific and effective than serological testing. In a normal carrier, EBV can only be detected in blood cells and not in plasma by PCR for residing primarily in B cells. However, when a large number of cell deaths occur in EBV-related cancers, and the contents of some cancer cells leak into the blood, it will be possible to detect EBV DNA in plasma. In some treatment centers, doctors use the detection of EBV DNA in plasma as part of the clinical management of NPC patients receiving radiotherapy. Plasma EBV DNA levels decrease after radiotherapy, once it rises again, it means that the tumor has recurred, and more therapy should be given. It has been found that similar methods can be used to monitor the treatment of EBV-related NK or T cell lymphoma and HL.

A Hong Kong study extended this method to screen and identify early nasopharyngeal cancer in normal people. Researchers used PCR to test the persistent plasma EBV DNA of more than 20,000 asymptomatic people, and followed up through endoscopy and magnetic resonance imaging in positive cases. A total of 34 people were found to have NPC, most of which are in stage I or II and could be cured successfully, which corresponds well to the expected incidence of NPC, and the sensitivity and specificity to NPC are both about 98%. Another study conducted in Zhongshan, China found the crude death rate of NPC in the EB screening group was 0.46-fold that of the control group, confirming that screening can indeed reduce the mortality of NPC patients. However, the cost of this test is high, so more economical ways that can provide this type of screening are being investigated [104].

Regardless of the role of EBV in carcinogenesis, there is an opportunity to use this connection to benefit patients. As the ultimate biomarker, EBV has been proved useful in detecting early disease, providing prognostic information, and monitoring patients after treatment and approaches may be further enhanced by the development of additional adjunctive tests [120]. In addition, as the development of novel therapeutic approaches including but not limited to using virus activation and gene therapy, it will provide more exciting opportunities for meaningful clinical intervention. The development, promotion, and application of economical and effective EBV vaccines will also bring great public health significance.

10.6 Human Herpes Virus Type 8 and Human Immunodeficiency Virus Infection and Kaposi's Sarcoma and Other Related Tumors

10.6.1 Biology of Human Herpes Virus Type 8 and Human Immunodeficiency Virus

Human herpesvirus type 8 (HHV-8) was also called Kaposi's sarcoma-associated herpesvirus (KSHV). It was first detected in Kaposi's sarcoma (KS) tissues in the 1990s and now is generally regarded as the pathogen of KS. It is a large, double-stranded DNA virus, one kind of rhadinoviruses (γ-2 herpesvirus). The HHV-8 capsid possesses a shell composed of 12 pentons, 150 hexons, and 320 triplexes arranged on a $T = 16$ icosahedral lattice. These units are constituted by four viral structural proteins, three of which were encoded by an open reading frame (ORF; ORF25, ORF26, and ORF 62). The HHV-8 genome consists of a unique coding region that is 140.5-kb long and flanked by a GC-rich terminal repeat region, which is 803 bp in length and is 85% G + C. There are around ninety ORFs in the long unique region. In addition, HHV-8 has many unique genes not present in other herpesviruses, namely K1-K15. Six subtypes of HHV-8 have been verified (A, B, C, D, E, and N) according to the differences in ORF K1 [121, 122].

There are two phases in the life cycle of HHV-8, namely latent and lytic replication. HHV-8 exists in latency as an episome and replicates with host cell DNA using host cell replication machinery after primary infection. Latency is essential for viral genome maintenance. The major reservoirs for HHV-8 latency are B lymphocytes and endothelial cells. Latency-associated nuclear antigen-1 (LANA) is the most consistently expressed viral protein. Thus it can be used as a sign of HHV-8 infection. In the lytic state, HHV-8 produces linear DNA molecules that are then encapsidated into infectious virions. Lytic replication plays a critical role in preserving, transmitting, and disseminating the virus and inducing an inflammatory microenvironment [122].

Human immunodeficiency virus (HIV) originated from multiple zoonotic transmissions of simian immunodeficiency virus from nonhuman primates. HIV belongs to the retroviruses, and the virion is about 100 nm in diameter. It comprises an envelope and a capsid enclosed by an associated matrix. The capsid encloses two copies of the single-stranded RNA (ssRNA) genome and several enzymes. The difference in structure from other retroviruses lies in the fact that there is a cone-shaped core including two copies of the ssRNA genome, the enzymes reverse transcriptase, integrase, and protease, the major core protein, and some minor proteins in the innermost region. The HIV genome contains nine genes encoding 15 viral proteins. These are synthesized as polyproteins producing proteins for virion interior [namely group-specific antigen (Gag)], the viral enzymes (polymerase), or the glycoproteins of the virion envelope. High rates of mutation and recombination of reverse transcriptase enzymes and virus replication contribute to HIV genetic variability. Circulating recombinant forms (CRFs) are the recombinants between subtypes. There have been 48 CRFs by now [123].

HIV attacks and destroys the CD4 cells of the immune system, which are white blood cells playing a significant role in protecting the body from infection. HIV multiplies and spreads throughout the body using the machinery of the CD4 cells. This process is called the HIV life cycle, and it is carried out in seven steps, including binding, fusion, reverse transcription, integration, replication, assembly, and budding [124].

10.6.2 Prevalence of Human Herpes Virus Type 8 and Human Immunodeficiency Virus

The prevalence of HHV-8 infection varies in geographical location and ethnic population. The infection rates in America and Northern Europe are relatively low (<10%), but rates in the African region (the Middle East and Sub-Saharan) are higher (>50%). The Mediterranean region (e.g., Italy and Spain) shows a relatively high prevalence of HHV-8 infection (10–30%). A systematic review showed that the pooled seroprevalence of HHV-8 in mainland China was around 11% among the general population. The prevalence was the lowest in Guangdong Province in South China (<6%) and the highest in Xinjiang autonomous region in South-west China (18–24%). The geographic discrepancy in KS incidence corresponds to the varied global seropositivity of HHV-8 infection [123].

According to the global burden of disease (GBD) 2017, global HIV incident cases peaked in 1999 (3.16 million) and then gradually decreased to 1.94 million in 2017. The increasing number of HIV infections and the scale-up of antiretroviral therapy (ART) contributed to the elevated prevalence. In 2017, 36.8 million individuals lived with HIV. Prevalence of HIV was highest in Southern Sub-Saharan Africa (≥10%), with about 1.21 million new cases occurring in 2017, whereas the annualized rate of change in new infections was −5.9% from 2007 to 2017. In China, there were 33.3 thousand new infections, and the prevalence was 0.025–0.50 per 1000 in 2017. A rapid decrease in the annual percentage change in new infections (−7.2%) was also shown. Joint United Nations Programme on HIV/AIDS (UNAIDS) set the goal of ending the epidemic by 2030. GBD 2017 HIV collaborators estimate that no more than ten countries could meet the UNAIDS 2030 incidence targets [125].

10.6.3 Kaposi's Sarcoma and Other Related Tumors

10.6.3.1 Kaposi's Sarcoma

According to the IARC, 22 cohort studies and 80 case-control studies have investigated the correlation between HHV-8 and KS, and consistent evidence demonstrated a correlation between HHV-8 and KS. All studies enrolled only immunosuppressed individuals. The relative risks for this association are generally greater than 10 in most of these studies. Among the 22 cohort studies, 13 were conducted among people with HIV infection and included 561 cases. Nine cohort studies enrolled transplant recipients, and included 48 cases. Evidence from cohort studies on "classical" or "endemic" KS is still lacking. Of the 80 case-control studies, about 50% of the included cases were not infected by HIV. Besides, studies conducted in HIV-uninfected subjects demonstrated elevated KS risk with increasing titers of anti-HHV-8 antibodies. Other studies showed that, among HHV-8-seropositive individuals, the presence of HHV-8 DNA in peripheral blood mononuclear cells (PBMCs) was correlated with an elevated risk of KS and increased risk of disease progression. In summary, given consistent results across all studies, IARC demonstrates a clear correlation between KS and HHV-8 infection [123].

Many cohort and case-control studies have confirmed the strong correlation between HIV-1 infection and KS [123]. The strength of association reported from Africa is remarkably lower than that reported in developed regions. Although the reasons remain unknown, this could reflect the discrepancy in background risk and competing mortality. Efficient ART for HIV-1-infected people usually substantially and rapidly reduces the KS risk. According to a calendar period meta-analysis on 47,936 HIV-1-positive individuals from North America, Europe, and Australia, compared to the era of the pre-highly the KS risk in the early post-HAART era (1997–1999) reduced by 68% (RR = 0.32, 95% CI: 0.26–0.40). Similar declines were also observed in Italy from 1986 to 1998 [126] and in America from 1989 to 2002 [127]. When the follow-up was prolonged to the late post-HAART period (2002), incidence rates for KS leveled off in the last study years.

10.6.3.2 Other Tumors

According to the IARC, there is adequate evidence in humans for the carcinogenicity of HHV-8. HHV-8 is the cause of KS and primary effusion lymphoma (PEL). Besides, a positive correlation is observed between HHV-8 infection and multicentric Castleman disease (MCD). HHV-8 is carcinogenic to humans (Group 1). PEL is a very rare subgroup of B-cell non-Hodgkin lymphomas. Given the rarity, much of the data regarding the association between HHV-8 and PEL are from case reports, along with several studies that inspected biopsy tissues, aspirates or cell lines. PEL was described primarily in HIV-immunosuppressed subjects or individuals with posttransplant immunosuppression. A total of 95 cases were identified as case reports in the published articles from 1996 to 2008. The majority of these were infected both with HHV-8 and HIV. Nineteen cases were HHV-8 negative and HIV negative; these were uncommon because they were elderly, with a genetic abnormality, or had cirrhosis, other idiopathic immunodeficiencies, or a renal transplant. These cases do not meet the diagnostic standard for PEL. Strictly speaking, MCD is not one type of cancer. Instead, it is a rare polyclonal lymphoproliferative disease that can develop into plasmablastic lymphoma. Several hospital-based studies showed a correlation between HHV-8 and MCD, although the detection way of HHV-8 and tissue type varied. For example, one study found the presence of HHV-8 in all 14 HIV-positive cases and 41% of HIV-negative cases (7/17), in comparison with 3% of the controls (1/34). Several studies have investigated the presence of HHV-8 sequences in other tumors, whereas the results are inconclusive. In 1999, an African study measured the seroprevalence of HHV-8 in 16 major cancers. Among people with all other cancers (e.g., esophagus, lung, and prostate), the seroprevalence was similar to the general population (about 20–30%). Nevertheless, a case-control study presented a significant negative correlation between HHV-8 and prostate cancer risk.

Studies have broadly investigated the correlation between HIV-1 and other cancer risks. According to the IARC, there is sufficient evidence in humans for the carcinogenicity of HIV-1-infection. Infection with HIV-1 causes several types of cancer, including cervix, anus, and conjunctiva, and KS, non-Hodgkin lymphoma, and Hodgkin lymphoma. Studies have observed a positive correlation between HIV-1 infection and tumors, including hepatocellular carcinoma (HCC), penis, vulva and vagina, and non-melanoma skin cancer. Infection with HIV-1 is carcinogenic to humans (Group 1). In 2007, a meta-analysis was conducted, including 12 prospective cohort studies on individuals with HIV/AIDS or transplant recipients. This study showed a considerably elevated incidence in both populations for 20 of the 28 types of cancer. Most of these were cancers with a known infectious cause, including all two types of EBV-related cancers (i.e., Hodgkin's lymphoma and Non-Hodgkin lymphoma), all three types of AIDS-defining cancer (i.e., KS, cervix uteri, and Non-Hodgkin lymphoma), all 10 HPV-related or possibly HPV-related cancers (i.e., cervix uteri, vulva and vagina, penis, anus, oral cavity and pharynx, non-melanoma skin, lip, esophagus, larynx, and eye), as well as liver cancer and stomach cancer. Standardized incidence ratios (SIRs) of these correlations ranged from 1.62 to 3640.0. SIRs also increased in other cancers, including kidney, multiple myeloma, and leukemia, ranging from 1.24 to 6.78. SIRs for three different types of cancer (bladder, thyroid, brain, and testis) were inconsistent among people with HIV/AIDS or transplant recipients. Most common epithelial cancers (breast, prostate, Colon and rectum, and ovary) did not occur at increased rates [128].

10.6.4 Future Perspectives

To date, the association of HHV-8 and HIV infection with many types of cancer has been verified by numerous studies, and infections with HHV-8 and HIV-1 are considered carcinogenic to humans (Group 1) according to IARC. HHV-8 causes KS and PEL. A positive correlation is found between HHV-8 infection and MCD. Infection with HIV-1 is the cause of cancer, including cervix, anus, and conjunctiva, KS, non-Hodgkin lymphoma, and Hodgkin lymphoma. In addition, a positive correlation is found between HIV-1 infection and cancer, including vulva and vagina, penis, HCC, and non-melanoma skin cancer. However, the occurrence and development of malignant tumors are still multifactor, multistage, and long-term complex processes. The specific carcinogenic mechanism of these infectious factors warrants further studies. Also, research on infection-related vaccines will be another challenge in reducing the disease burden of cancer. The development and application of cost-effective HHV-8 and HIV-1 vaccines will be significant to public health [129].

10.7 Summary

Presently a body of literature has identified that infectious agents, including HPV, HBV/HCV, *H. pylori*, EBV, and HHV-8, are highly correlated to human malignant tumors. Confirming infectious agents and early treatment could also prevent cancer development and optimize cancer control strategies. Cancer screening contributes to the early diagnosis of cancers. Over the past two decades, cancer screening in China has a wide range of implementation and extensive practice. The central government has financed several large-scale cancer screening programs, including the cancer screening program in Huai River Basin (started in 2007), the cervical and breast cancers screening program in rural areas (2009), and the Cancer Screening Program in Urban China (2012). HBsAg and *H. pylori* detections are also included in the liver and upper gastrointestinal cancers screening services, respectively. The programs mentioned above explore appropriate strategies for cancer screening and early diagnosis in rural and urban China, improve the early detection rate, and reduce cancer-related mortality. Novel screening techniques based on the early detection of infectious agents emerge. Persistent efforts should be devoted to tailoring a comprehensive and cost-effective screening program, which could strengthen early diagnosis and contribute to the Healthy China Blueprint.

Moreover, it is challenging to improve the removal rate and reduce drug resistance of infectious agents associated with malignant tumors. Since the development of malignant tumors occurs in a complex multistep process over a long-term period, the carcinogenesis mechanisms of infectious agents require further in-depth studies. Understanding these agents and their interaction with cancers are pressing issues. Additionally, it is critical to develop vaccines against infection-related malignant tumors. The HBV vaccination has extensively promoted liver cancer prevention and control for decades. China is the third country worldwide to achieve an independent supply of cervical cancer vaccine, with vaccination appointments expected to cover all provinces in China by the end of 2020. A growing number of cost-effective vaccines need to be developed.

References

1. Li K, Li Q, Song L, et al. The distribution and prevalence of human papillomavirus in women in mainland China. Cancer. 2019;125(7):1030–7.
2. Li N, Dai M. Human papillomavirus infection in China: a multi-centric cross-sectional study. Chin J Dis Control Prev. 2008;12(5):411–5.
3. de Martel C, Plummer M, Vignat J, et al. Worldwide burden of cancer attributable to HPV by site, country and HPV type. Int J Cancer. 2017;141(4):664–70.
4. Lu Y, Li P, Luo G, et al. Cancer attributable to human papillomavirus infection in China: burden and trends. Cancer. 2020;126(16):3719–32.
5. Brianti P, De Flammineis E, Mercuri SR. Review of HPV-related diseases and cancers. New Microbiol. 2017;40(2):80–5.
6. Yin J, Chen X, Li N, et al. Compartmentalized evolution of hepatitis B virus contributes differently to the prognosis of hepatocellular carcinoma. Carcinogenesis. 2020;42(3):461–70.

7. D'souza S, Lau KC, Coffin CS, Patel TR. Molecular mechanisms of viral hepatitis induced hepatocellular carcinoma. World J Gastroenterol. 2020;26(38):5759–83.
8. Shen S, Xie Z, Cai D, et al. Biogenesis and molecular characteristics of serum hepatitis B virus RNA. PLoS Pathog. 2020;16(10):e1008945.
9. Zhou X, Nakashima K, Ito M, et al. Prevalence and viral loads of polyomaviruses BKPyV, JCPyV, MCPyV, TSPyV and NJPyV and hepatitis viruses HBV, HCV and HEV in HIV-infected patients in China. Sci Rep. 2020;10(1):17066.
10. Li B, Wang Y, Yang M. Molecular mechanisms of hepatocellular carcinoma induced by the hepatitis C virus. Chin J Biochem Mol Biol. 2020;36(02):135–40.
11. Infectious Disease and Parasitic Disease Branch. The Chinese Liver Disease Association. Prevention and treatment of hepatitis C. Chin J Hepatol. 2004;22(2):131–6.
12. Li LM, Ye DQ, Zhang SY, et al. Epidemiology. Beijing: People's Medical Publishing House; 2007.
13. Wang L, Yin P, Liu Y, et al. Disease burden of liver cancer in the Chinese population during 1990–2013. Chin J Epidemiol. 2016;37(06):758–62.
14. Sha H, Du L, Wen L, et al. Epidemic dynamics and research progress of hepatitis B. J Prev Med Chin PLA. 2017;35(09):1149–53.
15. Jiang H, Chen Z, Fang R, et al. Epidemic analysis of hepatitis B in China during 2004–2012. Chin J Health Lab Technol. 2015;25(03):408–11.
16. Rao H. Epidemiology and natural history of the hepatitis C virus. J Mod Med Health. 2017;33(20):3059–63.
17. Chen Y, Zhao Y. Preliminary study on the infection status of HCV and HBV in cancer patients. Cancer Res Clin. 2002;04:280–1.
18. Li X, Wang J, Li Z, et al. Hepatitis B and hepatitis C virus infections in tumor patients. Chin J Nosocomiol. 2012;22(11):2342–4.
19. Beasley RP, Lin CC, Hwang LY, et al. Hepatocellular carcinoma and hepatitis B virus. A prospective study of 22707 men in Taiwan. Lancet. 1981;2(8256):1129–933.
20. Huang P, Wang N, Qian J, et al. A 22-year-follow-up cohort study on primary liver cancer in Haimen city of Jiangsu Province. Chin J Epidemiol. 2017;38(10):1376–9.
21. Sun Y, Chen T, Lu P, et al. Relationship between serum hepatitis B virus DNA load and hepatocellular carcinoma in Qidong, China: a cohort follow-up study of 14 years. Natl Med J China. 2012;92(027):1874–7.
22. Chen J, Lu J, Ni Z, et al. Follow-up study on the relationship between HBV carrying and malignant tumors. Chin J Prev Control Chronic. 2002;04:161–3.
23. Zou C, Nie J, Dai S, et al. A correlation factor analysis of clinical and virological charlatanistic on HBeAg negative and HBeAg-positive primary hepatic cancer. World Chin J Digestol. 2008;16(032):3696–9.
24. Cho J, Lee SS, Choi YS, et al. Occult hepatitis B virus infection is not associated with disease progression of chronic hepatitis C virus infection. World J Gastroenterol. 2016;22(42):9427–36.
25. Chien J, Liu J, Lee MH, et al. Risk and predictors of hepatocellular carcinoma for chronic hepatitis B patients with newly developed cirrhosis. J Gastroenterol Hepatol. 2016;31(12):1971–7.
26. Koike K, Tsutsumi T. The oncogenic role of hepatitis C virus. Recent Results Cancer Res. 2021;217:91–105.
27. Zeng Y. Oncology. 3rd ed. Beijing: People's Medical Publishing House; 2012.
28. Jiang M, Jiang R. The infection rate of HCV in patients with HBsAg-positive liver disease and its presence in blood. J China Med Univ. 1998;027(004):387–90.
29. Gao J. Summary of ten-year hepatitis C research in Taiwan, China. Chin Med Inf Guide. 2014;24:10.
30. Fusco M, Piselli P, Virdone S, et al. Infection with hepatitis viruses, FIB-4 index and risk of hepatocellular carcinoma in Southern Italy: a population-based cohort study. Infect Agent Cancer. 2016;11:54.
31. Lee MH, Hsiao TI, Subramaniam SR, et al. HCV genotype 6 increased the risk for hepatocellular carcinoma among Asian patients with liver cirrhosis. Am J Gastroenterol. 2017;112(7):1111–9.
32. Lee MH, Yang HI, Lu SN, et al. Hepatitis C virus genotype 1b increases cumulative lifetime risk of hepatocellular carcinoma. Int J Cancer. 2014;135(5):1119–26.
33. Shi J, Zhu L, Liu S, et al. A meta-analysis of case-control studies on the combined effect of hepatitis B and C virus infections in causing hepatocellular carcinoma in China. Br J Cancer. 2005;92(3):607–12.
34. Palmer WC, Patel T. Are common factors involved in the pathogenesis of primary liver cancers? A meta-analysis of risk factors for intrahepatic cholangiocarcinoma. J Hepatol. 2012;57(1):69–76.
35. Li H, Hu B, Zhou ZQ, et al. Hepatitis C virus infection and the risk of intrahepatic cholangiocarcinoma and extrahepatic cholangiocarcinoma: evidence from a systematic review and meta-analysis of 16 case-control studies. World J Surg Oncol. 2015;23(13):161.
36. Li L, Lan X. Association between hepatitis B virus/hepatitis C virus infection and primary hepatocellular carcinoma risk: a meta-analysis based on Chinese population. J Cancer Res Ther. 2016;12(Suppl):C284–7.
37. Oh JK, Shin HR, Lim MK, et al. Multiplicative synergistic risk of hepatocellular carcinoma development among hepatitis B and C co-infected subjects in HBV endemic area: a community-based cohort study. BMC Cancer. 2012;12:452.
38. Hassan MM, Li D, El-Deeb AS, et al. Association between hepatitis B virus and pancreatic cancer. J Clin Oncol. 2008;26(28):4557–62.

39. Sun W, Deng X. Research progress of pancreatic cancer and hepatitis B infection. J Surg Concepts Pract. 2020;25(02):171–3.
40. Saadi G, Kalantar-Zadeh K, Almasio P, et al. Hepatitis C virus infection and global kidney health: the consensus proceedings of the International Federation of Kidney Foundations. Afr J Nephrol. 2020;23(1):159–68.
41. Zhou J, Zhang Y, Lan Q. Analysis of hepatitis virus infection in tumor patients. Chin Foreign Med Res. 2014;12(35):73–5.
42. Zeng Y. Viruses and tumors. Sci Technol Eng. 2002;01:8–22.
43. Fiorino S, Bacchi-Reggiani L, de Biase D, et al. Possible association between hepatitis C virus and malignancies different from hepatocellular carcinoma: a systematic review. World J Gastroenterol. 2015;21(45):12896–953.
44. Shi YW, Yang RX, Fan JG. Chronic hepatitis B infection with concomitant hepatic steatosis: current evidence and opinion. World J Gastroenterol. 2021;27(26):3971–83.
45. de Mattos ÂZ, Debes JD, Boonstra A, et al. Current impact of viral hepatitis on liver cancer development: the challenge remains. World J Gastroenterol. 2021;27(24):3556–67.
46. Lemon SM, Thomas DL. Vaccines to prevent viral hepatitis. N Engl J Med. 1997;336(3):196–204.
47. Liu Y, Lu Y, Li J. Occult hepatitis B virus infection: a new challenge for hepatitis B vaccine to block mother-to-child transmission. Zhonghua Gan Zang Bing Za Zhi. 2016;24(2):157–60.
48. Zhu Q, Xie X. Immunoprevention of viral hepatitis B. Chin J Pract Pediatr. 2013;19:1452–4.
49. Jin J. Analysis on the control and prevention measures of viral hepatitis. China Rural Health. 2015;17:54.
50. Chen J, Zhu J, Zhang Y, et al. Analysis of the mortality trend of liver cancer in Qidong City, Jiangsu Province from 1958 to 2007. Chin J Oncol. 2012;07:532–7.
51. Wang G, Wang F, Zhuang H, et al. Guidelines for the prevention and treatment of chronic hepatitis B (2019 edition). Chin J Viral Dis. 2020;10(01):1–25.
52. Department of Medical Administration, National Health and Health Commission of the People's Republic of China. Standards for diagnosis and treatment of primary liver cancer (2019 edition). Electron J Compr Cancer Treat. 2020;6(02):55–85.
53. Guidelines for the prevention and treatment of hepatitis C (2019 edition). Chin J Viral Dis. 2020;10(01):26–46.
54. Marshall BJ, Warren JR. Unidentified curved bacilli in the stomach of patients with gastritis and peptic ulceration. Lancet. 1984;1(8390):1311–5.
55. Censini S, Lange C, Xiang Z, Crabtree JE, Ghiara P, Borodovsky M, Rappuoli R, Covacci A. cag, a pathogenicity Island of Helicobacter pylori, encodes type I-specific and disease-associated virulence factors. Proc Natl Acad Sci U S A. 1996;93(25):14648–53.
56. Hatakeyama M. Helicobacter pylori CagA and gastric cancer: a paradigm for hit-and-run carcinogenesis. Cell Host Microbe. 2014;15(3):306–16.
57. Peek RM Jr, Blaser MJ. Helicobacter pylori and gastrointestinal tract adenocarcinomas. Nat Rev Cancer. 2002 Jan;2(1):28–37.
58. Leja M, Axon A, Brenner H. Epidemiology of Helicobacter pylori infection. Helicobacter. 2016;21:3–77.
59. Hooi JKY, Lai WY, Ng WK, Suen MMY, Underwood FE, Tanyingoh D, Malfertheiner P, Graham DY, Wong VWS, Wu JCY, Chan FKL, Sung JJY, Kaplan GG, Ng SC. Global prevalence of Helicobacter pylori infection: systematic review and meta-analysis. Gastroenterology. 2017 Aug;153(2):420–9.
60. National Clinical Research Center for Digestive Diseases (Shanghai), National Early Gastrointestinal Cancer Prevention and Treatment Center Alliance (GECA), Helicobacter pylori Committee of Chinese Society of Gastroenterology, Gastric Cancer Committee of Chinese Society of Surgery, Chinese Health Management Association, Digestive Endoscopy committee of Chinese Endoscopist Association of Chinese Medical Doctor Association, Digestive Endoscopy Health Management & Physical Examination Committee of Chinese Endoscopist Association of Chinese Medical Doctor Association, Tumor Endoscopy Committee of China Anti-Cancer Association. Chinese consensus on eradication of Helicobacter pylori and prevention & control of gastric cancer (2019, Shanghai). Chin J Dig. 2019;39(5):310–6.
61. Wang KJ, Wang RT. Meta-analysis on the epidemiology of Helicobacter pylori infection in China. Zhonghua Liu Xing Bing Xue Za Zhi. 2003 Jun;24(6):443–6.
62. Zheng Y, Chen Z, Sai X, et al. Cross-sectional analysis of Helicobacter pylori infection in people undergoing physical examination. Chin J Clin. 2013;7:10044–7.
63. Jiang J, Chen Y, Shi J, Song C, Zhang J, Wang K. Population attributable burden of Helicobacter pylori-related gastric cancer, coronary heart disease, and ischemic stroke in China. Eur J Clin Microbiol Infect Dis. 2017 Feb;36(2):199–212.
64. International Agency for Research on Cancer. Helicobacter pylori eradication as a strategy for preventing gastric cancer. IARC Working Group Rep. 2014;20:5660.
65. The EUROGAST Study Group. An international association between Helicobacter pylori infection and gastric cancer. Lancet. 1993 May 29;341(8857):1359–62.
66. Nomura A, Stemmermann GN, Chyou PH, Kato I, Perez-Perez GI, Blaser MJ. Helicobacter pylori infection and gastric carcinoma among Japanese Americans in Hawaii. N Engl J Med. 1991 Oct;325(16):1132–6.
67. Forman D, Newell DG, Fullerton F, Yarnell JW, Stacey AR, Wald N, Sitas F. Association between

infection with Helicobacter pylori and risk of gastric cancer: evidence from a prospective investigation. BMJ. 1991 Jun 1;302(6788):1302–5.
68. Parsonnet J, Friedman GD, Vandersteen DP, Chang Y, Vogelman JH, Orentreich N, Sibley RK. Helicobacter pylori infection and the risk of gastric carcinoma. N Engl J Med. 1991 Oct 17;325(16):1127–31.
69. Hansen S, Vollset SE, Derakhshan MH, Fyfe V, Melby KK, Aase S, Jellum E, McColl KE. Two distinct aetiologies of cardia cancer; evidence from premorbid serological markers of gastric atrophy and Helicobacter pylori status. Gut. 2007 Jul;56(7):918–25.
70. Holleczek B, Schöttker B, Brenner H. Helicobacter pylori infection, chronic atrophic gastritis and risk of stomach and esophagus cancer: Results from the prospective population-based ESTHER cohort study. Int J Cancer. 2020 May 15;146(10):2773–83.
71. Charvat H, Sasazuki S, Inoue M, Iwasaki M, Sawada N, Shimazu T, Yamaji T, Tsugane S, JPHC Study Group. Prediction of the 10-year probability of gastric cancer occurrence in the Japanese population: the JPHC study cohort II. Int J Cancer. 2016 Jan 15;138(2):320–31.
72. Yoshida T, Kato J, Inoue I, Yoshimura N, Deguchi H, Mukoubayashi C, Oka M, Watanabe M, Enomoto S, Niwa T, Maekita T, Iguchi M, Tamai H, Utsunomiya H, Yamamichi N, Fujishiro M, Iwane M, Takeshita T, Ushijima T, Ichinose M. Cancer development based on chronic active gastritis and resulting gastric atrophy as assessed by serum levels of pepsinogen and Helicobacter pylori antibody titer. Int J Cancer. 2014 Mar 15;134(6):1445–57.
73. Inoue M, Sawada N, Goto A, Shimazu T, Yamaji T, Iwasaki M, Tsugane S, JPHC Study Group. High-negative anti-Helicobacter pylori IgG antibody titers and long-term risk of gastric cancer: results from a large-scale population-based Cohort Study in Japan. Cancer Epidemiol Biomark Prev. 2020 Feb;29(2):420–6.
74. Huang JQ, Sridhar S, Chen Y, Hunt RH. Meta-analysis of the relationship between Helicobacter pylori seropositivity and gastric cancer. Gastroenterology. 1998 Jun;114(6):1169–79.
75. Eslick GD, Lim LL, Byles JE, Xia HH, Talley NJ. Association of Helicobacter pylori infection with gastric carcinoma: a meta-analysis. Am J Gastroenterol. 1999 Sep;94(9):2373–9.
76. Huang JQ, Zheng GF, Sumanac K, Irvine EJ, Hunt RH. Meta-analysis of the relationship between cagA seropositivity and gastric cancer. Gastroenterology. 2003 Dec;125(6):1636–44.
77. Wang C, Yuan Y, Hunt RH. The association between Helicobacter pylori infection and early gastric cancer: a meta-analysis. Am J Gastroenterol. 2007 Aug;102(8):1789–98.
78. You WC, Zhang L, Gail MH, Chang YS, Liu WD, Ma JL, Li JY, Jin ML, Hu YR, Yang CS, Blaser MJ, Correa P, Blot WJ, Fraumeni JF Jr, Xu GW. Gastric dysplasia and gastric cancer: Helicobacter pylori, serum vitamin C, and other risk factors. J Natl Cancer Inst. 2000 Oct 4;92(19):1607–12.
79. Ma JL, Zhang L, Pan KF, Liu WD, Feng GS, You WC. Helicobacter pylori and the progression of gastric cancer: a 10-year cohort study. Zhonghua Yi Xue Za Zhi. 2005 Oct 19;85(39):2758–61.
80. Yuan Y. Comprehensive prevention and treatment for high risk population in high risk area with gastric cancer in Zhuanghe Region, Liaoning Province, China. Cancer. 2005;05:307–11.
81. Wang RT, Wang T, Chen K, Wang JY, Zhang JP, Lin SR, Zhu YM, Zhang WM, Cao YX, Zhu CW, Yu H, Cong YJ, Zheng S, Wu BQ. Helicobacter pylori infection and gastric cancer: evidence from a retrospective cohort study and nested case-control study in China. World J Gastroenterol. 2002 Dec;8(6):1103–7.
82. Yuan JM, Yu MC, Xu WW, Cockburn M, Gao YT, Ross RK. Helicobacter pylori infection and risk of gastric cancer in Shanghai, China: updated results based upon a locally developed and validated assay and further follow-up of the cohort. Cancer Epidemiol Biomark Prev. 1999 Jul;8(7):621–4.
83. Tran GD, Sun XD, Abnet CC, Fan JH, Dawsey SM, Dong ZW, Mark SD, Qiao YL, Taylor PR. Prospective study of risk factors for esophageal and gastric cancers in the Linxian general population trial cohort in China. Int J Cancer. 2005 Jan 20;113(3):456–63.
84. You WC, Zhang L, Gail MH, Ma JL, Chang YS, Blot WJ, Li JY, Zhao CL, Liu WD, Li HQ, Hu YR, Bravo JC, Correa P, Xu GW, Fraumeni JF Jr. Helicobacter pylori infection, garlic intake and precancerous lesions in a Chinese population at low risk of gastric cancer. Int J Epidemiol. 1998 Dec;27(6):941–4.
85. Cai Q, Zhu C, Yuan Y, Feng Q, Feng Y, Hao Y, Li J, Zhang K, Ye G, Ye L, Lv N, Zhang S, Liu C, Li M, Liu Q, Li R, Pan J, Yang X, Zhu X, Li Y, Lao B, Ling A, Chen H, Li X, Xu P, Zhou J, Liu B, Du Z, Du Y, Li Z. Gastrointestinal Early Cancer Prevention & Treatment Alliance of China (GECA). Development and validation of a prediction rule for estimating gastric cancer risk in the Chinese high-risk population: a nationwide multicentre study. Gut. 2019 Sep;68(9):1576–87.
86. Ji R. Gastric cancer screening and related risk factors analysis in the Wuwei natural population cohort. Lanzhou: Lanzhou University; 2018.
87. Xue FB, Xu YY, Wan Y, Pan BR, Ren J, Fan DM. Association of H. pylori infection with gastric carcinoma: a meta analysis. World J Gastroenterol. 2001 Dec;7(6):801–4.
88. Lee YC, Chiang TH, Chou CK, Tu YK, Liao WC, Wu MS, Graham DY. Association between Helicobacter pylori eradication and gastric cancer incidence: a systematic review and meta-analysis. Gastroenterology. 2016 May;150(5):1113–1124.e5.
89. Li WQ, Zhang JY, Ma JL, Li ZX, Zhang L, Zhang Y, Guo Y, Zhou T, Li JY, Shen L, Liu WD, Han ZX,

Blot WJ, Gail MH, Pan KF, You WC. Effects of Helicobacter pylori treatment and vitamin and garlic supplementation on gastric cancer incidence and mortality: follow-up of a randomized intervention trial. BMJ. 2019 Sep;11(366):l5016.
90. Ford AC, Forman D, Hunt RH, Yuan Y, Moayyedi P. Helicobacter pylori eradication therapy to prevent gastric cancer in healthy asymptomatic infected individuals: systematic review and meta-analysis of randomised controlled trials. BMJ. 2014 May;20(348):g3174.
91. Bray F, Ferlay J, Soerjomataram I, Siegel RL, Torre LA, Jemal A. Global cancer statistics 2018: GLOBOCAN estimates of incidence and mortality worldwide for 36 cancers in 185 countries. CA Cancer J Clin. 2018 Nov;68(6):394–424.
92. Malfertheiner P. Helicobacter pylori treatment for gastric cancer prevention. N Engl J Med. 2018 Mar 22;378(12):1154–6.
93. Crowe SE. Helicobacter pylori infection. N Engl J Med. 2019 Mar 21;380(12):1158–65.
94. Ford AC, Yuan Y, Moayyedi P. Helicobacter pylori eradication therapy to prevent gastric cancer: systematic review and meta-analysis. Gut. 2020 Dec;69(12):2113–21.
95. Yeh JM, Kuntz KM, Ezzati M, Goldie SJ. Exploring the cost-effectiveness of Helicobacter pylori screening to prevent gastric cancer in China in anticipation of clinical trial results. Int J Cancer. 2009 Jan 1;124(1):157–66.
96. Duan F, Song C, Zhang J, Wang P, Ye H, Dai L, Zhang J, Wang K. Evaluation of the epidemiologic efficacy of eradicating Helicobacter pylori on development of gastric cancer. Epidemiol Rev. 2019 Jan 31;41(1):97–108.
97. Chiang TH, Chang WJ, Chen SL, Yen AM, Fann JC, Chiu SY, Chen YR, Chuang SL, Shieh CF, Liu CY, Chiu HM, Chiang H, Shun CT, Lin MW, Wu MS, Lin JT, Chan CC, Graham DY, Chen HH, Lee YC. Mass eradication of Helicobacter pylori to reduce gastric cancer incidence and mortality: a long-term cohort study on Matsu Islands. Gut. 2021 Feb;70(2):243–50.
98. Liou JM, Malfertheiner P, Lee YC, Sheu BS, Sugano K, Cheng HC, Yeoh KG, Hsu PI, Goh KL, Mahachai V, Gotoda T, Chang WL, Chen MJ, Chiang TH, Chen CC, Wu CY, Leow AH, Wu JY, Wu DC, Hong TC, Lu H, Yamaoka Y, Megraud F, Chan FKL, Sung JJ, Lin JT, Graham DY, Wu MS, El-Omar EM. Asian Pacific Alliance on Helicobacter and Microbiota (APAHAM). Screening and eradication of Helicobacter pylori for gastric cancer prevention: the Taipei global consensus. Gut. 2020 Dec;69(12):2093–112.
99. Malfertheiner P, Megraud F, O'Morain CA, Gisbert JP, Kuipers EJ, Axon AT, Bazzoli F, Gasbarrini A, Atherton J, Graham DY, Hunt R, Moayyedi P, Rokkas T, Rugge M, Selgrad M, Suerbaum S, Sugano K, El-Omar EM. European Helicobacter and Microbiota Study Group and Consensus panel. Management of Helicobacter pylori infection-the Maastricht V/Florence Consensus Report. Gut. 2017 Jan;66(1):6–30.
100. Zeng M, Mao XH, Li JX, Tong WD, Wang B, Zhang YJ, Guo G, Zhao ZJ, Li L, Wu DL, Lu DS, Tan ZM, Liang HY, Wu C, Li DH, Luo P, Zeng H, Zhang WJ, Zhang JY, Guo BT, Zhu FC, Zou QM. Efficacy, safety, and immunogenicity of an oral recombinant Helicobacter pylori vaccine in children in China: a randomised, double-blind, placebo-controlled, phase 3 trial. Lancet. 2015 Oct 10;386(10002):1457–64.
101. Hu Y, Wan JH, Li XY, Zhu Y, Graham DY, Lu NH. Systematic review with meta-analysis: the global recurrence rate of Helicobacter pylori. Aliment Pharmacol Ther. 2017 Nov;46(9):773–9.
102. Robinson K, Atherton JC. The spectrum of helicobacter-mediated diseases. Annu Rev Pathol. 2020 Nov;16:123–44.
103. Nowalk A, Green M. Epstein-Barr virus. Microbiol Spectr. 2016 Jun;4:3.
104. Farrell PJ. Epstein-Barr virus and cancer. Annu Rev Pathol. 2019 Jan;24(14):29–53.
105. Elgui D, de Oliveira BG, Müller-Coan JS, Pagano. Viral carcinogenesis beyond malignant transformation: EBV in the progression of human cancers. Trends Microbiol. 2016 Aug;24(8):649–64.
106. Cesarman E. Gammaherpesvirus and lymphoproliferative disorders in immunocompromised patients. Cancer Lett. 2011 Jun 28;305(2):163–74.
107. Winter JR, Taylor GS, Thomas OG, Jackson C, Lewis JEA, Stagg HR. Predictors of Epstein-Barr virus serostatus in young people in England. BMC Infect Dis. 2019 Nov 28;19(1):1007.
108. Sharifipour S, Davoodi RK. Seroprevalence of Epstein-Barr virus among children and adults in Tehran, Iran. New Microbes New Infect. 2020 Mar;34:100641.
109. Xiong G, Zhang B, Huang MY, et al. Epstein-Barr virus (EBV) infection in Chinese children: a retrospective study of age-specific prevalence. PLoS One. 2014 Jun 10;9(6):e99857.
110. He YQ, Xue WQ, Xu FH, et al. The relationship between environmental factors and the profile of Epstein-Barr virus antibodies in the lytic and latent infection periods in healthy populations from endemic and non-endemic nasopharyngeal carcinoma areas in China. EBioMedicine. 2018 Apr;30:184–91.
111. Tsao SW, Tsang CM, Lo KW. Epstein-Barr virus infection and nasopharyngeal carcinoma. Philos Trans R Soc Lond Ser B Biol Sci. 2017 Oct 19;372(1732):20160270.
112. He YQ, Liao XY, Xue WQ, et al. association between environmental factors and oral Epstein-Barr Virus DNA loads: a multicenter cross-sectional study in China. J Infect Dis. 2019 Jan 9;219(3):400–9.
113. Cao SM, Liu Z, Jia WH, et al. Fluctuations of Epstein-Barr virus serological antibodies and risk

for nasopharyngeal carcinoma: a prospective screening study with a 20-year follow-up. PLoS One. 2011 Apr 22;6(4):e19100.

114. Jia WH, Zhang JB, Huang SY, et al. Identification of Epstein-Barr virus activation and lytic gene subtypes and the risk of nasopharyngeal carcinoma [C]. Chengdu, Sichuan, China: National Tumor Epidemiology and Tumor Etiology Academic Conference Proceedings; 2015. p. 27.
115. Shannon-Lowe C, Rickinson AB, Bell AI. Epstein-Barr virus-associated lymphomas. Philos Trans R Soc Lond Ser B Biol Sci. 2017 Oct 19;372(1732):20160271.
116. Lauren R, Teras I, Rollison DE, Pawlita M, et al. Epstein-Barr virus and risk of non-Hodgkin lymphoma in the cancer prevention study-II and a meta-analysis of serologic studies. Int J Cancer. 2015 Jan 1;136(1):108–16.
117. Cohen JI. Vaccine development for Epstein-Barr virus. Adv Exp Med Biol. 2018;1045:477–93.
118. Deng H, Zeng Y, Zheng YM, Liang JP, Liao J. Serological survey of 413164 nasopharyngeal carcinoma in natural population. Chin J Cancer. 2003;13(2):109–11.
119. Zeng YX, Li JZ, Jian SW, Li D, Li MZ, Song LB, Zhang L, Wang HM. The detection of EB virus antibody in saliva for early diagnosis of nasopharyngeal carcinoma. Chin J Cancer. 2001;20(3):2235–8.
120. Zeng Y. Epstein-Barr virus and nasopharyngeal carcinoma. Chin J Zoonoses. 1991;2(7):38–9.
121. Li S, Bai L, Dong J, et al. Kaposi's sarcoma-associated herpesvirus: epidemiology and molecular biology. Adv Exp Med Biol. 2017;1018:91–127.
122. Mui UN, Haley CT, Tyring SK. Viral oncology: molecular biology and pathogenesis. J Clin Med. 2017;6(12):111.
123. International Agency for Research on Cancer. Biological agents. Volume 100B: a review of human carcinogens. 2012. https://publications.iarc.fr/119. Accessed 20 Jan 2021.
124. HIV info. & NIH.gov. The HIV life cycle. https://hivinfo.nih.gov/understanding-hiv/fact-sheets/hiv-life-cycle. Accessed 18 Jan 2021.
125. GBD HIV collaborators. Global, regional, and national incidence, prevalence, and mortality of HIV, 1980–2017, and forecasts to 2030, for 195 countries and territories: a systematic analysis for the Global Burden of Diseases, Injuries, and Risk Factors Study 2017. Lancet HIV. 2019;6(12):e831–e59.
126. Franceschi S, Dal Maso L, Pezzotti P, et al. Incidence of AIDS-defining cancers after AIDS diagnosis among people with AIDS in Italy, 1986–1998. J Acquir Immune Defic Syndr. 2003;34(1):84–90.
127. Bedimo R, Chen RY, Accortt NA, et al. Trends in AIDS-defining and non-AIDS-defining malignancies among HIV-infected patients: 1989–2002. Clin Infect Dis. 2004;39(9):1380–4.
128. Grulich AE, Van Leeuwen MT, Falster MO, et al. Incidence of cancers in people with HIV/AIDS compared with immunosuppressed transplant recipients: a meta-analysis. Lancet (London, England). 2007;370(9581):59–67.
129. Liu Y, Li J, Zhu Y, Jia S, Fu G, Xu J, Tang F, Zhu F. Review for progress of vaccination for patients with HIV infection. Chin J Dis Control Prev. 2017;21(12):1187–90.

Check for updates

11 Progress of Lung Cancer Genomic Epidemiology in China

Meng Zhu and Hongbing Shen

Abstract

Lung cancer is one of the most common malignancies in China. Even though smoking was the most important risk factor of lung cancer, only a small fraction of smokers develop lung cancer, which suggested that genetic factors also play an important role in lung carcinogenesis. With the advancement of science and technology, the understanding of the human genome has been greatly improved during the past decades. The rapid improvements of genotyping and second-generation sequencing technology have facilitated the progress of lung cancer genomic epidemiology worldwide. In this paper, we will systematically summarize the latest findings of Chinese lung cancer genomic epidemiology with a particular focus on candidate gene studies, genome-wide association studies (GWAS), post-GWAS studies for germline variants, and genome sequencing studies for somatic mutations. In candidate gene studies and GWAS, dozens of lung cancer susceptibility variants have been identified in Chinese populations using pedigree analysis or large-scale case-control studies. Through integrated analysis and data mining in the post-GWAS era, researchers identified additional variants to fill the gap of missing heritability, revealed the biological mechanisms underlying lung cancer susceptibility loci, and assessed the potential clinical applications of these genetic variants. In the genome sequencing studies of lung cancer, the genomic characteristics of mutational landscapes and mutation burdens were revealed, and a group of key driver genes were identified in Chinese lung cancer patients. These findings deepen our understanding of the genetic basis of lung cancer in the Chinese population and provided a foundation for precision medicine of lung cancer in China.

Keywords

Lung cancer · Genetic susceptibility · GWAS · Genome sequencing · Somatic mutations

M. Zhu · H. Shen (✉)
Department of Epidemiology, School of Public Health, Nanjing Medical University, Nanjing, China
e-mail: hbshen@njmu.edu.cn

Lung cancer is one of the most common malignancies in the world. According to the World Cancer Report, there were 2.09 million incident lung cancer cases and 1.76 million lung cancer deaths worldwide in 2018, accounting for 11.6% and 18.4% of cancer morbidity and mortality [1]. The Cancer Statistics 2020 released by the American Cancer Society estimates that there were approximately 228,800 incident lung cancer cases and 135,700 lung cancer deaths

D.-Q. Ye (ed.), *Progress in China Epidemiology*, https://doi.org/10.1007/978-981-19-2199-5_11

in the United States in 2020, including 116,300 incident cases and 72,500 deaths in men and 112,500 incident cases and 63,200 deaths in women [2]. In China, Chen Wanqing and colleagues reported that there were about 733,000 incident lung cancer cases and 610,000 lung cancer deaths in 2015, among which 509,300 incident cases and 432,000 deaths were males and 224,000 incident cases and 177,800 deaths were females [3].

Epidemiological studies have indicated that the occurrence of lung cancer is the result of both environmental risk factors and genetic risks. Previous studies have shown that environmental factors, such as tobacco exposure, air pollution, radiation, and occupational exposure to asbestos, nickel, chromium, and other substances, are associated with the risk of lung cancer. Tobacco exposure is the most important risk factor of lung cancer, which accounts for 80% of lung cancer in men and at least 50% of lung cancer in women [4]. According to pathological types, lung cancer can be divided into small cell lung cancer (SCLC), adenocarcinoma (AD), squamous cell carcinoma (SqCC), large cell carcinoma, etc. Although all histopathological types of lung cancer are associated with tobacco exposure, lung SqCC is most closely related to tobacco exposure.

With the changes in tobacco products composition and smoking habits, the histological types of lung cancer changed gradually. For example, there was a gradual decrease in the proportion of SqCC, while increase in AD. There is an obvious dose-response relationship between smoking and lung cancer. With the extension of the year of quitting smoking, the risk of lung cancer in people who quit smoking gradually decrease and is equal to that of nonsmokers after more than 15 years [5]. As tobacco is the most important risk factor of lung cancer, the incidence and mortality trends of lung cancer are greatly affected by the change of tobacco exposure levels in population. According to the WHO, there are about 300–350 million smokers in China, and the smoking rate of adult men is as high as 52.9% [6]. Therefore, it is estimated that the incidence and mortality of lung cancer in China will continue to rise in the coming decades, which will seriously affect the life and health of the Chinese population. Air pollution is another important cause of lung cancer in nonsmokers [7]. Previous studies have shown that indoor air pollution and cooking fumes are important causes for the high incidence of lung cancer among women in China. The main components of air pollutants include atmospheric particulate matter (mainly $PM_{2.5}$), nitrogen oxides, CO, etc. A large cohort study in the United States showed that per 10 $\mu g/m^3$ increase of particulate matter in the atmosphere was associated with an increased risk of lung cancer by 19% [6]. In addition to tobacco exposure and air pollution, occupational exposure to asbestos, nickel and chromium are also revealed as important risk factors of lung cancer [8].

Although environmental exposures are important risk factors of lung cancer, only a small fraction of exposers develop lung cancer under similar exposure levels, which suggested that genetic factors are also involved in lung carcinogenesis. Among genetic factors, innate germline variants make the body show different resistance to external environmental exposures and affect the risk of tumorigenesis, which is the genetic basis of tumor susceptibility. The acquired somatic mutations can directly lead to the activation of oncogenes and the inactivation of tumor suppressor genes, which prompt tumor cells to gain selective growth advantages. Therefore, a comprehensive interpretation of the genetic and genomic characteristics will be essential for a comprehensive understanding of lung cancer. In the past 10 years, with the continuous development of science and technology, our understanding of the genome has made huge leap, which has greatly promoted the understanding of cancer etiology [9]. This chapter will introduce the latest research progresses in the genome epidemiology of lung cancer from the aspects of genome-wide association studies (GWAS), post-GWAS, and lung cancer genome sequencing in China.

11.1 Candidate Gene Study of Lung Cancer

The Human Genome Project provided a complete map of the human genome, which revealed the existence of a large number of genetic variations in the human genome. The subsequent HapMap

Project and 1000 Genomes Project based on chip or next-generation sequencing further established linkage information maps of genetic variations in different populations, which laid a foundation for revealing the genetic susceptibility of diseases [10]. After understanding the characteristics of human genetic variations, researchers began to identify genetic susceptibility loci for different diseases or traits with association studies.

In families with multiple lung cancer cases, genetic background may play a stronger role. Therefore, the genetic studies based on such family samples are more effective to identify lung cancer susceptibility genes. In 2004, Bailey-Wilson JE et al. conducted a multi-locus linkage analysis of 52 families with more than 3 lung cancer patients and found that the region of chromosome 6q23-25 may be involved in the susceptibility of lung cancer [11]. Then, You Ming et al. performed a fine mapping analysis of this region and identified three variants (rs6901126, rs4083914, and rs9479510) in the first intron of *RGS17*, which were significantly associated with the risk of lung cancer in the familial lung cancer patients [12]. Elevated expression of *RGS17* was observed in tumor tissues of lung cancer patients, and further functional studies showed that knockdown of *RGS17* significantly reduced the proliferation ability of lung cancer cell lines. These results suggested that *RGS17* in the 6q23-25 is significantly associated with the genetic susceptibility of familial lung cancer.

The accessible sample size is usually limited and hard to expand for familial lung cancer. Besides, the majority of lung cancer patients are sporadic. Therefore, case-control studies based on large sample of sporadic lung cancer patients can increase the power of study and identified more genetic variants with lower effects. With this strategy, researchers have found some new susceptibility genes of lung cancer, such as *GSTM1* and *CHEK2* [13, 14]. *GSTM1* plays an important role in the process of detoxification and metabolism of carcinogens. The protein encoded by *GSTM1* has a high affinity for the activation products of polycyclic aromatic hydrocarbon carcinogens (such as benzopyrene) and can catalyze its binding with glutathione. Studies have found that the deletion polymorphism in *GSTM1* was associated with the risk of lung cancer in the Chinese population. The tumor suppressor gene *CHEK2* plays an important role in the repair of DNA damage. Studies have found that the variants (rs2236141, G > A) in the promoter of the *CHEK2* can increase its expression by reducing methylation, thereby reducing the risk of lung cancer. Hundreds of studies focused on different key genes and pathways have been conducted in the past decades in the Chinese population. Although findings from these studies improved our understanding of lung cancer genetic susceptibility, such findings are often hard to be replicated in the following studies.

11.2 Genome-Wide Association Study of Lung Cancer in China

With the development of high-throughput genotyping technology, GWAS began to be gradually applied to the study of cancer susceptibility. GWAS was not based on prior assumptions but genotyped hundreds of thousands or even millions of variants simultaneously in the whole genome. GWAS usually adopts strict multiple comparison correction standards (i.e., 5×10^{-8}) and combines with a multi-stage design to control false-positive associations. As a result, the findings from GWAS are more reliable and can be verified by different studies. Since 2008, a number of GWAS studies have been reported for lung cancer in European, American, and Asian populations [15].

11.2.1 Genome-Wide Association Study of Lung Cancer in the Chinese Population

In 2011, our group organized the first lung cancer GWAS in the Chinese population. In this study, we genotyped 2383 lung cancer cases and 3160 controls (1473 cases and 1962 controls from Nanjing and Shanghai; and 858 cases and 1115 controls from Beijing and Wuhan) with

Affymetrix Genome-Wide Human SNP Array 6.0 [16]. The chip included 906,703 single-nucleotide polymorphisms (SNPs) in the whole genome. After systematic quality control, a total of 591,370 SNPs in 2331 lung cancer cases and 3077 controls were kept for further association analysis, and we identified 18 SNPs that were significantly associated with the risk of lung cancer at $P < 10^{-6}$. In addition, we further included another three reported lung cancer susceptibility loci (rs4488809 and rs10937405 in the 3q28 and rs2736100 in the 5p15.33) for the replication stage. As a result, a total of 21 SNPs were selected for replication in 2283 cases and 2243 controls, and consistent associations were further replicated in another 4030 cases and 4166 controls. Finally, we identified 4 susceptibility loci of lung cancer in the Chinese population, including rs4488809 in 3q28, rs2736100 and rs465498 in 5p15, rs753955 in 13q22, and rs17728461 and rs36600 in 22q12.

The rs4488809 located at the first intron of *TP63* and its isomer *TAP63* can transcribe and activate p53, which has been involved in the repair of DNA damage, cell growth and differentiation, and the development of tumors. The associations in 5p15 were consistent in Chinese and European or American populations, and these variants were also shown to be statistically interacted with smoking status and smoking amount. The rs753955 in 13q22 is located between the *MIPEP* and *TNFRSF19*. The former is an iron-sulfur cluster-associated protein Frataxin binding protein and involved in iron utilization, and the latter can activate the c-Jun N-terminal kinase pathway and mediate cell death independent of caspase. The rs17728461 in 22q12 is located at the downstream of *LIF*, which was shown to play an important role in the development of lung cancer through Janus kinase activation-transcription factor 3 activator sub-pathway. In addition, this susceptibility region also contains *HORMAD2* and *MTMR3*, the former may be involved in mitosis, chromosome synapses, and DNA repair, and the latter is responsible for encoding myostatin-related protein-3.

In order to further clarify the genetic susceptibility of lung cancer in the Chinese population, we selected the potential susceptibility loci from the previous GWAS ($1.0 \times 10^{-4} < P < 1.0 \times 10^{-6}$) and further replicated with an expanded sample of 7436 lung cancer cases and 7483 controls [17]. The results of the study showed that three novel SNPs in 5q32, 10p14, and 20q13.2 were significantly associated with the risk of lung cancer in the Chinese population at the genome-wide significance level ($P < 5.0 \times 10^{-8}$). The three SNPs were rs2895680 in 5q32, rs1663689 in 10p14, and rs4809957 in 20q13.2. In addition, we also found that rs9439519 at 1p36.32 and rs247008 at 5q31.1 were also associated with the risk of lung cancer in the replication stage but did not reach the level of genome-wide significance after combining with the results of GWAS.

Further stratification analysis showed that rs2895680, rs4809957, rs247008, and rs9439519 were interacted with the cumulative amount of smoking, which synergistically increased the risk of lung cancer. The rs2895680 is located in the second intron of *STK32A*, which is a member of the serine/threonine kinase (STK) family and involved in the stability of the intracellular environment, the phosphorylation of transcription factors, and the regulation of cell cycle. The rs1663689 is located about 908 kb downstream of *GATA3* in 10p14, which was a target gene of c-Myc and played an important role in the development of cancer. The rs4809957 in 20q13.2 is located in the 3′-untranslated region (UTR) of the *CYP24A1*, which is a member of the cytochrome p450 family and related to the metabolism of 1,25 $(OH)_2D_3$. Moreover, previous studies have reported that *CYP24A1* is overexpressed in the tumor tissues of lung cancer and acts as a potential diagnostic marker for NSCLC.

Although GWAS has achieved great success in the identification of lung cancer susceptibility loci, genetic factors associated with lung cancer risk have not been fully identified or validated, especially for the Chinese population. In 2019, we expanded the GWAS sample size and further genotyped 11,201 lung cancer cases and 10,251 controls with Infinium Global Screening Array (GSA) and Infinium OncoArray-500K BeadChip [18]. The participants were derived from four subsamples (the Nanjing GSA project: 4149 cases and 3198 controls from Nanjing and Shanghai; the Beijing GSA project: 2155 cases and 2035 controls from Beijing and Tianjin; the Guangzhou GSA project: 3944 cases and 4065 controls from Guangdong; and the NJMU OncoArray project: 953 cases and 953 controls from Nanjing). We then did a genome-wide meta-analysis of these GWASs with our published GWAS (the NJMU GWAS: 2126 lung cancer cases and 3077 controls) and those of European descent (13,793 cases and 14,027 controls). As a result, a total of 27,120 individuals with non-small cell lung cancer (NSCLC) and 27,355 individuals without NSCLC were included in the analysis. Finally, we identified 19 loci reached statistical significance in the meta-analysis of GWAS ($P \leq 5.0 \times 10^{-8}$) for overall NSCLC and histological subtypes (Fig. 11.1).

The study identified six novel susceptibility loci, including three loci that were associated with overall NSCLC risk (rs3769821 in 2q33.1, rs2293607 in 3q26.2, and rs1200399 in 14q13.1), two for lung adenocarcinoma (rs17038564 in 2p14 and rs35201538 in 9p13.3), and one for lung squamous cell carcinoma (rs4573350 in 9q33.2). Another 13 susceptibility loci have been previously reported, including 12 loci for overall NSCLC risk and 1 for lung adenocarcinoma. Some of the genes in the novel susceptibility loci have been reported to have important roles in carcinogenesis. For example, the index variant rs3769821 is located at an enhancer near *CASP8* in 2q33.1, and the risk alleles (rs3769821-C) exerted an increased enhancer activity by luciferase assays. The caspase-8, encoded by CASP8, is apical caspase acting in the death receptor-ligand interaction-induced apoptotic process and has been implicated in multiple cancer risk. Another example is the tag SNP rs2293607 at 3q26.2, which was located 8 kb upstream of *MYNN* and was confirmed to regulate its expression. MYNN encodes the myoneurin gene and belongs to BTB/POZ and zinc finger domain-containing protein family. Rs2293607 also maps within the promoter of TERC, the telomerase RNA component gene. Telomere length and activity maintained by telomerase are crucial for cancer initiation; and upregulation of telomerase is found in 90% of human tumors. The study provided a detailed map of the genetic susceptibility of lung cancer in the Chinese population, which further advanced the understanding of lung cancer susceptibility for the Chinese population.

11.2.2 Genome-Wide Association Study of Lung Cancer in Subgroup Population

11.2.2.1 Race

The genetic susceptibility of lung cancer in the Chinese population has both commonality and specificity compared with that in the Caucasian population. As described in the trans-ancestry meta-analysis of lung cancer [18], we observed that 2q33.1, 2p14, 3q26.2, 6p22.1, 8p12, 9p13.3, 9p21.3, 10q25.2, 11q23.3, 14q13.1, 15q21.1, and 17q24.2 were shared by Chinese and Caucasians with similar effects, while the effects of 3q28, 5p15.33, 8p12, 9q33.2, 15q25.1, and 19q13.2 were significantly different between the two populations (Fig. 11.2). For example, the rs55781567 at 15q25.1, which has been associated with smoking addiction, was a common variant and significantly associated with lung cancer risk in the Caucasian population. Although nominally significant, the frequency was relatively low and the effect was largely weaker in the Chinese population. In addition, two susceptibility loci in the 6p21.33 (rs3117582 in *BAT3* and rs3131379 in *MSH5*) were significantly associated with risk of lung cancer in Caucasians, while these variants were monogenic in the Chinese population [19]. However, follow-up studies found that low-frequency missense variants (rs9469031 in *BAT2* and rs200847762 in *FKBPL*) in this locus were significantly associated with the susceptibility of lung cancer in the Chinese population [20]. Therefore, it is of great significance to perform lung cancer GWAS in different ethnic groups.

11.2.2.2 Smoking Status

The clinicopathologic features of lung cancer showed significant differences between smokers and nonsmokers. Similarly, there were also dif-

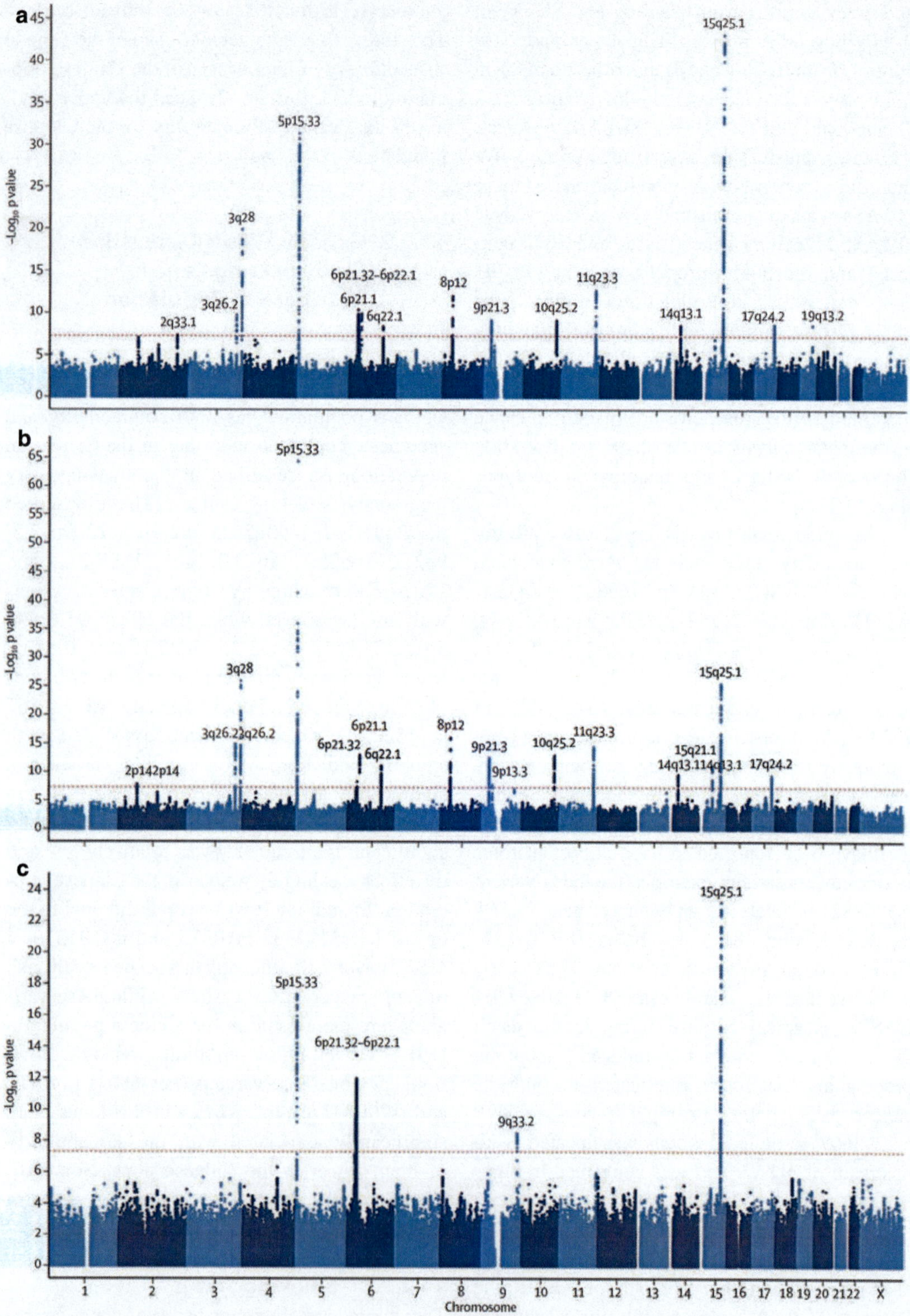

Fig. 11.1 Manhattan plots for trans-ancestry fixed-effects meta-analysis of lung cancer risk. (**a**) Non-small cell lung cancer, (**b**) lung adenocarcinoma, (**c**) lung squamous cell carcinoma

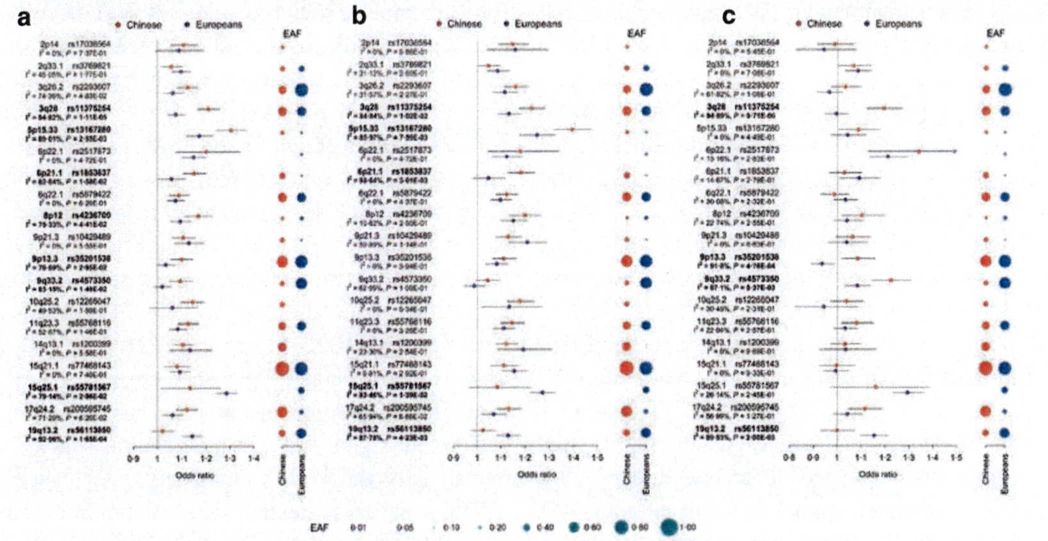

Fig. 11.2 Forest plot of lung cancer susceptibility loci between Chinese and European populations. (**a**) Non-small cell lung cancer; (**b**) lung adenocarcinoma; (**c**) lung squamous cell carcinoma

ferences in the genetic characteristics of smoking and nonsmoking lung cancer. The genetic variants of the nicotine choline receptor (nAChRs) gene cluster (*CHRNA3*, *CHRNA5*, and *CHRNB4*) have been associated with the risk of lung cancer in smokers but not in nonsmokers. Thorgeirsson et al. found that the SNPs of the nAChRs gene cluster were associated with daily smoking, smoking addiction, and lung cancer [21]. Therefore, it has been inferred that the association of the locus was mediated by smoking. In Asia, the incidence of nonsmoking lung cancer is much higher than that of Europeans and Americans. In 2010, a GWAS was performed in Asian nonsmoking female lung cancer patients. The study performed a whole-genome scan in 584 cases and 585 controls and then validated the promising associations in 1164 cases and 1736 controls [22]. The study confirmed that rs2736100 (*CLPTM1L-TERT*) in 5p15.33 was significantly associated with the risk of lung adenocarcinoma in nonsmoking females ($P = 2.60 \times 10^{-20}$). Subsequently, the research group further expanded the sample size and combined association results from 14 GWASs in Asia, which totally include 5510 female nonsmoking lung cancer patients and 4544 female controls [23]. Promising variants were further replicated in 1099 cases and 2913 controls. As a result, the study reported three novel genetic susceptibility loci in 10q25.2, 6q22.2, and 6p21.32. These results provide new evidences for revealing the genetic susceptibility of lung cancer in nonsmokers, but more studies were wanted to clarify why these genetic variants only affect lung cancer susceptibility in nonsmokers.

11.2.2.3 Histopathological Type

Lung cancer can be divided into small cell lung cancer (SCLC) and non-small cell lung cancer (NSCLC) according to histopathological type. The latter includes AD, SqCC, and other subtypes. Different histopathological types of lung cancer have both commonalities and specificities in genetic susceptibility. For example, although smoking has a dose-response association with different pathological types of lung cancer, it has a stronger effect on SqCC than on AD. In clinical practice, SqCC and AD have been regarded as different diseases and treated with different therapeutic schedules. Therefore, separate studies on different pathological types of lung cancer are of great significance for understanding the genetic susceptibility mechanism of lung cancer. In 2010, Miki et al. published the first GWAS study on lung adenocarcinoma in Asian populations and found that the genetic variations in 3q28 (*TP63*) were significantly associated with lung adenocarcinoma [24]. Based on the GWAS of lung cancer, our group also performed a subgroup analysis for lung SqCC, which included 844 cases and 3160 controls [25]. Promising loci with $P < 1.0 \times 10^{-4}$ were replicated in 822 cases and 2243 controls, as well as in 1401 cases and 4166 controls. The results of the study showed that rs12296850 in 12q23.1 was significantly associated with a reduced risk of lung squamous cell carcinoma, while not with lung adenocarcinoma ($P = 0.173$). Furthermore, in the following study with expanded sample size, we found that the genetic architecture of lung cancer risk varied markedly between lung AD and lung SqCC. Fewer genome-widely significant signals were found for lung squamous cell carcinoma (4 loci) compared with lung adenocarcinoma (17 loci) (Fig. 11.2).

11.2.3 Genome-Wide Association Study on the Prognosis of Lung Cancer

Besides susceptibility, GWAS has also made a series of achievements in exploring the prognosis-related genetic markers of lung cancer. In 2012, based on our previous GWAS data of lung cancer in the Chinese population, we further integrated clinical information of advanced non-small cell lung cancer patients who were treated with platinum chemotherapeutics and then conducted a GWAS on the prognosis of NSCLC in the Chinese population [26]. In the discovery stage, we included 535 cases from Nanjing and Beijing, and promising associations were further replicated in 340 cases from southeastern China. Finally, five SNPs (*P* value between $3.63 \times 10^{-5} \sim 4.19 \times 10^{-7}$) related to the prognosis of NSCLC were identified in the Chinese population. Of which, rs7629386 in 3p22.1, rs969088 in 5p14.1, and rs3850370 in 14q24.3 were associated with an increased risk of death in NSCLC patients, while rs41997 in 7q31.31 and rs12000445 in 9p21.3 were associated with a reduced risk of death in NSCLC patients. Furthermore, rs7629386 and rs3850370 were also significantly associated with the prognosis of NSCLC in the Caucasian population. In addition, a series of prognostic GWASs have been conducted for different tumor stages or treatment options. For example, a GWAS was conducted in early stage NSCLC patients who received surgical treatment [27]. The study included 365 early-stage NSCLC patients with surgery, followed by a fast-track replication in 327 NSCLC patients. As a result, rs10023113 (*CAMK2D*) was identified to be associated with an increased risk of death in NSCLC patients by 1.3 times. Wu et al. performed a genome-wide association study of overall survival in 245 small cell lung cancer (SCLC) patients treated with platinum-based chemotherapy, and the results were replicated in another independent set of 305 patients [28]. The study reported that rs1820453 T > G SNP within the promoter region of *YAP1* on chromosome 11q22 was associated with SCLC survival. Functional analysis showed that the rs1820453 T > G change created a transcriptional factor binding site and resulted in downregulation of *YAP1* expression. These results suggest that *YAP1* may play an important role in prognosis of small cell lung cancer patients treated with platinum-based chemotherapy. Besides prognosis, Cao et al. also found that rs2838566 at 21q22.3 was associated with platinum-induced hepatotoxicity in NSCLC patients; while rs13014982 at 2q24.3 and rs9909179 at 17p12 were proved to be associated with platinum-induced myelosuppression in NSCLC patients [29].

11.3 Post Genome-Wide Association Study in China

GWAS has achieved a great success in identifying genetic susceptibility loci of lung cancer, which provides a new perspective for explaining the development of lung cancer. These results also provide a new basis for optimizing lung cancer risk prediction models and promoting individualized prevention of lung cancer. Nevertheless, a number of challenges are needed to be solved in the study of genetic susceptibility to lung cancer. First, the susceptibility loci of lung cancer identified by now are still limited, and there is still a considerable degree of heritability that cannot be explained. Second, GWAS is usually focused on common variations, and low-frequency variations with stronger effect are difficult to be identified in GWAS. Third, although GWAS has identified many genetic susceptibility loci associated with lung cancer, we still know little about the molecular mechanisms underlying these susceptibility loci. In the post-GWAS era, we needed to carry out further data integration and functional study to explore the genetic susceptibility mechanisms of lung cancer.

11.3.1 Genome-Wide Meta-Analysis of Lung Cancer

Due to the limitations of the initial screening sample size and genotyping chip, it is difficult for GWAS to detect low frequency genetic variants (MAF < 0.05) or SNP with weak effect. Meta-analysis of multiple GWAS datasets can increase the sample size and improve the statistical efficacy, which can not only detect novel common variations with weak effects but also identify strong low-frequency variations. In 2014, 4 lung cancer GWAS datasets were combined by genome-wide meta-analysis, which results in a total of 11,348 lung cancer cases and 15,861 controls. The study identified *BRCA2* p.Lys3326X (rs11571833, OR = 2.47, $P = 4.74 \times 10^{-20}$) and *CHEK2* p.Ile157Thr (rs17879961, OR = 0.38, $P = 1.27 \times 10^{-13}$) were significantly associated with the risk of lung cancer [30]. In 2016, Wang et al. imputed data from 4 GWASs of Asian nonsmoking female lung cancer (6877 cases and 6277 controls) using the 1000 Genomes Project (Phase 1 Release 3) data as the reference and genotyped additional 5878 cases and 7046 controls for replication [31]. In the study, three novel loci achieved genome-wide significance were identified, including rs7741164 at 6p21.1, rs72658409 at 9p21.3, and rs11610143 at 12q13.13. These studies provided new clues for revealing the genetic susceptibility of lung cancer and confirmed the application value of whole-genome meta-analysis in the post-GWAS era.

11.3.2 Pathway Analysis

Genes do not exist in isolation. The molecular network composed of many genes affected cell function, metabolism, and biosynthesis processes and then participated in the occurrence and development of diseases. Integrating pathway information with GWAS summary statistics can improve statistical power and increase the interpretability of results. In 2013, Zhang et al. used BioCarta and KEGG databases to perform a gene set enrichment analysis (GSEA) based on the lung cancer GWAS data [32]. Finally, the nicotine acetylcholine receptor pathway (achPathway), angiotensin II-mediated JNK activation pathway (atlrPathway), hepatocyte growth factor receptor pathway (metPathway), and the Rac1 cell death signaling pathway (raclPathway) were identified to be significantly associated with the pathogenesis of lung cancer. In 2020, Qin et al. integrated large-scale genotype data of 15,581 lung adenocarcinoma (AD) cases, 8350 squamous cell carcinoma (SqCC) cases, and 27,355 controls and conducted pathway enrichment analysis and gene set enrichment analysis [33]. Finally, the study revealed that a total of 29 pathways were included in the development of NSCLC, of which 20 pathways related to immune function (such as PD-1 signaling and interferon gamma signaling pathway), 6 pathways in the neuronal system related to nicotinic acetylcholine receptors, and 3 pathways in the DNA repair system. Further subgroup analysis for lung AD and lung SqCC showed that lung AD related genes were specifically enriched in immune-related pathways, while lung SqCC genes were enriched in homologous recombination (HR)-related repair pathways, which suggested diverse mechanisms underlying the development of lung AD and SqCC.

11.3.3 Interactive Analysis

Most complex diseases or traits are not determined by pure genetic or environmental factors. Gene-environment interaction (G × E interaction) is of great significance in the pathogenesis of complex diseases including lung cancer. In addition, epistasis may also be an important mechanism underlying the disease susceptibility. In 2014, Chu et al. used the BOOST algorithm to analyze the paired gene (SNP-SNP) interaction of the 591,370 genotyping variants in 2331 lung cancer cases and 3077 controls and identified 4 candidate SNP pairs for replication in 2 cohorts (Beijing cohort: 1534 cases and 1489 controls; Shenyang, Guangzhou cohort: 2512 cases and 2449 controls) [34]. Finally, the study found that the interaction between rs2562796 and rs16832404 located in 2p32.2 was significantly associated the risk of lung cancer ($P_{LRM} = 1.03 \times 10^{-13}$). At the same time, Zhang et al. adopted a two-stage case-control design to explore gene-smoking interactions [35]. The preliminary screening stage included 2331 lung cancer cases and 3077 controls. The replication stage included 1534 cases and 1489 controls. Finally, two SNPs were found to have a significant interaction with smoking, where rs1316298 has an antagonistic effect with smoking and rs4589502 has a synergistic effect with smoking. In 2018, Wang et al. analyzed the associations between lung cancer risk SNPs and somatic alterations [36]. The study demonstrated that lung cancer driver genes are more likely to locate within cancer susceptibility regions. Both of lung cancer susceptibility genes and driver genes showed significant enrichment in pathways such as cell cycle and p53 signaling pathway. Gene-based analysis showed that rs36600 was associated with somatic mutations within *ARID1A*. Further analysis indicated that rs2395185 at HLA was associated with increased expression of APOBEC3A and elevated mutagenesis of APOBEC. These results indicated germline-somatic interactions were involved in the development of lung cancer.

11.3.4 Fine Mapping and Deep Sequencing Study

Multiple SNPs located in the same loci tend to be inherited as a whole. The GWAS chips selected tag SNPs for detection based on the linkage situation of each loci. As a result, the identified statistically significant SNP may not have biological function, and it only tagged the potentially functional SNP. In addition, the SNPs in GWAS chips usually contain less than 30% of the common SNPs in HapMap project. Therefore, fine-locating and deep sequencing of susceptible loci is one of the most important ways to clarify the biological functions of GWAS results. In 2017, Dong et al. conducted a two-stage fine-mapping analysis by targeted resequencing of 200 lung cancer cases and 300 controls individually and then validated in multiethnic lung cancer GWAS with 12,843 cases and 12,639 controls [37]. The study identified two independent variants in 5p15.33, including rs10054203 in *TERT* and rs397640 in *CLPTM1L*. Meanwhile, Cheng et al. performed a fine-mapping study of 15q25 using targeted resequencing of 200 lung cancer cases and 300 controls of Chinese descent [38]. The study identified two novel SNPs (rs6495304 and rs74733525) with independent effects in this locus, both of which were common in Chinese but rare or monomorphic in Caucasians. The rs6495304 was only significant in ever-smokers, and mediation analysis indicated that smoking behavior might mediate the effect of rs6495304 on lung cancer risk. These studies provided clues to reveal the potential molecular mechanisms of lung cancer susceptibility.

11.3.5 Association Analysis Based on Exon Chip

GWAS usually focus on common genetic variants and often ignore the low-frequency or rare variants. Although sequencing is an ideal method to explore low-frequency and rare variations associated with complex diseases, it is limited in population study due to its high cost. In order to make up the gap, Illumina launched a human "exon chip" (Illumina HumanExome BeadChip) for low-frequency genetic variation of the human exome in 2012. The chip selects >240,000 functional exon variants from the exome and whole-genome sequences of over 12,000 individuals. In order to explore the role of low-frequency and rare variants in the occurrence of lung cancer, our group performed a whole-exome microarray scanning on 1348 lung cancer cases and 1998 controls and promising variants were replicated in additional 4699 cases and 4915 controls [20]. Finally, three low-frequency missense variants were identified to be associated with the risk of lung cancer in the Chinese population, namely, rs9469031 (*BAT2*, c.1544C > T), rs200847762 (*FKBPL*, c.410C > T), and rs6141383 (*BPIFB1*, c.850G > A). Gene-based analysis further confirmed that *FKBPL* is associated with lung cancer susceptibility ($P = 1.29 \times 10^{-9}$). Furthermore, we also demonstrated that the rs9469031 and rs6141383 were also associated with the early onset of lung cancer patients. These results suggested that low-frequency variants are of great significance in the development of lung cancer, but more studies are needed to clarify the role of these low-frequency variants in the development of lung cancer due to the limited sample size of the previous studies.

11.3.6 Integration of GWAS with Other Omics

Epigenetics refers to the heritable changes in gene expression and function when the nucleotide sequence does not change. Epigenetic modification mainly includes DNA methylation and histone modification. Methylations of gene promoter, histone modification, non-coding RNA expression, chromosome modification complexes, etc. are considered to be important mechanisms in the development of cancer. Genetic variants can change sequence-specific allele methylation, which in turn affect gene expression and chromatin state. In 2012, Scherf et al. included 82 lung cancer cases to explore the differential expression of genes in known lung cancer susceptible regions (15q25.1, 5p15.33, and 6p21. 33) and analyzed the association between CpG islands and gene expression [39]. The study found that the expression of *CHRNB4* in lung cancer tissues was significantly increased and its promoter region was hypomethylated. In addition, the promoter regions of *CHRNA3* and *TERT* genes were hypermethylated, which led to changes in gene expression levels. Moreover, the author further included another 150 lung cancer cases and analyzed the association between SNP and DNA methylation. The genetic variants in the 5p15.33 and 15q25.1 were significantly associated with the methylation level of *TERT* and *CHRNB4* promoter regions, respectively. These results suggested that regulating the abnormal epigenetic modification of the nAChR genes might be one of the mechanisms of lung cancer susceptibility. However, there is still a lack of evidence that genetic variations regulated epigenetic changes affecting lung cancer susceptibility in the Chinese population.

Although GWAS has found a series of genetic susceptibility loci for lung cancer, the molecular mechanisms underlying these variants are still unclear. Regulating gene expression is one of the most important susceptibility mechanisms for many genetic variations. Construction of tissue-specific genotype-expression database (Expression Quantitative Trait Loci, eQTL) is essential to analyze the susceptibility mechanisms of GWAS. Recently, researchers have established a new strategy to systematically integrate GWAS and eQTL databases. The approach firstly constructed a reference panel with genome-wide genotype and expression data in a relatively large sample size and then predicted the expression with GWAS datasets to test the differences between cases and controls (transcriptome-wide association analysis, TWAS). This strategy can improve statistical power and help identify more potential pathogenic genes. On the basis of the strategy, Yohan Bossé et al. integrated summary statistics from 29,266 lung cancer cases and 56,450 controls of European descent with a large-scale expression quantitative trait loci (eQTL) mapping study in human lung tissues ($n = 1038$) to identify candidate causal genes for lung cancer and then replicated the results using lung data from the Genotype-Tissue Expression (GTEx) project [40]. The study confirmed the association in 15q25 and found the most significant gene was *IREB2*. Besides, higher predicted expression of *AQP3* was identified to be associated with lung adenocarcinoma susceptibility on 9p13.3. A total of 17 target genes were mapped among the 45 previously described lung cancer GWAS loci. These results located potential pathogenic genes in GWAS susceptible loci and deepen our understanding of lung cancer GWAS studies.

11.3.7 Polygenic Risk Score and Lung Cancer Risk Prediction

The genetic susceptibility loci of lung cancer identified by GWAS are a set of biomarkers. One of its important public health values is to identify high-risk populations through lung cancer risk assessment. Since the effect of a single susceptibility locus is generally weak, combining the effects of all identified variants and calculating a polygenic risk score (PRS) is a commonly used strategy for cancer risk assessment. In 2019, after combining association results from more than 13,327 cases and 13,328 controls of the Chinese descent population, we systematically evaluated the results of all SNPs that have been reported in GWAS (81 SNPs) [18]. After excluding those with minor allele frequency less than 0.01 in the Chinese population, in medium—high linkage disequilibrium ($r^2 > 0.1$), and association *P*-values ($P > 0.00125$, after multiple comparison at 0.05/40; 40 independent loci remained according to the abovementioned two criteria)—we selected 19 SNPs to construct a PRS by multiplying the genotype dosage of each risk allele for each variant by its respective weight (ln[OR]) of lung cancer for Chinese population. Then, we evaluated the PRS in the largest cohort study of China (the China Kadoorie Biobank, CKB), which included more than 0.5 million participants from ten regions across China. A total of 95,408 Chinese participants from the CKB cohort were included in the analysis, and 1316 patients were confirmed as incident lung cancer cases with a median follow-up time of 10.44 years. Based on the cohort, we found that incident lung cancer patients tended to have a higher PRS than other participants in the cohort. When dividing participants into ten groups according to deciles of PRS, a risk gradient across each grade of genetic risk was observed. Participants in the top tenth of the PRS were at significantly higher risk of lung cancer than those at the lowest tenth genetic risk. Participants at high genetic risk (top 5% of PRS) showed 137% higher relative risk of lung cancer compared to the low genetic risk (bottom 5% of PRS). A joint cumulative effect of the PRS and smoking was observed in incident lung cancer events according to the results from CKB. We used Pake-Year30 to define light and heavy smokers. The risk of lung cancer increased along with the amount of smoking and genetic risk categories, and light smokers at high genetic risk showed a comparable risk with heavy smokers at medium genetic risk (Fig. 11.3). These results indicated that PRS could be effectively used for lung cancer risk prediction, which potentially lead to a feasible lung cancer screening program for precision prevention in the future.

11.4 Research on Lung Cancer Genome Sequencing

Another hot spot in cancer genomics focuses on non-heritable somatic variations (such as mutations, copy number variations, chromatin remodeling, etc.). It has been pointed out that cancer is a type of "genomic disease" and somatic mutations directly drive tumor cells to gain evolutionary advantages. Therefore, identification of somatic mutations can help clarify the mechanisms of tumors and provide information for the precise treatment of lung cancer. In the past decades, the genomic landscapes of cancer have been gradu-

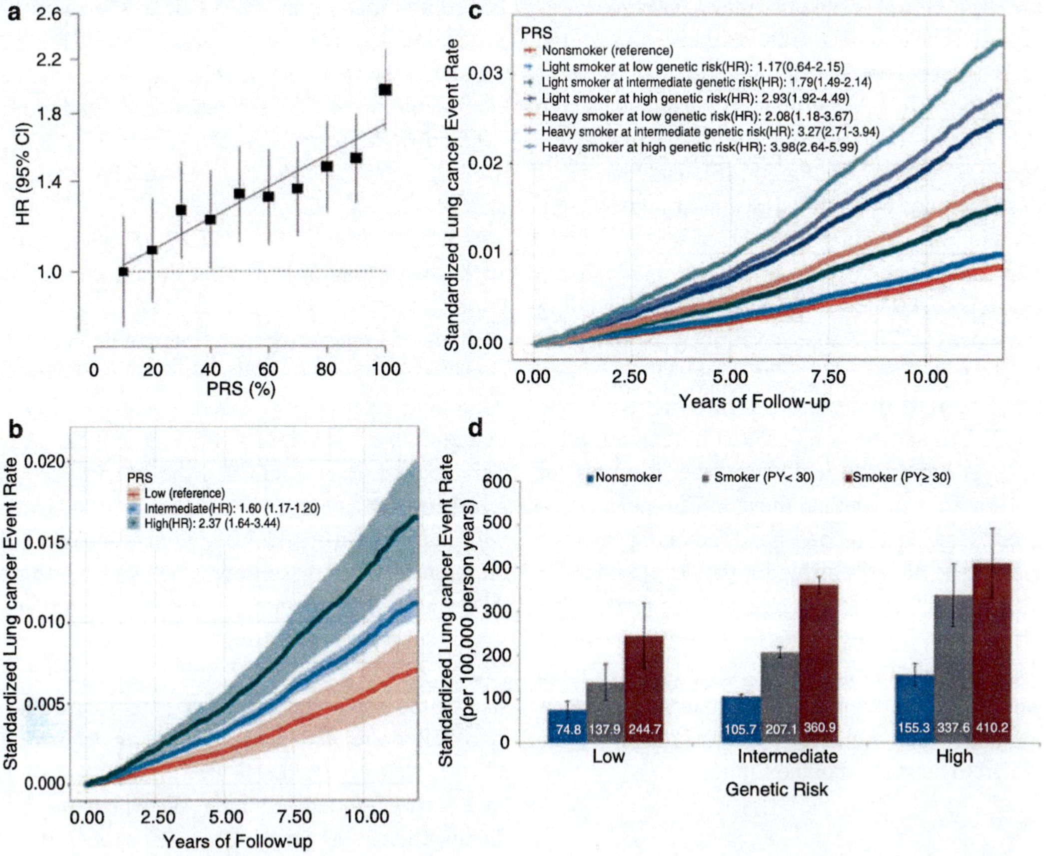

Fig. 11.3 Associations between PRS and lung cancer incidences in CKB. (**a**) Dose-response of PRS and lung cancer risk; (**b**) standardized rates of lung cancer events in low (bottom 5%), intermediate (5–95%), and high (top 5%) genetic risk groups in the CKB cohort; (**c**) cumulative effects of genetic risk and smoking status; (**d**) standardized cumulative lung cancer incidences in different degrees of smoking according to genetic risk categories

ally deciphered in the Caucasian population with the emergence of massively parallel sequencing (MPS) technology. In 2005, the National Cancer Institute of the United States organized the first large-scale research of cancer somatic cell variation, namely, the Cancer Genome Atlas (TCGA) [41]. More than 10,000 pairs of samples from different cancer types have been tested by whole-exome sequencing (WES) or whole-genome sequencing (WGS) before the end of 2013. In addition, the International Cancer Genome Consortium (ICGC) was formally established in London in April 2008 by research teams from multiple countries [42]. The organization planned to invest $1 billion over 10 years to sequence 25,000 tumor samples and to generate a catalog of cancer gene mutations of 50 common tumors.

11.4.1 Burden of Somatic Alterations in Chinese Lung Cancer Patients

After integrating the results of ICGC and the TCGA project, Ludmil et al. found that lung AD and lung SqCC had the highest mutation rate (8.7 mutations/Mb and 9.7 mutations/Mb for AD and SqCC, respectively) second only to melanoma, while the mutation rate of small cell lung cancer ranked fifth [43]. These mutations were characterized by high fractions of cytosine-adenine (C to A) nucleotide transversions, which was probably due to lung cancer patients commonly have a history of exposure to cigarette carcinogens. In East Asia, the mutation rate of lung SqCC was similar to that of the Caucasian population

[44, 45]. However, distinct mutation burden was reported for lung AD in the Chinese population. Li et al. reported that the mutation rate was 1.4 mutations/Mb in 271 lung AD patients, which was similar to that of our study (2.2 mutations/Mb in 84 lung AD patients) [46]. The reasons of the difference were probably due to study design, fraction of female patients, sequencing methods, and variant calling protocols. Through the analysis of 4,938,362 mutations and surrounding sequences in 7042 cancer samples, 20 mutation labels were identified. The lung AD and lung SqCC were both identified to be enriched of age, APOBEC, and smoking-related mutation signals [47]. The lung AD incidence rates were higher in Chinese women than those in European countries. However, second-hand smoking seemed unlikely to be responsible for the development of lung AD in Chinese women, because low burden of smoking-induced mutations were detected in these patients. Thus, the etiology of the female patients without smoking behavior and elevated mutation rate remained unclear and are warranted to be studied in the future.

11.4.2 Driver Genes in Chinese Lung Cancer Patients

Although a great number of alterations could be detected in lung cancer genomes, only a few somatic alterations have the potential to direct trigger of cancer. These alterations usually undergo positive selection in the evolution of cancer and could be accumulated in the essential genes. Thus, we usually regard genes with a significantly higher mutation rate (or amplification/deletion rate) than the backgrounds as potential driver genes.

In 2015, researchers from the BGI Institute and the First Affiliated Hospital of Guangzhou Medical University reported a large-scale sequencing study of primary and metastatic lung AD in Chinese patients [48]. The study performed whole-genome and transcriptome sequencing of 101 primary lung AD and 35 corresponding lymph node metastases and validated the promising mutations in an independent 234 samples in the Chinese population. The study identified 13 significantly mutated genes of lung adenocarcinoma in the Chinese population, including *TP53*, *EGFR*, *LRP1B*, *KRAS*, *PTPTD*, *STK11*, *SMAD2*, *PIK3CA*, *BRAF*, *FLT1*, *RHPN2*, *GLI3*, and *MRC2*, of which 6 genes (*TP53*, *EGFR*, *KRAS*, *STK11*, *PIK3CA*, and *BRAF*) were consistent with that from European and American populations. For mutations in *EGFR*, the proportions of Leu858Arg mutation and deletion of exon 19 accounted for 54% and 29% of the total mutations, respectively. Patients with these two mutations were sensitive to tyrosinase inhibitors. This result further confirmed the importance of screening for these two mutations in patients with lung AD in the Chinese population. Based on the results of transcriptome sequencing, lung AD can be divided into three subtypes, among which subtype 3 has a higher mutation rate of *KRAS*, *FLY1*, and *KEAP1* and a poor prognosis. At the same time, studies have found that cytoskeleton-related genes (including *IQGAP3*, *EPB41*, *CDC42*, *PARD6G*, *PTK2B*, and *KALRN*) have higher frequency in lung AD, which may be therapeutic targets for the Chinese population.

In 2018, we analyzed genomic events in 149 NSCLC cases (92 WGS and 57 WES) coupled with 100 NSCLC patients with WGS in TCGA data and comprehensively identified the genomic features of Chinese NSCLC patients [49]. The study included a total of 84 lung AD and 65 lung SqCC patients of the Chinese population. Overall, a total of 27 driven genes (*EGFR*, *PTEN*, *TP53*, *NFE2L2*, *RB1*, *CDKN2A*, *KRAS*, *KMT2D*, *STK11*, *TET2*, *FBXW7*, *ARID1A*, *SETD2*, *PBRM1*, *FLNC*, *ARHGAP35*, *CLASP2*, *WNK1*, *AGAP1*, *POLE*, *OBSL1*, *TDG*, *SEMA6B*, *ITGAL*, *EEF1D*, *NT5E*, *PFKM*) were identified in these NSCLC patients, of which 15 genes were reported in previous studies. Besides, *MARCA4* in lung AD, *FAT1*, and *SVEP1* in SqCC were identified as driver candidates in a histological subtype analysis. Notably, high *EGFR* mutations were identified in Chinese lung cancer patients (31.5%), especially for lung AD patients (52.0%); while smoking-related KRAS mutations were less common in our dataset (8.0%) compared with that in TCGA (31.3%). Most of the SqCC-specific driver genes were tumor suppressors, including *TP53*, *KMT2D*, *CDKN2A*, and *FBXW7*, indicating the highly disorganized status of SqCC cells. The study also revealed a mutational signature (MS3, 33.7%), which is associated with inflammatory tumor-infiltrating B lymphocytes. Moreover, we observed that the *EGFR* mutation rate is significantly increased with the proportion of the MS3 signature. These results indicated that inflammatory infiltration may contribute to the accumulation of *EGFR* mutations, especially in never-smokers of the Chinese population.

In addition, we have also completed a WES in 25 patients with normal adjacent tissue and matched tumor pairs, as well as 74 tumors tissue from Chinese SCLC patients [50]. The study found that T*P53* (82%), *RB1* (47%), *CSMD3* (47%), *NOTCH1* (18%), and *NOTCH3* (15%) were the most recurrent mutated genes. In addition, the study identified recurrent gains of *SRSF1* (50%) as well as concordant overexpression of mRNA for those patients with gains. Besides, overexpression of *SRSF1* was strongly associated with poor survival in Chinese patients, and further functional studies in vitro and in vivo demonstrated that SRSF1 play a key role in DNA repair and chemo-sensitivity. These results provided a rationale for personalized therapy of Chinese lung cancer patients.

11.5 Conclusion

In recent years, with the deepening of human genome research and the rapid development of technology, studies of lung cancer genomics have achieved unprecedented success. Based on GWAS, a series of susceptibility loci, potential causal genes, and functional SNPs related to lung cancer risk have been identified. Although there is still "missing heritability" of lung cancer, multi-center cooperation worldwide to increase sample size has been gradually carried out with the improvement of data transparency. With the completion of international large-scale functional genome databases (such as GTEx and ENCODE), we have ushered in a new opportunity to explore the underlying mechanisms of GWAS findings. The maturity of next-generation sequencing technology and the reduction of sequencing costs are opening up a new field of lung cancer genome research. Large-scale sequencing of tissues has identified a number of significantly mutated genes for lung AD and lung SqCC, which provided a foundation for precision medicine of lung cancer. However, more efforts are needed to translate these genomic research results to the clinical diagnosis and treatment of lung cancer to improve the clinical technology level of lung cancer in China.

References

1. Bray F, et al. Global cancer statistics 2018: GLOBOCAN estimates of incidence and mortality worldwide for 36 cancers in 185 countries. CA Cancer J Clin. 2018;68(6):394–424.
2. Siegel RL, Miller KD, Jemal A. Cancer statistics, 2020. CA Cancer J Clin. 2020;70(1):7–30.
3. Chen W, et al. Cancer statistics in China, 2015. CA Cancer J Clin. 2016;66(2):115–32.
4. Ozlü T, Bülbül Y. Smoking and lung cancer. Tuberkuloz ve Toraks. 2005;53(2):200–9.
5. Parascandola M, Xiao L. Tobacco and the lung cancer epidemic in China. Transl Lung Cancer Res. 2019;8(Suppl 1):S21–30.
6. Ekpu VU, Brown AK. The economic impact of smoking and of reducing smoking prevalence: review of evidence. Tob Use Insights. 2015;8:1–35.
7. Pope CA, et al. Lung cancer, cardiopulmonary mortality, and long-term exposure to fine particulate air pollution. JAMA. 2002;287(9):1132–41.
8. Mao Y, et al. Epidemiology of lung cancer. Surg Oncol Clin N Am. 2016;25(3):439–45.
9. Altshuler DM, et al. Integrating common and rare genetic variation in diverse human populations. Nature. 2010;467(7311):52–8.
10. Abecasis GR, et al. A map of human genome variation from population-scale sequencing. Nature. 2010;467(7319):1061–73.
11. Bailey-Wilson JE, et al. A major lung cancer susceptibility locus maps to chromosome 6q23-25. Am J Hum Genet. 2004;75(3):460–74.
12. You M, et al. Fine mapping of chromosome 6q23-25 region in familial lung cancer families reveals RGS17 as a likely candidate gene. Clin Cancer Res: An Official Journal of the American Association for Cancer Research. 2009;15(8):2666–74.

13. Yang H, et al. The association of GSTM1 deletion polymorphism with lung cancer risk in Chinese population: evidence from an updated meta-analysis. Sci Rep. 2015;5:9392.
14. Zhang S, et al. A variant in the CHEK2 promoter at a methylation site relieves transcriptional repression and confers reduced risk of lung cancer. Carcinogenesis. 2010;31(7):1251–8.
15. Bossé Y, Amos CI. A decade of GWAS results in lung cancer. Cancer Epidemiol Biomarkers Prev: A Publication of the American Association for Cancer Research, cosponsored by the American Society of Preventive Oncology. 2018;27(4):363–79.
16. Hu Z, et al. A genome-wide association study identifies two new lung cancer susceptibility loci at 13q12.12 and 22q12.2 in Han Chinese. Nat Genet. 2011;43(8):792–6.
17. Dong J, et al. Association analyses identify multiple new lung cancer susceptibility loci and their interactions with smoking in the Chinese population. Nat Genet. 2012;44(8):895–9.
18. Dai J, et al. Identification of risk loci and a polygenic risk score for lung cancer: a large-scale prospective cohort study in Chinese populations. The lancet. Respir Med. 2019;7(10):881–91.
19. Doherty JA, et al. DNA repair genotype and lung cancer risk in the beta-carotene and retinol efficacy trial. Int J Mol Epidemiol Genet. 2013;4(1):11–34.
20. Jin G, et al. Low-frequency coding variants at 6p21.33 and 20q11.21 are associated with lung cancer risk in Chinese populations. Am J Hum Genet. 2015;96(5):832–40.
21. Thorgeirsson TE, et al. Sequence variants at CHRNB3-CHRNA6 and CYP2A6 affect smoking behavior. Nat Genet. 2010;42(5):448–53.
22. Hsiung CA, et al. The 5p15.33 locus is associated with risk of lung adenocarcinoma in never-smoking females in Asia. PLoS Genet. 2010;6(8):e1001051.
23. Lan Q, et al. Genome-wide association analysis identifies new lung cancer susceptibility loci in never-smoking women in Asia. Nat Genet. 2012;44(12):1330–5.
24. Miki D, et al. Variation in TP63 is associated with lung adenocarcinoma susceptibility in Japanese and Korean populations. Nat Genet. 2010; 42(10):893–6.
25. Dong J, et al. Genome-wide association study identifies a novel susceptibility locus at 12q23.1 for lung squamous cell carcinoma in Han Chinese. PLoS Genet. 2013;9(1):e1003190.
26. Hu L, et al. Genome-wide association study of prognosis in advanced non-small cell lung cancer patients receiving platinum-based chemotherapy. Clin Cancer Res: An Official Journal of the American Association for Cancer Research. 2012;18(19):5507–14.
27. Tang S, et al. Genome-wide association study of survival in early-stage non-small cell lung cancer. Ann Surg Oncol. 2015;22(2):630–5.
28. Wu C, et al. Genome-wide interrogation identifies YAP1 variants associated with survival of small-cell lung cancer patients. Cancer Res. 2010;70(23):9721–9.
29. Cao S, et al. Genome-wide association study on platinum-induced hepatotoxicity in non-small cell lung cancer patients. Sci Rep. 2015;5:11556.
30. Wang Y, et al. Rare variants of large effect in BRCA2 and CHEK2 affect risk of lung cancer. Nat Genet. 2014;46(7):736–41.
31. Wang Z, et al. Meta-analysis of genome-wide association studies identifies multiple lung cancer susceptibility loci in never-smoking Asian women. Hum Mol Genet. 2016;25(3):620–9.
32. Zhang R, et al. Pathway analysis for genome-wide association study of lung cancer in Han Chinese population. PLoS One. 2013;8(3):e57763.
33. Qin N, et al. Comprehensive functional annotation of susceptibility variants identifies genetic heterogeneity between lung adenocarcinoma and squamous cell carcinoma. Front Med. 2021;15(2):275–91.
34. Chu M, et al. A genome-wide gene-gene interaction analysis identifies an epistatic gene pair for lung cancer susceptibility in Han Chinese. Carcinogenesis. 2014;35(3):572–7.
35. Zhang R, et al. A genome-wide gene-environment interaction analysis for tobacco smoke and lung cancer susceptibility. Carcinogenesis. 2014;35(7):1528–35.
36. Wang Y, et al. Interaction analysis between germline susceptibility loci and somatic alterations in lung cancer. Int J Cancer. 2018;143(4):878–85.
37. Dong J, et al. Fine mapping of chromosome 5p15.33 identifies novel lung cancer susceptibility loci in Han Chinese. Int J Cancer. 2017;141(3):447–56.
38. Cheng Y, et al. Targeted sequencing of chromosome 15q25 identified novel variants associated with risk of lung cancer and smoking behavior in Chinese. Carcinogenesis. 2017;38(5):552–8.
39. Scherf DB, et al. Epigenetic screen identifies genotype-specific promoter DNA methylation and oncogenic potential of CHRNB4. Oncogene. 2013;32(28):3329–38.
40. Bossé Y, et al. Transcriptome-wide association study reveals candidate causal genes for lung cancer. Int J Cancer. 2020;146(7):1862–78.
41. Weinstein JN, et al. The cancer genome atlas pan-cancer analysis project. Nat Genet. 2013;45(10):1113–20.
42. Hudson TJ, et al. International network of cancer genome projects. Nature. 2010;464(7291):993–8.
43. Alexandrov LB, et al. Signatures of mutational processes in human cancer. Nature. 2013;500(7463):415–21.
44. Cancer Genome Atlas Research Network. Comprehensive genomic characterization of squamous cell lung cancers. Nature. 2012;489(7417): 519–25.

45. Kim Y, et al. Integrative and comparative genomic analysis of lung squamous cell carcinomas in east Asian patients. J Clin Oncol. 2014;32(2):121–8.
46. Li S, et al. Comprehensive characterization of oncogenic drivers in Asian lung adenocarcinoma. J Thorac Oncol: Official Publication of the International Association for the Study of Lung Cancer. 2016;11(12):2129–40.
47. Alexandrov LB, et al. The repertoire of mutational signatures in human cancer. Nature. 2020;578(7793):94–101.
48. Wu K, et al. Frequent alterations in cytoskeleton remodelling genes in primary and metastatic lung adenocarcinomas. Nat Commun. 2015;6:10131.
49. Wang C, et al. Whole-genome sequencing reveals genomic signatures associated with the inflammatory microenvironments in Chinese NSCLC patients. Nat Commun. 2018;9(1):2054.
50. Jiang L, et al. Genomic landscape survey identifies SRSF1 as a key Oncodriver in small cell lung cancer. PLoS Genet. 2016;12(4):e1005895.

Progress in Epidemiology of Child Road Traffic Injury

12

Guoqing Hu

Abstract

First, this chapter introduces the definition and classification of external causes of child traffic injury and reports the current situation and trends in mortality, years of life lost, years lived with disability, and disability-adjusted life years from road traffic injuries among children over the world, based on the Global Burden of Disease (GBD) 2019 estimates and other published literature. We describe differences in child traffic injury burden across age group, year, month, date, time, and transportation method. Then, we systematically summarize the major influencing factors of child road traffic injury from three aspects: human factors, vehicle factors, and environment factors. Finally, we introduce intervention theories and basic strategies (including Haddon's ten basic strategies, 5Es intervention theory, active and passive intervention strategies) and summarize the published effective prevention interventions.

Keyword

Road traffic injury · Child · Influencing factor Intervention

12.1 Introduction

Road traffic injury (RTI) has become an important global public health issue, with accelerating industrialization and urbanization. *The Global Status Report on Road Safety 2018* by the World Health Organization shows that the number of road traffic deaths is approximately 1.35 million each year, yielding great impact on people's health.

RTI is currently a leading cause of global child mortality. According to *the World Report on Child Injury Prevention* by the World Health Organization (WHO), RTI accounts for approximately 262 thousand child deaths every year, and more than 10 million children suffer a non-fatal injury. RTI is the leading cause of deaths for young people aged 15–19 years.

Data in this chapter from online resources of the Global Burden of Disease Study 2019 (GBD 2019) and reports by the World Health Organization (WHO). Using the data, we regraphed all figures. Therefore, this chapter does not involve informed consent and ethical review.

G. Hu (✉)
Xiangya School of Public Health, Central South University, Changsha, China

D.-Q. Ye (ed.), *Progress in China Epidemiology*, https://doi.org/10.1007/978-981-19-2199-5_12

12.1.1 Definition

12.1.1.1 Children

We focus on road traffic crashes occurring on children younger than 18 years old according to the definition from *the Convention on the Rights of the Child*. Our analyses, however, were expanded to 19 years old because of data availability of GBD 2019 estimates.

12.1.1.2 Injury and Traffic Injury

According to *the World Report on Child Injury Prevention*, an injury event is defined as "the physical damage that results when a human body is suddenly subjected to energy in amounts that exceed the threshold of physiological tolerance—or else the result of a lack of one or more vital elements, such as oxygen."

Road traffic crash is defined as "a collision or incident that may or may not lead to injury, occurring on a public road and involving at least one moving vehicle."

Road traffic injury is defined as "fatal or non-fatal injuries incurred as a result of a road traffic crash."

12.1.2 Classification

Currently, the International Classification of Diseases, 10th Revision (ICD-10), is widely used to classify type of injuries over the world. Based on the ICD-10, the Centers for Disease Control and Prevention (CDC) in the United States develops an injury matrix by combining external cause and intent of injury which specifies the classification of traffic injury (Table 12.1).

12.2 Epidemiological Characteristics

12.2.1 Mortality

Data from GBD 2019 by the Institute for Health Metrics and Evaluation (IHME) was used to evaluate the latest epidemiological characteristics of road traffic injury. From 1990 to 2019, global RTI mortality rates all decreased substantially for children under 5, aged 5–15 years, and 15–19 years. During the study time period, children from low-income countries generally had much higher RTI mortality rates than those from high-income countries for under-5 children and children aged 5–14 years. The exceptional trend for children aged 15–19 years mainly reflects differences in motorization and prevention efforts across the four country income categories. In 2019, the child RTI mortality rates for three age groups were 5.80 (95% UI: 4.65–7.51), 4.26 (95% UI: 3.69–4.95), and 11.30 (95% UI 10.03–12.55) deaths per 100,000 people, respectively (note: UI, uncertainty interval) (Figs. 12.1, 12.2 and 12.3).

Road traffic injuries emerged as a leading cause of deaths for three age groups in both 1990 and 2019. Specifically, the rank of road injuries fell from the 13th place in 1990 to the 14th place in 2019 (Fig. 12.4). In 2019, the rank of road injuries was the second place for children aged 5–14 years and the first place for children aged 15–19 years, respectively (Figs. 12.5 and 12.6).

12.2.2 Years of Life Lost (YLLs)

Over the past three decades, YLLs per 100,000 population due to RTI all decreased in three age groups and four country income categories; but the rates were lowest among high-income countries. YLLs per 100,000 population were generally negatively correlated with country income, with higher country income corresponding to low rates. The trend for children aged 15–19 years in high-income countries was an exception; the YLLs per 100,000 population were higher than other country income categories before the early 2000s but then started to lower other categories; after 2013, it was lowest compared with the other three country income categories. In 2019, the YLLs per 100,000 population from RTI were 502.20 (95% UI: 402.39–650.27) among under-5 children, 337.82 (95% UI: 292.55–392.20) among children aged 5–14 years, and 806.69 (95% UI: 716.14–896.18) among children aged 15–19 years, respectively (Figs. 12.7, 12.8, and 12.9).

Table 12.1 ICD-10 classification of traffic injuries by external cause and intent

	Intent					
External cause	All injury	Unintentional	Suicide	Homicide	Undetermined	Legal intervention/ war
All transport	*U01.1, V01–V99, X82, Y03, Y32, Y36.1	V01–V99	X82	*U01.1, Y03	Y32	Y36.1
Motor vehicle traffic						
Occupant	[V30–V79] (0.4–0.9), [V83–V86] (0.0–0.3)	[V30–V79] (0.4–0.9), [V83–V86] (0.0–0.3)	…	…	…	…
Motorcyclist	[V20–V28] (0.3–0.9), V29 (0.4–0.9)	[V20–V28] (0.3–0.9), V29 (0.4–0.9)	…	…	…	…
Pedal cyclist	[V12–V14] (0.3–0.9), V19 (0.4–0.6)	[V12–V14] (0.3–0.9), V19 (0.4–0.6)	…	…	…	…
Pedestrian	[V02–V04] (0.1,0.9), V09.2	[V02–V04] (0.1,0.9), V09.2	…	…	…	…
Other	V80 (0.3–0.5), V81.1, V82.1	V80 (0.3–0.5), V81.1, V82.1	…	…	…	…
Unspecified	V87 (0.0–0.8), V89.2	V87 (0.0–0.8), V89.2	…	…	…	…
Pedal cyclist, other	V10–V11, [V12–V14] (0.0–0.2), V15–V18, V19 (0.0–0.3,0.8,0.9)	V10–V11, [V12–V14] (0.0–0.2), V15–V18, V19 (0.0–0.3,0.8,0.9)	…	…	…	…
Pedestrian, other	V01, [V02–V04] (0.0), V05, V06, V09 (0.0–0.1,0.3,0.9)	V01, [V02–V04] (0.0), V05, V06, V09 (0.0–0.1,0.3,0.9)	…	…	…	…
Other land transport	[V20–V28] (0.0–0.2), [V29–V79] (0.0–0.3), V80 (0.0–0.2,0.6–0.9), [V81–V82] (0.0,0.2–0.9), [V83–V86] (0.4–0.9), V87.9, V88 (0.0–0.9), V89 (0.0,0.1,0.3,0.9), X82, Y03, Y32	[V20–V28] (0.0–0.2), [V29–V79] (0.0–0.3), V80(0.0–0.2,0.6–0.9), [V81–V82] (0.0,0.2–0.9), [V83–V86] (0.4–0.9), V87.9, V88 (0.0–0.9), V89 (0.0,0.1,0.3,0.9)	X82	Y03	Y32	…
Other transport	*U01.1, V90–V99, Y36.1	V90–V99	…	*U01.1	…	Y36.1

Source: Fingerhut L. ICD Framework: External cause of injury mortality matrix. Hyattsville, MD: National Center for Health Statistics [EB/OL]. https://www.cdc.gov/nchs/data/ice/icd10_transcode.pdf (Accessed December 20, 2020)

12.2.3 Years Lived with Disability (YLDs)

During 1990–2019, YLDs per 100,000 population due to RTI demonstrated different trends in three age groups and four country income categories. The YLDs per 100,000 population were not strictly negatively correlated with country income, which probably reflected the effects of poor-quality non-fatal RTI data, varying prevention efforts and motorization levels. In 2019, the YLDs per 100,000 population due to RTI were 2.58 (95% UI: 1.64–3.88) among under-5 children, 19.57 (95% UI: 13.67–26.74) among children aged 5–14 years, and 60.59 (95% UI: 41.45–82.14) among children aged 15–19 years, respectively (Figs. 12.10, 12.11, and 12.12).

12.2.4 Disability-Adjusted Life Years (DALYs)

During 1990–2019, DALYs per 100,000 population showed roughly consistent trends as shown

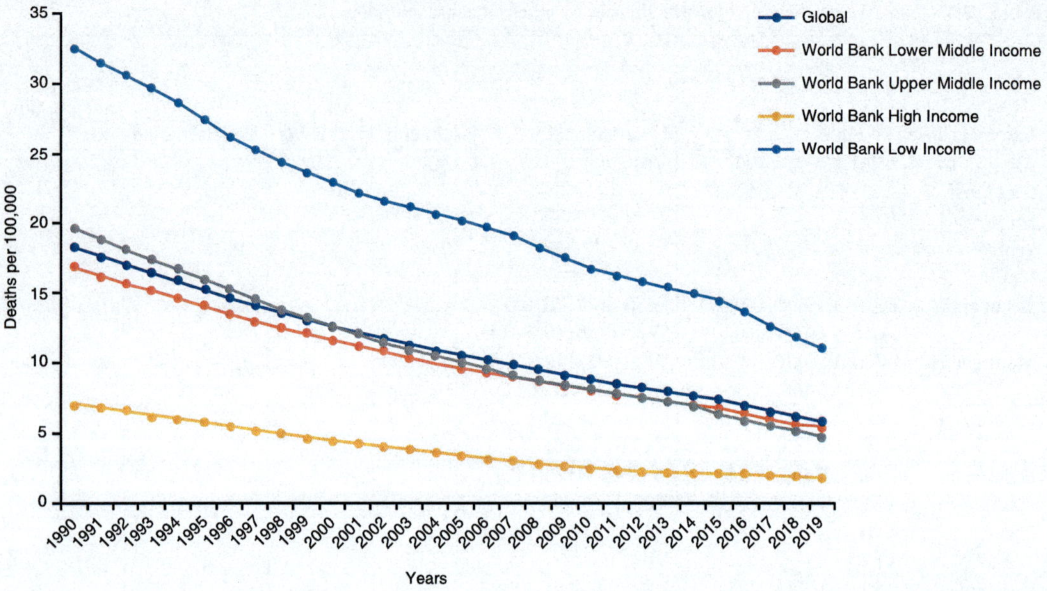

Fig. 12.1 Global road traffic injury mortality among under-5 children, 1990–2019. (Data source: GBD Compare, 2019)

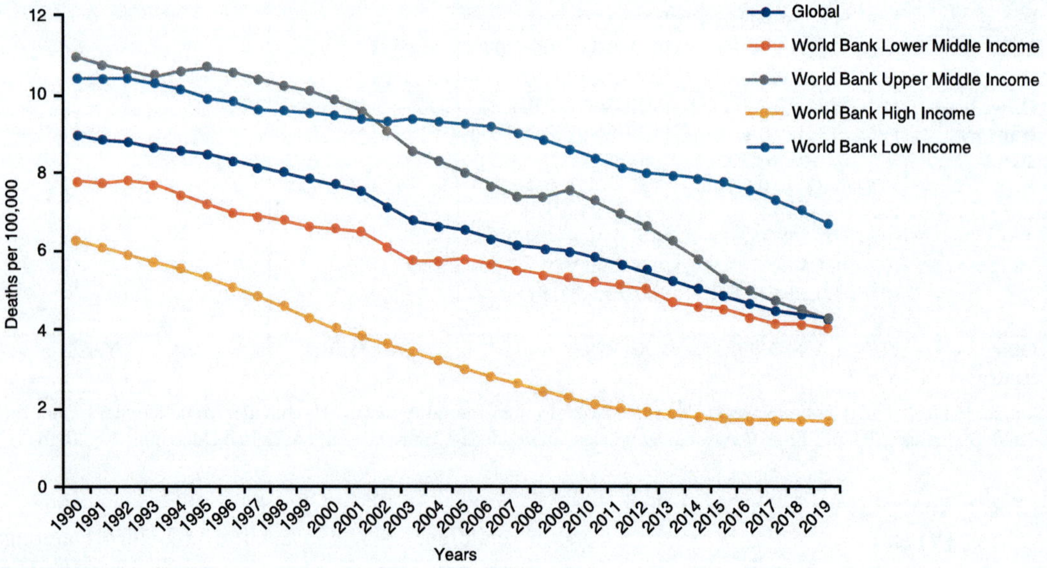

Fig. 12.2 Global road traffic injury mortality among children aged 5–14 years, 1990–2019. (Data source: GBD Compare, 2019)

for YLLs per 100,000 population in three age groups and four country income categories. In 2019, the DALYs per 100,000 population due to RTI was 504.78 (95% UI: 405.63–652.29) among under-5 children, 357.39 (95% UI: 312.38–410.73) among children aged 5–14 years, and 867.28 (95% UI: 775.85–960.48) among children aged 15–19 years, respectively. Low-income countries had the highest DALYs in all three age groups in 2019 (Figs. 12.13, 12.14, and 12.15).

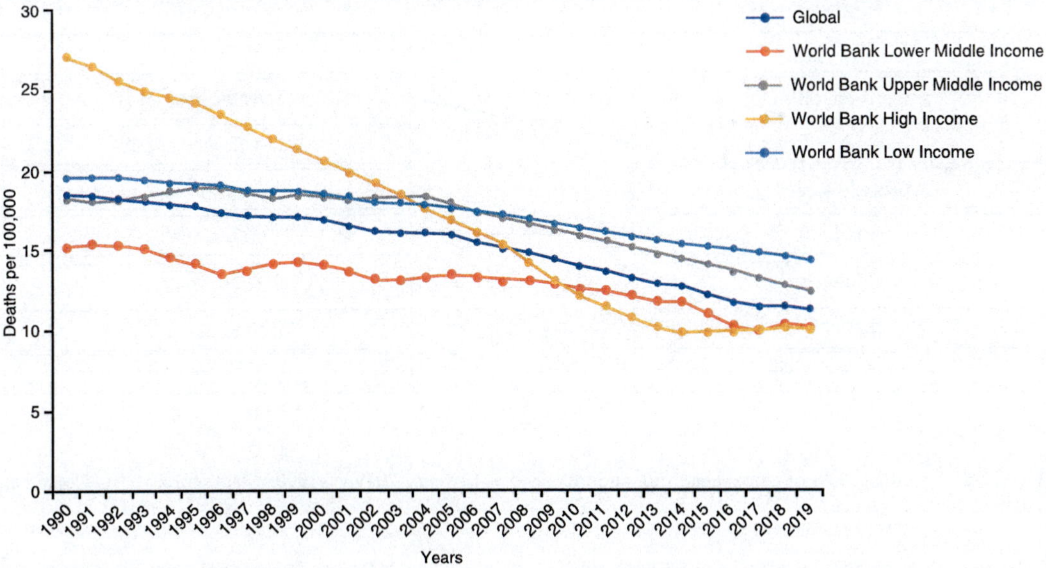

Fig. 12.3 Global road traffic injury mortality among children aged 15–19 years, 1990–2019. (Data source: GBD Compare, 2019)

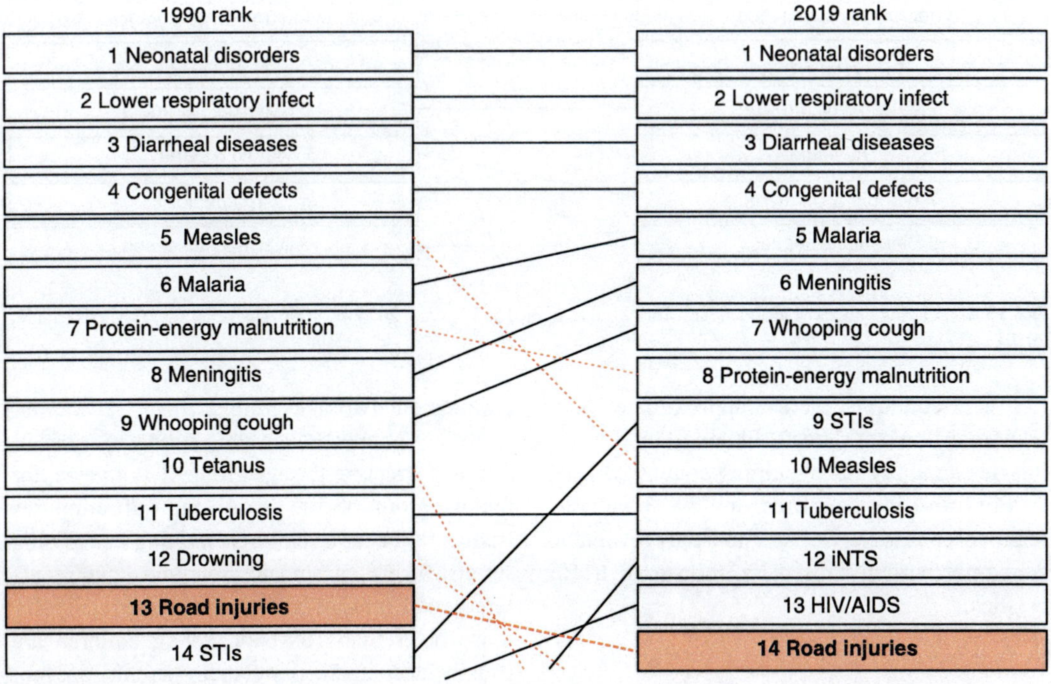

Fig. 12.4 Leading causes of global deaths for under-5 children, 2019 vs. 1990. (Data source: GBD Compare, 2019)

12.2.5 Economic Burden

Transport Research Laboratory [1], one of the most authoritative British institutions, reported that global road traffic injuries and deaths caused an economic loss of 518 billion dollars in 1997, which made up approximate 3% of GDP in most countries and had a great impact on global economic development. According to a study evaluating losses caused by road inju-

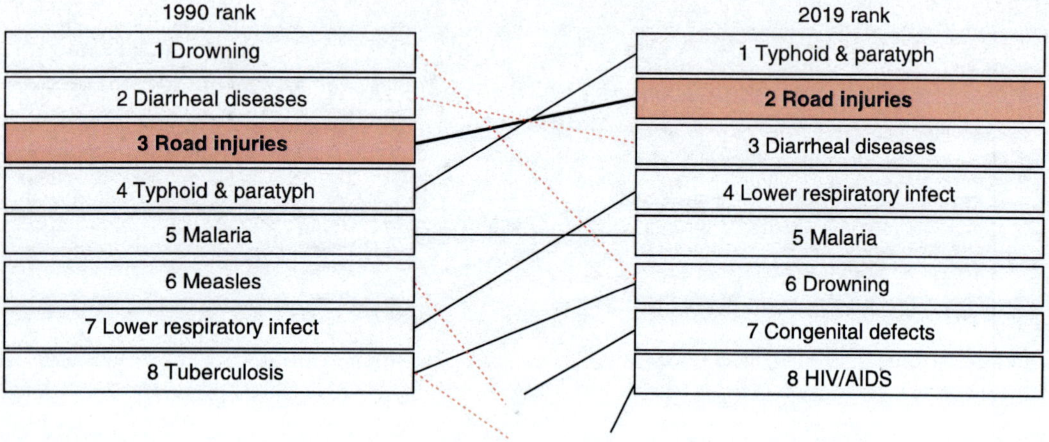

Fig. 12.5 Leading causes of global deaths for children aged 5–14 years, 2019 vs. 1990. (Data source: GBD Compare, 2019)

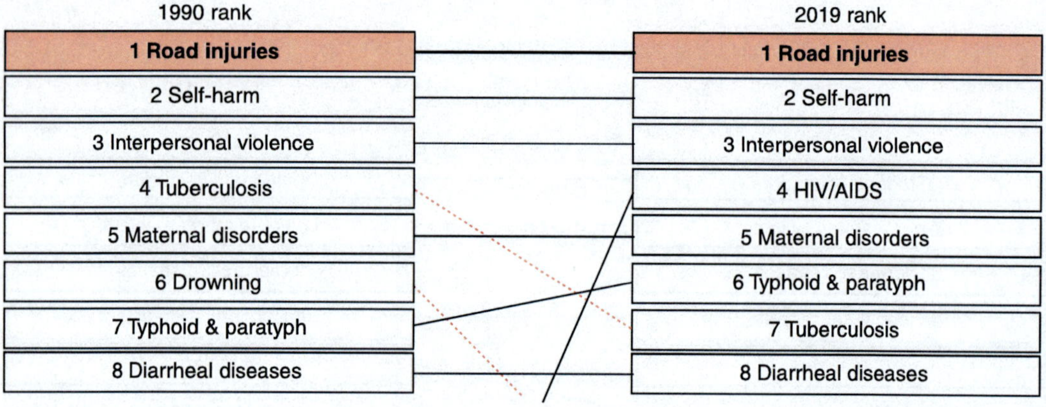

Fig. 12.6 Leading causes of global deaths for children aged 15–19 years, 2019 vs. 1990. (Data source: GBD Compare, 2019)

ries in 21 countries, there is approximate 1% of GDP loss that could be attributed to road traffic injuries annually in developing countries, 1.5% loss in transition countries, and 2% in vehicle-popular countries. So far, no study evaluates economic burden caused by child road traffic crashes.

12.2.6 Age Group

Several studies [2–4] showed a higher risk of RTI in 5–9 age group as well as 15–19 age group, which was possibly associated with individual behaviors and transportation methods of children for two age groups. Road traffic injuries often happen as children riding in a car or crossing streets at the age group of 1–4 years; for the age group of 5–9 years, road traffic injuries frequently occur as children walking or crossing streets. 58.3% of students reported having suffered road injuries while riding, especially for those older than 16 years. Young children are usually accompanied by their parents on foot and in motor vehicles. As children grow up, they become more active and independent and have requirements for school, with correspondingly less parental supervision and more transportation options either by bicycle or motorcycle, which accordingly increases the risk of road injuries.

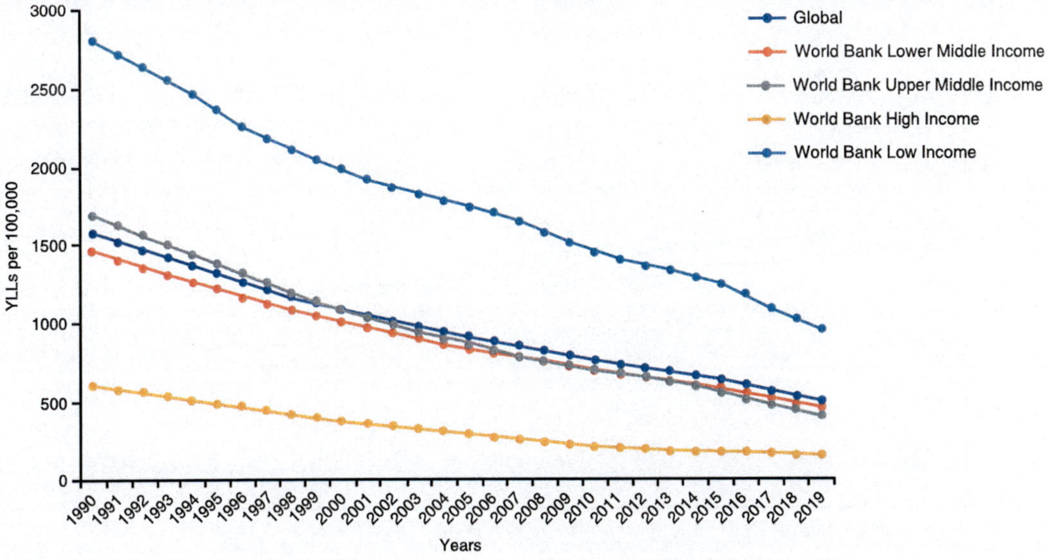

Fig. 12.7 YLLs per 100,000 population due to RTI among under-5 children, 1990–2019. (Data source: GBD Compare, 2019)

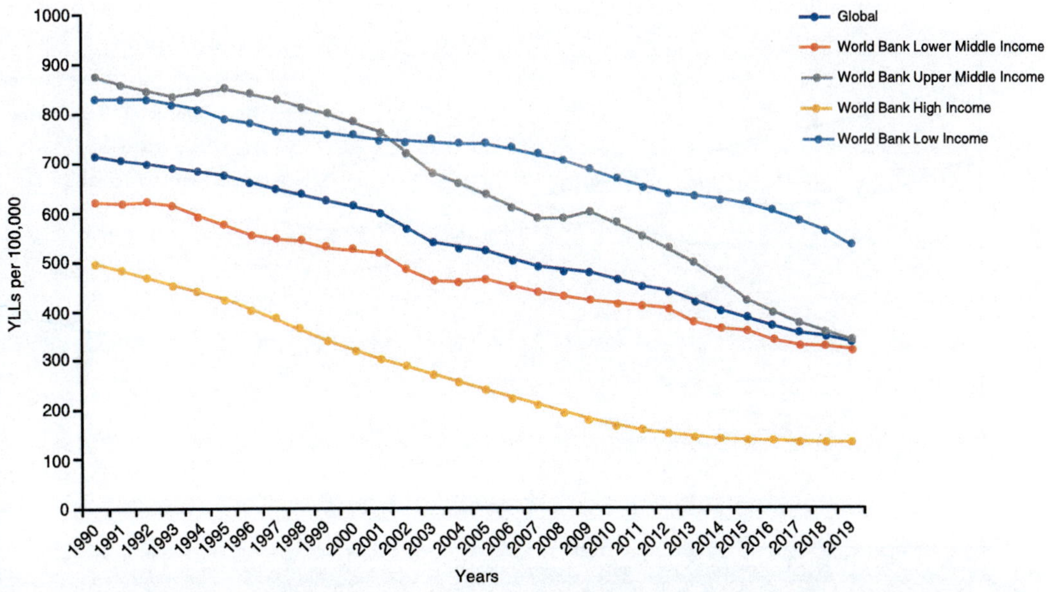

Fig. 12.8 YLLs per 100,000 population due to RTI among children aged 5–14 years, 1990–2019. (Data source: GBD Compare, 2019)

12.2.7 Region

Large child RTI morbidity and mortality variations exist across regions. At present, Africa has the highest child RTI mortality, followed by East Mediterranean. According to the WHO statistics [5], developing countries have higher rates of road traffic injuries, with 93% of fatalities occurring in low- and middle- income countries. Although Africa and East Mediterranean have the highest RTI mortality rates, two-thirds of global child road traffic deaths occur in Southeast Asia and West Pacific. Even in European Union countries where RTI mortality rates are comparatively low, 20% of total child deaths are caused by RTI.

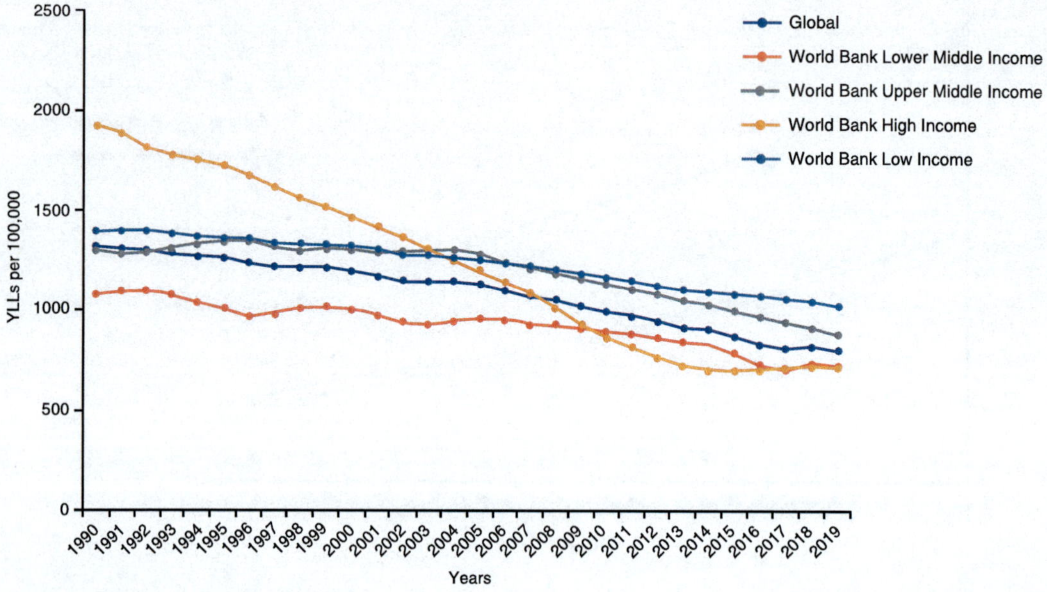

Fig. 12.9 YLLs per 100,000 population due to RTI among children aged 15–19 years, 1990–2019. (Data source: GBD Compare, 2019)

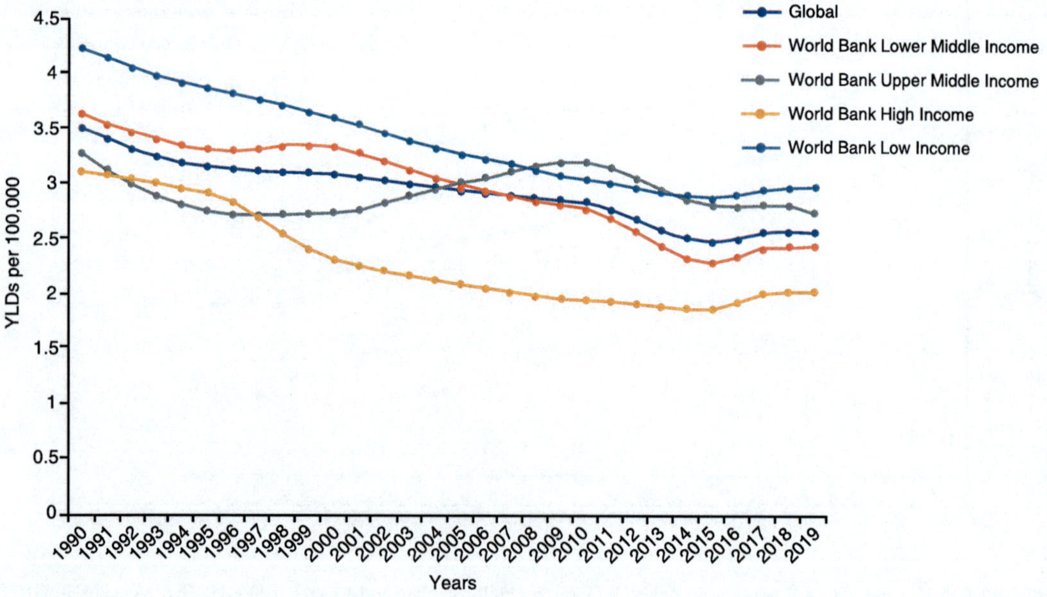

Fig. 12.10 YLDs per 100,000 population due to RTI among under-5 children, 1990–2019. (Data source: GBD Compare, 2019)

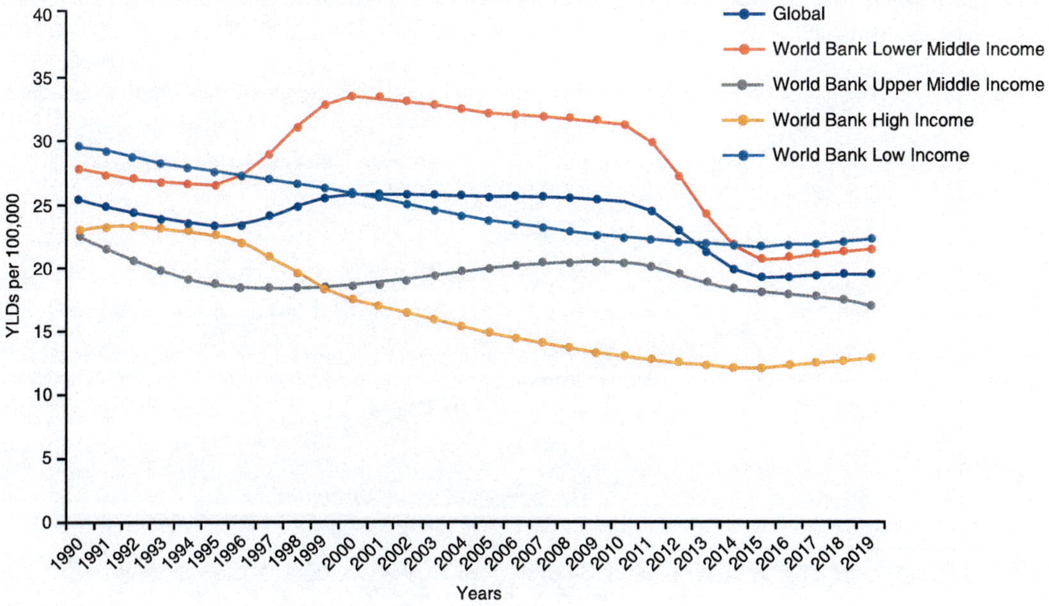

Fig. 12.11 YLDs per 100,000 population due to RTI among children aged 5–14 years, 1990–2019. (Data source: GBD Compare, 2019)

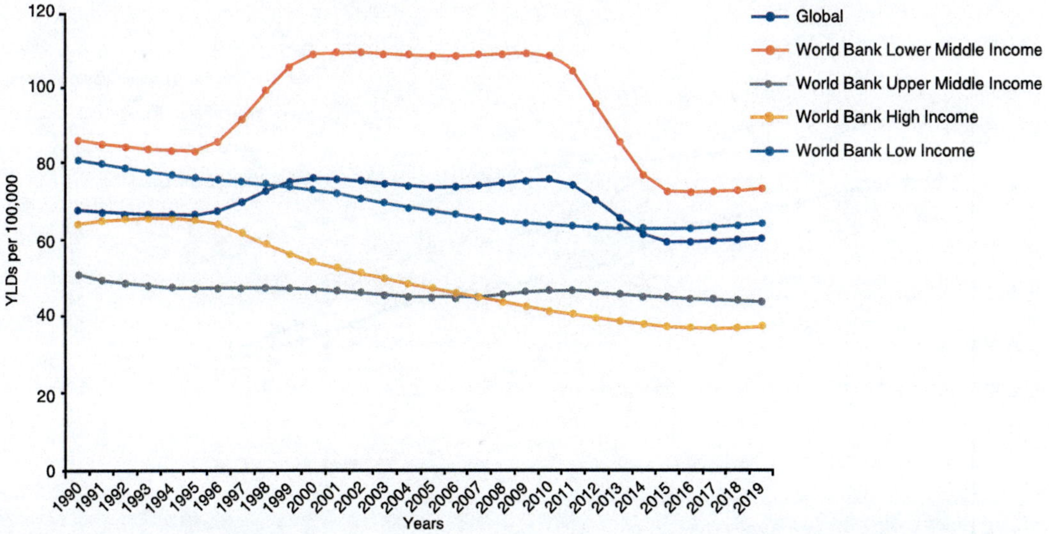

Fig. 12.12 YLDs per 100,000 population due to RTI among children aged 15–19 years, 1990–2019. (Data source: GBD Compare, 2019)

12.2.8 Date and Time

The occurring time of child RTI is closely related to pedestrian traffic density, children's activities, and parental supervision. A study by Duan et al. [6] on the traffic safety status of child pedestrians in three Chinese cities reported that most child RTIs occur in summer holiday in Chinese cities. A study from Romania [7] reported a higher child RTI incidence in summer and linked higher rates with lack of supervision, range of activity area, and time during summer vacation.

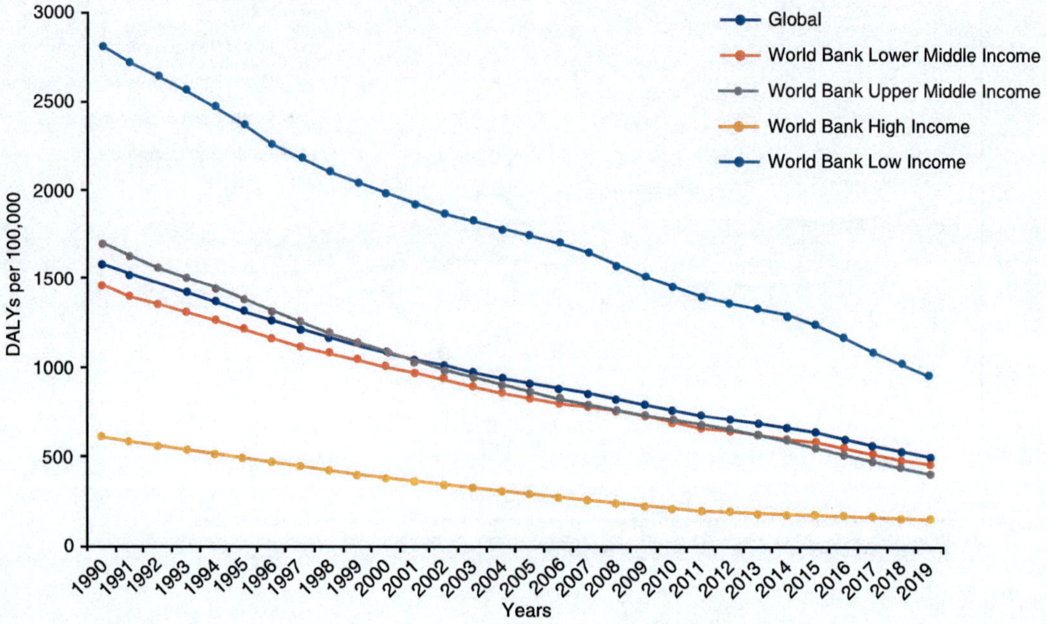

Fig. 12.13 DALYs per 100,000 population due to RTI among under-5 children, 1990–2019. (Data source: GBD Compare, 2019)

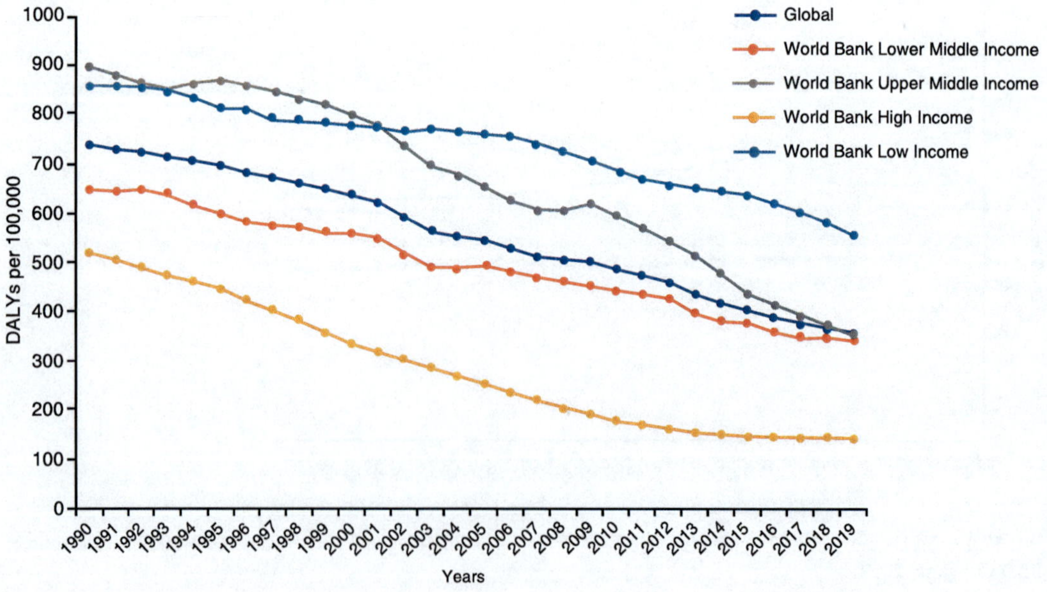

Fig. 12.14 DALYs per 100,000 population due to RTI among children aged 5–14 years, 1990–2019. (Data source: GBD Compare, 2019)

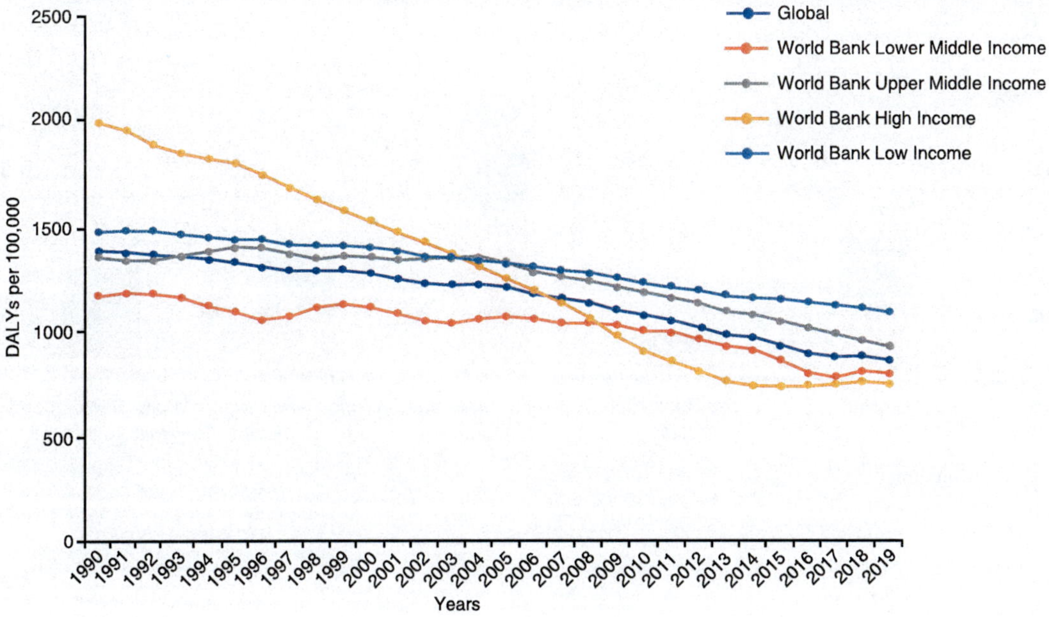

Fig. 12.15 DALYs per 100,000 population due to RTI among children aged 15–19 years, 1990–2019. (Data source: GBD Compare, 2019)

Child RTIs mainly occur at around 8 a.m., 11–12 a.m., and 15–18 p.m., corresponding with school hours and peak traffic hours.

12.2.9 Transportation Method

The severity and type of child RTIs are related to the choice of transportation method. According to statistics of 70 countries by the WHO, approximately 33% of child fatalities were pedestrians, other 65% of whom were vehicle passengers, bicyclists, or motorcyclists.

Transportation method related to fatal child RTIs varies greatly with countries with different economic levels. In low- and middle-income countries, the most common transportation methods of fatal RTIs are walking, cycling, and motorcycling; pedestrians, bicyclists, and motorcyclists have to share the road, raising the risk of RTIs. Due to high motorization, low legal driving age, and high proportion of junior drivers, motor vehicle occupant mortality is much high in high-income countries, especially among junior drivers.

In 2019, pedestrians and motor vehicle passengers were the most common road users of global RTI mortality among under-5 children, accounting for 44.2% and 41.9% of fatal RTIs for boys and 48.3% and 41.6% of fatal RTIs for girls. Generally, under-5 RTI mortality for pedestrians and for motor vehicle occupants substantially decreased as the country income increased, fastest in high-income countries and slowest in low-income countries. In high-income countries, pedestrian, motor vehicle, motorcyclist, and cyclist deaths accounted for 43.5%, 50.0%, 2.8%, and 2.3% for boys and 35.0%, 59.0%, 2.7%, and 1.9% for girls; the numbers were 40.5%, 45.2%, 9.0%, and 4.3% for boys and 48.3%, 42.9%, 5.8%, and 1.8% for girls in low-income countries (Fig. 12.16).

Among children aged 5–14 years old, pedestrian and motor vehicle road injuries remained as the two main contributors of child RTIs mortality, which explained 46.3% and 36.1% for boys and 48.5% and 39.5% for girls of child road traffic deaths. In high-income countries, motor vehicle road injuries made up 46.0% of fatal RTI deaths for boys and 59.1% of fatal RTI deaths for girls.

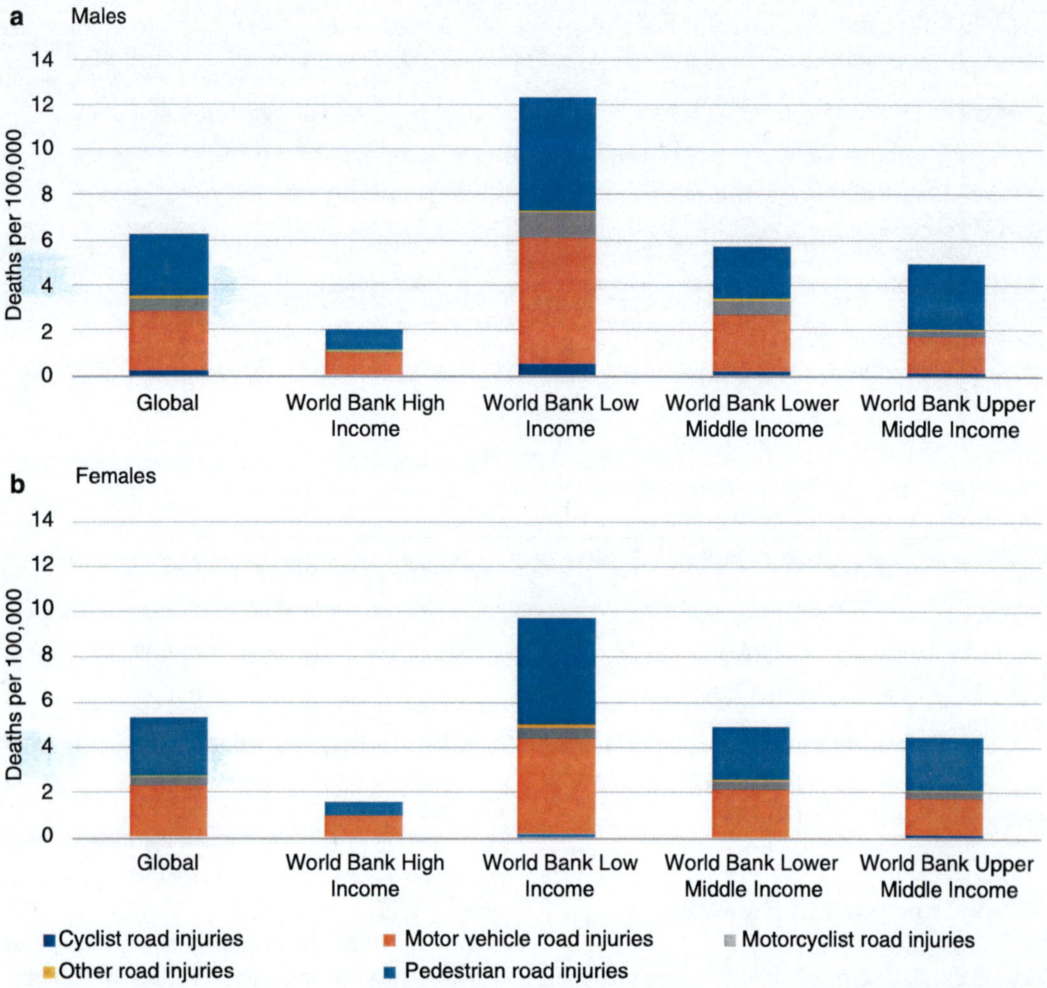

Fig. 12.16 Under-5 road traffic injury deaths per 100,000 population by sex, road user, and country income in 2019. (Data source: GBD Compare, 2019)

In addition, the proportion of cycling deaths rose in this age group, especially for boys (Fig. 12.17).

Among children aged 15–19 years old, riding in motor vehicles (excluding motorcycles), motorcycling and walking were the leading transportation methods of RTI deaths, accounting for 40.2%, 29.8%, and 24.6% of RTI deaths for boys and 50.8%, 14.6%, and 29.6% for girls, respectively.

In high-income countries, RTI mortality for motor vehicle occupants, motorcyclists, and pedestrians accounted for 64.7%, 18.9%, and 12.6% of fatal RTI deaths for boys and 78.5%, 6.6%, and 11.8% for girls, respectively. While in low-income countries, the proportions were 51.1%, 12.2%, and 32.5% for boys and 53.1%, 6.4%, and 36.7% for girls, respectively (Fig. 12.18).

12.3 Influencing Factors of RTI

The occurring mechanisms of injury change with external cause of injury. Based on the four-layer socio-ecological model proposed by Dahlberg et al [8], the US CDC divides the risk factors of injury individual, interpersonal, communal, and social levels.

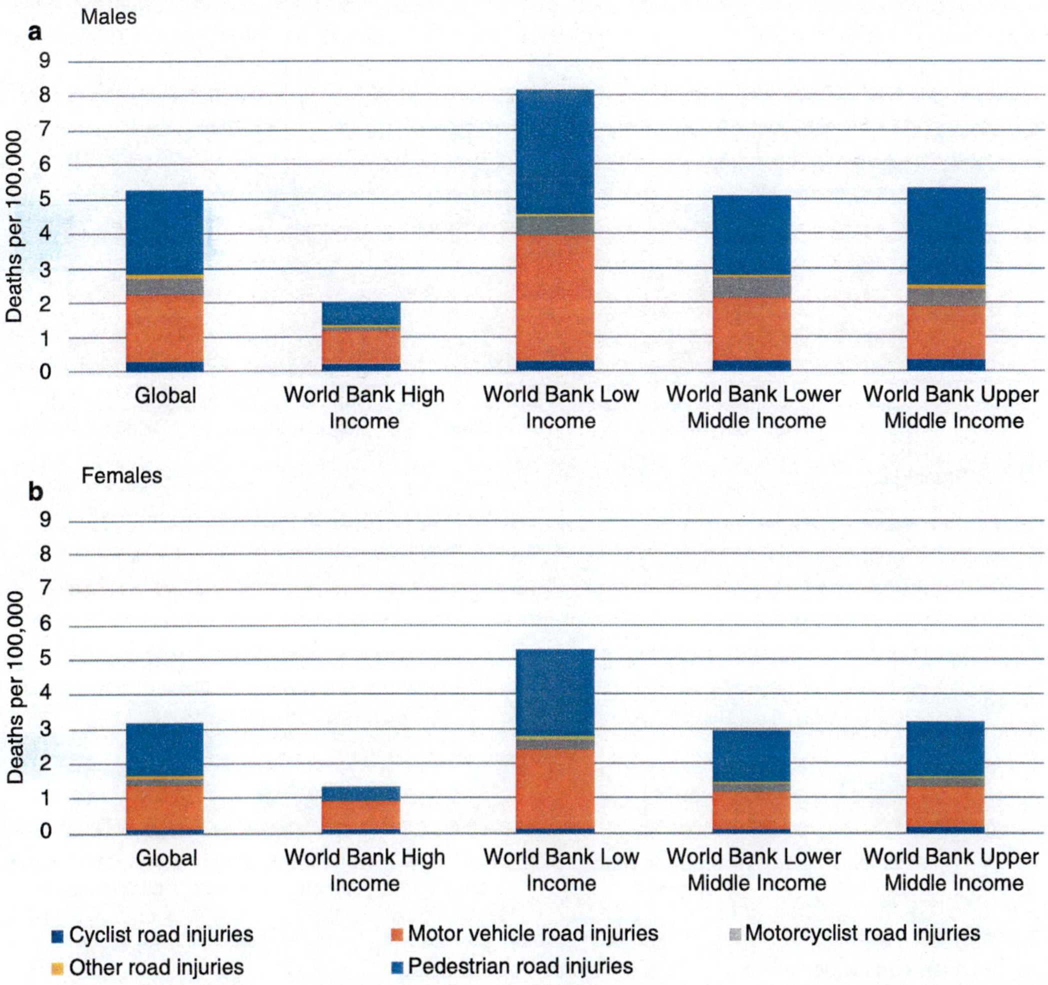

Fig. 12.17 Road traffic injury deaths per 100,000 population among children aged 5–14 years by sex, road user, and country income in 2019. (Data source: GBD Compare, 2019)

The Haddon matrix, developed by William Haddon [9], has been widely regarded as the most recognized model to explore the occurrence and prevention of a given injury event. The Haddon matrix is a grid with four columns and three rows, which describes four types of influencing factors (host, vehicle, physical environment, social environment) in three phases (pre-event, event, post-event). Table 12.2 illustrates an application of the Haddon matrix to child RTI. The influencing factors of child RTI are briefly introduced according to the stratification of host (human), vehicle (vector), physical environment, and social environment.

12.3.1 Host

12.3.1.1 Driver

People, vehicle, and road environment are three types of factors that cause traffic crashes. Epidemiological studies [10] show that around 95% of traffic crashes are attributed to human factors in China and 90% of which are caused by drivers. Research evidences show that accident-prone drivers and non-accident drivers differ in many aspects such as body shapes, physiological functions, night visions, dynamic visions, depth perceptions, attentions, complex reaction judgments, operational skills, hazard judgments,

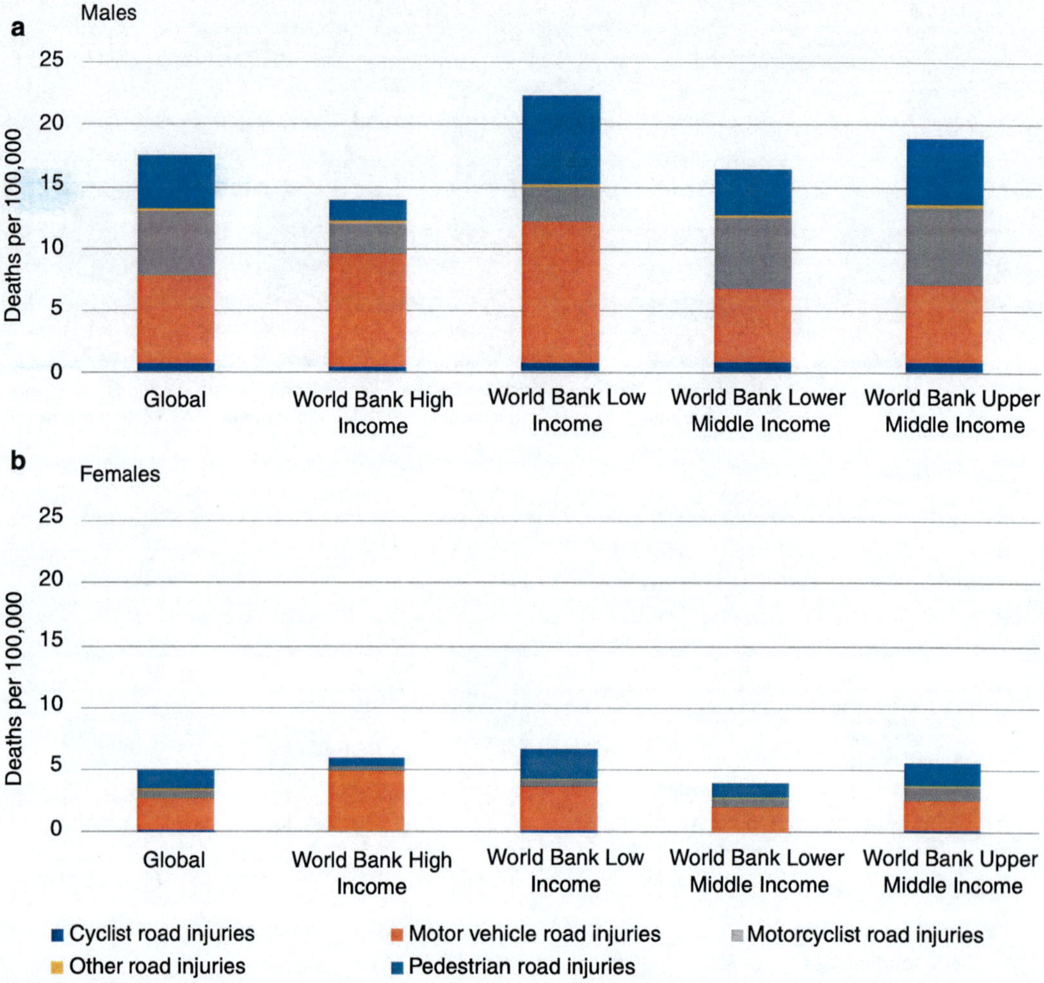

Fig. 12.18 Composition of deaths by transportation methods for children aged 15–19, categorized by World Bank income levels. (Data source: GBD Compare, 2019)

Table 12.2 Application of the Haddon matrix to child RTI prevention

Phase	Host	Vehicle	Physical environment	Social environment
Pre-event	Driver's ability and training, visual aids	Brakes, inspection, installation, and check of child safety seats	Suitable road signs, child safety seats with correct installment and suitable size	Attitude toward intoxicated driving, overspeed driving, and child safety seats
Event	Resistance to the crash, use of restraints (seat belts, child safety seats)	Invulnerability of vehicles and child safety seats	Crash-protective roadside objects, unsafe objects in vehicles	Mandatory seat belts and child safety seats
Post-event	Victim's health status	Fire risk	Effective and timely aids	Trauma treatment and rehabilitation

safety attitude, personality, aggressive personality, psychological disorders, etc. Driving a motor vehicle is a complex mission, which takes drivers a long time to improve their skills from basic level to proficient level. A study conducted in four countries (Australia, Japan, Malaysia, and Singapore) from 1986 to 1987 found that motorcyclists with provisional licenses had the highest risk of RTI, followed by motorcyclists with driving experience less than 1 year. Another study reported that motorists with riding experience less than 1 year had the highest risk of RTI.

12.3.1.2 Victim

As children are small in stature and thus have limited and imperceptible view of road traffic environment, they are more vulnerable to RTI. Immature cognitive development also affects children's ability to make judgments and decisions involving the safety of different transportation methods. Children have not yet developed a concept of traffic safety before 5–7 years old and cannot accurately identify road traffic hazards until they are 11 years old. Individuals are not mature in terms of competencies like drawing inferences, making decision, and controlling impulses before they are 20 years, making children tend to make incorrect judgments about traffic environment and have dangerous behaviors.

As children get older, especially when they enter puberty, their needs for independence and mobility increase. Driven by adolescent rebellion, impulsiveness, curiosity, and pursuit of excitement, children start to actively attempt some dangerous behaviors, which is more common among boys than girls; this is a major reason for the comparatively high road traffic injury risk among boys. Furthermore, children are susceptible to peer influence and attempting dangerous things encouraged by peers or performing dangerous behaviors to fill up self-vanity during puberty.

12.3.1.3 Seat Belt

Current research evidences show that the use of seat belt can reduce the risk of injury by 40–50%, serious injury by 43–65%, and fatalities by 40–60% for motor vehicle drivers and passengers. Because of differences in legislation and law enforcement, the use of seat belt in motor vehicles varies across countries. A research in Kenya [11] found that among drivers and passengers using seat belts, only 1% were injured in a crash. Another research in Argentina [12] reported that only 26% of drivers and front-seat passengers used seat belts in the city of Buenos Aires and 58% on national highways.

In the United States [13], the proportion of front passengers using seat belts rose from 58% in 1994 to 75% in 2002. A study [14] conducted in Guangzhou and Nanning of China found that the rate of seat belt use in the two cities was 72.2% and 71.9%, respectively.

12.3.1.4 Child Safety Seat

Child safety seats have an important role in preventing child RTI. It was reported [15] that proper installation and use of child safety seats can reduce the risk of death in crashes by about 70% for infants and 47–54% for children aged 1–4 years, respectively. Different types of safety seats should be considered for children with different ages. For infants aged 0–15 months and weighing less than 13 kg, rear-facing child safety seats provide better protection. The use of forward-facing child safety seats can reduce injuries by 34% and severe injuries by 60%, while rear-facing child safety seats can reduce injuries by 76% and severe injuries by 90%. Child safety seats are frequently utilized in developed countries, with 90% in Australia and 86% in the United States. However, incorrect installation and improper use of safety seats are common. Previous studies reported that incorrect use of safety seats ranged from 44% to 81%. A study conducted by the National Highway Traffic Safety Administration (NHTSA) [16] found that 72.6% of 3442 cases did not use safety seats correctly, and the most improper use of which were wearing adult seat belts and not fastening the belts on child safety seats. A study conducted among parents in Shanghai [17] showed that less than 30% of parents purchased safety seats for their children. The actual use of child safety seats was even lower due to children crying and the trouble of installation and disassembly.

12.3.1.5 Intoxicated Driving

Intoxicated driving raises the likelihood of both crashes and fatal or severe non-fatal injuries. A survey conducted in EU countries [18] showed that 1–3% of drivers reported having ever experienced an intoxicated driving. A study in low- and middle-income countries found that alcohol was detected in the blood of 33–69% of drivers killed in crashes and 8–29% of those injured. A study in New Delhi, India [19], reported that one-third of two-wheeled motorcyclists who were brought to hospital for treatment answered having drunk before driving. A similar risk exists in pedestrians consuming too much alcohol. A study in South Africa [20] revealed that over 61% of pedestrian dying in crashes had alcohol consumption. A recent British study [21] reported that 48% of pedestrians killed in car crashes had alcohol consumption.

12.3.1.6 Safety Helmet

Head trauma is a leading cause of death for two-wheeler motorcyclists and riders, explaining 75% of all-cause mortality in Europe and 55–88% in Malaysia. A study [22] by Kulanthayan et al. found that drivers not wearing safety helmets were three times more likely to suffer a head injury than those wearing safety helmets. Servadei [23] reported that safety helmets reduced fatal and severe head injuries by 20–45%. However, a US study found that nearly half of drivers and two-wheeled motorcycle riders using substandard safety helmets were at higher risk to suffer a head trauma than those not using safety helmets.

If children on bicycles wear safety helmets, the probability of experiencing a head injury in a crash would reduce by 63%, as well as loss of consciousness reduces by 86%. So far, legislative request that cyclists should wear safety helmets have been introduced in many countries like Australia, New Zealand, Sweden, and the United States.

12.3.1.7 Distracted Driving

Distracted driving behaviors involve all behaviors that interfere with driver's attention while driving, and endanger safety of drivers, passengers, and others. Common distracted driving behaviors include answering the phone, making a phone call, sending and receiving a text message, eating, drinking, talking to passengers, making up, looking at maps, using navigation, watching videos, and using a radio, CD, or MP3 player, using wireless communication devices to make and receive phone calls and text messages. Recent studies show that drivers' reaction time increases from 0.5 to 1.5 seconds while using mobile phone, making drivers difficult to keep in the right lane, maintain right speed, and make judgment for a safe distance. Drivers who use a mobile phone while driving are at four-time risk to suffer a crash than those not using mobile phone.

12.3.2 Vehicle

Vehicle design has a vital impact on RTI. Vehicle design defects lead to around 3–5% of traffic crashes. The design, testing, and maintenance of motor vehicles are closely correlated with the risk of RTIs. A British study reported that comprehensive improvements of vehicles, roads, legislation, and enforcement can reduce fatal or severe road traffic crashes by 33%, while the improvement of vehicle could reduce the number by 15.4%. Another study conducted in New Zealand drew a similar conclusion. It could reduce the hazards to pedestrians and cyclists if the front end of a vehicle is improved. The European Committee for the Promotion of Vehicle Safety [24] has designed performance tests for the front end of motor vehicles; the United States and the European Union has required to vehicles with forward crash prevention systems, and about 40 countries had agreed on the draft United Nations Regulation for cars with Advanced Emergency Braking Systems (AEBS) avoiding forward collision in 2019. Crashworthiness and immobilization devices need to be considered in the design of motor vehicles if we want to improve devices protecting passengers. In general, high-income countries adopt new test models of minibuses to ensure that the passenger compartment retains its shape and structure and the fixture devices function in a collision. Most high-income countries mandate that seat belts in cars and light trucks reach certain technical standards. In low- and middle-income countries, more than half of motor vehicles may not be equipped with reliable seat belts.

12.3.3 Natural Environment

About 2.9% of road traffic injuries can be attributed to road factors, and approximately 24.3% of road traffic injuries in China are associated with roads. Unsafe road environments increase the risk of child RTIs. Recently, the number of motor vehicles has increased rapidly in many countries and regions, but road construction and management lags in these countries. Lack of safe and efficient public transportation system not only causes road congestion but also raises the likelihood of RTIs. In addition, fast-traveling or slow-traveling motor vehicles and unreasonable road design are important risk factors of RTIs.

12.3.4 Socioeconomic Environment

12.3.4.1 Incidence of Traffic Crashes Among Children

Socioeconomic status is associated with the incidence of traffic crashes among children. The flourishing commercial economic activities increase people's travels and therefore raise the chances of road traffic crashes.

The World Bank analyzed the data of 88 countries between 1963 and 1999 and found that the mortality of RTIs rose sharply with the increase of gross domestic product (GNP) per capita; when the GNP per capita reached 1180 US dollars, RTI mortality began to decline as the GNP per capita grew.

12.3.4.2 Emergency Care

Pre-hospital emergency care is closely related to the treatment outcome of RTI patients. A review of European countries concluded that about 50% of road traffic deaths occurred within minutes of the collision, some of them died on the spot of car crashes and some died on route to hospital; about 15% of deaths occurred within 4 hours of crashes and died in hospital; and 35% of deaths occurred 4 hours later than crashes. In low- and middle-income countries, the majority of RTI deaths occur on the road to the hospital. Lack or low-level pre-hospital emergency care significantly delays the best time of treatment.

12.3.4.3 Trauma Treatment

Trauma care has developed rapidly recently. Unfortunately, many people in low- and middle-income countries still cannot access public health or individual commercial insurance in hospitals due to a large shortage of qualified surgeons. A study in Ghana reported that, of people who experience severe injuries in car crashes, only 38% in rural areas and 60% in urban areas were admitted to hospitals for treatment. Traumatic brain injury is the leading cause of RTI deaths. Because of lack of hospital admissions and qualified physicians, children who are seriously injured in road traffic crashes cannot receive timely treatment and probably die or have lifetime disabilities.

12.4 Interventions

12.4.1 Theories of Injury Intervention

The general intervention theories are also applicable to child road traffic injury prevention. Here, we briefly describe Haddon's ten strategies, the "5Es" intervention theory, and active and passive intervention strategies.

12.4.1.1 Haddon's Ten Strategies

Haddon proposed ten prevention strategies based on the Haddon matrix, including:

① Prevent the creation of the hazard in the first place, such as stopping the manufacture of some toxic substances.
② Reduce the amount of energy contained in the hazard, such as car speed limits.
③ Prevent or reduce the release of the hazard, such as the bathroom floor should not be too slippery.
④ Modify the rate or spatial distribution of the hazard from its source, such as the use of seat belts.
⑤ Separate people in time or space from the hazard and its release, such as bicycle and pedestrian pathways.

⑥ Separate people from the hazard by interposing a material barrier, such as the use of insulation to separate the cable and pedestrians.
⑦ Modify the relevant basic qualities of the hazard, such as eliminating the angles of objects in the kindergarten.
⑧ Make the person more resistant to damage.
⑨ Counter the damage already done by the hazard, such as setting up alarm telephone along roadside.
⑩ Stabilize, repair, and rehabilitate the injured person.

The ten strategies apply to the design of injury prevention interventions of all injury causes at all age groups.

12.4.1.2 "5Es" Intervention Theory

Interventions can be divided into five categories by their characteristics (5Es are the abbreviation of the initials of five types of interventions), including:

① Education strategy: to enhance people's awareness of the risk of injury through safety education and then reduce the dangerous behaviors
② Environmental modification strategy: to reduce the likelihood of injury to individuals by reducing environmental risk factors
③ Engineering strategy: to produce safer products through design and innovation
④ Enforcement strategy: to establish the laws and enforce the laws strictly to maintain certain behaviors and norms and also prohibit dangerous behaviors that increase the risk of injuries
⑤ Evaluation strategy: to evaluate the available interventions to prevent and control injuries and to determine the most effective interventions, programs, and policies

12.4.1.3 Active and Passive Intervention Strategies

Injury prevention strategies [25] can be divided into active interventions and passive interventions according to the behaviors that the host (individual) takes. Active interventions refer to intentional behavior changes through the choice of safety equipment or the adoption of safer behaviors to avoid injury, such as wearing a helmet correctly when riding a bicycle. Passive interventions refer to equipping the external environment with safety facilities to avoid injury or reduce the severity of injury when individuals are exposed to external intolerable energy such as installing airbags in a car, which will automatically open in the event of a crash.

12.4.2 Interventions

In 2010, the United Nations launched *the Global Road Safety 2011–2020 Action Plan*. The WHO released *the Global Status Report on Road Safety 2009* in the same year and regularly updates the report every 2 years since then. This report systematically assesses the legislation and enforcement of proven RTI interventions of the participating countries. In 2013, the WHO proposed ten strategies to prevent road traffic injury for children, including controlling speed, reducing drink and driving, using helmets for bicyclists and motorcyclists, improving children's ability to see and be seen, restraining children in vehicles, enhancing road infrastructure, adapting vehicle design, reducing risks for young drivers, providing appropriate care for injured children, and supervising children around roads.

Next, we present a brief summary of main interventions for child RTI based on the recent published literature.

12.4.2.1 Legislation

Legislation is a mandatory intervention. Legislation has the strongest public warning and enforcement power. Currently, the WHO recommends five legislative interventions to all WHO member states, including managing speeding, reducing drink-driving, increasing motorcycle helmet use, increasing seat belt use, and increasing child restraint use.

Between 2014 and 2017, 123 countries had laws meeting the best practice of at least one of five behavioral risk factors. However, only France, Hungary, Italy, Luxembourg, and Sweden had laws that meet the best practice of all five key risk factors (Fig. 12.19).

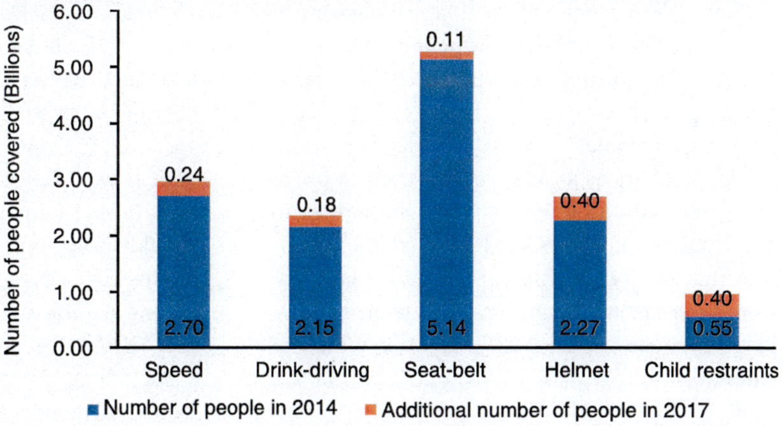

Fig. 12.19 Number of people covered by laws meeting the best practice, 2017 vs. 2014. (Data source: Global status report on road safety 2018. Geneva: World Health Organization, 2008.)

12.4.2.1.1 Speed Limits

A research by the WHO showed that high-speed driving accounted for about 1/3 of road traffic crashes in developed countries and up to 1/2 in developing countries. Driving at high speeds poses a significant threat to child road safety, especially on roads around schools, residential, and commercial areas. One study reported that a 5% reduction in average driving speed can reduce 30% of fatal crashes. Currently, the interventions for preventing high-speed driving include four categories: ① setting appropriate driving speeds according to use and quality of roads; ② setting maximum allowable speeds on roads with high occurring frequency of children (30 km/h is now recommended); ③ strengthening the control of road speed limits by installing automatic speed camera; and ④ separating pedestrians from speeding vehicles through establishing or improving urban sidewalks, street crossings, pedestrian underpasses, safety islands, and curb medians in road sections when needed.

(a) Speed limits supplemented by installation of pedestrian countdown signals: New York City in the United States installed pedestrian countdown signals at 1500 intersections throughout the city, set a maximum speed of 32 km/h for living areas and 75 school speed limit zones, enforced speed limits on major traffic arteries, and used mass media to inform the public about road safety and engage the public in road safety activities. Such efforts were followed by an around 25–51% decline in road traffic crashes involving pedestrians in New York City.

(b) Speed limits supplemented by pedestrian separation initiatives: London City in the United Kingdom has launched a "30 km/h" speed limit action in school zones and residential areas for a long time. The government has also built pedestrian segregation in the speed limit sections, such as street crossings, pedestrian underpasses, and safety islands. As a result of the comprehensive speed limit program, traffic safety has improved significantly among children aged 0–15 years old. Pedestrian fatality are reduced by 46% and bicyclist fatality reduced by 28% between 1987 and 2006.

(c) The use of red light camera to enforce speed limits: An analysis that compared crash data from 253 intersections in Flanders, Belgium, between 2002 and 2007 before and after the introduction of red light cameras to assist with speed limits, showed a 14% decrease in major road crashes, despite a 44% increase in rear-end crashes. In January 2011, a study that assessed the effectiveness of installing red light camera at high-crash intersections in Miami-Dade County, Florida, showed that the use of cameras reduced red light running crashes by 14% and injuries by 12% over 2 years, despite the fact that rear-end crashes increased 40% in the first year and rose 50% in 2 years.

Setting speed limits is an effective measure to reduce road traffic injuries. Although many countries have established national speed limit laws, few meet the best practice criteria for speed limit laws. As shown in Fig. 12.20, 95 countries set up speed limits equal to or under 50 km/h in urban areas, but only 84 empower local authorities to modify speed limits in local laws. 51% of countries that satisfy the three best practice laws are from high-income countries, 36% from middle-income countries, and 13% from low-income countries.

12.4.2.1.2 Restricting Drink-Driving

Laws and regulations for drink-driving mainly emphasize to raise the legal drinking age and set a maximum limit of blood alcohol concentration for drivers.

(a) Increasing the legal drinking age: The United States has an extremely strict limit for teenage drinking (current legal drinking age: 21 years old). Many states in the United States have set age limits for the purchasers who buy alcoholic beverages in supermarkets and other stores. Although China has not specified the rule, its law on *the Protection of Minors of the People's Republic of China* (article 11) requests that adult guardians should forbid people younger than 18 years old to drink alcohol beverages.

(b) Setting a limit of blood alcohol concentration (BAC) for drivers: Implementation of a BAC limit for motor vehicle drivers can reduce a number of road traffic fatalities related to drunk driving. The usual threshold of BAC is 20 mg/100 ml for drivers. Studies indicated that young drivers with a BAC of 50 mg/100 ml are twice as likely to have a road traffic crash than experienced drivers. The best practice is to set a lower BAC (20 mg/100 ml or lower) for young and novice drivers, which can dramatically reduce the number of alcohol-related traffic accidents.

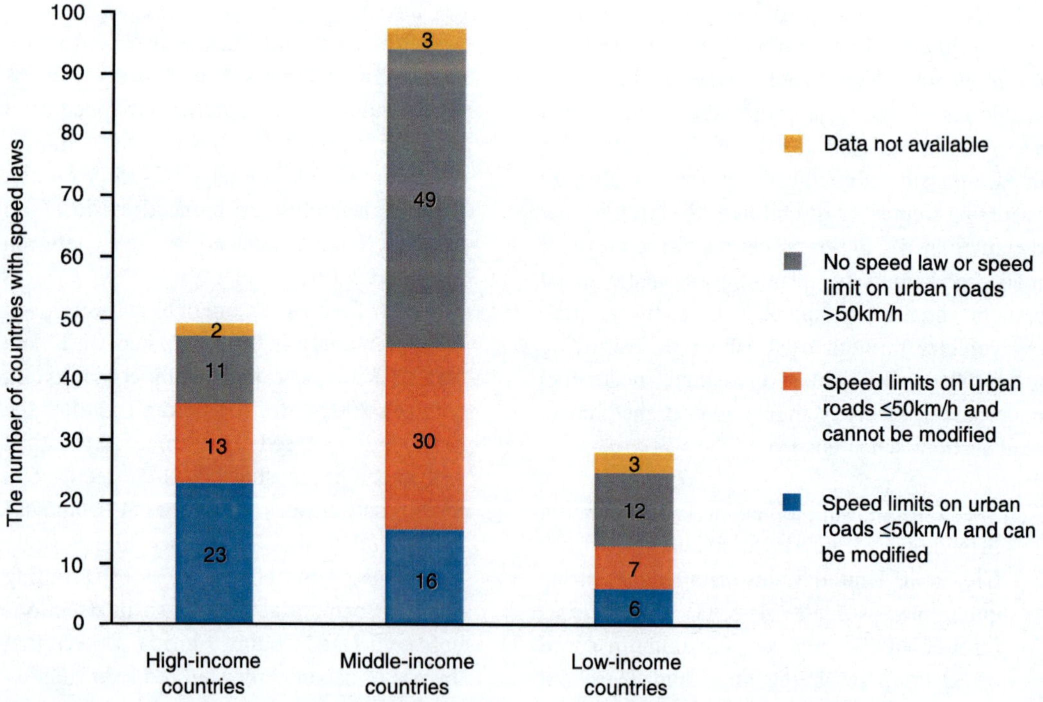

Fig. 12.20 Countries with speed laws meeting the best practice in 2017. (Data source: Global status report on road safety 2018. Geneva: World Health Organization, 2008)

A BAC of 50 mg/100 ml is acceptable. 174 countries have laws on drink-driving. Among these, 136 countries set up BAC limits; but only 45 countries both set specific limits for the general population (0.05 g/dl) and for young and novice drivers (0.02 g/dl). As shown in Fig. 12.21, 56% of countries that satisfy the three best practice laws are from high-income countries, 42% from middle-income countries, and 2% from low-income countries.

In addition, there are other interventions for drink-driving, but the effectiveness of these interventions is controversial, warranting further research to generate more solid evidence.

(a) Setting alcohol testing checkpoints: A study in the United States reported that frequent checkpoints with high publicity and visibility reduced road traffic injury crashes by about 18–24%. Alcohol testing checkpoints can easily detect drunk drivers and have a strong warning effect.
(b) Development and promotion the fitment of alcohol-locks: The American academic community has discussed the installation of alcohol concentration detection and lockout devices on motor vehicles since the 1960s. It contains an alcohol meter. Once the driver's blood alcohol level is detected to be high, the device will automatically lock the engine of motor vehicle. In 2009, Toyota Motor Corporation in Japan, together with its affiliated truck manufacturer Hino Motors, announced that they were designing an anti-drunk driving car with an alcohol interlock system in the car. The system includes a miniature alcohol meter and a digital camera, which are used to detect the alcohol level and take a picture of the driver's face to determine the identity. When the test result is positive (namely, the driver's blood alcohol concentration exceeds the law limit), the system will give a warning or lock the engine of car. Alcohol interlock systems have improved a lot recently. Several engineering studies in 2013 indicated that the conception of anti-drunk driving lockout system can be realized through integrating multiple technologies such as alcohol sensors, microcontrollers, and voice transmission.
(c) Mass media campaigns: Mass media is believed to be helpful for establishing cor-

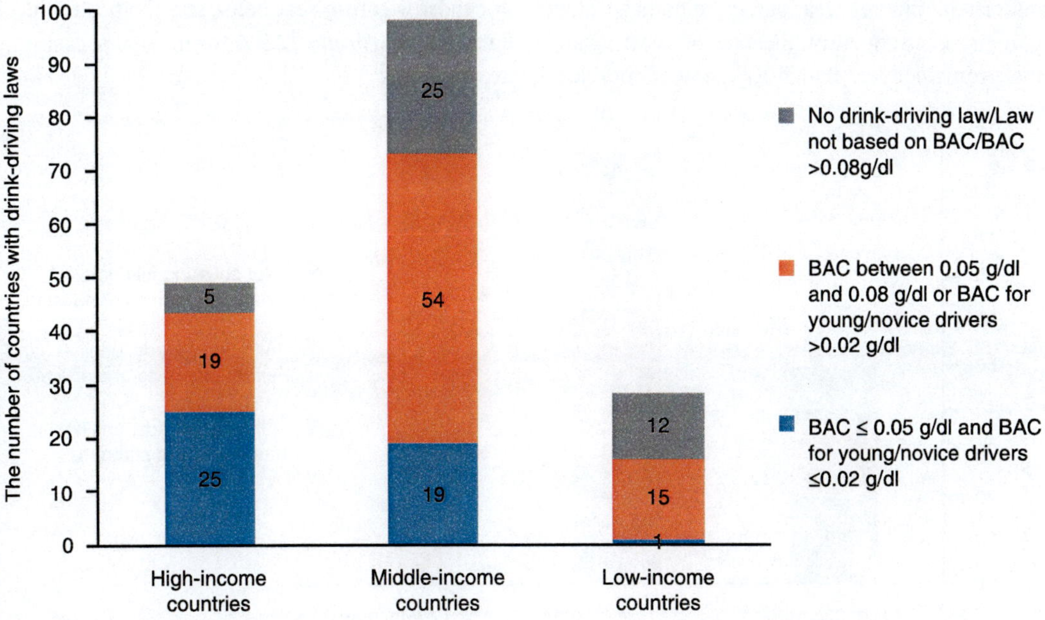

Fig. 12.21 Countries with drink-driving laws meeting the best practice in 2017. (Data source: Global status report on road safety 2018. Geneva: World Health Organization, 2008)

rect social norms against drunk driving. But implementation details must be considered.

(d) School safety education: School-based alcohol education programs were found to reduce drunk driving. Further studies showed that the success of school-based intervention programs is related to the length of time the intervention program implemented, the content of the program, and the extent of interaction with students.

12.4.2.1.3 Wearing Safety Helmets

Head and neck injuries are the leading cause of death and disability for motorcycle crashes. Substantial evidence suggests that the use of helmets effectively reduce motorcyclist injuries and fatalities. In motorcycle crashes, the rate of head injury for motorcyclists not wearing helmets is 2.19 times higher than those wearing helmets.

In late 2007, Vietnam had passed a law requesting all motorcyclists and passengers (including children) to wear a helmet. Following the law, the rate of wearing safety helmets quickly exceeded 90%, resulting in a dramatic decrease in head injury and fatality rates among motorcyclists and passengers. However, the law does not authorize traffic polices to penalize children aged 14 and under who did not wear safety helmets and their parents. Consequently, the rate of wearing helmets remained less than 40% among children.

In April 2010, the government amended the law to require children above the age of 6 to wear safety helmets when riding, which was a responsibility for their parents. After the regulation was implemented, the rate of wearing helmets in Vietnamese children rose to 56% by 2013.

Currently, the enforcement of helmet-wearing laws is generally weak. 167 countries have mandatory helmet laws for motorcyclists, but only 49 countries meet the overall best practice criteria. As shown in Fig. 12.22, 41% of countries that satisfy the overall best practice laws are from high-income countries, 53% from middle-income countries, and 6% from low-income countries.

12.4.2.1.4 Using Seat Belts

Substantial studies have proved that wearing seat belts is effective in protecting motor vehicle drivers and passengers of all age groups. It is estimated that the use of seat belt can reduce road traffic deaths and serious injuries by 60% in the United States, avoiding 18,000 deaths and an economic loss of more than 17 billion dollars. Rutledge et al. reported that the fatality rate of motor vehicle drivers and passengers was 7% for those not wearing seat belts and 3% for those wearing seat belts, and the head injury rate was 50.0% and 32.9% for the two occasions, respectively.

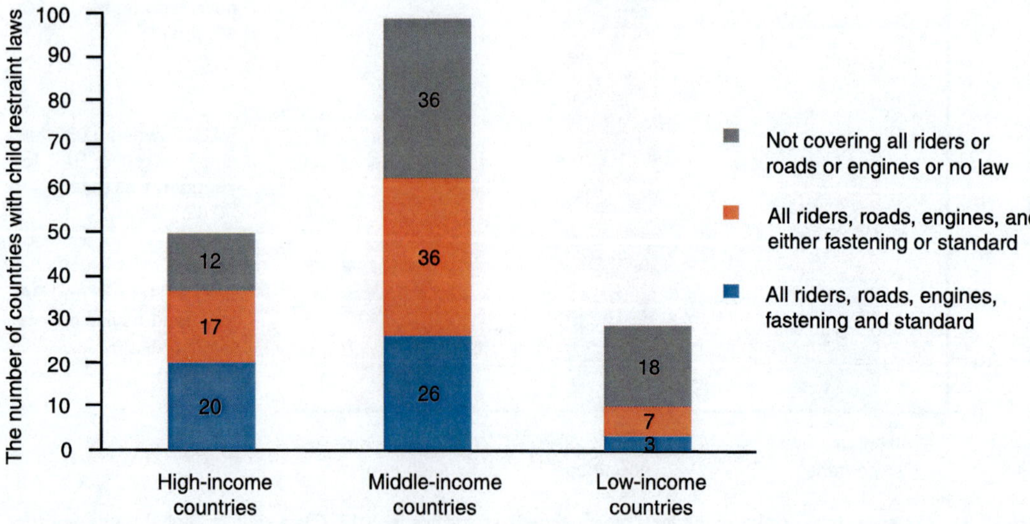

Fig. 12.22 Countries with helmet laws meeting the best practice in 2017. (Data source: Global status report on road safety 2018. Geneva: World Health Organization, 2008)

Of 161 countries with national seat belt laws in 2017, 105 countries have laws that met the overall best practice of mandating use of seat belts to all occupants, 41% of countries that are from high-income countries, 52% from middle-income countries, and 7% from low-income countries (Fig. 12.23).

12.4.2.1.5 Using of Child Restraints

Child car seats are effective in preventing non-fatal injuries and fatalities among child passengers. If correctly installed and used, child car seats can effectively protect children in vehicles and reduce the chance of hospitalization among under-5 children by 69%, the risk of road traffic deaths by 70%, and deaths of under-5 children by 54%. Compared with the use of seat belts alone, together using seat belts and child car seats can lead to a 59% reduction in the road traffic injury for children aged 4–7 years.

84 countries have national child restraint laws in 2017. Among these 33 countries, 9% of the world's population have laws that meet the overall best practice criteria, 85% of countries that are from high-income countries and 15% from middle-income countries (Fig. 12.24).

Research evidence showed that the use of child restraints was significantly associated with parental perception on its importance. In many developed countries, parents pay much more attention to the safety of children, with child safety seat use rate as high as 90%. Since July 1, 2012, the government of China implements a national standard for child safety seats (GB27887-2011); but the rate of using child car seats is still very low.

A study in Beijing [26] evaluated the effect of comprehensive interventions (including measures such as group discussions, showing child car safety promotional films, instruction and live demonstration of child booster seats, and free distribution of child car seats). The results found that 84.5% of children by car had never used a booster seat before the intervention, and 98% of children almost every day used the seat after 6 weeks, and 97% of parents indicated that they intended to continue using child car seats

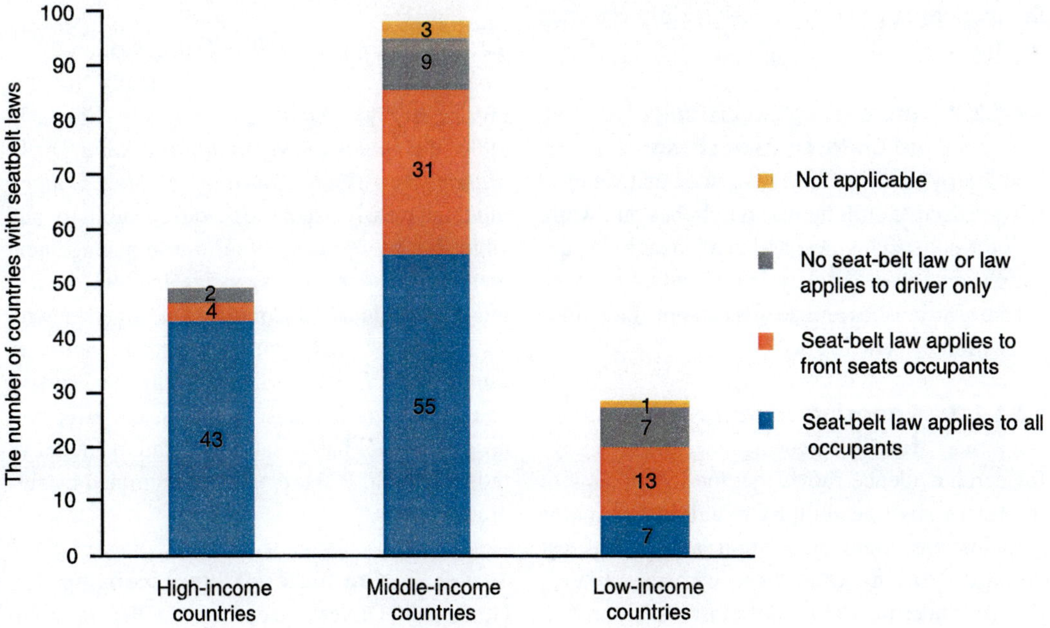

Fig. 12.23 Countries with seat belt laws meeting best practice in 2017. (Data source: Global status report on road safety 2018. Geneva: World Health Organization, 2008)

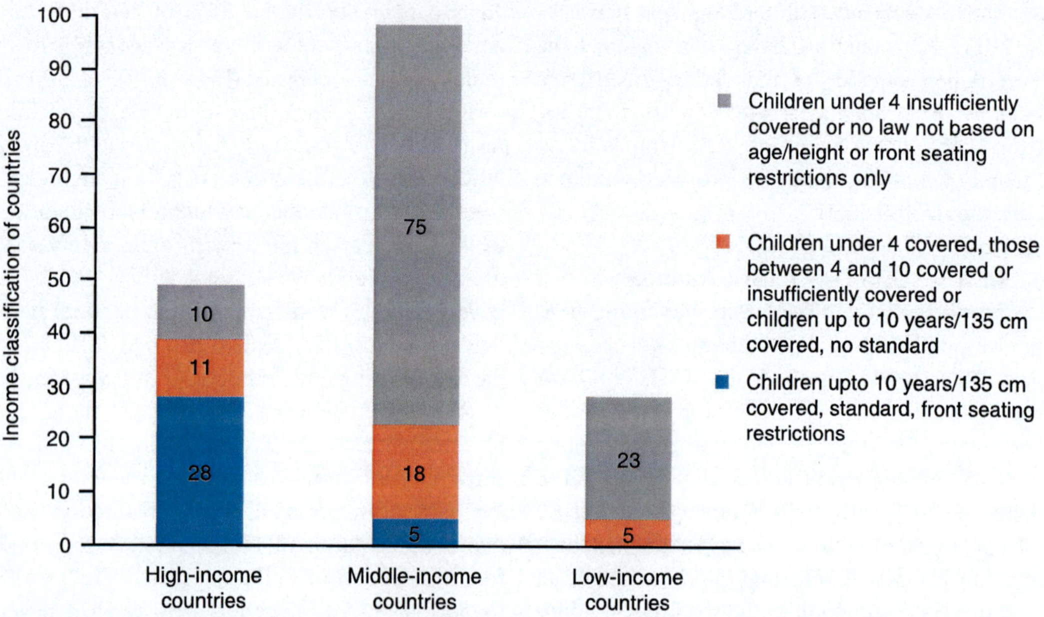

Fig. 12.24 Countries with child restraint laws meeting the best practice in 2017. (Data source: Global status report on road safety 2018. Geneva: World Health Organization, 2008)

for the next 6 months. The results of this study indicate that appropriate measures can increase the proportion of correctly using child car seats in China.

12.4.2.2 Increasing the Visibility of Children Pedestrians

A study by Wells et al. [27] showed that wearing retro-reflective and fluorescent clothes and white or light-colored helmets and using headlights are simple and practical ways to effectively reduce road traffic crashes and deaths and non-fatal injuries in motor vehicle crashes.

12.4.2.3 Choosing Suitable Car Seats for Children

Research evidence shows that the locations with the least risk of head injury to children in motor vehicles are braking position and crash test dummy position, while those with the greatest risk are innermost and outermost positions; the locations with the lowest risk of chest injury to children are medial position and crash test dummy position, while those with the highest risk are lateral position and braking position. Therefore, it is best for children to take the rear seats. Forbidding children sitting in the forward passenger seat can reduce the likelihood and severity of injuries to children during motor vehicle collisions.

12.4.2.4 School Safety Education

Road traffic safety education mainly focuses on primary and secondary schools in China. In 1986, the *Notice on Reforming the Road Traffic Management System* issued by the State Council of China clearly listed traffic safety publicity and education as a priority of all traffic management work of public security agencies. In 1996, the former State Education Commission, together with six ministries and commission issued a notice to establish the Safety Education Day for Primary and Secondary Schools. However, the effectiveness of school-based safety education model in reducing child RTIs remains unexamined by rigorous studies.

12.4.2.5 Graduated Driver Licensing

Graduated Driver Licensing (GDL) program involves three-level training according to the driver's age and driving experience:

(a) To obtain a learner's driver's license (G7, basic level), requesting that the applicants shall be above 14 years old, pass a written test and a vision test, have a valid identity document, and get parental consent if they are younger than 18 years old. If the applicants want to drive, they must be supervised by an adult driver with full license and cannot drive at midnight and early morning.

(b) To obtain an intermediate license (G5, trainee level), requesting that the applicants shall be above 16 years old and have held a G7 license at least 1 year. The applicants can drive alone but are ineligible to serve as an accompanying driver of a learner with a G7 license.

(c) To get a full or unrestricted license (G5, can instruct G7 holders to drive). The applicants must have held a junior G5 for 2 years and have no infraction record in the last year and pass an advanced road test.

In 2011, Russell et al. summarized 34 studies that evaluated the effects of 21 GDL cases and concluded that the implementation of GDL program resulted in a reduction of 8% to 27% in crash rate and of 2% to 46% in injury rate in the first year after 16-year-old teen drivers received their licenses, suggesting that GDL can significantly reduce road traffic crashes caused by lack of skills and experience of drivers.

12.4.2.6 Using Airbags with Caution

It has been proved that airbags pose a threat to child passengers in motor vehicles. Between January 1990 and January 2005, 157 children under the age of 13 were killed by the popped airbag in the non-fatal collision of low-speed vehicles in the United States. A study by the National Highway Traffic Safety Administration, with 3790 teenagers aged from 1 month to 18 years who seated in the right front seat while driving, found that children under 15 years old faced a great risk of injury when the airbag popped up. The strong impact of airbag popping up probably causes a serious injury or even lethal outcome to the children.

12.4.2.7 Improving Train for Young Drivers

Young drivers have been found to be a major cause of teenage car crashes. The results of many studies showed that underage drivers who get driving license prematurely upon the driver training are apt to cause road traffic crashes when driving.

12.4.2.8 Avoiding Distracted Driving

A review of 19 articles published between 2000 and 2013 examined the relationship between the use of a mobile phone while driving and the incidence of motor vehicle traffic crashes; the results suggested that drivers should take measures to avoid distractions (including using their mobile phones to access social media sites such as Facebook and Twitter), especially for young and inexperienced drivers. Texting and receiving messages during driving increase the risk of fatal road traffic crashes.

12.5 Conclusion

Currently, injury academic community in China and abroad has developed many effective interventions for child road traffic injury prevention. For most countries, the major challenge is how to strictly implement these interventions and monitor the progress of road traffic injury prevention interventions with reliable and valid data. Of course, necessary modifications or tailoring are needed when low- and middle-income countries like China translate the interventions proven in high-income countries. Each individual government should open child road traffic injury data to the researchers and encourage them to use the data to improve road traffic injury prevention. High-quality researches should be supported to assess the current status of child road traffic injury, identify new problems, and develop targeted interventions. Low- and middle-income countries may consider combining proven interventions with their national health initiatives to popularize these interventions.

Acknowledgments Author acknowledges Lei Yang and YouYou Wu from "Department of Epidemiology and Health Statistics, Xiangya School of Public Health, Central South University, Changsha, China" for their draft translating the chapter to English.

References

1. Jacobs G, Thomas AA, Astrop A. Estimating global road fatalities. 1st ed. Crowthorne: Transport Research Laboratory; 2000.
2. Chen RH, Zhang PB, Deng JY. An epidemiological survey of car accident injury deaths in children aged 0-14 years in Jiangsu Province. Chin J Pediatr. 1999;37(11):661–3.
3. Wang XX, He GS, Hao AH, et al. Epidemiological analysis of road traffic injuries among primary and secondary school students in Gansu Province. Disease Surveillance. 2004;19(9):353–5.
4. Chi GB, Wang SB. Analysis of long-term trends in road traffic injuries and the factors influencing them in the towel country. Chin J Epidemiol. 2007;28(2):148–53.
5. World Health Organization. Global burden of disease: 2004 update. Geneva: World Health Organization; 2008.
6. Duan LL, Sun YM, Deng X, et al. A retrospective study of road traffic safety among pedestrians in three cities in China. China Health Education. 2007;23(5):330–58.
7. Duma OO. Profile of service provided by an accident and emergency care department in connection with road traffic injuries involving children, 2003–2005. Cent Eur J Public Health. 2007;15(4):154–7.
8. Dahlberg LL, Krug EG. Violence-a global public health problem. Geneva: world health. Organization. 2002;1:56.
9. Haddon W Jr. A logical framework for categorizing highway safety phenomena and activity. J Trauma. 1972;12(3):193–207.
10. Jin HQ. Review and outlook of epidemiological studies on car accidents in China. Chin J Epidemiol. 2004;25(3):190–2.
11. Evans T, Whitehead M, Bhuiya A, et al. Challenging inequities: from ethics to action. 1st ed. Oxford: Oxford University Press; 2001.
12. Silveira AJ. Seat belt use in Argentina: a 10-year struggle. Traffic Inj Prev. 2003;4:173–5.
13. Glassbrenner D. Safety belt and helmet use in 2002: overall results. Washington DC: Department of Transport; 2002.
14. Li GL, Li LP, Mark S, Rebecca I, et al. A survey on the wearing status of seat belts in cars in Guangzhou and Nanning. Chin J Epidemiol. 2006;27(8):698–701.
15. Zaza S, Sleet DA, Thompson RS, et al. Reviews of evidence regarding interventions to increase use of child safety seats. Am J Prev Med. 2001;21(4S):31–7.
16. Lawrence ED, Kathy HL, Alan WB. Misuse of child restraints: results of a workshop to review field data results. Washington DC: NHTSA; 2005.
17. Wu XY, Yang L, Dong LP, et al. Analysis of the current situation of in-vehicle injuries among child occupants in China. J Jiamusi Univ. 2013;31(5):676–9.
18. European Transport Safety Council. Reducing injuries from alcohol impairment. Brussels: European Transport Safety Council; 1995.
19. Mishra BK, Banerji AK, Mohan D. Two-wheeler injuries in Delhi, India: a study of crash victims hospitalized in a neuro-surgery ward. Accid Anal Prev. 1984;16:407–16.
20. Peden M, Knottenbelt JD, van der Spuy J, et al. Injured pedestrians in Cape Town: the role of alcohol. S Afr Med J. 1996;16:1103–005.
21. Keigan M, Tunbridge R. The incidence of alcohol in fatally injured adult pedestrians. TRL REPORT TRL 579, 2003.
22. Kulanthayan S, Umar RS, Hariza HA, et al. Compliance of proper safety helmet usage in motorcyclists. Med J Malays. 2000;55:40–4.
23. Servadei F, Begliomini C, Gardini E, et al. Effect of Italy's motorcycle helmet law on traumatic brain injuries. Inj Prev. 2003;9:257–60.
24. European Road Safety Action Programme. Halving the number of road accident victims in the European Union by 2010: a shared responsibility. Brussels: Commission of the European Communities; 2003.
25. Liu XX, Si DM, Shi DH. Factors of childhood injury and its intervention control. Chin J Prev Med. 2000;34(4):250–2.
26. Cao RX, Zhang R. A study on parents' perceptions of car seats and interventions in Beijing. China School Health. 2015;05:548–9.
27. Wells S, Mullin B, Norton R, et al. Motorcycle rider conspicuity and crash related injury: case-control study. BMJ. 2004 Apr 10;328(7444):857.

13 Research Progress of Fracture Epidemiology

Yingze Zhang, Yanbin Zhu, Xin Xing, and Wei Chen

Abstract

Epidemiology of fracture is an essential part of epidemiological study, which consists of the incidence, proportion, risk factor analysis, and variation trend of fracture. As public requirements of health care develop, the precaution and management of fractures draw more attention. It's conducive to knowing the characteristics and the variation of each fracture and analyze the related risk factors to conduct epidemiological investigation. A thorough clinical epidemiology of fracture can be the foundation of national medical and health management policy. This epidemiologic system is the guideline of precaution and treatment management of fractures for clinical practice. This chapter mainly aims to introduce the definition, classification, epidemiological characteristics, and risk factors of fractures. And we also aim to summarize the current epidemiological characteristics and the prevention strategy development of fracture in China to help formulate prevention strategy of fractures. We hope that our data could provide the basis for clinical treatment and precaution management ultimately of our country.

Keywords

Fracture · Elderly · Prevention strategy and policy · Big epidemiologic data · Etiology and classification

Y. Zhang (✉) · Y. Zhu · W. Chen
Department of Orthopaedic Surgery, The Third Hospital of Hebei Medical University, Shijiazhuang, People's Republic of China

Orthopedic Research Institution of Hebei Province, Shijiazhuang, People's Republic of China

X. Xing
Orthopedic Research Institution of Hebei Province, Shijiazhuang, People's Republic of China

The Third Hospital of Hebei Medical University, Shijiazhuang, People's Republic of China

Fracture is one of the most common injuries in daily life, which seriously threatens human health and quality of life. With the improvement of modernization in today's society, the number and severity of fractures are increasing due to the increase of risk factors related to high violence such as traffic injuries and/or fall from a height, which has become an important public health concern. Countries around the world, especially developed countries, regularly carry out surveys on fracture incidence and risk factors and accordingly develop and evaluate corresponding social development policies to improve the national fracture status and promote the coordinated development of social economy [1–7].

China has a large population base, vast territory, complex terrain and geomorphology, and significant climatic differences, in addition to

D.-Q. Ye (ed.), *Progress in China Epidemiology*, https://doi.org/10.1007/978-981-19-2199-5_13

uneven economic development in various regions, resulting in a large number of fracture cases and the great variation in incidence rates. In recent years, with the rapid development of China's economy and the increasing aging trend of the population, the incidence of fractures caused by high-energy violence and osteoporotic fractures caused by low-energy injuries are also increasing. This not only seriously affects the quality of life of patients but also places a heavy burden on families and society. Carrying out fracture epidemiological study is helpful to understand the characteristics and changes of fracture injury in China, reveal the related risk factors of fracture, and develop targeted fracture prevention and treatment measures for the population, which has important practical significance for reducing the incidence of fracture, improving the therapeutic effect, reducing complications, reducing the disability rate, and improving the quality of life of patients.

This chapter will summarize the research progress related to epidemiology of fracture in order to provide the basis for the clinical diagnosis, treatment, and prevention and control measures of fractures in China.

13.1 Definition and Classification of Fractures

13.1.1 Definitions

A break in the integrity or continuity of bone is called a fracture. Its systemic manifestations are shock and fever; local general manifestations are pain, swelling, and dysfunction; and unique signs are deformity, abnormal activity, and bony crepitus.

13.1.2 Cause

1. Violence
   (a) Fractures occur at sites affected by direct violence. For example, after the lower leg is directly impacted by a heavy object, the tibiofibular shaft fractures at the site of impact.
   (b) Indirect violence fractures the distant site of limb through conduction, leverage, rotation, or muscle contraction. For example, when walking and slipping, palm supporting the ground, due to different angles between the upper limb and the ground, violence conducts upward, and distal radius fractures and supracondylar fractures of the humerus can occur. When an athlete strides abruptly, a torn fracture of the patella can occur due to sudden and violent contraction of the muscles.
2. Cumulative strain

   Long-term and repeated stress acts on a certain part of the bone to cause fracture. For example, fatigue fractures of the second metatarsal and lower third of the fibular shaft occur after long-distance marching or long-distance running exercises, also known as stress fractures. The fracture was not displaced but healed slowly.
3. Bone disorder

   The diseased bone is broken by slight external force, which is called pathological fracture. Such as osteomyelitis, bone tumors, severe osteoporosis, and other lesions of bone fractures.

13.1.3 Classification

There are many classification methods for fractures, and the more commonly used classification methods include traditional classification and Arbeitsgemeinschaft für Osteosynthesefragen (AO) fracture classification.

13.1.3.1 Traditional Classification Methods

1. According to whether the fracture site communicates with the outside environment, it can be divided into the following:
   (a) Closed fracture: the skin or mucosa at the fracture site is intact and does not communicate with the outside environment.
   (b) Open fracture: the skin or mucous membrane near the fracture ruptures and the fracture communicates with the outside environment.

2. According to the degree and shape of fracture, it can be divided into the following:
   (a) Incomplete fracture: the integrity or continuity of bone is only partially destroyed or interrupted. (1) Crack fracture: fractures like cracks on porcelain, without displacement, are more common in fractures of the skull, ilium, etc. (2) Greenstick fracture: fractures are similar to those in which young branches are broken and are more common in children.
   (b) Complete fracture: the integrity or continuity of bone is completely destroyed or interrupted, and tubular bone is rare. According to the direction of fracture line on X-ray, it can be divided into the following: (1) transverse fracture, the fracture line is almost perpendicular to the longitudinal axis of the shaft; (2) oblique fracture, the fracture line is not perpendicular to the longitudinal axis of the shaft; (3) spiral fracture, the fracture line was spiral; (4) comminuted fracture, if there are more than two fracture fragments, if the fracture line shows "T" type or "Y" type, it is also known as "T" type or "Y" type fracture; and (5) impacted fracture, it occurs mostly at the junction of dense bone and cancellous bone in the metaphysis of long tubular diaphyses. After fracture, dense bone is embedded in cancellous bone, which is more common in fractures of the femoral neck and surgical neck of the humerus; (6) compression fracture, bone deformation due to compression, more common in vertebral body and calcaneus fractures; (7) epiphysiolisthesis, through the fracture of epiphysis, the section of epiphysis may have different amounts of bone tissue. It occurs mostly in adolescents with patent epiphyses.
3. It can be divided into the following:
   (a) Stable fracture: the fracture end is not easy to be displaced or appropriate external fixation is not easy to be redisplaced, such as transverse fracture, twig fracture, impacted fracture, crack fracture, etc.
   (b) Unstable fracture: the fracture end is easy to be displaced or appropriate external fixation is still prone to redisplacement, such as oblique fracture, spiral fracture, comminuted fracture, and so on.

13.1.3.2 Arbeitsgemeinschaft für Osteosynthesefragen and the Association of Study of Internal Fixation (AO/ASIF) Classification

AO/ASIF fracture classification is to express the anatomical site, fracture type, and grouping of bones in Arabic numerals and English letters. A five-membered alphanumeric code was used to describe the fracture: ■■-□□.□, the first two digits represent the bone and bone segment, the next one with a letter represents the fracture type, and the last two digits represent the morphological characteristics of the fracture.

13.2 Epidemiological Characteristics of Fractures

13.2.1 Population Disposition

13.2.1.1 Age Distribution

1. Pediatric Fractures

   Children are lively and active, are curious, have poor safety awareness, are in the stage of growth and development, have incomplete bone development, and are prone to fractures. The incidence of fractures in children is strongly related to age, and the proportion of boys is high [8–11]. It has been reported that one-third of the population might have a fracture before the age of 17 years [8]. The predilection age is 3 and 11 years, the majority of boys, and supracondylar and clavicular fractures of the humerus are the most common [9].
2. Adult Fractures

   Adult fractures are complex. Different fracture types have their specific age of predilection and are related to the occupation, range of motion, and their own physiological conditions they engage in by people of this age group. The incidence of fractures in people over 50 years of age gradually increases with age [12]. Elderly osteoporotic fractures in the humerus, distal radius, spine, and hip are characterized by many complications, high mortality, long hospital stay, and high treatment costs. Studies have found that the mortality rate of hip fractures in the elderly is as high as 30% [13], and the annual cost for the treatment of osteoporotic fractures in the United States can reach 18 billion US dollars [14]. Osteoporosis in the elderly and the resulting fragility fractures are one of the major problems that seriously affect the quality of life and health of the elderly.

13.2.1.2 Gender Distribution

1. Age ≤ 50 years, incidence higher in men than in women

   Epidemiological surveys on fractures at home and abroad have shown that the incidence of fractures at all sites is almost more common in men than in women. For example, femoral shaft fractures, accounting for 24.2% of femoral fractures and 2.9% of total body fractures, are significantly more common in men than in women. And according to the AO classification, from 32A, 32B, to 32C, the number of fractures gradually decreases and the sex ratio gradually increases [15]. Studies have shown that the male to female ratio of spinal cord injury is 4.70:1 [16]. Adult thoracolumbar fractures are more common in men (51.67%) than in women (48.33%) [17].
2. Age > 50 years, higher incidence in women than in men

   After menopause in women, bone loss occurs rapidly with age; however, bone loss is not significant in men, which makes the incidence of fractures in elderly women significantly increase compared with men, and in people over 50 years of age, the prevalence of fractures gradually increases with age, significantly more in women than in men [12]. Among people aged >60 years in China, there are significantly more women than men with humerus fractures, radius and ulna fractures, femoral fractures, pelvic ring and acetabular fractures, vertebral fractures, and patellar fractures [18]. However, the incidence of tibiofibular fractures, hand fractures, foot and ankle fractures, clavicle fractures, and scapular fractures in elderly women is not much different from that in men [18].

13.2.2 Regional Distribution

13.2.2.1 Urban-Rural Distribution

There are significant differences in economic development and educational level between urban and rural areas, especially in developing countries, which are more significant, and their incidence of fractures is also significantly different. Data from an analysis in Sweden [19] showed that the incidence of fractures was lower in children and adults growing up in rural areas than in their urban counterparts. However, in China, there are also significant differences in urban and rural distribution between different provinces: the cumulative incidence of fractures in the elderly in Shanghai is as high as 16.5% in urban areas and 6.9% in rural areas [20]; for the resident population over 50 years of age in Chengdu, the risk of fractures in women is higher than that in men and higher in urban areas than in rural areas [21]; the standardized rate of falls in rural residents in Liaoning Province is 3.80%, higher than that in urban residents (3.26%) [22].

13.2.2.2 Geographic Distribution

1. Plains and Plateau

   There is a significant difference in the occurrence of fractures between plain and highland areas: studies have shown [23] that ankle injuries in both plain and highland areas are more common in males, with a high incidence age group of 21 to 30 years, and the types of injuries are mainly simple fractures (AO type 44-A); the proportion of male patients and the proportion of complex fractures (AO type 44-C injuries) in plain areas are lower than those in highland areas, but the average age and the proportion of young adult patients are higher than those in highland areas. Adult ulnar and radial fractures are more common in male patients than in females in highland areas, while female patients are more common in plain areas than in males; both areas have the highest constituent ratio in the age group of 51 to 60 years, and the high incidence types of fractures are simple fractures (AO type 23-A), and the left side is more than the right side [24].

2. Coastal and Inland

   There were also significant differences in the occurrence of fractures between coastal and inland areas: in the eastern coastal areas, the proportion of adult tibial shaft fractures accounting for adult tibiofibular fractures in this area and the proportion of adult systemic fractures were significantly lower than those in the western inland; the proportion of females, mean age, middle-aged, and elderly constituent ratio and constituent ratio of simple fractures (AO type 42A) in patients with tibial shaft fractures were higher than those in the western inland, while the constituent ratio of complex fractures, the constituent ratio of young adults, and the proportion of young adult males were lower than those in the western inland [25].

   There was no significant difference in the proportion of adult femoral neck fractures accounting for adult femoral fractures in this area between the eastern coast and the western inland, but the proportion of adult systemic fractures was significantly higher in the east than in the western inland; the proportion of females, mean age, and elderly constituent ratio of patients with femoral neck fractures were higher in the eastern coast than in the western inland, while the constituent ratio of young adults and the constituent ratio of Garden type III fractures were lower in the eastern coast than in the western inland [26].

13.2.3 Epidemiological Characteristics of Fractures in Different Countries

Many countries in the world are regularly monitoring the national fracture incidence, and the fracture incidence and population composition ratio vary in different countries, regions, and races [1, 2, 27], which may be related to the natural environment, socioeconomic development level, traffic architecture, and other industry-specific circumstances as well as customs culture and living habits in different countries, regions, or cities [3, 5].

An epidemiological survey of fractures completed by Donaldson et al. [6] in 1990 in the Leicestershire region of the UK showed 100 fractures per 10,000 men and 81 fractures per 10,000 women in the region. Johansen et al. [7] reported 23.5 fractures per 1000 men and 18.8 fractures per 1000 women. In 2000, British scholars reported [27] that the mean age of fracture patients was 49.1 years, the male-to-female ratio was 1:1, the incidence of fracture was 11.67/1000/year in males and 10.65/1000/year in females, and the age and gender curve of the whole population showed that the incidence of fracture increased dramatically during menopause in females, the highest age of fracture was 90 to 99 years in females, and the incidence of fracture was 49.7/1000/year; males showed a bimodal curve, and the high incidence age of fracture in males was 12 to 19 years and 90 to 99 years, with incidences of 23.2/1000/year and 21.9/1000/year, respectively, of which distal radius, metacarpal, phalanx, femur, and ankle fractures accounted for 60% of all fractures, but the peak fracture in the elderly was lower than that in females. In 2008, Donaldson et al. [13] conducted a national survey of fracture incidence in the United Kingdom, and this statistic included a total of 45,293 individuals nationwide in the United Kingdom, which contained 10,111 ethnic minorities. The reported data show that white people have a much higher incidence of fractures than other people of color (black and other ethnicities). The incidence of fractures in different countries such as Australia, the United Kingdom, Norway, and the United States is significantly higher than that reported in China (see Sect. 13.4 for details), which is related to different levels of socioeconomic development, transportation status, race, and lifestyle. The changes in the incidence of fractures in different years are shown in Fig. 13.1.

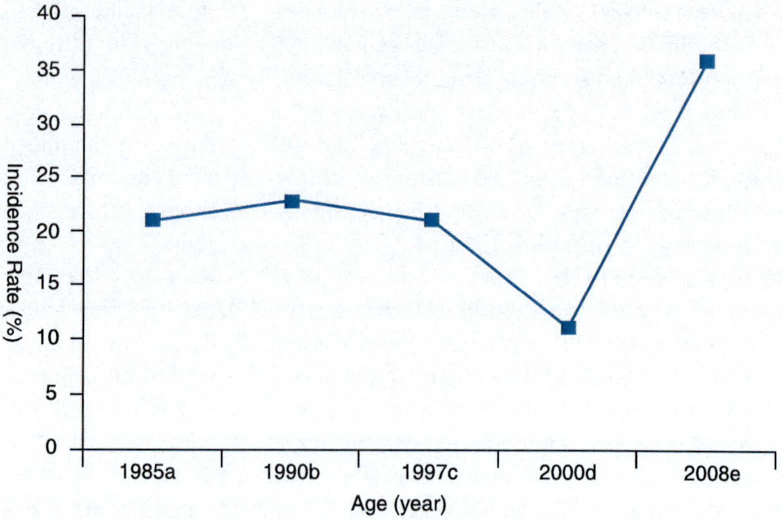

Fig. 13.1 Incidence of fractures varies over time. Note: a from Ref 28, b from Ref 29, c from Ref 7, d from Ref 27, e from Ref 13

13.3 Influencing Factors of Fracture

13.3.1 Influencing Factors of Fracture Occurrence

Understanding the risk factors of fracture occurrence and establishing a scientific management model for effective prevention of fracture occurrence can provide a basis for early clinical prevention and diagnosis.

13.3.1.1 Bone Density

Bone mineral density is an important marker of bone quality and an important indicator of bone strength. Numerous studies have found that there are many factors leading to increased risk of fracture, including low bone mineral density (BMD), age at menopause, long duration of menopause, taking diuretics and corticosteroids and other drugs affecting calcium intake and excretion, long-term smoking, suffering from long-term chronic diseases, low body mass index (BMI) or low body weight, family history of osteoporosis, and previous history of fracture [14, 30–37]. The effect of the above factors on elderly women with osteoporosis is more obvious, the lower the bone mineral density, the more risk of osteoporotic fractures, especially hip fractures. However, most of them are stable fractures, and the proportion of unstable fractures is relatively low. Du Wenwen et al. [38] evaluated 581 postmenopausal fracture women hospitalized from May 2010 to May 2012 by self-made questionnaire, self-rating anxiety scale, self-rating depression scale, and Pittsburgh Sleep Quality Index questionnaire and found that the incidence of refracture was 17.21%; the results of multivariate logistic regression analysis showed that osteoporosis, falls, fracture history, and depression were risk factors for refracture in postmenopausal fracture women.

13.3.1.2 Bad Habits

Smoking and alcoholism are risk factors for a variety of diseases. The big data study found that the risk of hip fracture was higher in smokers among 116,229 female nurses, and the risk of fracture was found decreased to 0.7% at 10 years of follow-up after smoking cessation [31]. Scholes et al. [32] and their team found that in people aged 55 years and older, maximum daily alcohol consumption during the week before fracture, > 8 units in men or > 6 units in women, was a risk factor for fracture.

13.3.1.3 Climate

Climate also has a significant impact on fracture occurrence. According to a group of emergency data containing 142,228 orthopedic patients, it was found that there was a direct correlation between orthopedic emergency volume and meteorological factors, with a number of meteorological factors such as air temperature, air pressure, precipitation, and wind speed having a high correlation with orthopedic emergency volume, with a higher emergency volume in April, May, and September and October, while the emergency volume was the lowest in January and February. The incidence of accidents during important holidays such as the Spring Festival generally decreased to the lowest level of the year, and blast injuries accounted for a high proportion of the causes of injuries. The incidence of fractures varies in different months of the same season, mainly during periods of weather changes. Zhang Chi et al. [39] analyzed the epidemiological data of ulnar and radial fractures in rain and snow weather in Shijiazhuang area and showed that the fractures were closely related to the weather, and ulnar and radial fractures and Colles fractures were likely to occur in rain and snow days.

13.3.1.4 Other Influencing Factors

1. Labor intensity

   Manual workers have a higher risk of fractures than mental workers [21].
2. Genetic factors

   Individuals also have a higher risk of fracture when they have VDR, collagen type I A1, and igf-1, il-6, TGF-β1, and LRP5 genes with bBsm polymorphisms associated with BMD [21].
3. Education or social class

   As education level increases, the risk of developing fractures decreases [40].

   Hedström et al. [19] found that the amount of activity at school could significantly affect the fracture incidence after 10 years and concluded that the living environment as well as the mode of exercise could significantly affect the fracture incidence. Tianjin Hospital and Hexi Orthopaedic Hospital analyzed the data of 1693 hospitalized patients with fractures and found that workers accounted for the largest proportion of fracture patients, 46.0%, and the rest were cadres and students. By location of fracture, 53.8% occurred on the way, followed by at work units and at home. Falls during cycling or walking, traffic accidents, and falls from height were the most common causes of injury, accounting for 31.8%, 27.6%, and 21.5%, respectively [41].
4. Injury

   It mainly includes traffic accidents and falls.

   Xinqiao Hospital Affiliated to Third Military Medical University and Southwest Hospital analyzed 3142 patients with traumatic spinal fractures and concluded that accidental falls and traffic accidents were the most common causes of injury, accounting for 58.9% and 20.9% of all causes of injury, respectively; accidental falls often occurred in elderly patients, with the highest incidence of lumbar fractures; traffic accidents occurred mostly in young patients, with cervical fractures being the most common [42]. A study in Taiwan included 653,386 hospitalized patients who were admitted due to traffic accidents, and there was a total of 391,197 patients with fractures, including 12.22% with upper limb fractures, 12.22% with lower limb fractures, and 6.10% with spinal and trunk bone fractures [43].

   In traffic accidents, the collision of motor vehicles is another important factor leading to fractures. Motor vehicle crash injuries are the third cause of potential life loss (YPLL) in people under 65 years of age in the United States (615.5 per 100,000). In 1995, the incidence of motor vehicle injury was 16.3 per 100,000 (1.8 per 100 million motor vehicle miles). In addition, motor vehicle injuries cause 523,000 hospitalizations each year. In China, 260,000 car accidents occur each year, more than 50,000 people die, and 150,000 people are disabled or injured [6].

13.3.2 Factors Influencing Fracture Healing

Fracture healing is also a complex process influenced by many factors, the main influencing factors of which include the following:

1. Systemic factors
   (a) Age: Fracture healing varies greatly at different ages, such as solid healing

of femoral fractures in neonates take 2 weeks, femoral fractures in adults generally 3 months, and fractures in the elderly longer.

   (b) Health status: poor health status, such as suffering from osteoporosis, diabetes, malnutrition, malignant tumors, and other chronic wasting diseases, the fracture healing time is significantly prolonged.

2. Local factors
   (a) Type and number of fractures: spiral and oblique fractures with large contact surface of the fracture section and rapid healing. Transverse fractures have a small cross-sectional contact surface and slow healing. Multiple fractures or multi-fragmentary fractures of one bone with slow healing.
   (b) Blood supply at the fracture site: It is an important factor affecting fracture healing, and the blood supply status of the fracture segment is also different with different fracture sites. Both fracture segments have rich blood supply and rapid fracture healing; one fracture segment has poor blood supply and slow fracture healing; and both fracture segments have poor blood supply or complete loss of blood supply to the fracture segment is prone to ischemic necrosis.
   (c) Degree of soft tissue injury: Severe soft tissue injury destroys the blood supply and affects the healing of fractures.
   (d) Soft tissue embedding: If there are muscles, tendons, and other tissues embedded between the two fracture ends, hindering the apposition and contact of the two fracture ends, the fracture is difficult to heal or even does not heal.
   (e) Infection: Local infection of open fractures can lead to suppurative osteomyelitis, which seriously affects fracture healing.
   (f) Bone defect: It is an important factor causing slow of fracture healing or nonunion.
   (g) Periosteal integrity: Fractures with intact periosteum heal faster than fractures with ruptured periosteum.
   (h) Nerves: Patients with paraplegia, polio, and nerve injury have slower fracture healing.
3. Treatment methods

   Improper treatment after fracture can lead to delayed union or even nonunion of fracture: (1) after repeated manual reduction, the local soft tissue and periosteum are injured, destroying the blood supply; (2) open reduction, excessive soft tissue, and periosteum stripping, affecting the fracture segment; (3) during debridement of open fracture, the fragment is removed too much, resulting in bone defect; (4) during continuous bone traction therapy for fracture, the traction force is too large, resulting in fracture segment separation and local blood supply deficiency due to vasospasm; (5) excessive pressure causes bone microfracture, local ischemia, bone resorption, and even osteonecrosis; (6) the fracture fixation is not firm, still affected by shear force and rotational force, interfering with callus growth; and (7) premature and inappropriate postoperative functional exercise, affecting fracture fixation.
4. Bad living habits

   Bad habits such as smoking and alcoholism can also cause significant prolongation of fracture healing and even lead to nonunion or necrosis of the bone.

Lv Hongzhi et al. [44] retrospectively analyzed the data of patients after internal fixation of supracondylar fracture of femur. Logistic regression model was performed for 22 related factors including age, gender, occupation, combined injury, length of hospital stay, and cause of injury that may affect the recovery of postoperative knee joint function. It was found that the effects on the recovery of knee joint function from largest to smallest were as follows: postoperative non-weight-bearing time, age, AO classification of fracture, combined injury, and osteoporosis.

In summary, a variety of factors, including temperature, topography, and terrain, have an impact on the incidence of fractures and the severity of injury; rehabilitation training, nursing, and psychological status of fracture patients also have a greater impact on their degree of functional recovery and the survival time of patients with severe fractures. The influencing factors of fracture occurrence and healing overlap with each other and have their own characteristics. Independent analysis cannot be performed for risk factors or protective factors of fracture occurrence and healing. Many factors interact with each other. The effect of synergistic effect of many factors, such as demographics, surgery, and environment, on the study results should be considered comprehensively.

13.4 Epidemiological Study of Fracture in China

China has a vast territory, numerous nationalities, cross-tropical temperate regions, complex and diverse terrain, coexistence of coastal inland areas, large differences in economic development levels, and different epidemiological characteristics of fractures in different regions of China. Similarly, it is difficult to carry out a nationwide epidemiological survey of fractures. However, in recent years, fracture epidemiological research has gradually attracted the attention of the majority of scholars, and we conducted a tabular analysis of fracture epidemiological surveys with geographical characteristics and a large amount of data after 2000 (Table 13.1). It can be seen that, at present, the epidemiology of fracture in China has developed rapidly, and people's attention to fracture, especially the attention of the fracture population, has been significantly improved; the epidemiological study of fracture carried out by all regions and units can guide the clinical work to a certain extent and also have a certain suggestive role in the prevention of ?? society and the masses.

At present, the largest and most comprehensive fracture epidemiological survey in China is the national fracture incidence epidemiological survey carried out by Zhang Yingze and his team [18]. The research group collected the data of 414,935 fracture patients (431,822 fracture sites) in 83 hospitals in 31 provinces, municipalities, and autonomous regions (except Hong Kong, Macao, and Taiwan) and conducted a detailed analysis according to AO/OTA fracture classification and other commonly used types of various sites. According to the statistics of anatomical sites, the patients were divided into 11 groups of fractures, namely, humeral fracture, radius and ulna fracture, femoral fracture, tibiofibula fracture, spinal fracture, pelvic ring and acetabular fracture, hand fracture, foot and ankle fracture, scapular fracture, clavicle fracture, and patellar fracture. Each site was more common in males than in females. The following compares the epidemiological characteristics of fractures in China with relevant domestic and foreign studies, which are listed as follows according to the fracture site:

1. Epidemiological characteristics of humeral fractures

   Humerus fractures: (1) accounted for 63.77% in males and 36.23% in females, with a male-to-female ratio of 1.76:1; (2) the left side (55.11%) was more than the right side (44.73%); (3) the high incidence age group was 0 to 10 years old (36.93%); (4) the middle and proximal (11%) fractures were the most common in adults (39.70%), while the middle and distal fractures were the most common in children (85.39%).

   Lind et al. [45] and Roux et al. [46] reported that the male-to-female ratio of adult patients with humeral fracture was 1:3 and 1:2, respectively; the annual incidence rate of humeral shaft fracture population was 12.9/100,000, accounting for 1.2% of adult systemic fractures, with a male-to-female ratio of 42:58 [27]; the male-to-female ratios reported by Tsai et al. [47] and Ekholm et al. [48] were 1.56:1 and 1.21:1, respectively. The annual population incidence of distal humerus fractures is 5.8/100,000, accounting for 0.5% of total body fractures in adults, with a male-to-female ratio of 29:71 [27].

2. Epidemiological characteristics of fracture of radius and ulna

   Radial and ulnar fractures: (1) male accounted for 60.95%, female 39.05%, male-to-female ratio 1.56:1; (2) left (53.97%) was

Table 13.1 List of fracture epidemiology with geographical characteristics and large data volume in China after 2000

Time	Institution	Article title	Study subjects
2000	School of Public Health, West China University of Medical Sciences	Epidemiological investigation and analysis of related factors of fracture in Chengdu population	Resident population ≥ 50 years of age 10,930
2000	Department of Orthopaedics, Zhongshan People's Hospital	Epidemiological characteristics of 1288 inpatients with traumatic fracture	Inpatients with traumatic fracture: a report of 1288 cases
2000	Department of Orthopaedics, the First Affiliated Hospital, Sun Yat-sen University	Epidemiological investigation and analysis of osteoporotic fracture and osteoarthrosis in the elderly population in Guangzhou	The elderly over 60 years of age, 630 in urban areas and 685 in rural areas
2000	Zhejiang Changxing Hospital of TCM	Epidemiological analysis of fracture in 2110 elderly patients	Elderly fracture: 2110 cases of this report
2001	Fujian Provincial Hospital	Epidemiological investigation of 3688 patients with bone and joint injury	3688 bone and joint damage patients
2001	Union Hospital, Tongji Medical College of HUST	Preliminary investigation on the incidence of osteoporotic fracture in the elderly population in Wuhan	1764 elderly residents over 60 years of age
2001	Epidemiology Laboratory, Beijing Hospital, Ministry of Health	Epidemiological study on the prevalence and risk factors of fracture in middle-aged and elderly population in some areas of China	48,165 men and women over 50 years of age
2002	Osteoporosis Treatment Center, the Fourth Affiliated Hospital of West China University of Medical Sciences	Epidemiological investigation and analysis of osteoporotic vertebral compression fractures	1081 middle-aged and elderly people aged ≥50 years
2004	Taishan Medical School	Epidemiological analysis of 1238 cases of traumatic fracture	1238 patients with traumatic fracture
2004	PLA Orthopaedic Research Institute, 304 Hospital of PLA	Epidemiological analysis of 661 patients with thoracolumbar fracture	661 patients with thoracolumbar fractures
2004	Henan Xiaoxian Orthopaedic Hospital	Epidemiological investigation of tibiofibula fracture in children	2603 children with tibiofibular fractures
2008	Trauma Emergency Center of the Third Hospital of Hebei Medical University	Clinical epidemiological analysis of spiral fracture of tibia combined with posterior malleolus fracture	1685 adult tibiofibular shaft fractures
2009	Yulin Orthopaedic Hospital of Guangxi Zhuang Autonomous Region	Enlightenment of epidemiological investigation of fracture in children aged 0–15 years to health education	3300 children with hospital fractures
2009	Peking University People's Hospital, Peking University Arthritis Clinical Research Center	Epidemiological investigation of hand fractures	5234 patients with hand injury
2009	Department of Orthopaedics, the First Staff Hospital of Yunnan Provincial Administration of Agricultural Reclamation	Preliminary epidemiological survey of osteoporotic fractures in the elderly in Xishuangbanna	Patients over 60 years of age with spinal and hip fractures
2009	School of Public Health, Central South University	Epidemiological study on 952 cases of traumatic vertebral fracture	Medical records of 952 cases of vertebral fracture caused by spinal trauma

2009	Department of Orthopaedics II, Ningxia Medical University People's Hospital	Study on the characteristics of senile hip fracture in some areas of Ningxia	608 elderly
2011	Department of Military Epidemiology, Third Military Medical University	Epidemiological distribution characteristics of 448 patients with hip fracture	448 patients with hip fracture
2011	Dali Affiliated Hospital of Dali University (Yunnan Dali Prefecture Hospital)	Enlightenment of epidemiological investigation of fracture in children to health education	1329 children with fracture
2012	Department of Orthopaedics, Xinqiao Hospital Affiliated to Third Military Medical University	Epidemiological analysis of patients with traumatic spinal fracture	1393 patients with spinal fracture
2012	Guangzhou Orthopedic Hospital	Epidemiological distribution characteristics of 1875 cases of distal radius fractures in the same institution in 1 year	1875 patients with distal radius fractures
2012	Wanzhou District People's Hospital of Chongqing	Statistical analysis of external causes of fracture inpatients in Wanzhou District from 2009 to 2011	9035 fractures in all age groups
2014	Dali Affiliated Hospital of Dali University	Epidemiological analysis of fractures caused by traffic injuries and falls from 2006 to 2012	8037 patients with fractures
2014	Gansu Provincial Hospital of TCM	Analysis of epidemiological characteristics of 1005 hospitalized patients with thoracolumbar fracture	1005 cases of thoracolumbar vertebral fracture
2014	Peking University Third Hospital	Analysis of 10,977 cases of fracture in children in Beijing	Fractures in children: 10,977 cases
2014	Affiliated Hospital of Guangdong Medical University	Epidemiological investigation and analysis of osteoporotic fractures in middle-aged and elderly people in Zhanjiang area	Middle-aged and elderly over 40 years old
2014	The First Affiliated Hospital, Zhejiang University	Incidence and epidemiological characteristics of 877 patients with hip fracture	877 patients with hip fracture
2015	The First Affiliated Hospital of Anhui Medical University	Epidemiological analysis of 1367 cases of traumatic fracture in Xiamen area	1367 patients with traumatic fractures
2015	The Third Hospital of Hebei Medical University	Epidemiological analysis of pelvic fracture Epidemiological analysis of metatarsal fractures in adults Analysis of epidemiological characteristics of spinal fracture in the elderly	Data of patients with fractures diagnosed and treated in the Department of Orthopaedics of the hospital during the 10 years from January 2003 to December 2012
2015	The Third Hospital of Hebei Medical University	Epidemiological comparison of distal radius and ulna fractures between northwest and northeast China from 2010 to 2011 Epidemiological analysis of intertrochanteric fractures in 1583 elderly patients in Beijing, Tianjin and Tang dynasties	Data of fracture patients in 83 hospitals nationwide
2015	The Third Hospital of Hebei Medical University	Epidemiological survey and design of fracture incidence among Chinese residents	National epidemiological survey of fracture incidence

more than right (45.06%); (3) high incidence age group was (22.56%); (4) adult distal radius and ulna (23) fractures were the most common (63.37%); and children were also the most common distal fractures (44.18%).

The literature in the United Kingdom showed [27] the annual incidence rate of ulnar and radial fractures was 55.5/100,000, accounting for 5.0% of adult systemic fractures, with a male-to-female ratio of 46:54; the annual incidence rate of ulnar and radial shaft fractures was 13.8/100,000, accounting for 1.2% of adult systemic fractures, with a male-to-female ratio of 64:36; and the annual incidence rate of distal radius and ulna fractures was 195.2/100,000, accounting for 17.5% of adult systemic fractures, with a male-to-female ratio of 31:69. Foreign literature reports that distal radius fractures are highly prevalent in children aged 6 to 10 years and the elderly population aged 60 to 69 years, and patients over 60 years of age are significantly more common in women than in men [49].

3. Epidemiological characteristics of femoral fractures

Femoral fractures: (1) male accounted for 64.44%, female 35.56%, male-to-female ratio 1.8:1; (2) left side (52.75) was more than right side (46.50%); (3) high incidence age group was 21 to 40 years old (30.13%); and (4) adult femoral fracture (31) was the most common (54.27%), while femoral shaft fracture was the most common in children (74.03%).

The annual incidence of femoral fracture is 129.4/100,000, accounting for 11.6% of adult systemic fractures, with a male-to-female ratio of 26:74; the annual incidence of femoral shaft fracture is 10.3/100,000, accounting for 0.9% of adult systemic fractures, with a male-to-female ratio of 36:64; and the annual incidence of distal femoral fracture is 4.5/100,000, accounting for 0.4% of adult systemic fractures, with a male-to-female ratio of 33:67 [27]. Martinet et al. [50] counted 2165 patients with distal femoral fractures in Europe in 2000, 1114 males and 1051 females, with a male-to-female ratio close to 1:1. Court-Brown et al. [27] reported in 2006 that the male-to-female ratio of patients with distal femoral fractures was 1:2, the mean age was 61 years, and more than half of the patients were over 65 years of age.

4. Epidemiological characteristics of spinal fractures

Spinal fracture: (1) male accounting for 54.99%, female 45.01%, male-to-female ratio 1.2:1; (2) high incidence age group was 31 ~ 60 years old (58.83%); and (3) high incidence was 52.12 (14.39%), 53.01 (17.37%), and 53.02 (15.08%).

Wang Hongwei et al. [42] investigated 1393 patients with traumatic spinal fractures and found that the number of male patients <59 years of age was higher than that of females, while patients ≥60 years of age showed a trend of higher number of female injuries than males. Among all age groups, the percentage of nerve injury was highest among patients with spinal fractures in the age group of 20 to 29 years (58.5%), followed by those in the age group of 40 to 49 years (54.1%). The proportions of cervical, thoracic, lumbar, and sacrococcygeal spine injuries were 23.8%, 31.9%, 43.9%, and 0.4%, respectively. The frequent site of spinal fractures was thoracolumbar (T10 to L2), accounting for 55.4%, of which L1, T12, and L2 were 22.5%, 5.4%, and 11.1%, respectively. The frequent sites of cervical spine fractures were C2, C5, and C6, which are 6.4%, 5.3%, and 4.0%, respectively.

5. Epidemiological characteristics of tibiofibular fractures

Tibiofibula fractures: (1) male accounting for 69.87%, female 30.13%, male-to-female ratio 2.32:1; (2) left (50.51%) was more than right (49.10%), fracture accounting for 0.39%; (3) high incidence age group was 21 to 50 years old (58.63%); and (4) adult diaphyseal (42) fractures were the most common (36.80%), followed by malleolar (44) fractures (36.69%), while in children diaphyseal fractures were the most common (48.46%), malleolar fractures accounting for only 27.42%.

Chen Xiao et al. [51] counted 1533 cases of adult distal tibial fractures from 2003 to 2012, accounting for 8.32% of adult tibial fractures and 1.42% of adult systemic fractures. 721 (47.03%) were young and 812 (52.97%) were middle-aged. The male-to-female ratio was 3.13:1. The proportion of young male patients was higher than that of middle-aged and elderly patients; young female patients were significantly lower than those of middle-aged and elderly patients. The proportion of extra-articular fractures in young people was lower than that in middle-aged and elderly people, while the proportion of intra-articular fractures was not significantly different from that in middle-aged and elderly people.

6. Epidemiological characteristics of pelvic ring and acetabular fractures

Pelvic ring and acetabular fractures: (1) male accounted for 56.14%, female 43.86%, male-to-female ratio was 1.28:1; (2) left (39.50%) was more than right (30.78%), accounting for 37.31%; (3) high incidence age groups were 21 ~ 30 years old (18.90%), 31 ~ 40 years old (24.67%), and 41 ~ 50 years old (20.91%); and (4) adults had the most 61 fractures (79.48%), and children had the most pelvic ring fractures (97.25%).

Yang Qing et al. [52] counted the data of 588 patients with pelvic fractures treated from November 2007 to May 2009, in which the male-to-female ratio was 1.24:1. The age ranged from 8 to 90 years, with an average of 38.5 ± 15.8 years. According to the age distribution, there were 5 cases under 10 years old, 44 cases between 10 and 19 years old, 145 cases between 20 and 29 years old, 143 cases between 30 and 39 years old, 118 cases between 40 and 49 years old, 78 cases between 50 and 59 years old, 25 cases between 60 and 69 years old, 16 cases between 70 and 79 years old, 10 cases between 80 and 89 years old, and 2 cases between 90 years old. A total of 384 patients (65.3%) were 20 to 59 years old. There were 340 cases (57.8%) of type 61-A. There were 95 cases (15.7%) of type 61-B. There were 33 cases (5.1%) of type 61-C. There were 54 cases (9.0%) of type 62-A. There were 38 cases (6.3%) of type 62-B. There were 14 cases (2.4%) of type 62-C. There were 14 cases (2.4%) of type 61 + 62.

7. Epidemiological characteristics of hand fracture

Hand fractures: (1) male accounted for 78.58%, female 21.42%, male-to-female ratio 3.67:1; (2) left side (47.15%) was less than right side (52.70%); (3) high incidence age group was 11 ~ 20 years old (23.81%), 21 ~ 30 years old (26.26%), and 31 ~ 40 years old (21.97%); and (4) adult phalangeal fractures were the most common (75.74%), and children phalangeal fractures were also the most (79.46%).

American scholar Frazier [53] studied 1164 emergency hand fracture patients and found that there were more males than females with hand fractures, the age group with high incidence of fractures was 21 to 25 years, and the number of phalangeal fractures was the highest. The British scholar Feehan [54] study also concluded that men had more hand fractures than women.

8. Epidemiological characteristics of foot fractures

Foot fractures: (1) accounting for 73.55% in males and 26.45% in females, with a male-to-female ratio of 2.78:1; (2) the left side (48.16%) was more than the right side (47.31%), accounting for 4.53%; (3) the high incidence age groups were 21 to 30 years (20.56%), 31 to 40 years (24.62%), and 41 to 50 years (21.02%); and (4) adult calcaneal fractures were the most common (34.15%), followed by metatarsal fractures (33.66%), while metatarsal fractures were the most common (48.83%) and calcaneal fractures accounted for 18.01% in children.

9. Fracture of other site

Patellar fracture: (1) male accounting for 71.38%, female 28.62%, male-to-female ratio 2.49:1; (2) left side (51.01%) was more than right side (48.43%); (3) high incidence age group was 31 ~ 40 years old (21.34%) and 41 ~ 50 years old (23.30%); and (4) patellar fracture had the most type 34-C fracture

(89.17%), and patellar fracture group had the most 34-C1 (62.70%).

Scapular fractures: (1) male accounting for 82.28%, female 17.72%, male-to-female ratio 4.64:1; (2) left side (47.36%) was less than right side (51.28%); (3) high incidence age group was 31 ~ 40 years old (31.18%) and 41 ~ 50 years old (25.55%); and (4) 14-A type fractures were the most common scapular fractures (56.46%), followed by 14-C type fractures (32.14%). The most frequent scapular fracture grouping was 14-A3 (43.54%) and 14-C1 (25.34%).

Clavicle fracture: (1) accounting for 73.28% in males and 26.72% in females; (2) accounting for 58.17% in the left side and 41.26% in the right side; (3) the high incidence age groups were 21 ~ 30 years old (17.69%), 31 ~ 40 years old (16.76%), and 41 ~ 50 years old (19.41%); and (4) 15-B fracture was the most common clavicle fracture (83.70%).

Liu Song et al. [55] studied patellar fractures in the Third Hospital of Hebei Medical University: more males than females; the age group with high incidence of fractures was 46 to 50 years; the type with high incidence of fractures was 34-C, with 34-C being the most common in both males and females. Liu Lei et al. [56] retrospectively analyzed the data of 424 patients with scapular neck fractures from January 2003 to December 2012, including 333 males and 91 females, with a male-to-female ratio of 3.66:1; the age group with high incidence of fractures was 41 to 50 years (24.53%); according to Miller classification, there were 144 cases (33.96%) of type I fractures, 230 cases (54.25%) of type II fractures, and 50 cases (11.79%) of type III fractures; there were 344 cases (81.13%) of stable fractures and 80 cases (18.87%) of unstable fractures. Zhu Xianghui et al. [57] analyzed the medical records of 363 patients with clavicle fracture admitted to Jinghu Hospital of Macao from February 1993 to November 2002 and performed epidemiological analysis of clavicle fracture in different age groups. It was concluded that the male-to-female ratio of patients with clavicle fracture was 2.85:1, and the age ranged from newborn to 96 years. The fracture site was 159 on the left and 204 on the right. There were 232 and 131 simple fractures and comminuted fractures, respectively; the fracture sites were divided into three segments, internal, middle, and external, 6, 328 and 29, respectively, and 78 cases were complicated with multiple injuries of fractures and dislocations at other sites, with concurrent rib fractures being the most common (31 cases).

Current problems in epidemiological surveys of fractures: The existing literature mainly reports the data of patients with fractures at a single site, in a specific area, in a single or several hospitals. The research content is mainly based on the basic demographic information of patients, fracture types, and injury factors, and there are few comparative studies on the investigation of fracture risk factors, especially the economic development level, climate, temperature, geography, terrain, and other related factors that have a potential impact on the incidence of fractures. Descriptive analysis is mostly used in the analysis, the methodology mainly uses cross-sectional studies in observational studies, and case-control studies with tracking and high-level prospective multicenter randomized controlled studies are rarely carried out. At present, there is an urgent need for a multi-part and multidisciplinary national fracture epidemiological survey with rigorous sampling design, large sample size, wide coverage, wide content, standardized methods, and rich information content in China.

13.5 Prevention and Treatment Strategies of Fractures

13.5.1 Prevention of Fractures

According to the risk factors of fracture, balanced nutrition, increased physical activity before the age of 18, adequate sleep, and the use of drugs or estrogens that increase bone mass can reduce the occurrence of fracture. In addition, obesity has been found to be a protective factor for reducing fracture risk in women over 55 years of age, and obesity has a protective effect in preventing osteoporosis and maintaining hormone levels at menopause [31]. Breastfeeding is also a protective factor for hip fracture in women.

13.5.2 Treatment of Fractures

13.5.2.1 Emergency Treatment of Fracture

The purpose of fracture first aid is to save the patient's life, protect it, and transport it safely and quickly in order to obtain proper treatment. Therefore, attention should be paid to ABC (airway, respiration, and circulation) and the blood circulation status of the limb before dealing with fractures.

13.5.2.2 Treatment Principles of Fracture

At present, AO tissue fracture treatment principles are often used internationally: ① reconstruct the anatomical relationship through fracture reduction and fixation; ② reconstruct stability with strong or elastic fixation (also known as splinting) according to the characteristics of fracture; ③ use meticulous operation and gentle reduction methods to protect the soft tissue and bone; and ④ early and safe activity training of the whole body and the affected area.

13.5.2.3 Management of Open Fractures

Open fracture is defined as a fracture in which the skin or mucosa near the fracture ruptures and the fracture communicates with the outside world. It is often caused by high-energy injury, with severe bone and soft tissue trauma, poor healing conditions, weak resistance to bacteria, and easy to cause infection. The key to management is thorough debridement to transform open contaminated wounds into near-sterile wounds, prevent infection, strive for rapid wound closure, and transform open fractures into closed fractures, thus creating favorable conditions for tissue repair and fracture treatment. Debridement of open fractures includes debridement, fracture reduction and soft tissue repair, and wound closure.

13.5.2.4 Treatment of Open Joint Injury

Open joint injury is the rupture of the skin and joint capsule, and the joint cavity communicates with the outside world. Its management principles are basically the same as those of open fractures, but it has its particularity due to the involvement of joints. The most common complications of open joint injuries are joint adhesions and malunion of intra-articular fractures, which affect joint function. Therefore, thorough debridement must be performed in the joint cavity to protect the articular cartilage and pay attention to repairing the articular surface.

13.5.3 Prevention and Treatment Strategy of Senile Fracture

Elderly fractures are not isolated orthopedic diseases, and it is accompanied by systemic multisystem pathophysiological changes. This requires the establishment of geriatric orthopedics based on orthopedic treatment, combined with multiple disciplines such as cardiovascular medicine, respiratory medicine, gastroenterology, neurology, endocrinology, and rehabilitation. Through multidisciplinary collaboration, individualized treatment plans are developed. At the same time, improving the understanding of the characteristics of osteoporotic fractures in the elderly, strengthening prevention and selecting the correct treatment, taking comprehensive measures, promoting osteoporosis publicity and education, and preventing the occurrence of osteoporotic fractures are important measures to improve and reduce the incidence of fractures and social burden.

1. Fall prevention

   One-third of older community-dwelling adults and 60% of older adults living in care facilities in the United States experience a fall each year. The incidence of falls among Australian community-dwelling adults ranged from 26% between 65 and 74 years of age, 40% between 75 and 85 years of age, to 48% in older adults over 85 years of age. The incidence of falls in elderly community residents over 60 years of age in China is about 22.6% (15.9% in males and 28.4% in females) in rural communities and 18.0% (14.9% in males and 20.1% in females) in urban communities [58].

Most of the falls are soft tissue injuries, and 10% to 15% of falls will lead to serious injuries, of which fractures are more serious injuries and the main cause of hospitalization after falls. Falls in the elderly are closely related to fractures, and studies have shown that 5% to 10% of the elderly who experience falls develop fractures; 90% of the elderly who experience fractures are due to falls [59].

Risk factors for falls are as follows: a history of one or more falls, cognitive impairment, chronic diseases, balance and gait disorders, low body mass index, female gender, fragility, taking diuretics or psychotropic drugs, and family risk factors for falls (such as slippery floors). According to the above risk factors, comprehensive intervention measures should be taken for the prevention of falls, including (1) stopping the drugs that induce falls; (2) eliminating or improving the factors that predispose to falls in families (such as anti-slip floor); (3) strengthening physical exercise; (4) performing gait training; (5) wearing clothing that meets personal needs and can reduce falls, such as wearing knee protection and underwear with pads; and (6) paying attention to the care and psychological concern of the elderly.

The study of balance training to prevent falls in Jing'an District, Shanghai, is to prevent the occurrence of falls by exercising through Tai Chi, yoga, or other modes of exercise that challenge balance, and their main benefits are to improve mobility and balance and reduce the risk of wrestling and fractures, while strengthening posture training, which can help the elderly protect the spine, reduce spinal pressure, and reduce the risk of wrestling and fractures, especially vertebral fractures [60].

2. Improve osteoporosis and prevent fracture

A survey of fracture treatment costs between 2000 and 2006 in a hospital in Beijing showed that the annual per capita treatment cost of a fracture was 20,477.2 yuan, with an average annual increase of 11.9%. However, after a vertebral fracture occurs in the elderly, the risk of other fractures within 1 year is increased by 2–5 times, which is 6–12 times higher than the risk of recurrent fractures in the normal population. The treatment and care of patients with severe osteoporosis poses a great economic burden on patients and their families, as well as society [61].

To prevent fractures in the elderly, we must first prevent or delay the occurrence of osteoporosis in the elderly. At present, there are three options for the treatment of osteoporosis. Basic treatment: calcium plus vitamin D, but the absorption rate of calcium is relatively low, so appropriate exercise and sun exposure should be combined [62]; taking osteoclast inhibitors can slow down calcium loss and delay the occurrence of osteoporosis; promote new bone growth, slow down calcium loss, and promote osteogenesis [63].

3. Reduce fractures caused by accidental injuries

Treatment of patients with fracture caused by traffic injury: It is necessary to strengthen the pre-hospital care of traffic injury, timely and correctly move, and give life-saving measures and appropriate treatment as soon as possible; then the lives of many injured can be saved or avoided from disability. Timely and correct diagnosis and rescue can improve the efficacy and prognosis [64]. Gao [65] emphasized that whether post-traumatic diagnosis and management are timely and accurate often affects survival more than the injury itself. The occurrence of fracture after trauma should be found in time and treated as early as possible to reduce misdiagnosis and missed diagnosis.

4. Strengthen physical exercise to prevent the occurrence of fractures

Adhering to one-legged jumps for 2 minutes a day can quickly increase bone mineral density within a year, thereby enhancing bone and reducing the risk of fractures, the Daily Mail reported on September 10, 2015. Researchers from the University of Loughborough investigated 34 men between the ages of 65 and

80 who adhered to one-legged jumping for a year while maintaining other physical activities or dietary habits unchanged. By CT scanning, there was a significant improvement in those body regions that were most prone to fracture when falling. The researchers say the findings have important implications for the prevention and response of osteoporosis [66]. In the United Kingdom, about three million people suffer from bone thinning each year, both because of old age and osteoporosis, and this new finding may effectively solve the current situation.

References

1. Johnell O, Kanis JA. An estimate of the worldwide prevalence and disability associated with osteoporotic fractures [J]. Osteoporos Int. 2006;17(12):1726–33.
2. Johnell O, Kanis J. Epidemiology of osteoporotic fractures [J]. Osteoporos Int. 2005;16(2):S3–7.
3. Madadi F, Vahid Farahmandi M, Eajazi A, et al. Epidemiology of adult tibial shaft fractures: a 7-year study in a major referral orthopedic center in Iran [J]. Med Sci Monit. 2010;16(5):CR217–21.
4. Cooper C. Epidemiology of osteoporotic fracture: looking to the future [Z]. Rheumatology (Oxford). 2005 Dec;44(Suppl 4):iv36–iv4.
5. Moayyeri A, Soltani A, Larijani B, et al. Epidemiology of hip fracture in Iran: results from the Iranian multicenter study on accidental injuries [J]. Osteoporos Int. 2006;17(8):1252–7.
6. Donaldson LJ, Cook A, Thomson RG. Incidence of fractures in a geographically defined population [J]. J Epidemiol Community Health. 1990;44(3):241–5.
7. Johansen A, Evans RJ, Stone MD, et al. Fracture incidence in England and Wales: a study based on the population of Cardiff [J]. Injury. 1998;28(9/10):655–60.
8. Cooper C, Dennison EM, Leufkens HG, et al. Epidemiology of childhood fractures in Britain: a study using the general practice research database [J]. J Bone Miner Res. 2004;19(12):1976–81.
9. Zhang T, Liu XG, Guo Y, et al. Analysis of 10,977 fractures in children in Beijing, Chinese. J Orthop Surg. 2014;22(24):2233–7.
10. Landin LA. Fracture patterns in children. Analysis of 8,682 fractures with special reference to incidence, etiology and secular changes in a Swedish urban population 1950–1979. Acta Orthop Scand Suppl. 1983;202:1–109.
11. Lyons RA, Delahunty AM, Kraus D, et al. Children's fractures: a population based study [J]. Inj Prev. 1999;5(2):129–32.
12. Li NH, Qu PZ, Zhu HM, et al. Prevalence of fracture in middle-aged and elderly Chinese population [J]. Chin J Clin Rehab. 2003;8(7):1284–5.
13. Donaldson LJ, Reckless IP, Scholes S, et al. The epidemiology of fractures in England [J]. J Epidemiol Community Health. 2008;62(2):174–80.
14. Ooms ME, Lips P, Van Lingen A, et al. Determinants of bone mineral density and risk factors for osteoporosis in healthy elderly women [J]. J Bone Miner Res. 1993;8(6):669–75.
15. Tao S, Wang HL, Zhu YB, et al. Epidemiological study on multi-center adult femoral shaft fractures in Beijing, Tianjin and Tang dynasties from 2010 to 2011 [J]. Chin J Orthopaedic Trauma. 2015;08(17):709–13.
16. Hao DJ, He BR, Yan L, etc. Epidemiological characteristics of patients with spinal cord injury in Xi'an Red Cross Hospital from 2011 to 2013 [J]. Chin J Trauma. 2015;07(31):632–6.
17. Sun JY, Cui YW, Liu L, et al. Epidemiological analysis of thoracolumbar fractures in adults in Xinjiang from 2010 to 2011 [J]. Chin J Orthopaedic Trauma. 2015;03(17):248–50.
18. Zhang YZ. Clinical trauma Orthopaedic epidemiology [M]. 2nd ed. Beijing: People's Medical Publishing House; 2014. p. 6–7.
19. Hedström IW, Waernbaum I. Incidence of fractures among children and adolescents in rural and urban communities - analysis based on 9,965 fracture events [J]. Inj Epidemiol. 2014;1(1):14.
20. Liu GP. Annual fracture incidence rate of osteoporotic fracture [J]. Chin J Osteoporosis. 2014;10:619–33.
21. Liu LK, Yuan P, An Z, et al. Epidemiological investigation of fracture and analysis of related factors in Chengdu population [J]. Modern Preventive Medicine. 2000;4:459–62.
22. Na J, Yu CY, Fu ZG, et al. Study on epidemic characteristics of injuries among urban and rural residents in Liaoning Province [J]. J Dis Control. 2007;11(4):352–4.
23. Liu L, Yang ZY, Sun JY, et al. Epidemiological comparative study of adult ankle joint injury between plain and highland areas from 2010 to 2011 [J]. Chin J Orthopaedic Trauma. 2015;17(12):1064–8.
24. Yin B, Li FA, Hao HY. Epidemiological comparison of distal radius and ulna fractures between Northwest China and Northeast China from 2010 to 2011 [J]. Chin J Anatomy Clinic. 2015;20(2):90–3.
25. Zhao HT, Chen W, Wang J, et al. Epidemiological comparative analysis of tibial shaft fractures between eastern coastal and western inland adults from 2010 to 2011 [J]. Chin J Orthopaedic Trauma. 2015;17(9):805–8.
26. Zhao HT, Chen W, Wang J, et al. Epidemiological comparative analysis of adult femoral neck fractures in eastern coastal and western inland areas from 2010 to 2011 [J]. Chin J Orthopaedic Trauma. 2015;8(17):704–8.
27. Court-Brown CM, Caesar B. Epidemiology of adult fractures: a review [J]. Injury. 2006;37(8):691–7.

28. Fife D, Barancik JI. Northeastern Ohio trauma study III: incidence of fractures [J]. Ann Emerg Med. 1985;14(3):244–8.
29. Sahlin Y. Occurrence of fractures in a defined population: a 1-year study [J]. Injury. 1990;21(3):158–60.
30. La Vecchia C, Negri E, Levi F, et al. Cigarette smoking, body mass and other risk factors for fractures of the hip in women [J]. Int J Epidemiol. 1991;20(3):671–7.
31. Cornuz J, Feskanich D, Willett WC, et al. Smoking, smoking cessation, and risk of hip fracture in women [J]. Am J Med. 1999;106(3):311–4.
32. Scholes S, Panesar S, Shelton NJ, et al. Epidemiology of lifetime fracture prevalence in England: a population study of adults aged 55 years and over [J]. Age Ageing. 2014;43(2):234–40.
33. De Laet C, Kanis JA, Odén A, et al. Body mass index as a predictor of fracture risk: a meta-analysis [J]. Osteoporos Int. 2005;16(11):1330–8.
34. Sharma S, Fraser M, Lovell F, et al. Characteristics of males over 50 years who present with a fracture: epidemiology and underlying risk factors [J]. J Bone Joint Surg Br. 2008;90(1):72–7.
35. Cummings SR, Melton LJ. Epidemiology and outcomes of osteoporotic fractures [J]. Lancet. 2002;359(9319):1761–7.
36. Ensrud KE. Epidemiology of fracture risk with advancing age [J]. J Gerontol A Biol Sci Med Sci. 2013;68(10):1236–42.
37. Lv HZ, Chen W, Zhang XL, et al. Survey design of the epidemiological study of traumatic fracture incidence in China residence [J]. J Hebei Medical Univ. 2015;36(4):485–7.
38. Du WY. Analysis of risk factors of refracture after fracture in postmenopausal women [J]. Chin J Gerontol. 2013;03(3):561–3.
39. Zhang C. Epidemiological characteristics of radius and ulna fractures in snow and snow in Shijiazhuang area [D]. Shijiazhuang: Hebei Medical University; 2015.
40. Fan F, Du SL, Xue WQ, et al. A case-control study of demographic and socioeconomic factors and the risk of hip fracture. Chin J Osteoporos. 2013;19(8):844–9.
41. Chen GZ, Lu WL, Wang W. Epidemiological investigation of inpatients with fracture [J]. J Tianjin Medical Univ. 2004;10(3):431–3.
42. Wang HW, Zhou Y, Li CQ, Wang C. Epidemiological analysis of patients with traumatic spinal fracture [J]. Chin J Trauma. 2012;11(28):988–92.
43. Pan RH, Chang NT, Chu D, et al. Epidemiology of orthopedic fractures and other injuries among inpatients admitted due to traffic accidents: a 10-year nationwide survey in Taiwan [Z]. Scientific World J. 2014;2014:637872.
44. Lv HZ, Xing X, Qin SJ, et al. From January 2008 to December 2011, the related factors of knee joint function after supracondylar fracture surgery in the third Hospital of Hebei Medical University were investigated and analyzed. Chin J Orthopaedic Trauma. 2014;16(11):978–82.
45. Lind T, Krøner K, Jensen J. The epidemiology of fractures of the proximal humerus [J]. Arch Orthop Trauma Surg. 1989;108(5):285–7.
46. Roux A, Decroocq L, El Batti S, et al. Epidemiology of proximal humerus fractures managed in a trauma center [J]. Orthop Traumatol Surg Res. 2012;98(6):715–9.
47. Tsai CH, Fong YC, Chen YH, et al. The epidemiology of traumatic humeral shaft fractures in Taiwan [J]. Int Orthop. 2009;33(2):463–7.
48. Ekholm R, Adami J, Tidermark J, et al. Fractures of the shaft of the humerus [J]. An epidemiological study of 401 fractures. J Bone Joint Surg Br. 2006;88(11):1469–73.
49. Alffram PA, Bauer GC. Epidemiology of fractures of the forearm a biomechanical investigation of bone strength [J]. J Bone Joint Surg Am. 1962;44:105–14.
50. Martinet O, Cordey J, Harder Y, et al. The epidemiology of fractures of the distal femur [J]. Injury. 2000;31(3):62–3.
51. Chen X, Yang ZY, Wang J, et al. Epidemiological study of adult distal tibial fractures in the third Hospital of Hebei Medical University from 2003 to 2012 [J]. Chin J Orthopaedic Trauma. 2015;17:314–7. https://doi.org/10.3760/CMA.J.ISSN.1671-7600.2015.05.012.
52. Qing Y, Wang QG, Pan FG, et al. Epidemiological characteristics and clinical analysis of 588 cases of pelvic fracture [J]. Chin J Joint Surg: Electronic Edition. 2013;01(7):64–9.
53. Frazier WH, Miller M, Fox RS, Brand D, Finseth F. Incidence and epidemiology in an emergency service. JACEP. 1978;7(7):265–8.
54. Feehan LM, Sheps SB. Demographics of hand fractures in British Columbia. Canada: a population-based study [J]. J Hand Surg Am. 2006;31(7):1068–74.
55. Liu S, Chen W, Wei W, et al. Epidemiological analysis of adult patellar fracture in the Third Hospital of Hebei Medical University from 2003 to 2012 [J]. Chin J Orthop Trauma. 2014;08(16):700–4.
56. Lei L, Sun JY, Zhang T, et al. Epidemiological study on scapular neck fracture in the third Hospital of Hebei Medical University from 2003 to 2012 [J]. Chin J Orthopaedic Trauma. 2015;04(17):318–21.
57. Zhu XH, Li WP, Chen ZJ. Epidemiological analysis of 363 cases of clavicle fracture [J]. Chin J Reparative Reconstr Surg. 2004;18(4):275–6.
58. Pulin Y, Zhaohui Q, Di W, et al. Investigation on the incidence of falls among the elderly in urban communities of Beijing [J]. Chin J Geriatrics. 2006;25:305–8.
59. Peeters G, van Schoor NM, Lips P. Fall risk: the clinical relevance of falls and how to integrate fall risk with fracture risk [J]. Best Pract Res Clin Rheumatol. 2009;23(6):797–804.
60. Chen XE, Zheng JJ, Shi HT, et al. Clinical study of cognitive attention and balance function dual-task training in the prevention of falls in the elderly [J], Chinese. Rehabilitation. 2016;3(2):215–7.

61. He L, Zhong W, Li N. Do orthopedic surgeons pay attention to the treatment and prevention of osteoporotic fractures [J]. J Pract Orthop. 2009;9(4):241–4.
62. Huang GY. Osteoporotic Fracture [J]. Geriatrics and Health Care, 79–81.
63. Wang SY. Injury epidemiology [M]. Beijing: People's Medical Publishing House. p. 51–5.
64. Tang H, Wang QG, Tan RX, et al. Analysis of 837 cases of fracture caused by traffic injury in hospital. Chin J Orthopaedic Trauma. 2003;5(3):254–5.
65. Gao JM. A clinical analysis of 94 cases with fatal trauma. Chin J Trauma. 1994;10:50–3.
66. Wang M. Two minutes of one-legged jumping a day can strengthen bones [J]. Health Care Life. 2016;1(1):55.

14 Extreme Weather and Mortality and Cardiovascular Diseases

Yonghong Zhang

Abstract

Since the twentieth century, the Earth on which humans live has been experiencing climate change, which is marked by warming of ground temperature and an increasing frequency of extreme weather. Climate change and extreme weather will cause not only changes of the human living environment but also many health problems. From a macro perspective, global warming is likely to be a common health challenge that humanity faces in the future. In recent decades, with the understanding of the impact of extreme weather on human health, people have begun to pay attention to the relationship between extreme weather and people's health, and some related research work has been carried out. This chapter will summarize and report the progress in epidemiology on the relationships between extreme weather and death and cardiovascular diseases. This chapter consists of three sections: first, an overview of global climate change; second, extreme weather and total mortality and cardiovascular mortality; and third, extreme weather or meteorological factor and myocardial infarction. At the end of the chapter, the limitations of previous research work and perspective in future are suggested.

Y. Zhang (✉)
Department of Epidemiology, School of Public Health, Medical College of Soochow University, Suzhou, China
e-mail: yhzhang@suda.edu.cn

Keywords

Extreme weather · Heat waves · Cold spell
Mortality · Cardiovascular diseases

14.1 Overview of Global Climate Change

14.1.1 Historical Record of Climate Change

The climate on Earth is an important environmental factor for human survival, production, and life. Although people always pay attention to the influence of meteorological factors on human production and life in the long history of humankind, some records of meteorological factors such as temperature have been available only in modern times. Due to the different sources of these records, their accuracy and reliability varied considerably. In the nearly 2000 years of history before 1850, the temperature on Earth was relatively stable for most of the period, although there were warm periods and small ice ages during the Middle Ages. After 1860, humans began to measure climatic temperatures with instruments, and the records on global temperatures became

D.-Q. Ye (ed.), *Progress in China Epidemiology*, https://doi.org/10.1007/978-981-19-2199-5_14

available. Relatively speaking, the records at that times were rough, and the impact of human activities on the Earth's temperature was rarely considered in these records, such as pollutant emissions from factories and mines, rapid urbanization, overconsumption of energy, and the urban heat island effect. Nevertheless, the records from that times were still very important historical sources for research on global climate change. Since the middle of the twentieth century, humans have had a more comprehensive and systematic records of the temperatures of both the Earth and ocean. With the development of satellite remote sensing technology, humans began to use satellite temperature measurement technology to measure and evaluate tropospheric temperatures. Some studies showed that the temperature of the troposphere increased by approximately 0.12 °C to 0.22 °C every 10 years. Based on the relevant records, the global average surface temperature increased by 0.85 °C between 1880 and 2012 [1]. According to the Intergovernmental Panel on Climate Change (IPCC), it was estimated that the average temperature of the Earth's surface would increase by 1.0–3.7 °C by the end of this century [2]. Global Climate 2001–2010: 10 Years of Extreme Climate Events released by the World Meteorological Organization (WMO) in 2013 claimed that the first decade of the twenty-first century was the hottest since 1850, at which data of modern measurements on climate temperature became available. The global average surface and sea surface temperature was 14.47 °C in 2001–2010 which was 0.21 °C warmer than that in 1991–2000. Among particular years, year 2010 was the warmest on record, followed by 2005. Based on separate reports from WMO member states, period of 2001–2010 was considered to be the warmest decade on record. Subsequently, in 2015, the WMO issued another communique, in which 2014 was listed as the hottest year since meteorological records, warning that the trend of global warming would continue. Furthermore, climate change has caused changes of extreme event frequency, intensity, and geographic distribution in the past years and will continue to be a driver for the change in the future, and some of these extreme weather events including heat waves, cold spells, droughts, flooding rains, storm surges, hurricanes, etc. will cause harmful effects for human health [3]. Globally, extreme weather events are becoming more frequent and more intense [4].

14.1.2 The Main Factors of Global Warming

Although the viewpoints of scholars from different countries on the factors contributing to global warming were not consistent, the following major factors are generally recognized.

Excessive Human Activities The rapid growth of the population on Earth is destroying or threatening the balance of natural ecological environment to a certain extent. The rapid growth of the population on Earth which would increase the Earth's load and overconsumption of natural resources would lead to the continuous increase in the contents of carbon dioxide and other related gases in the atmosphere, and the greenhouse effect caused by carbon dioxide directly affects the climate change on the Earth's surface. Due to the very large population load and neglect of environmental protection, the Earth has shown a tendency of desertification and soil erosion. As everyone knows, soil erosion decreases soil fertility and water retention, thereby reducing the biological productivity of the soil and its ability to maintain that productivity, and soil erosion may also cause large-scale floods and sandstorms and deteriorate the ecological environment. Good vegetation can preserve water and soil and avoid water and soil loss. Serious damage to vegetation has occurred through human activities such as excessive deforestation for timber, land reclamation for agricultural production, and overgrazing. Around the world, forest areas are decreasing dramatically due to natural and human-related factors, and the desertification of land is becoming increasingly serious due to excessive agricultural and livestock production.

Greenhouse Gas Emissions The ever-increasing amount of toxic chemicals not only poses a serious threat to the survival of humans but also poses a danger to the ecological environment of the Earth's surface [1]. The increasing seriousness of environmental pollution has become a major global problem, and environmental pollution is also one of the main factors leading to global warming. When people burn fossil fuels, such as oil, coal, etc., or cut down forests or burn wood, a large amount of carbon dioxide and other greenhouse gases are produced, which are highly permeable to visible light from the Sun and highly absorbent to longwave radiation emitted from the Earth and can strongly absorb infrared radiation from the ground, causing the Earth's temperature to rise, i.e., the greenhouse effect. The continued accumulation of greenhouse gases in the atmosphere results in an imbalance between the energy absorbed and emitted by the Earth's atmosphere, and energy continues to accumulate in the Earth's atmosphere, which leads to a rise in temperature, eventually resulting in the phenomenon of global warming. The temperature of the Earth's surface has been rising since the end of the last century.

The Earth's Climate Is Warming Due to Natural Factors The Earth's periodic rotation trajectory changes from an elliptical to a circular trajectory, with the Earth moving farther from and closer to the Sun. The Earth's temperature used to alternate between high and low with a certain regularity. In the past 100 years, the global average temperature has experienced four fluctuation periods, including cold, from cold to warm, from warm to cold, and back to warm; the general trend is upward, the global temperature has risen significantly since the beginning of the 1980s.

14.1.3 The Main Hazards of Climate Warming

Studies have shown that the Earth's climate has been changing significantly in the last hundred years, especially in recent decades, and the main feature of the change is global warming. The 2007 IPCC Fourth Assessment Report on Climate Change pointed out that the twentieth century might be the warmest 100 years in the last 1000 years. The report also clearly noted that most of the global warming in the past 50 years was related to greenhouse gas emissions generated by human activities [5, 6]. Climate change will cause not only changes in the human living environment but also many human health problems. From a macro perspective, global warming is likely to be the common challenge facing humanity in the future and probably the greatest health challenge. Understanding the relationships between climate change, environmental temperature, and population health is the basis for addressing climate change challenges and will help people develop long-term, efficient response strategies and specific measures.

In addition to affecting population health, climate change also affects changes of the environment that are highly related to environmental pollution. Therefore, apart from studying the relationship between climate conditions and population health, we should also study the relationships between climate change and environmental changes or environmental pollution and further understand the relationships between environmental pollution and population health related to climate conditions.

Since the Earth's climate change is progressive and global and the factors affecting human health as well as the disease spectrum are complex, it is difficult to study the relationship between climate change and human health from the perspective of global climate change. However, global climate change often brings drastic local temperature changes, the so-called extreme weather changes. In the context of global warming, the frequency of extreme weather conditions is becoming more frequent, which has attracted widespread concern in academia, and the study of the effects of extreme weather conditions on population health is becoming an important aspect in the field of environmental epidemiology. As a result, most scholars, when exploring the relationship between climate change and population health, often take extreme weather as the entry point to conduct research. The so-called extreme weather mainly refers to heat waves and cold waves, in addition to those that cause great catastrophes (tsunamis, typhoons, etc.). Internationally, there have been many research reports on the relationships between heat waves and cold spell and population health. In recent years, scholars in China have also begun to pay attention to these relationships and have also conducted fruitful studies.

14.2 Extreme Weather and Total Mortality or Cardiovascular Mortality

14.2.1 Heat Waves and Total Mortality or Cardiovascular Mortality

Heat Waves and Total Mortality A heat wave is an extremely hot weather that lasts for several days. However, there is no internationally unified definition. Definitions of heat waves vary widely from country to country. In fact, different countries are located in different geographical locations (longitude and latitude) on the Earth, geography and landforms are also different, and the daily climatic temperature varies greatly; residents living in different regions also have significantly different feelings about climatic temperature and adaptabilities to climatic temperature. Therefore, no universally accepted definition of a heat wave can be found worldwide. In general, heat waves can be defined in terms of local temperature levels (mean or maximum), thresholds, and durations, which are based on past local conventional and extreme temperature levels. Different temperatures during heat waves and large differences in the definitions of heat waves lead to a lack of comparability among different research results, which also affects the extrapolation of the results.

In the context of global climate change, the frequency and intensity of extreme hot weather events, such as heat waves, have increased with global warming in recent decades. Therefore, problems of health caused by heat waves and heat wave-associated mortality have become public health problem worldwide. In a special report released by the Intergovernmental Panel on Climate Change (IPCC) in 2012, heat waves are compared to "summer killers." In a study on the relationship between heat waves and population mortality, excess mortality or excess mortality risk was mainly used to evaluate the damage of heat waves to population health. Estimating the risk of heat wave-associated excess mortality has important social and public health implications.

There have been some studies on effects of heat waves on mortality in population [7–11]. American scholars [8] analyzed heat waves in duration of 14 years from 1987 to 2000 and the relationship between the time, duration, and intensity of the heat waves and the risk of death in the United States. In this study, a heat wave was defined as a continuous climate temperature above the heat threshold for 2 days or more. They used five heat cutoffs (95th–99th percentiles) and a two-stage model to estimate the excess risk of heat waves. During 14 years from 1987 to 2000, there were 115 heat waves with a total duration of 389 days. Among 115 heat waves, severe heat waves (taking 99th percentile as cutoff value) occurred 9 times with a total duration of 19 days. The results showed that heat waves, especially the hottest heat wave, could significantly increase the risk of death. Their findings showed that the hottest heat wave increased the risk of death by 1.6% [95% confidence interval (CI): 1.1%–2.1%]. They further analyzed deaths in different age groups during heat waves, which showed a significant increase in mortality among aged people during heat waves, as defined by all thresholds. The excess deaths of elderly individuals due to the hottest waves were mainly attributed to cardiovascular disease. Their analysis also showed that heat waves were more harmful in the early part of the warm season [8].

Anderson et al. [9] analyzed characteristics of heat wave (intensity, duration, start time) and heat wave-associated health effects in 43 American cities (communities) over 19 years (1987–2005). They defined heat waves as ≥2 days with temperatures ≥95th percentile of the community for 1st of May through 30th of September. The risk of death during each heat wave period (compared to non-heat wave periods) was estimated after controlling for potential confounding factors in each city (community). They analyzed the effects of characteristics of heat wave on mortality based on effect estimates of combined individual heat wave using Bayesian hierarchical model to generate overall effects at the city, regional, and national levels. Table 14.1 presents a summary of characteristics of heat wave for 43 cities and different regions in the United States.

Table 14.2 lists excess deaths during heat waves in 43 American cities and other areas. The results showed that there was a 3.74% [95% posterior interval (PI): 2.29%–5.22%] increase in mortality during the heat wave period compared to the non-heat wave period across the country (43 cities combined). The mortality rate increased by 6.76% (95% PI: 1.79%–11.98%), 5.62% (95% PI: 3.36%–7.93%), and 1.84% (95% PI: −0.11%–3.84%) in the Northeast, Midwest, and South, respectively.

For a total of 43 cities, the risk of death increased by 2.49% and 0.38% for every 1 °F increase in heat wave intensity and for each additional day of heat wave duration, respectively. In the Northeast, Midwest, and South, the risk of death increased by 4.39%, 3.22%, and 0.43%, respectively, for every 1 °F increase in heat wave intensity, and the effect of heat wave on risk of death was significant in the Northeast and Midwest. The risk of death increased by 2.50%, 0.09%, and 0.08% in the Northeast, Midwest, and South for heat wave duration increasing by 1 day, respectively. Both nationally and regionally, the impacts of heat wave on death decreased with every delayed 1 day of the start time of heat wave (Table 14.3). Throughout the summer, the earlier a heat wave occurs, the greater the risk of death, and the risk of death from a lagging heat wave (before the end of the warm season) was lower. As shown in Table 14.4, the risk of death

Table 14.2 Summary of excess mortality effects due to heat wave

Region (*n* = number of city)	Excess mortality, % (95% PI)
Nationwide (*n* = 43)	3.74 (2.29, 5.22)
Northeast (*n* = 7)	6.76 (1.79, 11.98)
Midwest (*n* = 12)	5.62 (3.36, 7.93)
South (*n* = 19)	1.84 (−0.11, 3.84)

The heat wave effect is the increase in non-accidental mortality risk for heat wave days compared with non-heat wave days, controlling for daily temperature (the added heat wave effect described by Hajat et al. 2006)
Anderson and Bell, Environ Health Perspect, 2011, 119:210–218

Table 14.3 Percentage (%) of increased relative risk of mortality during a heat wave per unit increase in heat wave characteristics (1987–2005)

Region (*n* = number of city)	Increase of 1 °F in average T_{mean}	One-day increase in duration of heat wave	One-day increase in timing in season (1 May = 1)
Nationwide (*n* = 43)	2.49 ***	0.38	−0.063 **
Northeast (*n* = 7)	4.39 ***	2.50 **	−0.227 **
Midwest (*n* = 12)	3.22 ***	0.09	−0.071
South (*n* = 19)	0.43	0.08	−0.022

Data are percent increase in the relative risk of non-accidental mortality on heat wave days compared with non-heat wave days, controlling for daily temperature, for a unit increase in the heat wave characteristic
**$p < 0.05$; ***$p < 0.01$
Anderson and Bell, Environ Health Perspect, 2011, 119:210–218

Table 14.1 Summary of heat waves characteristics (1987–2005)

Region	Heat waves characteristics Number/year/community	Intensity (°F)	Duration (day)	Start time
Nationwide (*n* = 43)	1.9	86.4	3.3	21 July
Northeast (*n* = 7)	1.9	84.4	3.1	21 July
Midwest (*n* = 12)	1.9	83.3	3.2	18 July
South (*n* = 19)	1.8	88.1	3.4	23 July

For each characteristic shown, community-specific averages were calculated and then averaged nationally or by region
Anderson and Bell, Environ Health Perspect, 2011, 119:210–218

Table 14.4 Average mortality effects of the first heat wave in a summer versus later heat waves (1987–2005)

Region (n = number of city)	Average effect of heat waves (95% PI) First in season, %	Not first in season,%
Nationwide (n = 43)	5.04 (3.06, 7.06)	2.65 (1.14, 4.18)
Northeast (n = 7)	11.08 (4.05, 18.58)	3.45 (−1.16, 8.28)
Midwest (n = 12)	5.29 (1.76, 8.94)	5.42 (2.46, 8.46)
South (n = 19)	3.29 (0.12, 6.56)	0.68 (−1.60, 3.02)

The heat wave effect is the increase in non-accidental mortality risk for heat wave days compared with non-heat wave days, controlling for daily temperature [the added heat wave effect described by Hajat et al. (2006)]
Anderson and Bell, Environ Health Perspect, 2011, 119:210–218

was increased by 5.04% (95% PI: 3.06%–7.06%) for the first heat wave in summer and by 2.65% (95% PI: 1.14%–4.18%) for the later heat waves (Table 14.4). The effect of heat waves on mortality in the early warm season may be related to the low adaptability of humans to heat. These results suggested that the effects of heat waves on mortality should be influenced by different characteristics of heat waves, and the different characteristics of heat waves had a more significant impact on mortality in the Northeast and Midwest than in the South.

It is very important to study the effect of heat waves on human health because it is helpful for us to explore strategies to address the impact of climate change on human health. It can be predicted that the Earth will be hit by heat waves more frequently in the future, their durations will be longer, and their intensities will be stronger due to the excessive activities of humans and the drastic changes in the natural ecology. This was one of some systematic studies to date on the effects of heat waves on mortality in the United States. It examined the effects of heat waves and their characteristics on mortality of population from a national, regional, and city perspective. They reported not only the effect of heat waves on excess deaths but also the effect of different characteristics of heat wave on deaths in different regions, providing an important reference for other countries to research the effect of heat wave on human health and formulate countermeasures.

Guo et al. [10] investigated the impacts of heat waves on mortality with lag effects in 400 communities in 18 countries/regions internationally. This was the largest and first multi-country study of heat waves to examine effect modification by heat wave duration and intensity. They collected daily data of temperature and mortality systematically from the 1980s to the 2000s. The 12 types of heat waves were defined by combining community-specific daily mean temperature ≥ 90th, 92.5th, 95th, and 97.5th percentiles of temperature with duration ≥2, 3 and 4 days. Time series analyses were used to estimate relationship between the community-specific heat wave and mortality over lags of 0–10 days. Then, a meta-analysis was applied to pool heat wave effects at the level of country for cumulative and lag effects for each type of heat wave definition. The findings showed significant cumulative associations between heat waves of all definitions and mortality in all countries, but varied by community. They found that heat waves of all types of definitions were associated with increased risk of death in all countries/regions. The estimated effects of heat wave on mortality were higher when using higher temperature thresholds (e.g., 97.5th vs 95th percentile of temperature). Furthermore, heat waves had stronger associations with mortality in areas of moderate cold and moderate hot than those of cold and hot. They believed that people living in areas of moderate cold and moderate hot were more sensitive to heat waves than those living in areas of cold and hot.

In 2003, Shanghai experienced the hottest summer in 50 years. Huang et al. [11] analyzed the variation in mortality during the 2003 heat wave in Shanghai using meteorological and population mortality data. The heat wave lasted for 19 days from 19th of July to 6th of August 2003. They chose 28th of June to 9th of July and 16th of August to 22nd of August as the roughly comparable non-heat wave period, which also lasted 19 days. Excess mortality and relative risk (RR) were calculated during the heat wave period compared to the non-heat wave period. The results showed that the RR of total mortality during the heat wave period was 1.13 (95% CI: 1.06–1.20) compared with the non-heat wave period. The average daily maximum temperature during the heat wave period was 36.3 °C, the average daily maximum temperature during the non-heat wave period (28 June–9 July; 16 August–22 August) was 32.3 °C, and the hottest day during the heat wave period was 25 July, with a temperature of 39.0 °C. The total number of excess deaths during the heat wave period was 258 cases. Their study suggested that the 2003 heat wave in Shanghai had a substantial effect on the increase of mortality rate (Table 14.5).

The results also showed that there was no significant difference between males and females but a significant difference between age groups in the effects of heat wave on mortality; people aged over 65 years were the most sensitive to heat wave, and the risk of death among people aged over 65 years increased by 13% during heat wave period compared with non-heat wave period (Table 14.6).

The impact of heat waves on population health was affected by many factors, such as the local socioeconomic development level, building heatstroke prevention facilities, rate of air-conditioning utilization, rate of city afforestation, and income level of residents. With the deepening understanding of the relationship between heat waves and population health, researchers began to explore the impact of heat waves on population health with the concept of multiple factors. Along with meteorological data on heat waves and their effects on health, such as deaths, they also focused on collecting other relevant data affecting the health effects of heat waves, such as latitude, air-conditioning use rate, greenery rate, and income levels.

Ma et al. [12] from Fudan University in Shanghai, China, carried out a multicenter study on the impact of urban heat waves on health of population in 16 typical cities in China to assess the effects of seasonal first heat waves on health in population and to assess the modification of urban characteristics on the health risks associated with heat waves. Relatively speaking, their research was a more systematic and comprehensive study on the impact of heat waves on the health of population in China.

Table 14.6 Sex- and age-stratified total mortality during the 2003 Shanghai heat wave period (July 19–August 6, 2003), versus the summer time reference period (June 28–July 9 and August 16–August 22)

	Reference period	Heat wave period	RR (95% CI)
Sex			
Male	1053	1217	1.16 (1.06, 1.26)
Female	972	1066	1.10 (1.01, 1.20)
Age (year)			
0–4	9	6	0.67 (0.24, 1.87)
5–44	62	71	1.15 (0.81, 1.61)
45–64	292	325	1.11 (0.95, 1.30)
≥65	1662	1881	1.13 (1.06, 1.21)

Huang W, Kan H and Kovats S, Science of the Total Environment, 2010, 408: 2418–2420

Table 14.5 Total and cause-specific death number during the 2003 Shanghai heat wave period (July 19–August 6, 2003), versus the summer time reference period (June 28–July 9 and August 16–August 22)

	Reference period death number	Heat wave period death number	RR (95% CI)[a]
Total	2025	2283	1.13 (1.06, 1.20)
Cardiovascular	691	825	1.19 (1.08, 1.32)
Stroke	371	450	1.21 (1.06, 1.39)
CHD	283	339	1.20 (1.02, 1.40)
Respiratory	201	247	1.23 (1.02, 1.48)
COPD	167	199	1.19 (0.97, 1.46)
ARI	18	15	0.83(0.42, 1.65)

[a]RRs were calculated as ratios between the death numbers in the heat-wave period and in the reference period
Huang W, Kan H and Kovats S, Science of the Total Environment, 2010, 408: 2418–2420

The cities chosen for their research included Beijing, Taiyuan, Tangshan, Tianjin, Shenyang, Anshan, Nanjing, Shanghai, Suzhou, Hangzhou, Lanzhou, Xi'an, Wuhan, Fuzhou, Guangzhou, and Hong Kong. These cities are widely distributed in all geographical regions of China (except the southwest region). The city at the highest latitude was Shenyang (41 degrees 48 minutes north latitude), and the city at the lowest latitude was Hong Kong (22 degrees 15 minutes north latitude). This study included three temperature zones, subtropical, warm temperate, and moderate temperate, and covered three types of climate: subtropical monsoon climate, temperate monsoon climate, and temperate continental climate. The 16 selected cities basically reflected the different geographical locations and social and economic development levels of the Chinese Pearl River Delta, Yangtze River Delta, Beijing-Tianjin-Hebei, and Northeast China provinces. According to the 2008 population statistics in China, the urban population of these 16 studied cities was approximately 69.7 million, and the geographical distribution of these 16 cities could basically reflected the climate characteristics and regional socioeconomic development levels in China. The 16 cities in the study were divided into southern and northern cities based on whether they had centralized heating in winter. The southern cities in China had no centralized heating in winter, while northern cities had centralized heating.

Data for these cities were collected from the China Statistical Yearbook, using the median year of the study period to represent characteristics such as latitude, air conditioning rate, age structure, greening rate, and per capita disposable income.

These cities had established a relatively comprehensive mortality monitoring system, and the daily data about mortality for residents in each city were collected by the staff at the Centers for Disease Control and Prevention. The data on death for residents in the study were coded according to the International Classification of Diseases (ICD-10). The ICD codes for total deaths (non-accidental deaths) were A00-R99, and the ICD codes for cardiovascular deaths were I00-I99. Data on disease-specific deaths were available in 15 of these cities.

Average daily temperature, daily maximum temperature, daily minimum temperature, and the data on daily average relative humidity were collected from meteorological bureaus in various cities for the study period. Data on daily air pollution were collected from the national air quality automatic monitoring system, including particulate matter smaller than 10 microns (PM_{10}), sulfur dioxide (SO_2), and nitrogen dioxide (NO_2). During the heat wave period, the daily maximum temperature was above 37 °C (81%) in 13 cities, the daily maximum temperature was above 35 °C (19%) in 3 cities, the daily maximum temperature in Xi'an was 41.7 °C, and the daily maximum temperature in both Lanzhou and Shenyang was 34 °C [12].

A total of 137 heat waves occurred in 16 cities, with an average of approximately 2 heat waves per year (Table 14.7). The average duration of heat waves was 6 days, with a maximum

Table 14.7 Number of heat wave and average days of heat wave duration in 16 cities in China

	Number of heat wave	Average days of a heat wave duration
Northern city	66	6
Beijing	5	5
Tianjin	6	4
Tangshan	5	6
Taiyuan	12	6
Shenyang	10	6
Anshan	5	4
Lanzhou	11	6
Xi'an	12	6
Southern city	71	7
Wuhan	6	8
Nanjing	10	8
Suzhou	8	7
Shanghai	7	9
Hangzhou	6	7
Fuzhou	8	7
Guangzhou	6	7
Hong Kong	20	6

Ma W, et al. A study on temperature-related mortality in 16 Chinese cities, PhD dissertation, Fudan University (2014), from Wanfang data of 9 days in Shanghai and a minimum of 4 days in Anshan and Tianjin.

The study showed that the RR of overall mortality associated with heat waves was statistically significant in 9 of the 16 studied cities: Beijing, Taiyuan, Shenyang, Lanzhou, Xi'an, Wuhan, Nanjing, Suzhou, and Shanghai. The RR of total mortality from heat waves was highest in Wuhan and Suzhou, with RRs of 1.10 (95% CI: 1.03–1.18) and 1.10 (95% CI: 1.04–1.16), respectively [12] (Table 14.8).

The total risk of death was analyzed in 11 cities by age subgroup. The results showed that the overall risk of death associated with heat waves in residents aged ≥65 was higher than in those aged <65 in 9 cities: Beijing, Guangzhou, Lanzhou, Shanghai, Shenyang, Suzhou, Taiyuan, Tianjin, and Xi'an. In Xi'an, the overall risk of death for residents aged 65 or older was 1.06 (95% CI: 1.02–1.11) during the heat wave period, which was a 6% increase compared with that during the non-heat wave period. In Suzhou, the overall RR of death for residents aged 65 or older was 1.09 (95% CI: 1.03–1.17), which was 9% higher in the heat wave period than in the non-heat wave period.

Table 14.8 The relative risk (RR) of non-accidental mortality associated with heat waves in 16 cities of China

City	Average RR	95% CI
Northern city		
Beijing	1.03	1.00, 1.06
Tianjin	1.00	0.91, 1.08
Tangshan	1.01	0.92, 1.12
Taiyuan	1.04	1.00, 1.08
Shenyang	1.05	1.03, 1.07
Anshan	1.04	0.95, 1.15
Lanzhou	1.04	1.01, 1.08
Xi'an	1.05	1.02, 1.09
Southern city		
Wuhan	1.10	1.03, 1.08
Nanjing	1.03	1.01, 1.06
Suzhou	1.10	1.04, 1.16
Shanghai	1.06	1.03, 1.09
Hangzhou	1.02	0.96, 1.08
Fuzhou	0.90	0.90, 1.07
Guangzhou	1.03	0.96, 1.10
Hong Kong	1.01	1.00, 1.02

Ma W, et al. A study on temperature-related mortality in 16 Chinese cities, PhD dissertation, Fudan University (2014), from Wanfang data

The results stratified by sex showed that the overall risk of mortality associated with heat waves was higher in women than in men in Guangzhou, Lanzhou, Shanghai, Suzhou, and Hong Kong. In Beijing, Fuzhou, Shenyang, Taiyuan, Tianjin, and Xi'an, the total risk of death during the heat wave period was lower for women than for men [12].

From the results above, it could be seen that the impact of heat waves on the health of residents differed significantly among different residents in different cities. There were many factors affecting the results. The differences among cities may be due to different characteristics of the cities. The differences among residents may be caused by factors such as different living habits, physiological reactions, and local socioeconomic conditions. In addition, the characteristics of the heat wave, such as the severity, duration, and occurrence time of the heat wave, were also important factors in the different mortality risks.

Recently, Sun et al. [13] conducted a multicenter study nationally on characteristics of heat wave, mortality, and modification of effect by temperature zones in 130 counties of China. They defined heat waves as ≥2 days with a temperature ≥ 99th percentile for the county from May 1 to September 30. Within each county, the total non-accidental mortality during each heat wave were estimated by comparing with duration of non-heat wave and adjusting for potential confounders in summer. They combined effect estimates of individual heat wave using a random-effects model to compute overall effects at the temperature zone and national levels. Across the 130 counties, the risks of non-accidental mortality were substantially increased during heat waves; they found that heat waves increased the risk of total non-accidental death by 15.7% (95% CI: 12.5%–18.9%) in the periods of heat wave compared with periods of non-heat wave. There was a significant timing effect in the season on the associations between heat wave and mortality. The first heat wave in the season was associated with the greatest risk of non-accidental mortality. The risk of non-accidental mortality during the first heat wave of the season increased by 16.3% (95% CI: 12.6%–20.2%), and the risks decreased substantially for the second heat wave (6.3%) and the subsequent heat waves (−2.1%). Thus, early heat waves were associated with a greater risk of mortality than later waves. The effect sizes of the first day, and second to third days, of the heat wave on total non-accidental mortality appeared to be larger than that of the fourth and subsequent days of the heat wave [13] (Table 14.9).

The risk of non-accidental mortality associated with heat waves in Model A increased by 18.2% (95% CI: 11.4%–25.4%), 17.6% (95% CI: 11.7%–23.9%), and 13.6% (95% CI: 9.4%–17.9%) in the mid-temperature zone, warm temperature zone, and subtropical zone, respectively. Mid- and warm temperature zones showed greater risk of non-accidental mortality than subtropical zone, although there were non-significant differences in the risks of heat wave-associated mortality across mid-, warm, and subtropical temperature zones. In the present study, they concluded that heat waves increased the risks of mortality, and characteristics of heat waves, including intensity levels and duration as well as timing, played important roles in risks of heat wave-associated mortality. They also suggested that national early warning systems about heat wave should be developed, as well as precautions and protection warranted according to characteristics of heat waves [13].

Heat Waves and Cardiovascular Mortality The Czech scholar Kyselý [14] studied the effect of heat waves on cardiovascular mortality using meteorological and mortality data from 1986 to 2006 in the Czech Republic. During the 21 years, the Czech Republic experienced a total of 29 heat waves that met the study's definition, lasting a total of 83 days, with an average duration of 4 days per heat wave. The results showed that heat waves were associated with excess cardiovascular mortality, and excess cardiovascular mortality caused by heat waves might be a direct effect that occurred mainly during the heat wave period. In both the general population and males, excess mortality occurred between the first and third days of the heat waves. In females, excess mortality occurred between the first and fourth days of the heat waves. There was a significant difference between males and females in the effect of excess mortality caused by heat waves. The excess mortality rate of females was higher than that of males and was twice as high as that of males on the second day of heat waves. Their study also showed that the effect of heat waves on excess mortality from cardiovascular disease varies with age, with the largest effect in the over 80 age group. Study by Son et al. [15] in seven cities in South Korea also showed that heat waves increased the all-

Table 14.9 Percent increase (95% CI) in total non-accidental mortality risk due to heat waves in 130 counties

Heat wave		Total non-accidental mortality	
		% increase (95% CI)	P^a
Model A[b]	Heat wave	15.65 (12.47, 18.92)	/
Model B[b]	The first heat wave	16.30 (12.58, 20.15)	Ref
	The second heat wave	6.28 (2.76, 9.92)	$P < 0.05$
	Additional heat waves	−2.14 (−4.60, 0.38)	$P < 0.05$
Model C[b]	The first day of the heat wave	11.67 (7.58, 15.92)	Ref
	The second-third days of the heat wave	16.95 (13.07, 20.96)	$P > 0.05$
	The fourth and subsequent days of the heat wave	6.34 (2.35, 10.49)	$P < 0.05$

Sun, et al. Int J Epidemiol. 2021 Jan 23;49(6):1813–1822

[a]The Wald test P-values are the mortality risk of the second heat wave vs the first heat wave (Model B), additional heat waves vs the first heat wave (Model B), the second-third days of the heat wave vs the first day of the heat wave, and the fourth and subsequent days of the heat wave vs the first day of the heat wave

[b]Model A: percent increase (95% CI) in the mortality risk associated with heat waves across the 130 counties. Model B: percent increase (95% CI) in the mortality risk associated with the timing of the heat wave in the season across the 130 counties. Model C: percent increase (95% CI) in the mortality risk associated with the day of the heat wave across the 130 counties

cause mortality, with cardiovascular and respiratory diseases being the most affected.

In 2003, Shanghai experienced the hottest summer in past 50 years. The heat wave lasted for 19 days from 19 July to 6 August in 2003. Huang et al. [11] analyzed the variation in mortality during the 2003 heat wave in Shanghai using meteorological and population mortality data. The results showed that the RR of total mortality during heat waves was 1.13 (95% CI: 1.06–1.20) compared with that during non-heat waves. Among various diseases leading to deaths, cardiovascular disease and respiratory disease had the greatest impact on mortality, the RR of cardiovascular death caused by heat waves was 1.19 (95% CI: 1.08–1.32), and the RR of respiratory disease death was 1.23 (95% CI: 1.02–1.48) (Table 14.5).

A study conducted in 16 typical Chinese cities by Ma et al. [12] at Fudan University in Shanghai, China, also found that cardiovascular diseases accounted for a large proportion of the mortality caused by heat waves. However, the risk of cardiovascular death varied greatly among cities. For example, Wuhan, Shanghai, and Suzhou had the highest risk of cardiovascular death during the heat wave period compared with the reference period, and the corresponding RRs were 1.14 (95% CI: 1.04–1.24), 1.08 (95% CI: 1.05–1.11), and 1.11 (95% CI: 1.01–1.21), respectively. Residents in Wuhan, Shanghai, and Suzhou had excess cardiovascular mortality of 14%, 8%, and 11%, respectively.

Sun et al. [13] reported that heat waves increased the risk of cardiovascular-related death in their study, a multicenter study of 130 counties in China. Across the 130 counties, the risk of cardiovascular deaths was substantially increased in periods of heat waves, with an increase of 22.0% (95% CI: 16.9%–27.4%) compared with periods of non-heat wave. They also observed a significant timing effect in the season on the associations between heat wave and cardiovascular mortality. The first heat wave in the season was associated with the greatest risk of cardiovascular mortality with 23.83% increase (95% CI: 18.17%–29.77%) and the risks of cardiovascular mortality decreased for the second heat wave (6.28%) and the subsequent heat waves (−0.03%). The effect sizes of the first day, and second to third days, of the heat wave on cardiovascular mortality were larger than those of the fourth and subsequent days of the heat wave [13] (Table 14.10). These findings suggested that the effect of heat waves on cardiovascular disease-associated mortality could be more pronounced in the death association, and cardiovascular death could be more sensitive to high temperature.

Table 14.10 Percent increase (95% CI) in cardiovascular mortality risk due to heat waves in 130 counties

Heat wave		Cardiovascular mortality	
		% increase (95% CI)	P[a]
Model A[b]	Heat wave	22.02 (16.91, 27.35)	/
Model B[b]	The first heat wave	23.83 (18.17, 29.77)	*Ref*
	The second heat wave	9.73 (3.76, 16.05)	*P < 0.05*
	Additional heat waves	−0.03 (−4.02, −4.12)	*P < 0.05*
Model C[b]	The first day of the heat wave	15.38 (8.83, 22.33)	*Ref*
	The second-third days of the heat wave	24.26 (18.15, 30.68)	*P > 0.05*
	The fourth and subsequent days of the heat wave	12.01 (5.69, 18.70)	*P > 0.05*

Sun, et al. Int J Epidemiol. 2021 Jan 23;49(6):1813–1822

[a]The Wald test P-values are the mortality risk of the second heat wave vs the first heat wave (Model B), additional heat waves vs the first heat wave (Model B), the second-third days of the heat wave vs the first day of the heat wave, and the fourth and subsequent days of the heat wave vs the first day of the heat wave

[b]Model A: percent increase (95% CI) in the mortality risk associated with heat waves across the 130 counties. Model B: percent increase (95% CI) in the mortality risk associated with the timing of the heat wave in the season across the 130 counties. Model C: percent increase (95% CI) in the mortality risk associated with the day of the heat wave across the 130 counties

14.2.2 Cold Spell and Total Mortality or Cardiovascular Mortality

Notably, with more and more heat waves, there is also a cold spell; the impact of a cold spell on the health of the population is also worthy of in-depth study. A cold spell is a kind of catastrophic weather in winter. A so-called cold spell refers to cold air from high latitudes rapidly intensifying and invading middle and low latitudes in a specific weather situation, causing severe cooling, wind, rain, and snow in the areas along the way. When this cold air invasion reaches a certain standard, it is called a cold spell. As defined by China's meteorological department, when a cold air invasion causes the temperature to drop by more than 10 °C per day and the minimum temperature is lower than 5 °C, the cold air outbreak process will be called a cold spell.

A cold spell can cause great harm to human health. Windy and cold weather can easily cause colds, bronchitis, asthma, pulmonary heart disease, coronary heart disease, stroke, myocardial infarction, and other severe diseases and can sometimes aggravate patients' conditions. As a result, when a cold spell arrives and a sudden drop in temperature occurs, it is more harmful to elderly and weak patients, especially to those with a history of the abovementioned diseases and those who are sensitive to temperature changes. The results of several domestic and international studies have shown that cold spells are associated with an excess risk of death in the population and that cold spells can lead to an increased risk of total mortality [8, 16–18] and cardiovascular disease mortality [12, 19, 20] in the population.

Kyselý et al. [14] found that the risks of cardiovascular disease-related deaths during cold spells were the highest among residents aged between 25 and 59 years old. The effect of cold spells on the risk of total mortality in the population was studied by scholars in Russia who analyzed the excess mortality rate of total deaths in all age groups in a city during 2 cold spells [20]. Their results showed that the effect of cold spells on the total mortality of the population was significant only in the group of elderly people over 75 years of age. Compared with the mortality rate during the same period without cold spells, the excess total mortality rates for the population over 75 years of age during the two cold spells were 9.9% (95% CI: 8.0%–12%) and 8.9% (95% CI: 6.7%–11.0%), while the excess total mortality rates for all age groups under 75 years of age were not significant. However, the excess risk of death due to cold spell-related cardiovascular disease in the total population was significant [20].

Barnett et al. [8] conducted a similar study in which they statistically analyzed the change in mortality in total population during cold spells in 99 US cities over a 14-year period (1987–2000), comparing the mortality rates during cold spells with those during normal cold weather conditions. Their results showed that cold spells did not significantly increase the risk of mortality. In contrast to the results of Barnett et al. [8], Ma et al. [21] from Japan found a significant increase in the risk of residential mortality due to cold spells, which mortality was significantly higher during cold spell days vs other days for all causes of death. Associations between cold spells and mortality from all causes and several more specific outcomes were stronger for longer and more intense cold spells and for cold spells earlier in the cold season.

Scholars from India [22] investigated effects of heat and cold on mortality in India by using a nationally representative study for 2001–2013. Nonlinear models of distributed-lag with case-crossover models were applied to estimate the effects of heat and cold on all medical death causes for all ages from birth ($n = 411{,}613$) as well as on stroke ($n = 19{,}753$), ischemic heart disease ($n = 40{,}003$), and respiratory diseases ($n = 23{,}595$) among adults of 30–69 years. They computed the attributable risk fractions by death cause for extremely cold (0.4 to 13.8 °C), moderately cold (13.8 °C to cause-specific minimum mortality temperatures), moderately hot (cause-specific minimum mortality temperatures to 34.2 °C), and extremely hot temperatures (34.2 to 39.7 °C). Mortality from all medical causes, stroke, and respiratory diseases showed excess risks at moderately cold temperature and hot temperature. For all examined causes, moderately cold temperature had higher attributable risks [6.3% (95%

CI: 1.1%–11.1%) for all medical deaths, 27.2% (95% CI: 11.4%- 40.2%) for stroke, 9.7% (95% CI: 3.7% –15.3%) for ischemic heart disease, and 6.5% (95% CI: 3.5%–9.2%) for respiratory diseases] than extremely cold, moderately hot, and extremely hot temperatures [22]. Their findings suggested that moderately cold temperature should be more harmful effects for health than moderately hot and extremely hot temperatures in India. Therefore, public health interventions for detrimental effects of ambient hot and cold temperatures on population health need to focus on not only extremely hot temperatures but also moderately cold temperatures in India.

The findings on the effects of cold spells on the risk of non-accidental death in the population varied considerably among studies, and there were multiple reasons for this variability. First, there was no a unified international standard for the definition of a cold spell, different countries were located in different geographical regions, and different definitions or temperature criteria for cold spells were used in different studies, in which case, the results obtained were also different. Second, different countries or different regions had different levels of socioeconomic development, resulting in different precautions and protection levels to cold spells when they struck, and this might also be the main reason for the differences in results among different studies. In China, some scholars analyzed the effects of cold spells on cardiovascular and cerebrovascular disease-related death in the population. The results showed that cold spells with large temperature drops and accompanying high pressure might cause an increased risk of death from cardiovascular and cerebrovascular diseases. During such cold spells, the daily risks of death from cardiovascular and cerebrovascular diseases in the population increased significantly [23, 24]. Previous findings also suggest a higher overall risk of death during cold spells in older age groups than in younger age groups. Most of the studies conducted in China on cold spells, total mortality, and cardiovascular mortality in the population were conducted only for individual cities and restricted to studies in a few regions or cities.

Ma et al. [12] at Fudan University in Shanghai, China, conducted a multicenter study on the effects of urban cold spells on residents' health in 16 typical cities in China, and the risks of death due to cold spells in these 16 cities were shown in Table 14.11. Overall, the RR of total non-accidental deaths due to cold spells was 1.07 (95% CI: 1.05–1.09), and the RR of cardiovascular death was 1.10 (95% CI: 1.07–1.13); the city with the highest total risk of death was Tianjin (RR: 1.24; 95% CI: 1.08–1.41), and the city with the lowest risk was Fuzhou (RR: 0.90; 95% CI: 0.79–1.02), which was not statistically significant. The total risk of death among residents due to cold spells was statistically significant in six of the eight southern cities, and the cities with higher RRs were Hangzhou (RR: 1.14; 95% CI: 1.07–1.21), Guangzhou (RR: 1.13; 95% CI: 1.09–1.18), and Hong Kong (RR: 1.13; 95% CI: 1.10–1.17). Among the eight northern cities, only two cities had statistically significant RRs, namely, Tianjin (RR: 1.24; 95% CI: 1.08–1.41) and Xi'an (RR: 1.05; 95% CI: 1.00–1.11) (Table 14.11). In comparison to cities by geographic region, the total residential mortality risk due to cold spells was higher in the eight southern cities, where the

Table 14.11 Total relative risk (RR) of death associated with cold spell in 16 cities in China

Cities	RR	95% CI
Beijing	1.14	0.92, 1.41
Tianjin	1.24	1.08, 1.41
Tangshan	0.99	0.90, 1.09
Taiyuan	1.05	0.96, 1.15
Shenyang	1.06	0.97, 1.06
Anshan	1.00	0.94, 1.06
Lanzhou	1.04	0.98, 1.13
Xi'an	1.05	1.00, 1.11
Wuhan	1.00	0.95, 1.17
Nanjing	1.06	1.03, 1.10
Suzhou	1.07	1.00, 1.16
Shanghai	1.01	0.92, 1.10
Hangzhou	1.14	1.07, 1.21
Fuzhou	0.90	0.79, 1.02
Guangzhou	1.13	1.09, 1.18
Hong Kong	1.13	1.10, 1.17
China	1.07	1.05, 1.09

Ma W, et al. A study on temperature-related mortality in 16 Chinese cities, PhD dissertation, Fudan University (2014), from Wanfang data

Table 14.12 Relative risk (RR) of cardiovascular mortality associated with cold spell in 16 cities in China

Cities	RR	95% CI
Beijing	1.13	0.84, 1.51
Tianjin	1.44	1.20, 1.73
Tangshan	1.07	0.94, 1.21
Taiyuan	1.02	0.97, 1.08
Shenyang	1.07	0.99, 1.16
Anshan	1.01	0.93, 1.09
Lanzhou	–	–
Xi'an	1.04	0.97, 1.11
Wuhan	1.05	1.01, 1.10
Nanjing	1.10	1.02, 1.18
Suzhou	1.09	1.00, 1.20
Shanghai	1.03	0.95, 1.11
Hangzhou	1.12	0.93, 1.34
Fuzhou	0.87	0.75, 0.99
Guangzhou	1.18	1.10, 1.28
Hong Kong	1.23	1.17, 1,29
China	1.10	1.05, 1.09

Ma W, et al. A study on temperature-related mortality in 16 Chinese cities, PhD dissertation, Fudan University (2014), from Wanfang data

residents seemed to be more sensitive to cold spells, than in the northern cities [12].

As shown in Table 14.12, the risk of death from cardiovascular disease due to cold spells among residents varied significantly among the 15 cities; the city with the highest RR was Tianjin (RR: 1.44; 95% CI: 1.20–1.73), and the city with the lowest RR was Fuzhou (RR: 0.87; 95% CI: 0.75–0.99). Among the eight southern cities, five cities had statistically significant RRs: Wuhan (RR: 1.05; 95% CI: 1.01–1.10), Nanjing (RR: 1.10; 95% CI: 1.02–1.18), Suzhou (RR: 1.09; 95% CI: 1.00–1.20), Guangzhou (RR: 1.18; 95% CI: 1.10–1.28), and Hong Kong (RR: 1.23; 95% CI: 1.17–1.29). Among the seven northern cities, only Tianjin had a statistically significant RR (1.44; 95% CI: 1.20–1.73). When comparing cities by region, the risk of death from cardiovascular disease due to cold spells among residents was higher in the eight cities in the south than in those in the north, and the difference was not statistically significant. The study also analyzed the mortality effects due to cold spells in 11 of these cities on residents stratified by age. In southern cities, residents aged ≥65 years had a higher overall mortality risk than residents aged 0–64 years; in northern cities, such as Xi'an, Lanzhou, and Beijing, residents aged ≥65 years had a higher mortality risk [12].

14.3 Extreme Weather or Meteorological Factor and Myocardial Infarction

In recent years, extreme weather occurred frequently and had an impact on the incidence and mortality of cardiovascular diseases. During extreme weather conditions, such as heat waves, the incidence, mortality, emergency visits, and case-fatality rate of cardiovascular diseases had increased significantly. The main reason might be that extreme weather or some meteorological factors induced the onset of cardiovascular diseases or promoted the aggravation of diseases. Meteorological factors are mainly manifested in changes in temperature, atmospheric pressure, air humidity, wind speed, and other factors. Some meteorological factors may also be related to the incidence and mortality of cardiovascular diseases [25, 26]. Some meteorological factors not only manifest as changes in temperature, atmospheric pressure, air humidity, wind speed, and other factors but also affects air quality and even aggravates air pollution [27]. Therefore, the effects of some meteorological factors on incidence and mortality of cardiovascular diseases may be the result of the dual effects of meteorological factors and the aggravation of pollution. In field of research on the relationships between extreme weather or some meteorological factors and the incidence and mortality of cardiovascular diseases in past years, one of the hotspots was the effect of extreme weather or meteorological factors on acute myocardial infarction (AMI) or heart failure. Data of extreme weather or meteorological and hospital admission and death due to AMI or heart failure were often used to carry out relevant research.

In recent years, researchers had placed increasing emphasis on studying and exploring the effects of extreme weather or meteorological factors on cardiovascular disease, and a larger number of studies emerged. Among these studies, a special attention had been given to the effects of extreme weather or meteorological factors on AMI because it was the most serious cardiovascular disease with a high mortality rate. Methodologically, studying AMI as a representative cardiovascular disease could help elucidate the effects of extreme weather or meteorological factors on cardiovascular disease.

Loughnan et al. [25] investigated the relationships between summer temperature, family socioeconomic status, and the incidence and hospitalization of AMI in Melbourne, Australia. They took acute patients hospitalized in 37 hospitals as their research subjects. These patients were 35 years old and over, and the main diagnosis on admission was AMI. These patients included 99.2% of all patients hospitalized with AMI. They found that the rate of hospital admissions due to AMI increased significantly during a short-term (3 days) hot period in summer compared with that during the regular temperatures in summer. During the 3-day hot period, the rate of admissions due to AMI approached or exceeded that of the whole summer.

However, the results of Bhaskaran et al.'s study [26] in 15 large cities in England and Wales seemed to be contrary to those of Loughnan et al.'s study [25]. Bhaskaran et al. [26] used relevant data from the National Ischemic Heart Disease Survey Project from 2003 to 2006 to analyze the relationship between weather and temperature changes and AMI. There was no standard for the rise or fall of temperature in this study and having AMI admission as study outcome. A total of 84,010 patients with AMI were admitted to the hospital during this period. The results showed a wide linear relationship between temperature and AMI onset. Within 28 days, the daily average temperature dropped by 1 °C, and the cumulative risk of AMI increased by 2.0% (95% CI: 1.1%–2.9%). The study of Bhaskaran et al. [26] did not show that elevated temperature increased the risk of AMI. The completely different conclusions of the two studies may be related to the large geographical differences between the two countries and the different definitions of hyperthermic weather.

In another study by Bhaskaran et al. [27], they found that high temperature significantly increased the risk of AMI. In that study, they defined a clear temperature cutoff (20 °C), and they found that for per 1 °C increase in temperature exposure on the basis of the 20 °C cutoff, the risk of AMI was increased by 1.9% (95% CI: 0.5%–3.3%).

In another survey, Loughnan et al. [28] investigated the seasonal distribution of AMI. Their results showed that the rate of hospital admissions due to AMI showed obvious seasonal distribution characteristics throughout the year, with a significant increase from April to November, and the peak month was July. Further analysis of the seasonal characteristics by age and sex showed that the admission rate of men aged 65–74 increased significantly in October. After careful inspection, they found that the weather in October was often extremely hot or cold. Their results suggested that the occurrence of AMI had obvious characteristics of seasonal distribution with the lowest and highest incidences of AMI seasonally, and the high incidence of AMI often occurred in the hottest season. Dramatic temperature changes could lead to significant increases in the incidence of AMI and hospital admissions. A study described the ICU hospitalization rates due to acute coronary syndrome (unstable angina pectoris, ST-elevation MI, non-ST-elevation MI) in different climatic seasons in a hospital in Pakistan. Among the 428 patients hospitalized for acute coronary syndrome during the same period, 158 cases (36.9%) were admitted in winter, 130 (30.3%) in summer, 80 (18.69%) in spring, and 60 (14.02%) in autumn [29]. The rate of hospital admissions due to acute coronary syndrome was related to the season. The admission rates in summer and winter were higher than that in spring and autumn, and the admission rate in winter was the highest. Their study also found that the incidence of non-ST-elevation AMI in winter is more seasonal characteristics with temperature changes than that of ST-elevation AMI [29]. A study in New Zealand also calculated statistics on the seasonal changes in the hospitalization rate of patients with ST-elevation AMI. Their results showed that the hospitalization rate of patients with AMI in winter was significantly higher than that in summer ($P < 0.02$); especially in elderly patients over 70 years old, the incidence in winter was 8.5% higher than that in summer [30].

Liu et al. [31] investigate the association between extreme temperature and hospital admission due to AMI from 2013 to 2016 in Beijing, China. Indicators of extreme temperature included daily maximum temperature (Tmax), the apparent temperature of the daily maximum temperature (ATmax), daily minimum temperature (Tmin), and the apparent temperature of the daily minimum temperature (ATmin). The study outcome was defined as AMI by the tenth edition of International Classification of Diseases (ICD-10). They obtained a total of 81,029 patients with AMI and data of daily temperature from January 1, 2013, to December 31, 2016. Time series design and nonlinear model of distributed lag were employed to analyze effects of temperature on daily AMI patients. In this large population-based study, they found statistically significant association between short-term exposure to cold temperatures and hospital admissions due to AMI. For example, compared with the tenth percentile temperature measured by daily mean temperature (T mean), daily minimum temperature (Tmin), and daily minimum apparent temperature (ATmin), the cumulative relative risks (CRR) associated with first percentile of Tmean, Tmin, and AT min for AMI hospitalization were 1.15 (95% CI: 1.02–1.30), 1.24 (95% CI: 1.11–1.38), and 1.41 (95% CI: 1.18–1.68), respectively. However, no associations were found between high temperature and AMI risk.

Lam et al. [32] used nonlinear models of distributed lag to estimate the short-term association between daily mean temperature and admissions due to AMI, stratified by diabetes mellitus (DM) status among 53,769 admissions for AMI to all public hospitals in Hong Kong of China from 2002 to 2011, adjusting for other meteorological variables and air pollutants. The number of admissions for AMI generally increased when the temperature dropped. Admissions for AMI among patients with DM increased sharply and linearly with decreasing temperatures throughout the range of temperatures observed in the cold season [cumulative relative risk: 2.10; 95% CI: 1.62–2.72 in lag 0–22 days (12 °C versus 24 °C)], while admissions among the patients without DM increased linearly only when the temperature dropped below 22 °C to 24 °C [cumulative relative risk: 1.43; 95% CI: (1.21–1.69)]. Their findings suggested that admissions for AMI increased during extreme temperatures, while admissions for AMI increased more sharply for DM patients relative to non-DM patients.

14.4 Summary

In the last century and especially in recent decades, the Earth's climate has changed significantly, and the main feature of this change was global warming. In the context of global warming, extreme climatic conditions (e.g., heat waves or cold spells) are occurring with increasing frequency. In fact, the impact of extreme climatic conditions on population health has become the subject of preventive medicine and public health research, especially environmental epidemiology research. While exploring this subject, descriptive and analytical epidemiological research methods are generally adopted, and meteorological and health surveillance information (morbidity, mortality, and hospital records) are often used for statistical analysis. Due to the limitations in data availability, primarily extreme weather records, mortality data, and hospital record data have been used in evaluating the relationship between climate conditions and population health to understand the linkages between extreme weather and population mortality and between extreme weather and cardiovascular mortality or hospital admissions for cardiovascular disease. There is a convergence of findings that dramatic climate change is associated with all cause and cardiovascular mortality and that the increase in all cause and cardiovascular mortality due to dramatic climate change has become a global public health issue that should be taken seriously by governments.

Current studies on the relationships between extreme climates and all-cause mortality and between extreme climates and cardiovascular mortality in the population had some limitations. First, there was no standard international definition of relevant extreme weather, making it difficult to compare the results of studies from different countries and to generalize them. Second, the quality of the studies depended on the accuracy of meteorological data and health surveillance data. Satisfactorily obtaining complete and representative health surveillance information was very difficult in most countries, except for a few developed or developing countries. Furthermore, the occurrence of cardiovascular disease was the result of complex effects of multiple factors, and climate change was also complicated and may cause other environmental changes (e.g., environmental pollution) in addition to changes in climate-related variables. Climate change was related to the severity of air pollution, which was already a widespread public health problem, and epidemiological data showed that adverse health effects could be induced even with air pollution levels below the World Health Organization (WHO) standards. In addition, another limitation of many studies was that they used the data on temperature from fixed sites to define heat waves or cold spell, rather than the data on individual exposure to extreme temperatures, which could introduce exposure error to some extent. Obviously, methodology in studies on the relationships between extreme weather and mortality and cardiovascular disease need to be further improved in the future.

References

1. Gray SB, Brady SM. Plant developmental responses to climate change. Dev Biol. 2016 Aug 9. pii: S0012-1606(16)30264-0. https://doi.org/10.1016/j.ydbio.2016.07.023. [Epub ahead of print].
2. IPCC. Climate change 2014: synthesis report. Contribution of working groups I, II and III to the fifth assessment report of the intergovernmental panel on climate change [Core Writing Team, R.K. Pachauri and L.A. Meyer (Eds.)]. Geneva: IPCC; 2014. p. 151.
3. Bell JE, Brown CL, Conlon K, Herring S, Kunkel KE, Lawrimore J, et al. Changes in extreme events and the potential impacts on human health. J Air Waste Manag Assoc. 2018 Apr;68(4):265–87.
4. Zhao C, Chen J, Du P, Yuan H. Characteristics of climate change and extreme weather from 1951 to 2011 in China. Int J Environ Res Public Health. 2018;15:2540.
5. Metz B, Davidson O, Bosch P, et a1. Climate change 2007: mitigation of climate change; Contribution of Working Group III to the 4th Assessment Report of the intergovernmental Panel on Climate Change. 2007.
6. Solomon S. Climate Change 2007: the physical science basis: contribution of working group I to the fourth assessment report of the intergovernmental panel on climate change [M]. Cambridge: Cambridge University Press; 2007.
7. Pascal M, Le Tertre A, Saoudi A. Quantification of the heat wave effect on mortality in nine French cities during summer 2006 [J]. PLoS Curr. 2012;4:N1307.
8. Barnett AG, Hajat S, Gasparrini A, Rocklöv J. Cold and heat waves in the United States [J]. Environ Res. 2012;12:218–24.
9. Anderson B, Bell ML. Heat Waves in the United States: mortality risk during heat waves and effect modification by heat wave characteristics in 43 U.S. communities. Environ Health Perspect. 2011;119(2):210–8.
10. Guo Y, Gasparrini A, Armstrong BG, Tawatsupa B, Aurelio T, Lavigne E, et al. Heat wave and mortality: a Multicountry, Multicommunity study. Environ Health Perspect. 2017 Aug; 125(8):087006. Published online 2017 Aug 10. https://doi.org/10.1289/EHP1026.
11. Huang W, Kan HD, Kovats S. The impact of the 2003 heat wave on mortality in Shanghai. China Sci Total Environment. 2010;408(11):2418–20.
12. Ma W, Kan H, Chen B, et al. A study on temperature-related mortality in 16 Chinese cities. PhD Thesis, Fudan University (2014), from WANFANG DATA.
13. Sun Z, Chen C, Yan L, Shi W, Wang J, Ban J, et al. Heat wave characteristics, mortality and effect modification by temperature zones: a time-series study in 130 counties of China. Int J Epidemiol. 2021 Jan 23;49(6):1813–22.
14. Kysely J, Plavcova E, Davidkovova H, et al. Comparison of hot and cold spell effects on cardiovascular mortality in individual population groups in the Czech Republic. Clim Res. 2011;49(2):113–29.
15. Son JY, Lee JT, Anderson GB, Bell ML. The impact of heat waves on mortality in seven major cities in Korea. Environ Health Perspect. 2012;120(4):566–71.
16. Miron IJ, Montero JC, Criado-Alvarez JJ, Linares C, Díaz J. Intense cold and mortality in Castile-La Mancha (Spain): study of mortality trigger thresholds from 1975 to 2003 [J]. Int J Biometeorol. 2012;56(1):145–52.
17. Ma W, Kan H. The impact of the 2008 cold spell on mortality in Shanghai, China [J]. Epidemiology. 2011;22(1):S17.
18. Kysely J, Pokorna L, Kyncl J, Kriz B. Excess cardiovascular mortality associated with cold spells in the Czech Republic [J]. BMC Public Health. 2009;9:19.
19. Monteiro A, Carvalho V, Góis J, Sousa C. Use of "Cold Spell" indices to quantify excess chronic obstructive pulmonary disease (COPD) morbidity during winter

(November to March 2000—2007): case study in Porto[J]. Int J Biometeorol. 2013;57:857–70.
20. Revich B, Shaposhnikov D. Excess mortality during heat waves and cold spells in Moscow, Russia [J]. Occup Environ Med. 2008;65(10):691–6.
21. Ma C, Yang J, Nakayama S F., Iwai-Shimada M, Jung C-R, Sun X-L, Honda Y. Cold spells and cause-specific mortality in 47 Japanese prefectures: a systematic evaluation. Environ Health Perspect. 2021 Jun; 129(6):067001. Published online 2021 Jun 15. https://doi.org/10.1289/EHP7109.
22. Fu S, Gasparrini A, Rodriguez PS, Jha P. Mortality attributable to hot and cold ambient temperatures in India: a nationally representative case-crossover study. PLoS Med. 2018 Jul; 15(7):e1002619. Published online 2018 Jul 24. https://doi.org/10.1371/journal.pmed.1002619.
23. Zhou M, Wang L, Liu T, Zhang Y, Lin H, Luo Y, Xiao J, et al. Health impact of the 2008 cold spell on mortality in subtropical China: the climate and health impact national assessment study (CHINAs). Environ Health. 2014 Jul 24;13:60. https://doi.org/10.1186/1476-069X-13-60.
24. Xie H, Yao Z, Zhang Y, Xu Y, Xu X, Liu T, et al. Short-term effects of the 2008 cold spell on mortality in three subtropical cities in Guangdong Province, China. Environ Health Perspect. 2013 Feb;121(2):210–6.
25. Loughnan ME, Nicholls N, Tapper NJ. The effects of summer temperature, age and socioeconomic circumstance on acute myocardial infarction admissions in Melbourne, Australia. Int J Health Geogr. 2010 Aug 11;9:41. https://doi.org/10.1186/1476-072X-9-41.
26. Bhaskaran K, Hajat S, Haines A, Herrett E, Wilkinson P, Smeeth L. Short term effects of temperature on risk of myocardial infarction in England and Wales: time series regression analysis of the Myocardial Ischaemia National Audit Project (MINAP) registry. BMJ. 2010 Aug 10;341:c3823. https://doi.org/10.1136/bmj.c3823.
27. Bhaskaran K, Armstrong B, Hajat S, Haines A, Wilkinson P, Smeeth L. Heat and risk of myocardial infarction: hourly level case-crossover analysis of MINAP database. BMJ. 2012 Dec 13;345:e8050. https://doi.org/10.1136/bmj.e8050.
28. Loughnan M, Tapper N, Loughnan T. The impact of "unseasonably" warm spring temperatures on acute myocardial infarction hospital admissions in Melbourne, Australia: a city with a temperate climate. J Environ Res Public Health. 2014;2014:483785. https://doi.org/10.1155/2014/483785. Epub 2014 Jun 4
29. Lashari MN, Alam MT, Khan MS, Bawany FI, Qayoom M, Soomro K. Variation in admission rates of acute coronary syndrome patients in coronary care unit according to different seasons. J Coll Physicians Surg Pak. 2015;25:91–4.
30. Swampillai J, Wijesinghe N, Sebastian C, et al. Seasonal variations in hospital admissions for ST-Elevation myocardial infarction in New Zealand. Cardiol Res. 2012;3:205–8.
31. Liu X, Kong D, Fu J, Zhang Y, LiuY ZY, Lian H, Zhao X, Yang J, Fan Z. Association between extreme temperature and acute myocardial infarction hospital admissions in Beijing, China: 2013–2016. PLoS ONE. 2018;13(10):e0204706. https://doi.org/10.1371/journal.pone.0204706.
32. Lam H, Chan J, Luk A, Chan E, Goggins W. Short-term association between ambient temperature and acute myocardial infarction hospitalizations for diabetes mellitus patients: A time series study. PLoS Med. 2018;15(7):e1002612. https://doi.org/10.1371/journal.pmed.1002612.

15

Twin Research in China and Worldwide

Wenjing Gao, Hexiang Peng, Songjian Chen, and Liming Li

Abstract

Twins provide a unique opportunity for epidemiological research by investigating the role of genetic predisposition vs. environmental factors. The Chinese National Twin Registry (CNTR) is relatively young compared with those of western countries. Twin research, however, grows fast in China. The CNTR has registered 61,566 twin pairs including 31,705 monozygotic and 28,591 dizygotic pairs. These twins are important resources for examining genetic and environmental contributions to common diseases in China. With the development of novel technologies, twin studies will have substantial value in exploring the molecular mechanisms of complex diseases with multiple genetic and/or environmental risk factors. This review will introduce history of twin research, the value of twin studies, twin registries in the world, and the advances of twin research in exploring the etiology of chronic diseases using Chinese twins, including heritability estimation of single trait, genetic correlation among multiple phenotypes, as well as the modification of heritability and multi-omics studies particularly focusing on DNA methylation, DNA methylation age, and metabolomics. Despite the progress made in twin studies of China, there is still a long way to go for the CNTR in exploring the mysteries of the human organism in the future. At last, the short-term and long-term goals of the CNTR will be presented.

Keywords

Twin studies · Chronic disease · Environment Genetics · China

15.1 Brief History of Twin Research

Twin study was first proposed in 1875 by Francis Galton (1822–1911), an English social scientist, hereditarian, selectionist, and a founder of biometrics. He hypothesized that the life history of twins would help to distinguish the genetic and environmental effects on human development in the article "*The history of twins, as a criterion of the relative powers of nature and nurture*" [1]. In 1924, Hermann Werner Siemens and Curtis Merriman used twins to study the genetic predisposition in nevus and intelligence quotient (IQ) independently [2]. By comparing phenotypic resemblances between monozygotic (MZ) twins and dizygotic (DZ) twins, the genetic contributions to the variances of these two phenotypes were estimated. For the first time, the above two

W. Gao · H. Peng · S. Chen · L. Li (✉)
Department of Epidemiology & Biostatistics, School of Public Health, Peking University, Beijing, China
e-mail: lmlee@bjmu.edu.cn

D.-Q. Ye (ed.), *Progress in China Epidemiology*, https://doi.org/10.1007/978-981-19-2199-5_15

studies introduced the basic theory of comparison between MZ and DZ twins. Therefore, Siemens and Merriman were regarded as the pioneers of the classical twin study.

The classical twin study is based on the fact that MZ twins arise from a split of fertilized egg and thus share all of their genes, while DZ twins develop after a dual ovulation and share on average half of genes. In contrast, MZ and DZ twins share their intrauterine and part of their childhood environment. This implies that differences between MZ twins are due to their specific environmental factors, whereas how MZ twins are more alike than DZ twins reflects genetic influences [3]. By comparing the phenotypic similarity of MZ and DZ twins, researchers are able to analyze the phenotypic variation contributed by genetic effects, that is, to calculate the heritability. High heritability represents that it is much more feasible for researchers to map genes for diseases or phenotypes successfully, while low heritability indicates that it might not be a good choice for gene finding. Over the past century, twin research has laid a solid foundation for genetic epidemiology by providing the heritability for different phenotypes or diseases.

15.2 The Value of Twin Studies

Owing to the natural advantages of limited individual variability, twins are excellent subjects for studying the effects of genetic and environmental factors on their discordance of diseases or phenotypes. Though the emphasis of twin studies at initial stage may have been on founding the heritability of phenotypes and diseases, twin studies also offer many other unique chances to improve understandings of the mechanisms that trigger individual differences. The discordant MZ design provides the ultimate case-control matching for genes, age, sex, intrauterine, and childhood environment. The discordant MZ design could minimize sample size and improve statistical power. Li et al. confirmed that the disease-discordant case-control twin design presents better statistical power over the classical case-control study [4]. Epigenetic disease research had particularly benefitted from this special disease-discordant MZ twins design [5]. These studies not only provide phenotypic information but also shed light on the effects of epigenetic modifications that occur across the entire lifespan, including but not limited to DNA methylation and histone modifications. Moreover, many of the genetic adaptations to environments may be driven by genes, and the multi-level, phenotypic, and genetic data collection provides chances for an in-depth investigation of the gene-environment interaction in disease development [6]. It is promising that the established twin studies worldwide would continue to contribute significantly to our knowledge in the causes of individual differences. Moreover, many emerging studies are being carried out in twins, such as intestinal microbiology research. Therefore, twin studies are a burgeoning field of research and are worth further exploration in the methodology and research content.

15.3 Twin Registries in the World

Twins are scattered in the population. During the period from 2007 to 2014, for instance, the overall twinning rate was 18.8 per 1000 births in China [7]. Compared to the general population, it is much more difficult for researchers to recruit twins for specific research. Thus, twin registry is commonly used by researchers for twin recruiting around the world. As of 2019, twin registries have been established in at least 25 countries in the world and over 1.3 million twins and their family members have joined the registration system [6].

Table 15.1 lists the top 10 twin registries ranked by sample size, age, and phenotype of their twin participants. Many of the current twin registries were developed from specific research projects, usually in psychology or medicine. Thus, most of the twin registries focus on the phenotypes of behavior or psychological variables. Twin research was first developed in Europe, with the oldest twin registry in Denmark. The Nordic countries registered the most twins based on their technically advanced population register

Table 15.1 The Top ten twin registries ranking by sample size in the world [6, 8]

	Twin registry	Sample size	Age (years)	Phenotypes	Websites
1	The Netherlands Twin Register	255,785 twins	All ages	Psychological variables, mental health, physical growth	http://www.tweelingenregister.org/en
2	Swedish Twin Registry	216,258 twins	All ages	Mental and somatic disease, behavior	http://ki.se/en/research/the-swedish-twin-registry
3	Danish Twin Registry	175,518 twins	10 to 100+	Diseases, lifestyle/health-related behaviors, aging, psychological data, socioeconomic status	https://www.sdu.dk/en/Om_SDU/Institutter_centre/Ist_sundhedstjenesteforsk/Centre/DTR.aspx
4	The Chinese National Twin Registry	61,566 twin pairs	All ages	Lifestyles, chronic diseases	
5	The Cuban Twin Registry	58,000 twin pairs	All ages	Mental and somatic disease, behavior	
6	The Finnish Twin Cohort Study	105,149 twins and family members	10–100	Health and related behaviors, environment, morbidity, and mortality	http://www.twinstudy.helsinki.fi
7	The Russian School Twin Registry	Approximately 50,000 twin pairs	7–18	Cognition, emotion, motivation, achievement	
8	Twins Research Australia	45,000 pairs	All ages	Health, psychological traits	http://www.twins.org.au
9	California Twin Program	36,965 twin pairs	>16	Medical history, lifestyle	http://twins.usc.edu/
10	Mid-Atlantic Twin Registry of Virginia Commonwealth University	54,042 twins	All ages	Developmental psychopathology	http://www.matr.vcu.edu

systems. The most twin study groups are in the USA compared with other countries. The total sample size of the USA is very impressive despite the small sample size of the individual twin registry. In Asia, Sri Lanka was the first country to establish the twin registration system, while the current top three registries with the most sample sizes are China, Japan, and South Korea.

In China, the main sources of twin research are from the Chinese National Twin Registry (CNTR), Guangzhou Twin Eye Study, and Beijing Twin Study. CNTR, established in 2001, is a population-based twin registry in both north and south of China, including urban and rural areas. In contrast to other twin registries emphasizing on behavioral genetics, CNTR was designed primarily to investigate the genetic and environmental influences on complex diseases. With 20 years of growth, CNTR has not only helped understandings of cardiovascular and cerebrovascular diseases but also served as a valuable database for research of other diseases or phenotypes. As of 2020, CNTR has collected data of 61,566 twin pairs, including 31,705, 15,060, and 13,531 pairs which are MZ, same-sex DZ, and opposite-sex DZ pairs, respectively, categorized by sex and intra-pair similarity from questionnaires. Details for study designs and twin recruitment have been described elsewhere [9, 10].

15.4 Advances in Twin Research

Twin registries worldwide have collected abundant phenotypic data on large sample sizes of twins, providing a treasured resource for studying complex traits and their underlying mechanisms. As a classical methodology of genetic epidemiology, twin studies have been focusing on the estimation of genetic contribution to the variance of complex traits or phenotypes for decades. In recent years, with the expansion of epidemiological research methods and the development of bioinformatics, the classical twin research joint with new technologies represent a powerful tool toward detecting the molecular paths that underlie complex traits [11].

15.4.1 Heritability Estimation of Single Trait

The variance of a target phenotype can be divided into four components: additive genetic effects (A), non-additive genetic effects (D), common environmental effects (C), and unique environmental effects (E) [12]. A represents the sum of all individual allele effects that influence the trait. D represents the interplays between alleles at the same locus or at different loci. C refers to environmental influences shared by family members, such as socioeconomic status. E refers to different environmental influences experienced by each family members and measurement errors. The difference between the biology of MZ and DZ twins makes them a valuable resource for estimating heritability, the contribution of genes to phenotypic variance. The variance explained by additive genetic factors (A) is named the narrow-sense heritability (h^2) of a trait; while the variance explained by additive genetic factors (A) and non-additive genetic factors (D) is termed the broad-sense heritability (H^2).

MZ twin pairs share nearly all genes, whereas DZ twin pairs share an average of 50% genes. If we assume that environment factors contribute equally to the variance of the target phenotype in MZ and DZ twins, the difference of phenotypic correlation between MZ and DZ pairs must come from genetic factors. Therefore, Falconer's formula is applied to estimate the broad-sense heritability (H^2) by doubling the phenotype correlation difference between MZ and DZ twins: $H^2 = 2(rMZ - rDZ)$, where r is the intraclass correlation coefficient. Although the Falconer's formula is conceptually simple and easy to calculate, it's not suitable for multivariable data as well as testing the effect of covariates and model fitting. Structural equation models (SEM) are more advanced and more widely used than the Falconer's formula. Using the maximum likelihood approaches, the SEM estimates parameter values by minimizing the goodness-of-fit function between observed and predicted covariance matrices while the goodness-of-fit can be compared by the likelihood ratio test between models [3].

In 2003, Ren et al. conducted the heritability calculation in CNTR for the first time [13]. They analyzed the heritability of the metabolic syndrome-related characters including blood pressure, body mass index, fasting plasma glucose, and several index of plasma fat with the twin sample data collected from Weihai City and Lishui City. Since then, the heritability of over 30 phenotypes, mainly including risk factors for chronic diseases, has been estimated from the CNTR participants (Table 15.2). Obesity-related phenotypes appeared most frequently in the heritability estimation. There were six studies [13–18] that analyzed the heritability of body mass index (BMI), height, weight, waist circumference, waist-hip ratio, and waist-height ratio. Differences in analytical methods, the city where subjects came from, and the age of subsets sample resulted in differential heritability estimation. The heritability of BMI was estimated to be 0.88 with Falconer's formula; however, in another twin sample from the same cities, it was calculated to be 0.61 with SEM [13, 14]. In participants who came from two eastern cities, the heritability of waist circumference was estimated to be 0.75, while it was calculated to be 0.53 in participants who were from nine western, eastern, northern, and southern cities, which indicates that the genetic effect on waist circumference varied across study locations [14, 18]. The heritability of some phenotypes may vary with age. A study conducted by Liu et al. showed that the heritability for weight, height, and BMI increased over time for boys under 18 years [16]. This finding indicates that the expression of related genes may alter at different ages and the emphasis of interventions should be changed accordingly with age. The heritability estimations for the rest of the phenotypes are also listed in Table 15.2 and Fig. 15.1.

Table 15.2 Heritability of phenotypes in the Chinese National Twin Registry [9]

Phenotype	Heritability estimated in CNTR
BMI (≥18 years)	0.88, 0.61, 0.74 (0.71, 0.77), 0.70 (0.66, 0.74), 0.54–0.76 in different birth cohorts
BMI (<18 years)	
Girls	0.07–0.30 in different age groups
Boys	0.15–0.58 in different age groups
Height (<18 years)	
Girls	0.07–0.32 in different age groups
Boys	0.13–0.72 in different age groups
Weight (<18 years)	
Girls	0.13–0.35 in different age groups
Boys	0.28–0.63 in different age groups
Smoking behavior (yes/no)	0.69 (0.65, 0.73), 0.26 (0.19, 0.34)
Age at starting smoking	0.00, 0.05 (0.00, 0.14)
Physical activity	0.78 (0.35, 0.96), 0.59 (0.00, 0.94)
Sedentary behavior	0.68 (0.59, 0.75), 0.32 (0.07, 0.62)
Systolic blood pressure	0.78, 0.46 (0.30, 0.62)
Diastolic blood pressure	0.67, 0.30 (0.14, 0.48)
Insulin sensitivity (Homeostasis model assessment)	
Men	0.35
Women	0.46

Of note, the phenotype may have different heritability estimates in different subsets of the CNTR

These heritability estimations have not only guided future gene mapping efforts and given insights into the mechanisms to target phenotype-related genes but also provided evidence for the feasibility of environmental interventions that modify risk behaviors. Smoking is a moderate to high heritable trait if we target the variable of "whether twins smoke or not." However, it is also controlled by environment if we analyze "the age on which twins start smoking." This difference reminds that it is feasible to prevent smoking by postponing the onset age although smoking behavior is genetically contributed. It has been proposed that common environmental factors account for 80% of the smoking onset age variation, indicating that family environments such as parental smoking behavior and parenting style might be the key points to postpone the smoking onset age [21]. Nevertheless, genetic factors play a quite limited role in smoking cessation, which guides us to conduct the tobacco control by targeting environmental factors.

Apart from the original study based on the Chinese twins, we also used meta-analysis

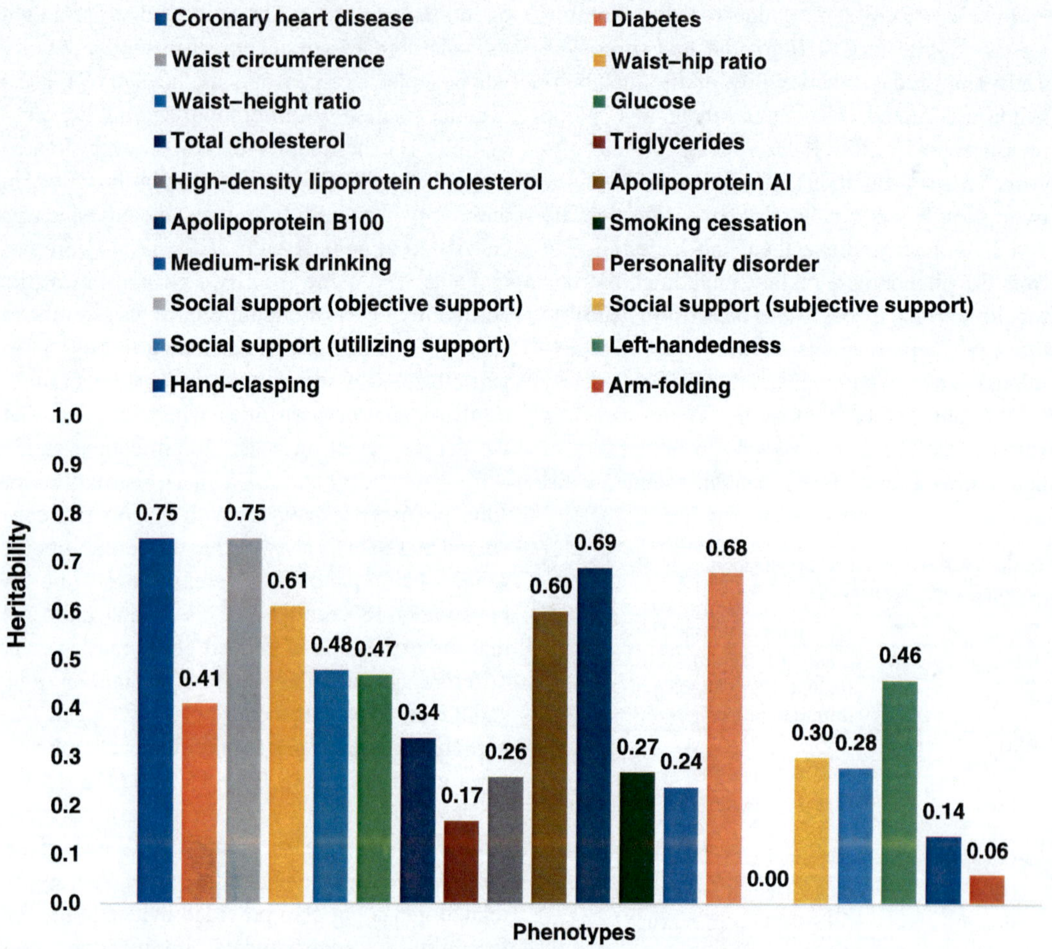

Fig. 15.1 Heritability of phenotypes in the Chinese National Twin Registry [9, 19, 20]

to improve the statistical power of heritability estimation. By pooling 10,163 participants from 17 studies, we estimated that the heritability for systolic blood pressure (SBP) and diastolic blood pressure (DBP) was 0.54 (95% CIs 0.48–0.60) and 0.49 (95% CIs 0.42–0.56), respectively [22]. The CNTR also participated in the Collaborative project of Development of Anthropometrical measures in Twins (CODATwins), in which the height and weight of 87,782 complete twin pairs between 0.5 to 19.5 years of age from 45 cohorts were pooled to explore the genetic and environmental contributions to body mass index [23].

15.4.2 Genetic Correlation Among Multiple Phenotypes

An important extension of the SEM introduced above is to be used in the analysis of multiple phenotypes. By analyzing bivariate or multivariate phenotypes, the genetic and environmental overlap in correlated phenotypes can be estimated. The etiology of the association between phenotypes can be investigated by testing whether similar environmental variables explain for the correlation or whether the same genetic background affects correlated traits [3]. In a series of bivariate analyses from the CNTR, the relationship among the risk factors of chronic diseases including smoking, alcohol consumption, body composition measurements, serum lipid, glucose, insulin profiles, obesity indicators, and blood pressure was investigated [9], to test the hypothesis that the co-morbidity of these factors is due to shared genetic background (Fig. 15.2).

The genetic correlation between current tobacco use and alcohol use in Chinese adult male twins was 0.32, which indicates that cigarette smoking and alcohol drinking share a common genetic vulnerability [24]. Due to this genetic correlation, tobacco users are more likely to be alcohol consumers. Therefore, efforts should be made to prevent non-drinking smokers becoming drinkers and vice versa. The genetic correlation also provides a clue to seek genes that are common to tobacco use and alcohol use. If the specific genetic variations shared by these behaviors are characterized, interventions for tobacco and alcohol control could be improved at the same time. Genetic correlations between body composition measurements with serum metabolites ranged from 0.303 (WC-LDL-C) to 0.795 (PBF-TG), demonstrating that common genes play a vital role in these phenotypes [25]. This result provides evidences to explain why obesity is one of the most important risk factors for metabolic syndrome, cardiovascular disease, and type 2 diabetes mellitus. A study conducted by Liao et al. revealed that there was a high genetic correlation between SBP and DBP, indicating that genes affecting SBP may overlap with those associated with DBP [26]. The genetic correlation between obesity indicators and blood pressure components ranged from 0.309 (WC-SBP) to 0.457 (WHtR-DBP), suggesting that there are genes exerting pleiotropic effects on obesity and blood pressure [26].

15.4.3 Heritability Modification

Heritability may differ for males and females or in different age groups. In the CNTR, the heritability for BMI was less than 20% at 0–2 years old for both sexes but increased with age increasing,

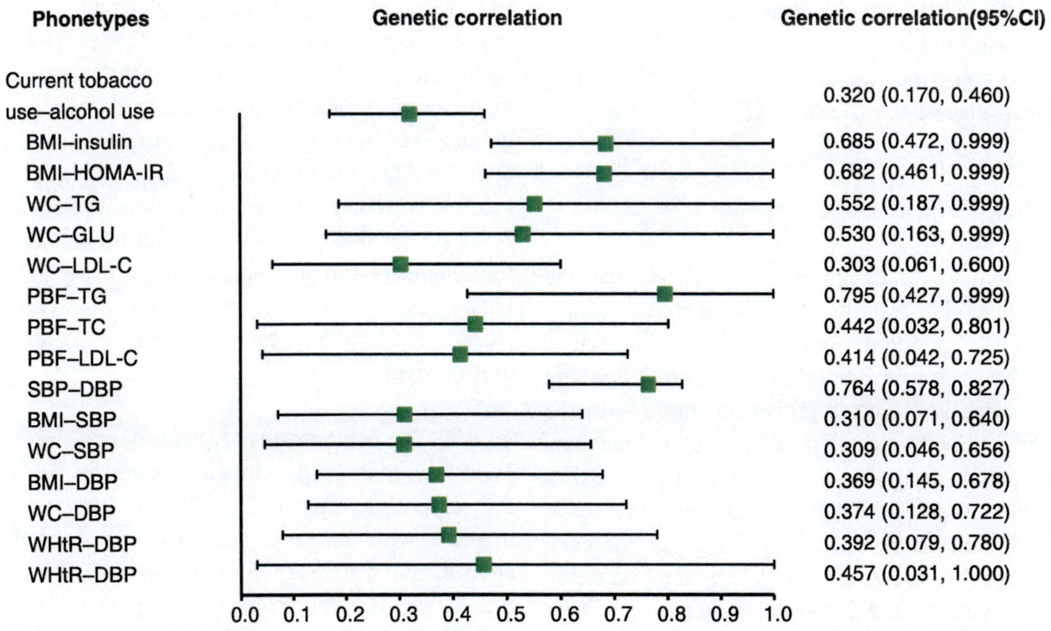

Fig. 15.2 Genetic correlations based on the Chinese National Twin Registry [9]. *CI* confidence interval, *BMI* body mass index, *HOMA-IR* homeostatic model assessment of insulin resistance, *WC* waist circumference, *TG* triglycerides, *GLU* glucose, *LDL-C* low-density lipoprotein cholesterol, *PBF* percentage body fat, *TC* total cholesterol, *SBP* systolic blood pressure, *DBP* diastolic blood pressure, *WHtR* waist-height ratio

accounting for 50% or over of the variance in 15–17 years for boys. For girls, heritability was maintained at around 30% after puberty [16]. One hypothesis to explain the observed difference in heritability is that the genetic variance can differ between males and females as well as different age groups. Another hypothesis is that the genetic variance may be the same while the environmental variance is larger in some groups since heritability is expressed as a ratio of genetic variance over total variance [3]. The modification of heritability provides evidences for potential gene-environment interaction. For example, physical activity was found to attenuate the genetic effects on BMI [27] and heritability of BMI increased with age in a Chinese adult twin cohort born in 1959–1961 [17]. The genetic effects of type 2 diabetes can be modified by physical activity. The modification coefficient of sufficient physical activity on the genetic effects of type 2 diabetes was −0.34, suggesting that sufficient physical activity could weaken the genetic effects on type 2 diabetes [28]. In addition, the heritability of type 2 diabetes in twins with sufficient physical activity was 0.46, which was lower than that in twins with insufficient physical activity. Another study in CNTR found that higher BMI could reduce the genetic effects of coronary heart disease in male twins [29].

15.4.4 Multi-omics Study

Systematic epidemiology emphasizes that the organic integration of traditional epidemiology and modern high-throughput multi-omics technology is an important direction of etiology research and precise prevention [30]. With the rapid growth of modern biotechnology, the classical twin design has been extended from the simple heritability estimation to the complex traits at molecular level. In the initial level of the gene mapping, researchers might prefer recruiting DZ twins since MZ twin data do not contribute toward detecting linkage. With the development of functional genomics, however, discordant MZ twin design, which offers unique opportunity to control the influences of DNA sequence, has become more attractive in gene expression exploration. Therefore, MZ twins play a more prominent role in the study of newly emerging fields, including epigenome, transcriptome, metabolome, proteome, and microbiome. During the past 5 years, we have carried out omics studies on DNA methylation and metabolomics. The following sections present our progress in different omics studies.

15.4.4.1 Epigenome Study-DNA Methylation

15.4.4.1.1 Introduction of DNA Methylation

Epigenetics refers to the phenomenon that gene expression changes heritability without changes in nucleotide sequence. DNA methylation is the most widely studied branch of epigenetics at present. It is regarded as a covalent modification of the nucleotide cytosine at the 5′ position, which is generally associated with gene silencing [31]. It is also the best-understood epigenetic modification and plays an important role in occurrence and development of human diseases and aging [32]. Many studies have been conducted to evaluate the effects of environment factors on DNA methylation. In the meantime, the significance of methylation as a biomarker for the prediction and diagnosis of human diseases has attracted lots of attention [33]. Finding in novel epigenetic associations with diseases has implications in identifying potential targets of drugs and biomarkers for diagnosis and prognosis. Twins, especially phenotypic and disease discordant MZ twin pairs, were used to explore epigenetic profiles during development, aging, and disease.

15.4.4.1.2 Advantages of Discordant Twin Design in Epigenome Studies

Phenotypic and epigenetic differences in twins increase with age, especially with non-shared environment difference [5]. Fraga et al. [34] first found that MZ twin pairs exhibited epigenetic differences by comparing their methylcytosine and histone acetylation levels in peripheral lymphocytes. A simulation study revealed that disease discordant twin design had higher statistical power over the classic case-control design in epigenome-wide association studies. For heritability over 0.3, the disease-discordant twin design allowed for large sample size reduction compared with the ordinary case-control design [4]. Furthermore, both population-based and discordant twin-based epigenetic studies may be biased by potential confounders and need replication to reduce false-positive findings, while twin studies perform better in controlling those unmeasurable confounders.

15.4.4.1.3 Research Progress of DNA Methylation in CNTR

In the CNTR, discordant MZ twin resources have been used in analyzing epigenetic mechanism underlying BMI, blood pressure, and diabetes-related phenotypes. Table 15.3 summarized CpG markers found to be significantly correlated with the target traits. Results of the twin studies provided insight to the mechanism of methylation from a unique perspective. However, due to the high cost of DNA methylation test and limited funds, the studies mentioned above were performed with a cross-sectional study design. Therefore, further studies conducted with large sample size or perspective studies are needed to validate the foregoing results and to clarify the causal relationship between DNA methylation and target phenotypes.

Table 15.3 The main findings from DNA methylation study in the CNTR [9]

Phenotypes	Suspected markers correlated
BMI (7–16 years)	cg05684382, cg26188191
BMI (adults)	cg15053022 in *ATP4A* gene
SBP, DBP, mean arterial pressure (adults)	cg07761116
Fasting plasma glucose [35]	cg19693031, cg01538969, cg08501915, cg04816311, ch.8.1820050F, cg06721411, cg26608667
HbA1c [35]	cg19693031, cg04816311, cg01538969, cg01339781, cg01676795, cg24667115, cg09029192, cg20697417, ch.4.1528651F, cg16097041
Alcohol drinking [36]	cg07326074

BMI body mass index, *SBP* systolic blood pressure, *DBP* diastolic blood pressure

15.4.4.1.4 DNA Methylation Age and Its Related Progress

In addition, epigenetic patterns also change over the lifespan, suggesting that epigenetic changes may constitute an important component of the aging process. The DNA methylation levels of certain CpG sites are thought to reflect the pace of human aging [37]. DNA methylation is a promising biomarker of epigenetic aging, which could show the actual aging stage of human, better than chronological age calculated by calendar. The epigenetic clock is a complicated mechanism of aging that can be influenced by both genetic and environment factors and is also closely associated with the occurrence, development, and prognosis of cancer and other diseases [38]. When discordant epigenetic aging occurred in twins with the same age, sex, genes, and early environment factors, environmental factors might play an important role in the process of aging. In CNTR, we first generated a chronological age model that could accurately predict between 6 and 17 years old using the 83 CpG sites [39]. Moreover, as a validation population on behalf of twins, we validated the accuracy of the methylation age predictor developed by Li et al [40]. To explore the relationship between lifestyle factors and DNA methylation age, twins discordant for combined lifestyle factors (consisting of smoking, drinking, intake of vegetable and fruit, and physical activity) were applied to detect the differential epigenetic aging rate [41]. Our results revealed that healthy lifestyle factors like active physical activity and adequate intake of vegetable and fruit could alleviate epigenetic aging, but the influence of smoking and drinking on epigenetic aging is unclear. In addition, the number of healthy lifestyle factors was negatively correlated with epigenetic aging. Future studies conducted in large sample sizes and longitudinal design are needed in CNTR, to better elucidate the mechanism of epigenetic senescence based on the special advantages of twin population.

15.4.4.2 Metabolomics Study

With the traditional epidemiology reaching its mature stage, the omics studies have inevitably become a hot research trend in epidemiology in recent years. Metabolomics, the metabolite profiling in biological matrices, is regarded as a key tool for biomarker discovery and personalized medicine and has great potential to elucidate the ultimate product of the genomic processes [42]. The concept of metabolomics was raised in 1999 by Nicholson et al [43]. The research related to metabolomics has shown an explosion trend [42]. In addition to genomics, metabolomics studies are an important way to identify biomarkers of future risk of cardiovascular disease and other chronic diseases [44, 45]. Moreover, microbiome-correlated metabolomics pipeline and interactive metabolomics profile explorer could become a powerful tool to characterize microorganisms and interplays between microorganisms and their host [46]. Interaction between metabolic and epigenetic remodeling might be crucial to pathogenic potential in inflammation [47]. In the context of rapid development and growth of traditional epidemiology, genetic epidemiology, and genomics, metabolomics has its unique advantages.

In CNTR, with the accumulation of the number of samples for metabolomics detection, metabolomics-related studies have been carried out in twins. A metabolomics study was also conducted in obesity-discordant twin pairs and 11 metabolites were found to be correlated with obesity measures. The major pathways relating the 11 metabolites included tyrosine metabolism, pyrimidine metabolism, and purine metabolism [48]. We also found that metabolically healthy overweight/obesity (MHO) and metabolically unhealthy non-obesity (MUNO) phenotypes accounted for a large proportion in Chinese twin population. The two metabolic phenotypes were significantly associated with elevated insulin resistance and high sensitivity C-reactive protein, which may culminate in serious health concerns [49]. Metabolomics research in CNTR is in the ascendency, and further research in this area will be carried out in the future.

15.5 Future of the Twin Research in China

Despite the progress made in twin studies, there are still plenty of opportunities for future CNTR research and data mining. As a short-term goal, the CNTR is going to test additional 1000 twins on genotyping, DNA methylation, and metabolites data. Multi-omics studies, combining genomics with metabolomics, transcriptomics, and proteomics, will help a significantly improved understanding of the mechanisms and the pathophysiology of diseases in a systematic perspective. Besides, multi-omics studies have potential in discovering novel biomarkers and identifying high-risk populations to guide precision intervention. For the long-term goal, the CNTR will continue to follow those twins recruited and design matched case-control studies in discordant twin pairs. The previous studies conducted in CNTR were mostly cross-sectional design, which could not judge the temporal sequence or make causal inference. Causal inference methods, such as longitudinal study design, Mendelian randomization, and Inference about Causation through Examination of FAmiliaL CONfounding (ICE FALCON) [50], are also being explored in CNTR to obtain causal relationships. Ultimately, longitudinal data will be necessary to determine the timing of the epigenetic modification with respect to disease onset and investigate the role of epigenetic alteration in disease susceptibility or progression. Moreover, gut microbiome, which may soon be included in multi-omics studies in CNTR, is also a hotspot in the field of twin studies in recent years. As mentioned before, the CNTR initially aims to investigate the genetic and environmental influences on complex diseases. At present, the average age of the population cohort of twins is still young and the accumulated cases of chronic diseases and cancers are relatively limited. As the number of cases increases, the CNTR will further explore the etiology of these diseases. Moreover, with the extensive use of artificial reproductive technologies, twins have been increased rapidly across the world. The implications of the rise of artificial reproductive technologies are unknown, and the CNTR will monitor future developments and research in this area. It is important to mention that the CNTR has developed cooperation with researchers from several countries, including joint application for international cooperative projects and joint consortia. The CNTR will continue to promote collaboration with scholars and teen registries around the world.

References

1. Galton F. The history of twins, as a criterion of the relative powers of nature and nurture (1,2) [J]. Int J Epidemiol. 2012;41(4):905–11.
2. Teo T, Ball LC. Twin research, revisionism and metahistory [J]. Hist Human Sci. 2009;22(5):1–23.
3. Boomsma DI. Twin, association and current "omics" studies [J]. J Matern Fetal Neonatal Med. 2013;26(Suppl 2):9–12.
4. Li W, Christiansen L, Hjelmborg J, et al. On the power of epigenome-wide association studies using a disease-discordant twin design [J]. Bioinformatics. 2018;34(23):4073–8.
5. Castillo-Fernandez JE, Spector TD, Bell JT. Epigenetics of discordant monozygotic twins: implications for disease [J]. Genome Med. 2014;6(7):60.
6. Hur YM, Bogl LH, Ordonana JR, et al. Twin family registries worldwide: an important resource for scientific research [J]. Twin Res Hum Genet. 2019;22(6):427–37.
7. Deng C, Dai L, Yi L, et al. Temporal trends in the birth rates and perinatal mortality of twins: a population-based study in China [J]. PLoS One. 2019;14(1):e209962.
8. Hur YM, Craig JM. Twin registries worldwide: an important resource for scientific research [J]. Twin Res Hum Genet. 2013;16(1):1–12.
9. Gao W, Cao W, Lv J, et al. The Chinese National Twin Registry: a 'gold mine' for scientific research [J]. J Intern Med. 2019;286(3):299–308.
10. Huang T, Gao W, Lv J, et al. The Chinese National Twin Registry: a unique data source for systems epidemiology of complex disease [J]. Twin Res Hum Genet. 2019;22(6):482–5.
11. van Dongen J, Slagboom PE, Draisma HH, et al. The continuing value of twin studies in the omics era [J]. Nat Rev Genet. 2012;13(9):640–53.
12. Rijsdijk FV, Sham PC. Analytic approaches to twin data using structural equation models [J]. Brief Bioinform. 2002;3(2):119–33.
13. Ren T, Wu D, Hu Y, et al. The heritability analysis of the metabolic syndrome related characters in twins. Chin J Prev Contr Chron Non-Commun Dis. 2003;11:4. (in Chinese)
14. Lee J, Chen L, Snieder H, et al. Heritability of obesity-related phenotypes and association with adiponectin gene polymorphisms in the Chinese national twin registry [J]. Ann Hum Genet. 2010;74(2):146–54.
15. Wu T, Snieder H, Li L, et al. Genetic and environmental influences on blood pressure and body mass index in Han Chinese: a twin study [J]. Hypertens Res. 2011;34(2):173–9.
16. Liu Q, Yu C, Gao W, et al. Genetic and environmental effects on weight, height, and BMI under 18 years in a Chinese population-based twin sample [J]. Twin Res Hum Genet. 2015;18(5):571–80.
17. Zhao Q, Gao W, Yu C, et al. Association between birth cohort and the heritability of body mass index. Chin J Epidemiol. 2017;38(08):1043–9. (in Chinese)
18. Zhou B, Gao W, Lv J, et al. Genetic and environmental influences on obesity-related phenotypes in Chinese twins reared apart and together [J]. Behav Genet. 2015;45(4):427–37.
19. Wang D, Gao W, Lv J, et al. Heritability of coronary heart disease, based on the data from the Chinese adult twins. Chin J Epidemiol. 2020;41(5):700–4. (in Chinese)
20. Meng L, Gao W, Cao W, et al. Heritability of alcohol intake among adult twins, calculate by the structural equation model. Chin J Epidemiol. 2020;41(06):819–23. (in Chinese)
21. Bao ZQ, Yu CQ, Wang BQ, et al. Influences of genetic and environmental factors on smoking related behaviors among male twin adults in China [J]. Zhonghua Liu Xing Bing Xue Za Zhi. 2016;37(5):618–23.
22. Wang B, Liao C, Zhou B, et al. Genetic contribution to the variance of blood pressure and heart rate: a systematic review and meta-regression of twin studies [J]. Twin Res Hum Genet. 2015;18(2):158–70.
23. Silventoinen K, Jelenkovic A, Sund R, et al. Genetic and environmental effects on body mass index from infancy to the onset of adulthood: an individual-based pooled analysis of 45 twin cohorts participating in the collaborative project of development of anthropometrical measures in twins (CODATwins) study [J]. Am J Clin Nutr. 2016;104(2):371–9.
24. Zhang T, Gao W, Cao W, et al. The genetic correlation between cigarette smoking and alcohol drinking among Chinese adult male twins: an ordinal bivariate genetic analysis [J]. Twin Res Hum Genet. 2012;15(4):483–90.
25. Liao C, Gao W, Cao W, et al. Associations of body composition measurements with serum lipid, glucose and insulin profile: a Chinese twin study [J]. PLoS One. 2015;10(11):e140595.

26. Liao C, Gao W, Cao W, et al. Associations between obesity indicators and blood pressure in Chinese adult twins [J]. Twin Res Hum Genet. 2017;20(1):28–35.
27. Wang B, Gao W, Lv J, et al. Physical activity attenuates genetic effects on BMI: results from a study of Chinese adult twins [J]. Obesity (Silver Spring). 2016;24(3):750–6.
28. Chen S, Gao W, Lv J, et al. Modification of physical activity on genetic effects of type 2 diabetes mellitus: a twin pairs cohort study in China. Chin J Epidemiol. 2021;42(7):1167–73. (in Chinese)
29. Xi Y, Gao W, Lv J, et al., Gene-body mass index interaction on coronary heart disease in the Chinese adult twins. Chin J Epidemiol. 2021; 42(9):1573-9. (in Chinese).
30. Huang T, Li L. Systems epidemiology. Chin J Epidemiol. 2018;39(05):694–9. (in Chinese)
31. Feinberg AP. The key role of epigenetics in human disease prevention and mitigation [J]. N Engl J Med. 2018;378(14):1323–34.
32. Klutstein M, Nejman D, Greenfield R, et al. DNA methylation in cancer and aging [J]. Cancer Res. 2016;76(12):3446–50.
33. Dor Y, Cedar H. Principles of DNA methylation and their implications for biology and medicine [J]. Lancet. 2018;392(10149):777–86.
34. Fraga MF, Ballestar E, Paz MF, et al. Epigenetic differences arise during the lifetime of monozygotic twins [J]. Proc Natl Acad Sci U S A. 2005;102(30):10604–9.
35. Wang Z, Gao W, Wang B. Correlation between fasting plasma glucose, HbA1c and DNA methylation in adult twins. J Peking Univ (Health Sciences). 2020;52(3):425–31. (in Chinese)
36. Meng L, Qin X, Peng H. Genome-wide associations between alcohol consumption and blood DNA methylation: evidence from twin study [J]. Epigenomics. 2021;13(12):939–51.
37. Jones MJ, Goodman SJ, Kobor MS. DNA methylation and healthy human aging [J]. Aging Cell. 2015;14(6):924–32.
38. Declerck K, Vanden BW. Back to the future: epigenetic clock plasticity towards healthy aging [J]. Mech Ageing Dev. 2018;174:18–29.
39. Li C, Gao W, Gao Y, et al. Age prediction of children and adolescents aged 6-17 years: an epigenome-wide analysis of DNA methylation [J]. Aging (Albany NY). 2018;10(5):1015–26.
40. Li J, Zhu X, Yu K, et al. Exposure to polycyclic aromatic hydrocarbons and accelerated DNA methylation aging [J]. Environ Health Perspect. 2018;126(6):67005.
41. Peng H, Gao W, Cao W, et al. Combined healthy lifestyle score and risk of epigenetic aging: a discordant monozygotic twin study [J]. Aging (Albany NY). 2021;13(10):14039–52.
42. Jacob M, Lopata AL, Dasouki M, et al. Metabolomics toward personalized medicine [J]. Mass Spectrom Rev. 2019;38(3):221–38.
43. Nicholson JK, Lindon JC, Holmes E. 'Metabonomics': understanding the metabolic responses of living systems to pathophysiological stimuli via multivariate statistical analysis of biological NMR spectroscopic data [J]. Xenobiotica. 1999;29(11):1181–9.
44. Wang Z, Klipfell E, Bennett BJ, et al. Gut flora metabolism of phosphatidylcholine promotes cardiovascular disease [J]. Nature. 2011;472(7341):57–63.
45. Mardinoglu A, Stancakova A, Lotta LA, et al. Plasma mannose levels are associated with incident type 2 diabetes and cardiovascular disease [J]. Cell Metab. 2017;26(2):281–3.
46. Han S, Van Treuren W, Fischer CR, et al. A metabolomics pipeline for the mechanistic interrogation of the gut microbiome [J]. Nature. 2021;595(7867):415–20.
47. Shi H, Chi H. Polyamine: a metabolic compass for T helper cell fate direction [J]. Cell. 2021;184(16):4109–12.
48. Liao C, Wang B, Gao W, et al. Associations of obesity measurements with serum Metabolomic profile: a Chinese twin study [J]. Twin Res Hum Genet. 2021;24(1):14–21.
49. Liao C, Gao W, Cao W, et al. Associations of metabolic/obesity phenotypes with insulin resistance and C-reactive protein: results from the CNTR study [J]. Diabetes Metab Syndr Obes. 2021;14:1141–51.
50. Li S, Wong EM, Bui M, et al. Inference about causation between body mass index and DNA methylation in blood from a twin family study [J]. Int J Obes. 2019;43(2):243–52.

16 Development of Active Surveillance System for Drug Safety in China

Yu Yang, Yang Xu, and Siyan Zhan

Abstract

Drug safety surveillance is crucial for patient safety. Passive surveillance has been broadly applied, but there are still shortcomings. The active surveillance system based on the electronic health database has gradually attracted various countries' regulatory authorities' attention. China's electronic healthcare data sources are suggested to be feasible for active post-market surveillance of drug safety. The China Hospital Pharmacovigilance System (CHPS) and the first version of China's active surveillance system, the China ADR Sentinel Alliance (CASSA), had been established 5 years ago. Researchers have begun to build relevant data models for active surveillance and evaluate the applicability and feasibility of active surveillance-related statistical analysis methods in China's electronic healthcare databases. In the future, the development of active surveillance of drug safety in China needs to incorporate more electronic healthcare databases and conduct quality assessments. It also needs to evaluate further the application conditions of active surveillance-related methods and tools and establish good cooperation and a win-win mechanism to encourage more stakeholders to be involved in active surveillance.

Keywords

Adverse Drug Reactions (ADRs) · Active surveillance · Prescription Sequence Symmetry Analysis (PSSA) · Tree-Based Scan Statistic (TBSS)

Y. Yang (✉)
National Institute of Health Data Science, Peking University, Beijing, China
e-mail: yangyu@bjmu.edu.cn

Y. Xu
Peking University Clinical Research Institute, Peking University First Hospital, Beijing, China
e-mail: xuyang_pucri@bjmu.edu.cn

S. Zhan
School of Public Health, Peking University, Beijing, China

Research Center of Clinical Epidemiology, Peking University Third Hospital, Beijing, China
e-mail: siyan-zhan@bjmu.edu.cn

16.1 Passive Surveillance and Active Surveillance

Drug safety has been well considered during the highly complex process of drug development, including phase I to phase III trials. However, premarketing trials lack sufficient power to detect crucial adverse drug reactions (ADRs) reliably. ADRs are defined by the World Health Organization (WHO) as a response to a drug that is harmful and unintended and occurs at doses typically used commonly for the prevention, diagnosis, or therapy of disease or physiological modification function.

D.-Q. Ye (ed.), *Progress in China Epidemiology*, https://doi.org/10.1007/978-981-19-2199-5_16

Due to the limited number of participants in the pre-marketing trial, it is difficult to observe some adverse reactions with an incidence of 1/10,000 or less. There was also an insufficient follow-up to detect ADRs widely separated in time from the delayed consequences associated with initial or long-term use. In addition, particular groups that may have a unique risk of ADRs or an increased frequency of ADRs compared with the general population, such as pregnant women or children, are usually not included in the pre-market trial. Post-marketing surveillance for ADRs is indispensable since the possibility of rare but severe ADRs or common delayed ADRs cannot be excluded even after approval to further ascertain safety for patient consumption [1, 2].

For decades, post-marketing drug safety surveillance mainly depends on the spontaneous data of adverse event (AE) reporting system, which depends on the voluntary reports of medical professionals, pharmaceutical companies, health authorities, or patients and their families. A spontaneous report system is the fundamental approach of passive surveillance, such as the Food and Drug Administration (FDA) Adverse Event Reporting System (FAERS) in the United States and the WHO Programme for International Drug Monitoring. These systems were established to improve post-marketing surveillance for ADEs [2, 3]. The passive ADR reporting system also has been established in China since 1989. However, this spontaneous reporting system is hampered by its nature and has some limitations, including serious insufficient reporting [4], incomplete information, lack of denominator to estimate the incidence of suspected adverse reactions, and over-reporting and selective reporting of drug-related events that have attracted media attention [5–7].

Given the inherent pitfalls of spontaneous reporting systems, active or intensive surveillance programs were introduced to address ADRs successfully [8]. Active surveillance for adverse effects of the therapeutic drug was first mentioned in 1994 regarding adverse events of digitalis in elderly patients. Primarily, active surveillance comprises case-control networks, hospital-based intensive monitoring systems, record linkage systems, and epidemiological studies [9]. Since electronic medical record (EMR), as well as other databases, have been well used for epidemiological researches, for instance, the General Practice Research Database (GPRD) in the United Kingdom. The interest in developing an active surveillance system by incorporating and using existing electronic data such as administrative claims and electronic health record (EHR) data was raised [10].

Drug regulatory agencies and the pharmaceutical industry in many countries have established active surveillance systems for drugs [11]. The Sentinel system is a good example of an active surveillance system using electronic data of health. The US FDA Sentinel program began more than a decade ago to establish a national system to actively monitor the safety and performance of FDA-regulated medical products (including drugs). Sentinel initiative is the FDA's response to the 2007 FDA Amendment Act (FDAAA) requiring the FDA to use electronic medical databases (EHDs) to quickly and reliably evaluate the safety of approved drugs and other medical products. As of 2014, Mini-Sentinel (MS), the pilot project of the Sentinel Initiative, has covered 380 million person-years of data, and nearly 180 million people are actively accumulating. It prospectively surveils the safety of listed medical products from more than 17 data partners [12–15]. The MS system was transitioned into the Sentinel system, becoming an integral part of routine safety surveillance for the FDA. The Sentinel system leverage distributed data network, a common data model (CDM), curated real-world data (RWD), and distributed analytic tools in signal generation, signal refinement, and signal evaluation of drug safety to support FDA decision-making [16–18].

16.2 Development of Active Surveillance in China

16.2.1 Available Data Sources for Active Surveillance

Data is the fundamental elements for constructing post-marketing active surveillance systems such as the Sentinel system, Exploring and Understanding Adverse Drug Reactions

Table 16.1 General characteristics of three databases [19]

Database name	Source type	Starting date	Estimated no. of individuals	Age group	Coverage area
Yinzhou database	Regional EHRs	2005	1.19 million (2015)	All ages	Yinzhou District in Ningbo City
National claims database	Claims data	Resampled annually (started in 2008)	5.4 million (2014)	All ages	All the country
CACMS database	60 hospitals' EMRs	2003	3.0 million (2015)	All ages	Cities: BJ, SZ Provinces: GD, SX, FJ, HB, JL

BJ Beijing, *CACMS* China Academy of Chinese Medical Sciences, *FJ* Fujian Province, *EHR* Electronic Health Record, *EMR* Electronic Medical Record, *GD* Guangdong Province, *HB* Hebei Province, *JL* Jilin Province, *SX* Shanxi Province, *SZ* Shenzhen

by Integrative Mining of Clinical Records and Biomedical Knowledge (EU-ADR), or Observational Medical Outcomes Partnership (OMOP) [19]. Take the Sentinel system as an example: the Sentinel Distributed Database (SDD), as the collection of harmonized datasets from 17 data providers (such as Aetna, Medicare Fee-for-Service data, Harvard Pilgrim Health Care Institute, Anthem, Inc. data, Kaiser Permanente, Optum, Tennessee Medicaid data, etc.), acts as the data source for active surveillance. The SDD has a total of 351.8 million unique patient identifiers spanning the 2000 to 2020 time period. And 228.7 million patients have at least 1 day of drug and medical coverage. The data of SDD comes from electronic healthcare databases (EHDs) in national health insurance plans, large integrated delivery systems, and healthcare organizations.

Yang and colleagues [19] conducted a study to describe the availability, characteristics, and structure for post-marketing active surveillance of drug safety and pharmacoepidemiology by EHDs in China. Through literature review, expert suggestions, and contacts, three examples of the main types of EHD in China were determined:

- National claim database (national claim database)
- Yinzhou database of Yinzhou District of Ningbo City (regional community database)
- Database of Chinese Academy of traditional Chinese medicine (CACMS) (EMR database)

Table 16.1 list the general characteristics of the three databases. In short, the national claims database collects data from the urban employees' basic medical insurance (UEBMI), which is one of the three major insurance plans in China; The national claims database is the only national claims database available for research purposes. Yinzhou database is one of the best databases based on regional communities, covering more than 95% of the resident population in the region. CACMS database is from the hospital information systems (HIS), including 60 hospitals in two cities and five provinces.

Another cross-sectional study using a questionnaire conducted by Yu and her colleagues in 17 children's hospitals of Beijing Children's Hospital Group investigated the feasibility of active surveillance of pediatric medicine in the EMR database. The questionnaire contained database features, degree of computerization, degree of structuring, data type, data encoding, degree of linkage on information systems, and data sharing willingness. The result demonstrated that it is feasible to conduct active surveillance of adverse events for pediatric drugs, despite the fact that the EMR data from children's hospital need to be further linked and standardized [20].

In conclusion, EHDs from health insurance, regional data platform, or hospitals is feasible for active surveillance of drug safety. However, further evaluation and standardization is still needed.

16.2.2 Specific System for Active Surveillance

In 2012, the 12th Five-Year Plan for Drug Safety decided that drug safety surveillance should be updated and that evaluation and alerts regarding ADRs should be strengthened [21]. On July 30, 2020, China National Medical Products Administration (NMPA) issued "the Opinions on Reinforcing ADR Monitoring & Evaluation System and Capacity Building" and claimed to build active monitoring and evaluation system based on big data in healthcare. The China National Center for Adverse Drug Reaction Monitoring (CNCAM) has established the China Hospital Pharmacovigilance System (CHPS) in 2016 and established the China ADR Sentinel Alliance (China ADR Sentinel Surveillance Alliance, CASSA).

The sentinel hospitals in CASSA refer to medical institutions that have been approved by the National Adverse Drug Reaction Monitoring Center and can use CHPS to achieve strong drug-device adverse reaction/event monitoring capabilities and the ability to carry out critical drug monitoring and re-evaluation capabilities. In the 13th 5-year plan period, the number of sentinel hospitals ve surveillance in China will be 300 [22–25].

CHPS is connected to sentinel hospitals' information system, which can automatically obtain medical data and connect with CASSA's coordination center. The medical data of sentinel hospitals can be directly extracted through CHPS and uploaded to the CASSA coordination center. CHPS assists CASSA in carrying out post-market safety monitoring and evaluation research with CDM and distributed data network (DDN). At present, the CDM of CHPS is relatively primary and solves the problem of unified transmission standards. In monitoring and research, it is still necessary to establish a CDM at the research project level to facilitate final analysis and utilization. CHPS realizes the virtual integration and management of data by establishing a distributed data network. Each data partner's data is converted into general data according to a unified data standard and stored in a free environment. The ownership and control rights are in the data partner (e.g., Sentinel hospital). This approach addresses the security concerns of data partners, including data security (data leakage, use for non-cooperative purposes), operational security (response to the ordinary operation of partner application systems), and personal privacy.

Besides, CHPS can also realize the online generation, review, reporting, feedback, and ADR information analysis in sentinel hospitals. It has functions such as the auxiliary report of adverse drug reactions, intelligent search for underreported cases, and sharing of drug safety information to assist sentinel hospitals. Therefore, CHPS has a potential to solve the problem of underreporting adverse drug reaction reports, improving the efficiency and quality of reports and providing references for the physician to use drugs safely. For example, the number of reports of severe adverse reactions is an important quality indicator for measuring adverse drug reaction data. In 2018, the number of severe reports of medical institutions using CHPS increased by 98% [26].

16.2.3 Feasibility Studies

Differences in data models and coding systems of various heterogeneous data sources are bottleneck issues that constrain the analysis of electronic health data in active surveillance systems. Most of the previous data analysis is only suitable for a particular database's data structure and data standard. While conducting cross-database analysis, a customized modification of the analysis procedure for different data structures and data standards is often required. Moreover, that would increase the cost of the analysis. CDM is the practical approach to harmonize and incorporate different data sources that differ in data structure and data standards [27].

CDM can be used to create a typical structure and framework to organize and standardize observational data, which allows researchers to develop various analysis methods that can be run on any data source in their format without altering the original data's content. CDM has been applied to distributed networks and centralized databases, playing a central role in data access, transformation, and normalization. CDM enables the active surveillance system to centrally develop and share the analytic code with each data partner and run in the data stored in a standard format, which can reduce the potential for logical inconsistency and ensure that the results from those data sources are comparable. Using CDM may avoid differences in interpretation of protocols by separate data sources and maximize efficient use of analyst effort. All active surveillance systems, including the Sentinel system, OMOP, and EU-ADR, have developed their own CDMs.

However, there are challenges while mapping EHDs in China into these CDMs. The result of the earlier research revealed that only part of the variables in the Yinzhou database and CACMS database were available or could be derived/transferred from the original data to harmonize with those variables in either MS CDM or OMOP CDM. Comparing with the Sentinel and OMOP common data model, part of the core data elements (55–85%) potentially valuable for post-market drug safety surveillance were collected in these three databases (Table 16.2). The result showed that the three major types of EHDs (regional community database, EMR database, and national claim database) in China are feasible for active surveillance and pharmacoepidemiology [19].

Developing Chinese-based CDMs may be a practical way to integrate a variety of EHDs in China [19]. Wu and Zhang constructed CDM of multidrug-resistant tuberculosis (MDR-TB) and evaluated its validity of ADR signal detection in EMR of 1318 MDR-TB patients. The MDR-TB CDM included demographic table, visit table, vital signs table, diagnostic table, dispensing table, laboratory results table, adverse events table, and discharge table, with 90 variables. The result suggested that the MDR-TB CDM can help analyze existing data from specialized hospitals in China and improve the timeliness of adverse event surveillance [28, 29].

Active surveillance of vaccine safety using EHDs is also in its infancy in China as part of pharmacovigilance. Very little is known about EHD capacity for active surveillance of adverse events following immunization, making feasibility assessment an essential work. Taking the human papillomavirus (HPV) vaccine as an example, Liu and his colleagues [30] designed and conducted a feasibility study to evaluate Ningbo regional health data platform, including the description of database stakeholders and components, evaluate the integrity of data related to the safety of HPV vaccine, and check the data links between different data sources. Ningbo's regional health data platform covers almost all health-related activities of the city's residents. By 2015, more than 87% of residents had registered in the database and had proper healthcare registers. In order to study the feasibility of active monitoring after HPV vaccination, a structured questionnaire and an open-ended interview guide were developed. The questionnaire is sent to the data manager by email, and face-to-face interviews are performed to confirm details or resolve differences. Their research results show that the Ningbo regional health data platform integrates the fundamental data source for active surveillance of the HPV vaccine and links it with a unique ID or coding identifier. These essential data sources include immunization program registration, EMR, resident health records, and death records. Moreover, the database can sensitively recognize the interest results through ICD-10 coding and actively monitor the risk after HPV vaccination by linking HPV vaccination records with EMR, death, or adverse events from other data sources. Therefore, the database is convenient and workable in the active surveillance of adverse events after HPV vaccination.

16.3 Some Practices of Active Surveillance

16.3.1 Signal Generation

16.3.1.1 Prescription Sequence Symmetry Analysis (PSSA)

Petri first proposed the PSSA in 1988, a method for judging whether there is an association between a drug and an event by measuring the

Table 16.2 Core variables in three databases[a] [19]

Variable name	Yinzhou database	National claims database	CACMS database
Source type	Regional community-based database	Claims database	EMR database
Patient ID	Numeric	Numeric	Numeric
Demographics			
Gender	Numeric	String	String
Birthdate	Date	Date	Date
Ethnicity	String	N	String
Residency	String	String	N
Death information			
Date of death	Date	N	D
Cause of death	String	N	D
Diagnosis information			
Symptom description	N	N	N
Start date of symptom	N	N	N
End date of symptom	N	N	N
Reason for symptom disappearance	N	N	N
Diagnosis description	String	String	String
Diagnosis date	Date	Date	Date
Drug exposure			
Trade name of drug	D	N	D
General name of drug	String	String	String
Drug specification	String	String	String
Dosage form of drug	String	String	String
Drug manufacturer	String	N	String
Batch number of drug	N	N	N
Prescription start date	Date	Date	Date
Prescription stop date	Date	N	Date
Prescription stop reason	D	N	D
Single dose of drug use	Numeric	N	Numeric
Dose unit of drug	String	String	String
Drug frequency	String	N	String
Route of administration	String	String	String
Total dose	D	Numeric	D
Drug history	N	N	N
Laboratory test			
Name of laboratory test	String	String	String
Date of laboratory test	Date	Date	Date
Type of laboratory test	D	D	D
Qualitative laboratory result	String	N	String
Quantitative laboratory result	Numeric	N	String
Quantitative unit of laboratory result	String	N	String
Other information of hospital visits			
Visiting date (clinic/emergency)	Date	Date	N
Admission date	Date	Date	Date
Discharge date	Date	Date	Date

Table 16.2 (continued)

Variable name	Yinzhou database	National claims database	CACMS database
Procedure name	String	String	String
Date of procedure	Date	Date	Date
Counts of procedure	Numeric	Numeric	Numeric

Reprinted with permission from Springer Nature

[a]Numeric = the variable is stored as digits (e.g., 25.6); date = the variable is stored as date; string = the variable is stored as characters or text; N = the variable was unavailable; D = explicit information of the variable is not available, but it may be derived or transformed through other variables in the same database, for example, "Trade name of drug" can be derived by combining other variables including "General name of drug," "Drug manufacturer," and "Drug specification"

symmetry of events distribution before and after administering the study drug. For example, drug A may have some adverse reactions and need to be treated with drug B. The first step is to determine the patients who have prescribed both A and B within a period of time in the database. In the absence of a causal relationship, the order of the two drugs is equal. The number of people who were prescribed A first and then prescribed B is equal to the number of people who were prescribed B first and then prescription A. However, if A causes adverse reactions that require treatment with B, then the prescription of drug A will increase prescription B, that is, an asymmetric order distribution. The second step is to divide the number of patients in the related group by the number of patients in the non-related group yielding sequence ratio (SR), the statistical effect size for prescribing sequence analysis, which measures the magnitude of timing asymmetry. The lower limit of the confidence interval of the SR greater than one was considered to indicate statistical relevance for the drug is causing the adverse effect [31].

The essence of PSSA is a self-contrasted research design. Its advantage is that those confounding factors that do not change over time, such as gender and genetic traits, will not affect the time sequence of prescriptions and therefore does not introduce bias to the analysis results of PSSA [32]. Therefore, unlike traditional epidemiologic studies that require a large amount of information related to confounders to be collected, the minimal dataset required to conduct a PSSA study contains only three variables: patient number, drug name (or code), and date of drug prescription [33]. The highly streamlined data requirements facilitate the development of standardized analytical procedures on the one hand and make PSSA suitable for integrative analysis of heterogeneous data sources on the other. At present, PSSA has become one of the routine active surveillance methods in the Asia Pacific Pharmacoepidemiology Network (ASPEN) [34]. Besides, the PSSA, which only enrolled patients who developed adverse reactions and used exposed drugs, had effect estimates that were not affected by the incidence of adverse reactions, and it also identified significant asymmetry with a small sample size [35]. PSSA was first introduced in the Chinese journal in 2012. After that, studies used the PSSA method to investigate drug safety issue in EHDs of China. Fang et al. [36] and Zhou et al. [37] used PSSA in medical insurance data to study the liver safety of statins (Fig. 16.1) and the allergic reaction of Xiyanping injection. In the electronic medical record data warehouse, PSSA combined with nested case-control (NCC) design was used to study the influencing factors of Shuxuening injection-related allergic reactions [38].

16.3.1.2 Tree-Based Scan Statistic (TBSS)

Scan statistic is one of the spatial statistical methods, and the basic principle is to probe local, temporal, and spatial increases in the number of certain events and test whether the increase is not due to random variation. Tree-based scan statistic (TBSS) is an ADR signal mining method for longitudinal electronic medical database and has

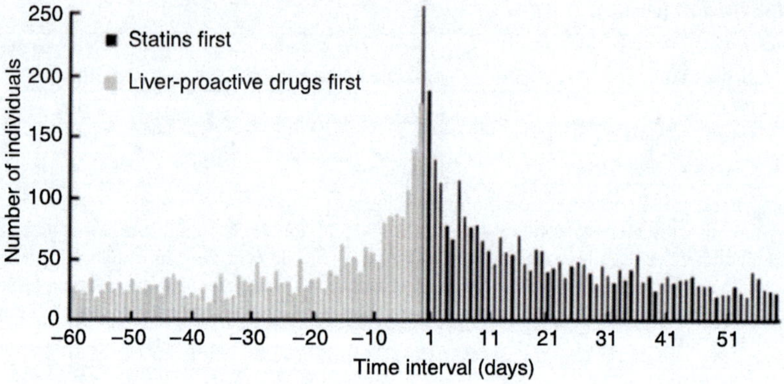

Fig. 16.1 Distribution of statins and liver-proactive drugs users [36]

been used to monitor occupational diseases [39]. TBSS enables active surveillance with minimal prior assumptions about adverse events caused by drugs and adjusts for multiple testing (which refers to increased false-positive rates due to the need to compare multiple, mutually overlapping regions, or time intervals) issues arising from the overlap between adverse events.

Kulldorff applied the TBSS method in the monitoring of adverse drug reactions for the first time in 2013 [40]. In 2016, researchers used the diagnosis of angioedema as the outcome event to construct the study drugs into a tree structure and excavate the drugs associated with the outcome [41]. Their researches showed fewer false positives in TBSS results, and the method was able to be applied to drug safety active surveillance with disease diagnosis as a lead.

Li et al. [42] conducted a study to explore the feasibility of applying TBSS in EHD of China. Based on the prescription data and diagnostic data of outpatients and hospitalizations from 2010 to 2016 in the Yinzhou regional medical database, they mined the statins' ADR signals by using the TBSS method. They also established the standard signals by searching relevant systematic reviews of the literature and drug instructions and compared the TBSS results with the standard signals to evaluate the signal detection ability of the TBSS method. They compared the difference in performance between the TBSS method and three commonly used ADR signal detection methods, the crude cohort, Bayesian Confidence Propagation Neural Network (BCPNN), and Gamma Poisson Shrinker (GPS) (Fig. 16.2). Also, they analyzed the applicability of the TBSS method in the context of a Poisson model, data on new drug users, and matched data. The findings suggested that the TBSS approach can effectively unearth the adverse effect signals of statins as candidate drug event pairs to be further validated. The TBSS method achieved high specificity while maintaining sensitivity, and the all-around performance was at the medium to a high level. The TBSS method applies to raw data, data of new drug users, and matched data simultaneously. The TBSS approach enables the simultaneous detection of many adverse events with different levels and mutual coincidence and effectively addresses multiple hypothesis testing [43, 44].

16.3.2 Signal Evaluation

Signal evaluation means conducting a formal epidemiological analysis to determine or refute the causal relationship between drug exposure and ADE. Signal evaluation may include the following aspects: (a) collecting evidence that can be used to determine the relationship between drugs and adverse events; (b) determining whether the signal represents the known or unknown risk; and (c) if the risk is known, it is necessary to propose practical measures to reduce the risk.

Regional health databases in China have been leveraged to evaluate drug safety signals. Yang et al. [45] used the Yinzhou database to establish a cohort study, comparing new sulfonylureas users and acarbose users to assess the

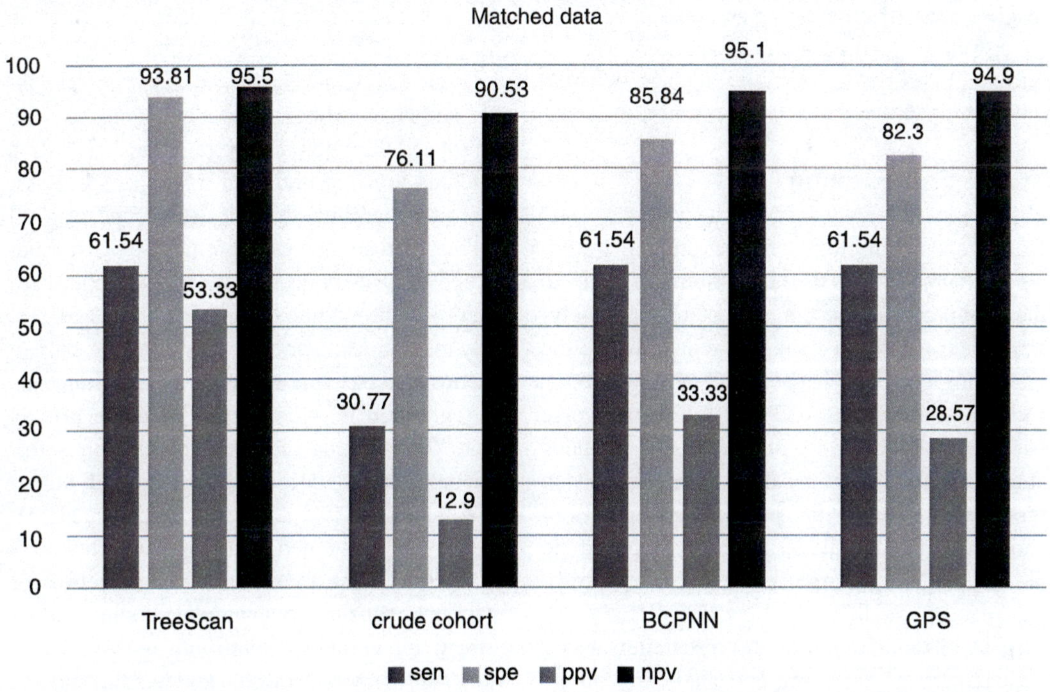

Fig. 16.2 Sensitivity, specificity, positive predictive value, and negative predictive value of four mining methods under propensity score matching data* [42]. * *sen* sensitivity, *spe* specificity, *ppv* positive predictive value, *npv* negative predictive value

association between sulfonylureas and heart failure (HHF) in Chinese patients with type 2 diabetes mellitus (T2DM). They enrolled 15,752 adult T2DM patients newly exposed to sulfonylurea monotherapy (n = 12,487) or acarbose monotherapy (n = 3265) from January 2010 to September 2016. They assessed the balance of these covariates between the two groups by standardized mean difference (SMD) and estimated each patient's propensity score (PS) by fitting the logistic regression model to predict the probability of receiving sulfonylurea monotherapy and acarbose monotherapy as a function of baseline covariates. Cox proportional hazard model was used to compare the HHF risk between sulfonylurea and acarbose initiator with the inverse probability weighting of treatment weight. Their results showed that sulfonylurea monotherapy for about 0.5 years of initial treatment of T2DM was significantly associated with a high risk of HHF compared with acarbose monotherapy. Another study is a retrospective cohort study of patients with hypertension conducted from January 1, 2010, to August 31, 2016, using the Yinzhou database, conducted by Li et al. [46] to discover the association between statin use and diabetes new-onset. Patients aged 30–90 years without T2DM are eligible. They used the prescription records of inpatients and outpatients to identify new statin initiators and non-users. A multivariate Cox model and propensity score method were used to adjust for potential confounding factors, including age, gender, body mass index, comorbidities, lifestyle characteristics, and baseline antihypertensive drug use. The Cox proportional hazard model was used to estimate the risk of T2DM between the initiators and non-users of statins. Then logistic regression was used to establish a statin use propensity score. According to the propensity score, the nearest neighbor matching method was used to match statin initiators and non-users at a ratio of 1:1 within 0.2 caliper width, and then Cox regression was performed again. The study results by Li and colleagues show that there is an association between the use of statins and the increased risk of new-onset diabetes.

16.3.3 Confounding Control

Pharmacoepidemiology observational studies are subject to bias and confounding due to the inappropriate design and statistical analysis, which results in wrong conclusions. As the increasing use of pharmacoepidemiology observational studies, the condition is getting worse [47]. To handle this problem, many methods about design or statistical analysis have been proposed. However, the problem has not been completely fixed until Hernan et al. proposed the idea of emulating a target trial when conducting a pharmacoepidemiology observational study [2]. Target trial emulation provides researchers a systematic way of designing and analyzing observational study, which aims to eliminate bias and decrease confounding.

In an ideal world, every pharmacoepidemiology study should be conducted by an RCT, but in practice, it is impossible. Therefore, pharmacoepidemiologic observational studies should be designed and analyzed to simulate pragmatic clinical trials that we wish but cannot or will not perform, which we call the targeted trial [48]. The successful target trial emulation of a pharmacoepidemiology observational study can be done in two steps, correct setup of time zero at design phase and full adjustment of confounders at time zero at analytical phase.

In RCT, time zero is the time of specification of eligibility, assignment of treatment, and initiation of follow-up, which are aligned by researchers. Thus, when emulating a target trial by observational data, we should follow the same rule, i.e., making specification of eligibility, assignment of treatment, and initiation of follow-up coincide, otherwise immortal time bias or selection bias will arise [49]. Based on different research questions, different study designs should be used to correctly define time zero. For example, Li et al. [42, 46] investigated the risk of statins in people with hypertension in mainland China in the Yinzhou database. They conducted new user and new T2DM designs to exclude patients taking statins or who have been diagnosed with T2DM and through prescription time distribution matching to avoid immortal time bias and better determine baseline characteristics. The original and matched cohorts used multivariate Cox models and propensity scoring methods to adjust for potential confounding factors, including age, sex, body mass index, comorbidities, lifestyle characteristics, and baseline antihypertensive drug use.

Regression is widely used what we usually did to control unbalanced confounders in observational studies a decade ago, just put all unbalanced confounders into the regression model. It is easily implemented, but what we obtain by regression is just a conditional causal effect of treatment/exposure, for example, the causal effect of treatment in male patients with age > 65 years, when confounders sex (male and female) and age category (≤65 and > 65 years) are adjusted in the regression model. To get the marginal causal effect of treatment/exposure directly, we should choose the matching method. In a study of Yang et al. "causal association between sulphonylurea initiation and heart failure" [45], inverse probability weighting was used as a matching method to control confounding and to obtain marginal effect of sulphonylurea versus acarbose to heart failure. After the two steps of target trial emulation, observational data is close to data from RCT. Thus the causal effect of treatment can be estimated to some degree.

16.4 Discussion

16.4.1 Enrolling Data Sources

The data source is the decisive factor in establishing an active surveillance system for drug safety. Therefore, to establish an adequate active surveillance system, it is first necessary to have a comprehensive and in-depth understanding of China's existing data sources for active post-marketing drug safety surveillance. Common data resources in developed countries for active surveillance systems include registration information, electronic medical records, and medical insurance data, which have been well used. China has also accumulated many valuable health and medical data resources, including electronic medical record systems at all hospitals, regional medical information platforms in some cities or regions, and medical insurance data covering the whole country. The hospital electronic medical record warehouse established by the Chinese Academy of Medical Sciences includes 60 hospitals in 7 provinces and cities across the country. As of 2015, it has accumulated three million electronic medical records. The information system of 17 children's hospitals in China stores about 60 million children's medical information. The medical information platform of Yinzhou District, Ningbo City, links the electronic diagnosis and treatment data of medical service institutions at all district levels. In 2015, it covered the entire district's population of 1.19 million. These data resources have significant potential value for post-market safety surveillance of drugs. However, only a few data are used for active post-marketing safety surveillance of drugs, and the understanding of various health and medical data resources nationwide is minimal. There is lack of in-depth analysis on the data characteristics, accessibility, and applicability of various data resources. CASSA's sentinel hospitals are currently only dominated by tertiary medical institutions. Although tertiary medical institutions have a high degree of information technology and strong research capabilities, they also have limited data and incomplete drug coverage. It is necessary to conduct a comprehensive and systematic survey of all kinds of existing health and medical data resources in China as soon as possible to identify and evaluate the data resources that can be used for active monitoring of the safety of drugs after the market is launched. As a result, it will speed up establishing an active monitoring system for the safety of Chinese drugs after the market is launched and formulate an active monitoring model that meets the characteristics of China's health and medical data resources [19, 20, 26].

16.4.2 Developing Methods and Tools

Methods and technologies are the key factors that affect the active surveillance of drug safety after marketing. The active surveillance system's core is analysis and mining based on real-world data, whether it is signal discovery, signal enhancement, and signal evaluation; advanced data extraction, conversion, cleaning, standardization, storage, transmission, and statistical analysis technologies are required. Since active surveillance was proposed and developed by developed countries, as far as developing countries are concerned, there is a general lack of understanding of advanced methods and technologies for active surveillance. Only some active surveillance methods have been used in China's EHDs. The application conditions, application modes, and application effects of active surveillance methods in China's EHDs still need to be studied in depth. For example, CDM, Sentinel system, and OMOP in the United States, although they have relatively mature versions, have also played an essential role in the active surveillance of drug safety after the market. However, due to the characteristics of China's EHDs, these CDMs cannot be directly applied. Although the CDM developed by CASSA can realize data exchange between different sentinel hospitals, it cannot make the data research-ready. It still needs to be further updated and iterated to adapt to the EHDs in China for active post-market surveillance of drug safety.

16.4.3 Encouraging Stakeholders

The mutually beneficial and win-win cooperation model is the basis for the active safety surveillance system's excellent functioning after the drug is marketed. The effective operation of the active surveillance system depends on the cooperation willingness of each stakeholder in the system. On the one hand, it is necessary to expand the scale of data sources (data partners) in the active surveillance system, explore new types of data-sharing partnerships, and dispel data partners' concerns about data security and privacy protection, so that they can get a certain profit after getting on board. For example, data management systems with free deployment and authorization will help data partners obtain more drug safety information and improve data quality. On the other hand, it requires the participation of multidisciplinary teams of different natures. Regulators should cooperate with high-level universities or scientific research institutions to act as the coordinating center of the active surveillance system and jointly promote administrative supervision and scientific research cooperation. At the same time, pharmaceutical manufacturers should also be encouraged to participate actively. Combine the multidisciplinary teams of pharmacy, epidemiology, clinical medicine, informatics, statistics, and data science to develop the tools and technologies required by the active surveillance system.

In general, post-market safety surveillance of drugs in China has entered an era where active surveillance and passive surveillance coexist. However, China's active surveillance system is still in its infancy compared with the relatively mature active surveillance systems of other developed countries. And many barriers and obstacles still need to be overwhelmed. With the continuous investment in active surveillance from the government, medical institutions, research institutions, and pharmaceutical companies, establishing a high-level and effective active post-market safety surveillance system in China is just around the corner.

References

1. Raj N, Fernandes S, Charyulu NR, et al. Postmarket surveillance: a review on key aspects and measures on the effective functioning in the context of the United Kingdom and Canada [J]. Ther Adv Drug Saf. 2019;10:584407365.
2. Brewer T, Colditz GA. Postmarketing surveillance and adverse drug reactions: current perspectives and future needs [J]. JAMA. 1999;281(9):824–9.
3. Lindquist M, Edwards IR. The WHO Programme for international drug monitoring, its database, and the technical support of the Uppsala monitoring center [J]. J Rheumatol. 2001;28(5):1180–7.
4. Wadman M. Strong medicine [J]. Nat Med. 2005;11(5):465–6.
5. Stephenson WP, Hauben M. Data mining for signals in spontaneous reporting databases: proceed with caution [J]. Pharmacoepidemiol Drug Saf. 2007;16(4):359–65.
6. Molokhia M, Tanna S, Bell D. Improving reporting of adverse drug reactions: systematic review[J]. Clin Epidemiol. 2009;1:75–92.
7. Goldman SA. Limitations and strengths of spontaneous reports data [J]. Clin Ther. 1998;20(Suppl C):C40–4.
8. Aronson JK, Hauben M, Bate A. Defining 'surveillance' in drug safety [J]. Drug Saf. 2012;35(5):347–57.
9. WHO. The importance of pharmacovigilance [J]. Who Drug Information, 2002.
10. Chen RT, Destefano F, Davis RL, et al. The vaccine safety datalink: immunization research in health maintenance organizations in the USA [J]. Bull World Health Organ. 2000;78(2):186–94.
11. Huang YL, Moon J, Segal JB. A comparison of active adverse event surveillance systems worldwide [J]. Drug Saf. 2014;37(8):581–96.
12. Platt R, Wilson M, Chan KA, et al. The new sentinel network--improving the evidence of medical-product safety [J]. N Engl J Med. 2009;361(7):645–7.
13. Behrman RE, Benner JS, Brown JS, et al. Developing the sentinel system--a national resource for evidence development [J]. N Engl J Med. 2011;364(6):498–9.
14. Platt R, Carnahan RM, Brown JS, et al. The U.S. Food and Drug Administration's Mini-Sentinel program: status and direction [J]. Pharmacoepidemiol Drug Saf. 2012;21(Suppl 1):1–8.
15. Curtis LH, Brown J, Platt R. Four health data networks illustrate the potential for a shared national multipurpose big-data network [J]. Health Aff (Millwood). 2014;33(7):1178–86.
16. Maro JC, Platt R, Holmes JH, et al. Design of a national distributed health data network [J]. Ann Intern Med. 2009;151(5):341–4.
17. Brown JS, Holmes JH, Shah K, et al. Distributed health data networks: a practical and preferred approach to multi-institutional evaluations of comparative effectiveness, safety, and quality of care [J]. Med Care. 2010;48(6 Suppl):S45–51.
18. Curtis LH, Weiner MG, Boudreau DM, et al. Design considerations, architecture, and use of the Mini-Sentinel distributed data system [J]. Pharmacoepidemiol Drug Saf. 2012;21(Suppl 1):23–31.
19. Yang Y, Zhou X, Gao S, et al. Evaluation of electronic healthcare databases for post-marketing drug safety surveillance and Pharmacoepidemiology in China [J]. Drug Saf. 2018;41(1):125–37.
20. Yu Y, Yang Y, Xu Y, et al. Feasibility of post-marketing active safety surveillance for pediatric medication based on big medical data: a survey on information systems in 17 children's hospitals in China [J]. Adverse Drug React J. 2017;19(3):168.

21. Council CS. Notice on the issuance of national 12th five-year plan for drug safety [Z]. 2012:2021.
22. Council CS. Notice on the issuance of national 13th five-year plan for food safety and drug safety [Z]. 2017.
23. Li L, Yin J. Drug safety evaluation in China [J]. Curr Allergy Asthma Rep. 2019;19(9):39.
24. Li X, Li H, Deng J, et al. Active pharmacovigilance in China: recent development and future perspectives [J]. Eur J Clin Pharmacol. 2018;74(7):863–71.
25. Zhao Y, Wang T, Li G, et al. Pharmacovigilance in China: development and challenges [J]. Int J Clin Pharm. 2018;40(4):823–31.
26. Hou Y, Song H, Liu H, et al. Practice and discussion on active surveillance by China hospital pharmacovigilance system[J]. Chin J Pharmacovigilance. 2019;16(4):212–4.
27. Overhage JM, Ryan PB, Reich CG, et al. Validation of a common data model for active safety surveillance research[J]. J Am Med Inform Assoc. 2012;19(1):54–60.
28. Wu S. Methodology study of adverse drug reactions and construction of common data model in MDR-TB patients (in Chinese) [D]. 2015.
29. Zhang Y. Construction of common data model for active surveillance of adverse drug reaction in multidrug-resistant tuberculosis treatment (in Chinese) [D]. 2017.
30. Liu Z, Zhang L, Yang Y, et al. Active surveillance of adverse events following human papillomavirus vaccination: feasibility pilot study based on the regional health care information platform in the City of Ningbo, China [J]. J Med Internet Res. 2020;22(6):e17446.
31. Petri H, de Vet HC, Naus J, et al. Prescription sequence analysis: a new and fast method for assessing certain adverse reactions of prescription drugs in large populations [J]. Stat Med. 1988;7(11):1171–5.
32. Hallas J. Evidence of depression provoked by cardiovascular medication: a prescription sequence symmetry analysis [J]. Epidemiology. 1996;7(5):478–84.
33. Lai EC, Yang YH, Lin SJ, et al. Use of antiepileptic drugs and risk of hypothyroidism [J]. Pharmacoepidemiol Drug Saf. 2013;22(10):1071–9.
34. Lai EC, Pratt N, Hsieh CY, et al. Sequence symmetry analysis in pharmacovigilance and pharmacoepidemiologic studies [J]. Eur J Epidemiol. 2017;32(7):567–82.
35. Maclure M, Fireman B, Nelson JC, et al. When should case-only designs be used for safety monitoring of medical products?[J]. Pharmacoepidemiol Drug Saf. 2012;21(Suppl 1):50–61.
36. Fang RF, Li JH, Zhang J, et al. Association between statins use and liver injury based on prescription sequence symmetry analysis [J]. Zhonghua Liu Xing Bing Xue Za Zhi. 2016;37(7):935–9.
37. Zhou Y, Cheng Y, Gao S, et al. Study of Xiyanping injection and allergic reaction based on prescription sequence symmetry analysis [J]. Chin J Pharmacoepidemiol. 2019;28(6):376–9. 388
38. Yang W, You L, Xie Y, et al. Discussion on influencing factors of suspected allergic reaction caused by Shuxuening injection based on combination with prescription sequence analysis and nested case-control design [J]. China J Tradit Chin Med Pharmacy. 2015;30(5):1417–20.
39. Lieu TA, Kulldorff M, Davis RL, et al. Real-time vaccine safety surveillance for the early detection of adverse events [J]. Med Care. 2007;45(10 Supl 2):S89–95.
40. Kulldorff M, Dashevsky I, Avery TR, et al. Drug safety data mining with a tree-based scan statistic [J]. Pharmacoepidemiol Drug Saf. 2013;22(5):517–23.
41. Maro JC, Dal Pan GJ, Dashevsky I, et al. Monitoring all drugs for a specific outcome in the sentinel system [C]. Hoboken: Wiley-Blackwell; 2016.
42. Li H. The application of tree-based scan statistic method in active surveillance for statins [D]. 2018.
43. Hailong L, Houyu Z, Yifan Z, et al. Data mining methods for adverse drug reaction signals detection in healthcare databases: a literature review [J]. Chin J Pharmacoepidemiol. 2018;27(8):541–9.
44. Hailong L, Houyu Z, Siyan Z. The application of tree-based scan statistic in drug safety surveillance [J]. Chin J Pharmacoepidemiol. 2018;27(3):209–13.
45. Xu Y, Wang T, Yang Z, et al. Sulphonylureas monotherapy and risk of hospitalization for heart failure in patients with type 2 diabetes mellitus: a population-based cohort study in China [J]. Pharmacoepidemiol Drug Saf. 2020;29(6):635–43.
46. Li H, Lin H, Zhao H, et al. Statins use and risk of new-onset diabetes in hypertensive patients: a population-based retrospective cohort study in Yinzhou district, Ningbo city, People's Republic of China [J]. Ther Clin Risk Manag. 2018;14:823–32.
47. Prada-Ramallal G, Takkouche B, Figueiras A. Bias in pharmacoepidemiologic studies using secondary health care databases: a scoping review [J]. BMC Med Res Methodol. 2019;19(1):53.
48. Hernan MA, Robins JM. Using big data to emulate a target trial when a randomized trial is not available [J]. Am J Epidemiol. 2016;183(8):758–64.
49. Hernan MA, Sauer BC, Hernandez-Diaz S, et al. Specifying a target trial prevents immortal time bias and other self-inflicted injuries in observational analyses [J]. J Clin Epidemiol. 2016;79:70–5.

17 Research Advances in Epidemiology of Autoimmune Diseases in China

Xin-yu Fang and Dong-Qing Ye

Abstract

Autoimmune diseases (ADs) are a group of chronic diseases, including systemic lupus erythematosus, rheumatoid arthritis, multiple sclerosis, type 1 diabetes, etc., which are characterized by loss of immunological tolerance to autoantigens, resulting in damage to specific target organs or multiple organ systems. The chronic nature of these diseases imposes a significant disease burden on the utilization of medical care, direct and indirect financial costs, and quality of life. The etiology of ADs has not been fully elucidated yet. Thus, epidemiological studies of ADs can help us better understand the potential risk factors for the development of ADs and enable us to plan health services to cope with a significant disease burden. In the past few decades, there are outstanding achievements in the epidemiology of ADs in China. This chapter aims to summarize the epidemiological characteristics and key risk factors of some common ADs in China, so as to provide some new insights for understanding these diseases.

Keywords

Autoimmune diseases · Chinese Epidemiology

17.1 An Overview of Autoimmune Diseases

17.1.1 A Brief Introduction of Autoimmune Diseases

Autoimmune diseases (ADs) are a heterogeneous group of diseases characterized by the activation of immune cells and excessive production of autoantibodies. To date, there is still a lack of formal and consensus diagnostic criteria for ADs. The modified version of Witebsky's postulates is the most widely accepted standard for diagnosing ADs [1], which include (1) the specific adaptive immune response is directed to the affected organ or tissue; (2) autoreactive T cells and/or autoantibodies are present in the affected organ or tissue; (3) autoreactive T cells and/or autoantibodies can transfer the disease to healthy individuals or animals; (4) immunization with the autoantigen induces the disease in animal models; and (5) elimination or suppression of the autoimmune response prevents disease progression or even lessens the clinical manifestation. According to the modified version of Witebsky's postulates, 81

X.-y. Fang · D.-Q. Ye (✉)
School of Public Health, Anhui Medical University, Hefei, China
e-mail: ydq@ahmu.edu.cn

D.-Q. Ye (ed.), *Progress in China Epidemiology*, https://doi.org/10.1007/978-981-19-2199-5_17

ADs have already been identified, including 64 likely and 17 probable ADs.

Among them, some of which are organ-specific and some reflect a variety of immunological dysfunction involving multiple organs. Here we list some typical ADs in Table 17.1.

17.1.2 The History of Autoimmunity

The development and recognition of the concept of autoimmunity paralleled the history of immunology. The oldest traditional Chinese medicine literature on immunology and auto-

Table 17.1 List of some typical autoimmune diseases

Autoimmune disorders	Classification	Tissue autoantibody
Pernicious anemia/atrophic gastritis	Organ-specific	Anti-H/K
Autoimmune hemolytic anemia	Organ-specific	Anti-erythrocyte I/i
Immune thrombocytopenic purpura	Organ-specific	Anti-GpIIb/IIIa
Alopecia areata	Organ-specific	Anti-hair follicle antibodies
Dermatitis herpetiformis	Organ-specific	Anti-TGase3
Pemphigus foliaceus	Organ-specific	Anti-desmoglein I
Pemphigus vulgaris	Organ-specific	Anti-desmoglein III
Vitiligo	Organ-specific	Anti-MCHR1, anti-SOX-10
Graves' disease	Organ-specific	TSIg
Diabetes mellitus, type 1	Organ-specific	Anti-GAD, anti-insulin, anti-ICA512
Autoimmune polyglandular syndrome I	Organ-specific	Anti-candidal enolase, anti-pituitary, anti-calcium sensing receptor protein, anti-aromatic L-amino acid decarboxylase, anti-tyrosine hydroxylase
Myasthenia gravis	Organ-specific	Anti-AChR, MuSK
Addison's disease	Organ-specific	Anti-21-hydroxylase, Anti-17 alpha-hydroxylase, anti-P450scc
Stiff-person syndrome	Organ-specific	Anti-GAD, anti-amphiphysin
Rheumatic fever	Organ-specific	Anti-streptolysin O, anti-DNase B
Systemic lupus erythematosus	Systematic	Anti-dsDNA, anti-U1A, anti-U2B, anti-PCNA, anti-smith, anti-SSA, anti-SSB
Sjögren's syndrome	Systematic	ANA, SSB, SSA
Scleroderma	Systematic	Anti-Scl70, anti-PM/Scl, anti-RNA polymerase III, anti-centromere
Wegener's granulomatosis	Systematic	cANCA
Antiphospholipid syndrome	Systematic	Anti-cardiolipin, lupus anticoagulant, anti-b2GPI
Rheumatoid arthritis	Systematic	Rheumatoid factor, anti-CCP
Polymyositis/dermatomyositis	Systematic	Anti-Jo1, anti-Mi-2, anti-CADM140

immunity dates back more than 1700 years. Around 303 AD, Ge Hong put forward the idea of "prophylactic immunization" to prevent the recurrence of rabies by "covering the people with the sick dog's brain" in his book. It may be the earliest recorded vaccination practice in the world. The idea of inhaling powders made from patient's crusty skin lesions to prevent children's smallpox has been widely accepted since the Ming Dynasty in ancient China. The practice then spread along the "Old Silk Road" connecting China with the Western Country and then facilitated the discovery of a vaccine against smallpox in 1798 by Edward Jenner, who is often regarded as the founder of immunology.

In the 100 years following 1789, Jules Bordet first discovered antibodies in the blood, which marked the concept of autoimmunity were really taken shape. In fact, people were already developing vaccines and treating autoimmune diseases before antibodies were discovered. In 1901, Paul Ehrlich in Germany had introduced his famous "horror autotoxicus" that the body must have a system to protect against the dangers posed by autoantibodies. Only 3 years later, Donath and Landsteiner reported their discovery that antibodies could destroy one's own red blood cell. It was really a landmark observation, the first time we knew about autoimmune diseases. Shortly thereafter, August Wassermann showed that sera from syphilis patients could react not only with extracts of syphilitic tissue but also with extracts of normal tissue. Namely, some autoantibodies directly target human tissues. Then, more hints of autoimmunity began to surface, with autoimmune diseases of the eyes, thyroid, testicles, brain, and other organs discovered. However, autoimmune research entered the Dark Ages from 1911 to the end of World War II. Nothing much happened during this period, the concept of autoimmunity failed to take hold.

The period from 1945 to 1965 was the golden age when the concept of autoimmunity took off. Philip Hench recognized the effectiveness of Compound E in a rheumatoid arthritis patient. The cellular effect of lupus erythematosus (LE) was eventually reported in 1948 by Hargraves. Rheumatoid factor (RF) was "incidentally" discovered in 1948. In 1951, Harrington et al. described a remarkable experiment. He transfused serum from patients with idiopathic thrombocytopenic purpura (ITP) into volunteers and found an immediate decrease in levels of circulating blood platelets. This phenomenon indicated a serum agent, presumably an autoantibody, passively transferred to volunteers and reacting with platelets, thus causing their destruction. In 1956, Ivan Roitt and colleagues in London proved that levels of anti-thyroglobulin antibodies in patients with Hashimoto's thyroiditis were extremely high compared with controls. Interestingly, at the same time (1956), endocrinologists Purves and Adams from New Zealand had demonstrated that thyrotoxicosis sera contained a long-acting thyroid stimulator (an autoantibody) that stimulated the excessive release of thyroid hormone in Graves' disease. Three years later, Marianne and Felix Bielschowsky from Dunedin, New Zealand, successfully established the first murine model of autoimmunity and reported their observation of inbred mice with spontaneous autoimmune hemolytic anemia. Another technological innovation that significantly promoted advances in autoimmunity was fluorescence microscopy. It prepared the way for autoantibodies detection by using frozen sections of tissues or serum of patients, thus leading to the confident nomination of diverse diseases as autoimmune in the early 1960s. Together, these studies established the prototype of human autoimmune diseases and went far toward inculcating an acceptance of autoimmunization as a general cause of human disease.

In retrospect, although China has a very early understanding of the immune system and autoimmune diseases, it has stagnated since the Ming Dynasty. In 1959, the Rheumatology Association was established in China, marking the beginning of China's research on autoimmune diseases. Unfortunately, the system of rheumatology was not really established in our country because China at that time was in a difficult economic period and affected by the subsequent "cultural revolution." But we still have made some achievements, such as Yunde Hou finding a novel type of IFN-α and identifying its potential role in treating autoimmune disease. After the Cultural Revolution (1966–1976), China experienced rapid economic growth.

The benefit of the Economic Reform and Open Up in China is that the government has invested a lot of money in scientific research. The first rheumatology department in China was founded in Peking Union Medical College Hospital in 1980. Since then, the study of autoimmune diseases in China has entered a golden age.

Considering the classification of autoimmune diseases and the major research directions in China in recent years, four major autoimmune diseases, namely, systemic lupus erythematosus (SLE), rheumatoid arthritis (RA), multiple sclerosis (MS), and type 1 diabetes (T1D), are introduced in this chapter, with emphasis on the epidemiological characteristics in Chinese population and the contributions made by Chinese researchers to the identification of risk factors of these diseases.

17.2 Epidemiological Characteristics of Autoimmune Diseases in China

Although rare disease study has attracted more and more attention in recent years, the exploration of rare disease epidemiology still lacks in China. However, studying the epidemiology of ADs allows us to identify and explore changes in potential risk factors for the disease and allows planning of health services in response to the overall disease burden. This part aims to summarize the epidemiological studies of ADs (mainly in SLE, RA, MS, and T1D) conducted in China to clarify its epidemiological characteristics. More detailed information can be seen in Table 17.2.

17.2.1 Systemic Lupus Erythematosus (SLE)

SLE is a representative systemic autoimmune disease characterized by aberrant production of autoantibodies that are direct or indirect against nuclear and cytoplasmic antigens, thus resulting in variable clinical symptoms. It also has a significant disease burden among different countries, racial, and age groups. Studies on SLE epidemiology are relatively few, and most of them focused on Europe and North America. The incidence and prevalence rate of SLE fluctuate worldwide, with the highest estimates in North America (241/100,000 person-years, compared with 23.2/100,000 person-years in Europe) and the lowest estimates in Northern Australia (0 cases in a sample of 847 people). Moreover, women had a higher incidence and prevalence rate of SLE than men among every age group, ranging from 2:1 [2] to 15:1 [3]. Furthermore, there is usually a peak age of incidence before declining both in female and male patients, which often occurs in middle-aged adults.

In China, good estimated epidemiological studies of SLE are mainly lacking. In the 1990s, three studies estimated the prevalence rate of SLE in Shanghai, Guangzhou, and Shandong, and the obtained prevalence rates of SLE were 70.1/100,000, 31.1/100,000, and 46.5/100,000, respectively [4–6]. The significant difference in prevalence between the three cities may be due to the choice of participants. The study in Shanghai was conducted among textile factory workers who were predominantly females and may have occupational exposure and thus may obtain an overestimated prevalence rate. In 2014, our team conducted an extensive population-based epidemiological survey including 1,253,832 participants to explore the prevalence of SLE in rural areas of Anhui Province of China. We reported a prevalence rate for SLE of 37.56/100,000. Gender difference in the prevalence of SLE was significant, and the prevalence rate was higher in females than in males, with a ratio of 10.99:1. The distribution of SLE prevalence also varied by age group, and the peak prevalence was observed at 40–50 years. In addition, the estimated point prevalence of SLE in Hong Kong is around 58.8/100,000 (rates for men and women are 11.7/100,000 and 104/100,000, respectively [7]).

In recent years, there is a trend of improvement in SMR for SLE in China. A longitudinal cohort study of Chinese patients with SLE found a decreasing SMR of 7.88 in 2000 and 2.17 in

Table 17.2 List of studies on SLE, RA, MS, and T1D in China between 1980 and 2020

Site of survey	Disease	Age (years)	Ethnic	Time	Number	Prevalence	Incidence
Shanghai	T1D	<15	Han	1980–1991	54,990		0.61/100,000
Shanghai	SLE	–	Han	1985	32,000		70.41/100,000
China	T1D	<15	Han	1985–1994	20,654,990		0.51/100,000
Hong Kong	MS	–	Han	1981–1987	4,900,000	0.88/100,000	
Shanghai	T1D	<15	Han	1989–1993	54,990		0.96/100,000
Ningxia	RA	≥18	Hui	1990	10,420	360/100,000	
Harbin	T1D	<15	Han	1990–2000	1,286,154		0.73/100,000
Shanghai	RA	≥16	Han	1992	2010	200/100,000	
Hong Kong	RA	≥16	Han	1992	1988	350/100,000	
Guangzhou	SLE	–	Han	1992	3000		31.1/100,000
Anhui	SLE	–	Han	1993	204,345		4.4/100,000
Taiwan	RA	≥16	Han	1994	3000	930/100,000	
Taiwan	RA	≥20	Han	1994	3000	780/100,000	
Taiwan	RA	≥20	Han	1994	3000	200/100,000	
Shandong	RA	≥20	Han	1996	5055	360/100,000	
Beijing, Shantou	SLE		Han	1997	9247		41/100,000
Shanghai	T1D	<15	Han	1997–2011	54,990		3.1/100,000
Hong Kong	MS	–	Han	1999	6,883,116		0.77/100,000
Hong Kong	SLE	–	Han	2001	5055		58.8/100,000
Taiwan	MS	–	Han	2000–2005	22,770,000		0.63/100,000
Taiwan	SLE	–	Han	2000–2007	22,182		8.1/100,000
Shandong	SLE	–	Han	2001	1988		46.5/100,000
Shandong	SLE	–	Han	2001	1988		46.5/100,000
Taiyuan	RA	<15	Han	2004	3915	280/100,000	
Hong Kong	SLE	–	Han	2006	3915		6.7/100,000
Shanghai	MS	–	Han	2007	8,860,000		1.39/100,000
Zhejiang	T1D	<19	Han	2007–2013	44,789		2.02/100,000
Beijing	RA		Han	2011	10,556	410/100,000	
Hong Kong	SLE	–	Han	2011	3000		6.7/100,000
Beijing	SLE	–	Han	2011	14,642		30/100,000
Anhui	SLE	–	Han	2013	1,253,832		37.56/100,000
Shandong	MS	–	Han	2013	95,792,719	5.2/100,000	
Shantou	RA	≥16	Han	2015	5504	350/100,000	

2006 compared to the general population [8]. The SMR was higher in men than in women and significantly increased in younger patients, indicating a greater effect of the disease on young women individuals. Meanwhile, SLE also leads to considerable disease costs, with an average outpatient cost of US$71.5 and an average inpatient cost of US$1922.3 [9].

17.2.2 Rheumatoid Arthritis (RA)

RA is a chronic inflammatory disorder characterized by irreversible joint damage and significant disability that can cause substantial societal effects in cost, disability, and lost productivity. To date, approximately 20 surveys in China have reported the prevalence rate of RA. The prevalence rate ranged from 200/100,000 to 370/100,000 in mainland China. The prevalence rate of RA is relatively higher in Taiwan Island (930/10,000) than that in other areas of China. In addition, a population-based cross-sectional survey conducted in Tibet have reported that the overall prevalence of RA was 486/100,000, and the age-standardized prevalence of RA was 630/100,000 [10]. There was no significant difference in prevalence rate of RA between Han and

Zhuang nationality population [11]. Compared to males, females had a five times higher prevalence of RA. Studies in China do not indicate a growing trend in the prevalence rate of RA; however, the total RA cases increased considerably with time, especially in children and adolescents aged <15 years old. In addition, due to China's large population base, even a slightly 0.1% increase in prevalence would translate to approximately four million additional RA cases. It is evident that RA has had a substantial disease burden in China. For example, RA imposes a magnificent financial burden on patients and their families, classified as direct and indirect costs. The direct cost consists of medications, hospital stays and visits, caregivers and aides, and the indirect costs including lost productivity through absenteeism or early retirement and intangible costs measured in their impact on quality of life. In the United States, the direct cost of RA was nearly US$ 13,500 per affected per person-year, and indirect costs could range from US$ 1000 to US$ 33,000 per affected person per year. Unfortunately, no evidence exists to date about the costs of RA in China. It is also noteworthy to point out the lack of morbidity data of RA from China. Given that estimating the incidence of RA is intended to be a first step toward raising awareness among policy makers and healthcare workers, further research should be specifically orientated toward RS, with greater attention on the mortality and disease burden.

17.2.3 Type 1 Diabetes (T1D)

T1D is an autoimmune, metabolic disease characterized by autoimmune-mediated destruction of beta cells and subsequent severe deficiency of endogenous insulin and hyperglycemia. Initially, it was recognized as one of the most common chronic pediatric diseases, but over time, its occurrence at any age was widely accepted.

The epidemiological characteristics of T1D have been studied extensively in China in the past few decades. In 1991, Chinese IDDM (insulin-dependent diabetes mellitus) was established based on the WHO Diamond Project to evaluate the T1D incidence rate in China. A total of 20,654,990 children <15 years old were enrolled from 1985 to 1994 in this study. The overall adjusted T1D incidence rate was 0.51/100,000 person-years, and sex-specific incidence rates were 0.47/100,000 person-years for boys and 0.59/100,000 person-years for girls [12]. With the rapid change in lifestyle in China, studies have revealed continuously increasing incidence trends of T1D. For example, the average incidence rate of childhood T1D was 0.61/100,000 person-years in Shanghai City during 1980–1991 and has risen to 0.96/100,000 person-years from 1989 to 1993 and then increased to 3.1 /100,000 person-years during 1997–2011 [13]. The average annual age-standardized incidence of T1D in children and adolescents aged 0–19 years old was 2.02/100,000 (95% CI: 1.92–2.12) person-years during 2007–2013 in Zhejiang Province, with a mean annual increase of 12.0% [14].

The incidence of type 1 diabetes also varied in different sex, different ages, and different regions. The risk for T1D in girls was 1.25 times higher than that in boys. The incidence rate of T1D was associated with age. For instance, compared with T1D patients aged<5 years, the rate ratios were 2.06 and 4.1 for those aged 5–9 and 10–14 years, respectively [15]. The incidence was higher in urban than in suburban regions. Besides, the prevalence of T1D among adults was also estimated in China. A recent large cross-sectional study involved 17,349 newly diagnosed adult T1D patients was conducted in 2010 and identified the prevalence of T1D was 5.49% (5.14% in males and 6.16% in females [16]).

17.2.4 Multiple Sclerosis (MS)

Multiple sclerosis is a chronic, rare, immune-mediated disease that mainly affects the central nervous system and results in a disabling condition with devastating social and economic impacts. MS is considered rare in China, and reports on MS are few. The first case of MS in China was reported from Peking Union Medical College Hospital in 1926. Since then, surveys on MS have been developed gradually, but until now there is still a lack of sizeable national-based surveillance on MS frequency in the Chinese population. In recent years, few population-based surveys on MS were conducted in a few areas. A population-based study in Shanghai has reported that the crude MS prevalence rate was 1.39/100,000 and higher in females than in males (female-to-male ratio of 1.8 [17]). The prevalence of MS in Hong Kong was estimated to be from 0.77 to 4.8 per 100,000 population [18, 19]. The incidence rate of MS among the Taiwan population was 0.79/100,000, and female MS patients outnumbered males by a ratio of 2.5: 1 [20]. Another study in Shandong Province based on the hospitalization data has indicated that the incidence of MS was estimated to be 0.2 /100,000 and 0.12/100,000 for females and males [21].

MS is increasing in incidence and prevalence in China, which is considered as a traditionally low-prevalence region of the world. The prevalence of MS increased in Taiwan island in recent decades from 0.84/100,000 in 1975 and 1.9/100,000 in 1999 to 2.96/100,000 in 2005 [20–23]. In the last three decades, the mean age at disease onset also ranged from 46.4 in 1993 and 32.6 in 2006 to 33.7–36.0 in 2013 [21, 24, 25]. As an essential cause of neurologic disability among the working-class population, MS patients had a significant disease burden in China. Studies have shown that the disease burden in disability-adjusted life years of MS was 3316, including 903 (27.2%) years of life lost (YLL) and 2413 (72.8%) years lived with disability (YLD [21]).

In conclusion, there is a large number of ADs patients with a high disease burden in China. However, China currently lacks important epidemiological data (e.g., disease burden data) of most ADs, especially in large-scale and national-based data. A specific registration system for rare diseases should be considered to solve this problem in the future.

17.3 Risk Factors for Autoimmune Diseases

Despite the advent of disease classifications, monitoring strategies, and therapeutic options, the survival rate of SLE, RA, and MS patients has not improved much further since the 1980s. The heterogeneous nature of the disease and the lack of complete understanding of its pathogenesis are major hurdles to further improving the current management strategies for autoimmune diseases. Hence, it is important to identify risk factors for the development of autoimmune diseases to encourage prevention and early diagnosis and reduce the disease burden. Here, we review relevant knowledge on the etiology of autoimmune diseases and particularly describe important work done by Chinese researchers.

17.3.1 Genetic Factors of Autoimmune Diseases

17.3.1.1 Familial Aggregation and Twin Studies

Our early understanding of the familial aggregation of the disease is derived from the high rate of autoimmune disease concordance in twins, siblings, and family members compared to the general population. For example, the prevalence of MS in the general population is approximately 0.1%, while the risk for monozygotic twins and first-degree relatives (such as siblings) is about 2–5% and 25–30%, respectively. The degree of clustering of disease in families can be demonstrated by calculating the ratio of the risk for relatives of patients with an illness and the overall population prevalence of that disease [26]. This ratio is referred to as λ_s, and if it has a value of 1.0, then there is no evidence for familial aggregation. Namely, if the value of λ_s exceeds 1.0, then relatives of patients are at higher risk of disease. For example, the value of λ_s ratio in RA in monozygotic twins and siblings of affected individuals are 12 to 62 and 2 to 17, respectively [27].

However, what causes familial aggregation of autoimmune diseases? It cannot be assumed that genes are fully responsible because similar environmental factors are also shared among family members that might explain such familial aggregation. To distinguish the relative contribution of genetic and environmental factors in the clustering of disease in families, thus twin studies were conducted. The comparison of concordance rates between monozygotic and dizygotic pairs is generally considered to measure the influence of genetic factors. For instance, the proportion of concordance in MS for monozygotic twins is approximately 25–30%, whereas the concordance percentage for dizygotic twins is 3–5%. Because twins share the same intrauterine environment and similar postnatal environments, the large difference in concordance between monozygotic and dizygotic twins must, at least in part, be due to genetic factors [28]. Moreover, adopted children studies also showed that the frequency of MS among first-degree non-biological relatives living with the case was no greater than expected from population prevalence data and significantly less than for biological relatives, again implying familial aggregation of MS is genetically determined [29]. Taking all the data together, environmental factors are probably not a major cause of familial aggregation. Evidence indicates that familial aggregation has been observed in some AIDs, including type 1 diabetes, rheumatoid arthritis, MS, and SLE. The concordance rate in AIDs is ranging from 15% to 60%. However, the fact that the majority of AID patients have no family history suggests either that environmental factors take precedence over genetic risks or that genetic risk is owing to the effect on multiple genetic traits that, by themselves, result in low disease penetrance. Indeed, the majority of autoimmune diseases, including type 1 diabetes, RA, MS, and SLE, are not monogenic but rather have multiple genetic factors working together.

17.3.1.2 Linkage Analysis

Human leucocyte antigen (HLA) region, the major histocompatibility complex (MHC) in humans, is the first associated locus identified in autoimmune disease. It is located on the short arm of chromosome 6 and harbors critical genes encoding molecules involved in viral antigen presentation pathway and therefore play essential roles in distinguishing self from non-self (foreign) entities. By using sera typing and microlymphocytotoxicity technique, early studies have found certain peripheral blood mononuclear cell surface antigens were overrepresented in patients with autoimmune diseases compared to healthy controls. For example, such cell surface antigens including HLA-A3, HLA-B7, and HLA-DR2 have been reported in MS. These studies established an association between autoimmunity diseases and specific variations in genes encoding HLAs. However, due to the extensive linkage disequilibrium in the chromosomal region that encodes these antigens, it was difficult to clarify which linkage genes in HLA were responsible for disease susceptibility, thus requiring modern molecular techniques.

With the advent of new DNA-based in the 1980s, dissection of linked genes at the HLA locus and screening of the entire genome enabled. The new DNA-based technologies use restriction fragment length polymorphisms (RFLPs) and microsatellite repeats which are unique variations in DNA sequence, to determine whether the DNA locus that harbors the variant has more than a chance to link with an inherited trait of interest. DNA markers near the disease-causing gene are more likely to inherit together with the disease trait due to the linkage disequilibrium. Thus, it is possible to detect the chromosomal location of causing genes through exploring the linkage between an inherited trait and DNA markers in familial members with autoimmune disease. It is in this context that many linkage studies have conducted and identified HLA variants associated with autoimmune diseases such as SLE (HLA-DR3, HLA-DR2 and HLA-DR8), RA (HLA-DR4, HLA-TNF), and T1D (HLA-DQ2, HLA-DQ8, HLA-A, and HLA-DQB1*0602).

However, follow-up studies have found that all HLA alleles are commonly discovered in healthy controls, though they are overrepresented among patients with autoimmune diseases. Moreover, genetic risks of autoimmune diseases have been observed in some families that lack the HLA alleles. Namely, none of the HLA alleles associated with autoimmune diseases is disease-causing variations. Indeed, as mentioned above, the majority of autoimmune diseases have complex multigenic traits, so it is difficult to identify the genetic basis for these traits since the penetrance of each gene may be very low. Thus, it was hypothesized that non-MHC loci could be accounted for disease inheritance, which might contribute more to autoimmune disease risk than the HLA locus. In this context, a series of genomic linkage screens using several hundred microsatellite repeats in families affected by autoimmune diseases were undertaken in the 1990s to identify novel loci. Unfortunately, no statistically significant novel loci were discovered. The main reason is that identifying novel genetic mutations associated with autoimmune diseases requires not only ideal DNA markers but also a substantially increased number of families to attain sufficient statistical power. It is obviously that using linkage analysis to analyze tens of thousands of families to identify novel loci was effectively not possible. A new genetic analysis called GWAS was thus developed to overcome these barriers.

17.3.1.3 Genome-Wide Association Study (GWAS)

With further technological innovations, identifying single-nucleotide polymorphisms (SNPs) across the entire genome has become possible. After the completion of Human Genome Sequencing in 2001, researchers realized that despite 99.9% of the human genome is invariant, there are still many millions of SNP variants, some of which are quite common (present in at least 5% of the general population). If heritable traits are commonly associated with SNP variants, genotyping of these mutations in both affected individuals and unaffected controls will help identify those loci related to the genetic traits.

Genome-wide association study (GWAS) is a commonly used study design that uses chip technology to genotype hundreds of thousands of common SNPs in both case and control populations and then compares the frequency and distribution of SNPs between the two groups to further identify associations between variations and human traits. Autoimmune diseases were one of the first diseases to be studied using this GWAS technique and many non-MHC loci have been identified. For example, the first GWAS for TID was published in 2006, reporting an association with the innate immunity viral RNA receptor gene region, *IFIH1*. The IMSGC conducted the first GWAS for MS in 2007 and identified two non-MHC loci that encode genes involved in immune regulation: the interleukin-2 receptor (*IL2Rα*) and the interleukin-7 receptor (*IL7Rα*). It was followed rapidly by a number of other GWAS that increased the number of loci demonstrating association. Over the past two decades or so, thousands of autoimmune disease susceptibility loci have been identified, greatly improving our understanding of the genetic basis of autoimmune diseases.

GWAS in Chinese has contributed significantly to the advance in the genetics of autoimmune diseases. Here, we list some large and representative studies. For example, Xue-Jun Zhang and his group firstly performed SLE GWAS in the Chinese Han population in 2009, which genotyped 1047 SLE patients and 1205 healthy controls by using Illumina Human610-Quad Bead Chips; identified nine new susceptibility loci consisting of *ETS1*, *IKZF1*, *RASGRP3*, *SLC15A4*, *TNIP1*, 7q11.23, 10q11.22, 11q23.3, and 16p11.2; and replicated seven loci including *BLK*, *IRF5*, *STAT4*, *TNFAIP3*, *TNFSF4*, 6q21, and 22q11.21, which have been reported in previous European studies [30]. Another large GWAS, including total of 3300 SLE cases and 4200 controls, was conducted in mainland and Hong Kong Chinese populations. Two genetic variants in ETS1 and WDFY4 were found and several European loci, including *TNFSF*, *STAT4*, *BLK*, *BANK1*, *IRF5*, and *HLA* locus were again confirmed [31]. One year later, Lin et al. performed a two-stage GWAS to identify susceptibility loci for ankylosing spondylitis (AS). The study analyzed 1,356,350 autosomal SNPs in 1837 individuals with AS and 4231 controls and found 2 new loci between *EDIL3* and *HAPLN1* at 5q14.3 and within *ANO6* at 12q12. Also, the results showed that rs13202464 within the MHC region mainly represents the risk effect of HLA-B*27 variants in the Chinese Han population. Subsequently, in 2013, a three-stage GWAS in Han Chinese was conducted to identify new genetic susceptibility loci for primary Sjögren's syndrome. The study identified a new locus, *GTF2IRD1-GTF2I* at 7q11.23 (rs117026326), associated with primary Sjögren's syndrome and confirmed associations of variants in the *STAT4*, *TNFAIP3*, and MHC regions in Han Chinese [32]. These results provide new insight into the pathogenesis of autoimmune diseases.

It is unquestionable that GWAS has greatly improved our understanding of complex human diseases, such as autoimmune diseases, by revealing the polygenic basis of genomic risk. However, GWAS had two important consequences. First, the majority of the GWAS associations fall into non-coding regions, proposing a possible regulatory effect of the variants in the etiology of the disease. Second, the associated genes and loci appear to explain only a small fraction of the overall heritability of the diseases, while most remain unexplained. Thus, a new area of intense study such as the expression quantitative trait loci (eQTLs) mapping studies has emerged.

17.3.1.4 Rare Variants as the Heritability of Autoimmune Diseases

GWAS has proven to be a powerful tool for identifying risk loci in common diseases. However, it is increasingly apparent that common variants explain only a small proportion of the heritability of these diseases. For example, the total contribution to MS heritability by the polymorphisms identified in GWAS was only 25%, suggesting that 75% of MS genetic risk would be due to mutations that SNP chips could not identify. Thus, the missing heritability might be explained by the effects of rare variants, usually defined as minor allele frequencies <1%. The signals from rare variants are difficult to detect in a conventional GWAS because genetic markers used in this study are mainly common variants. However, the development of next-generation sequencing technologies has enabled the re-sequencing of the entire genome. The contribution of each variant to disease development would be potentially higher for a rare missense variant than a common missense variant, fascinating the sequencing of protein-coding regions.

The largest-ever effect size in non-HLA loci was identified as a missense variant (g.74779296G > A; p.Arg90His; ORs of 3.35, 2.45, and 3.27, respectively) encoded in *NCF1* in Chinese as a novel risk variant for SLE, Sjögren's syndrome, and rheumatoid arthritis. In addition, the reduced copy number of *NCF1* (5:1 ratio) was found to be independently associated with an increased risk of SLE in Chinese ($P = 0.011$ [33]). TLR7 3′UTR SNP, rs3853839 (G/C) was identified as a functional polymorphism in the Chinese population which can confer upregulation of type I IFN pathway gene TLR7 expression and thus predisposes to the development of SLE, especially in male individuals [34]. Another nonsynonymous SNP (Q412R) in *IRF7* was identified, which regulates IFN-7 response and is associated with the development of SLE in multiple ethnic groups, including Chinese [35].

To sum up, the rare variants identified to date appear to be associated with gene products involved in both innate and adaptive immune responses. In detail, these mutations enhance the positive selection of autoreactive B cells and the production of autoantibody, which is accompanied by increases in T cell numbers, and increases in activation of dendritic cells, and impairs B cell signaling.

17.3.1.5 Epigenetics in Autoimmune Diseases

Epigenetic modification is also proposed to explain somewhat part of this missing inheritability. Moreover, epigenetic modification is a dynamic link between genotype, environment, and phenotype. The most important epigenetic modifications include DNA methylation, histone modification, microRNA, and non-coding RNA, which play important roles in the regulation of immunological functions and the prevention of autoimmunity. Published epigenetic studies of autoimmune diseases in China mainly involve DNA methylation, microRNA, and long non-coding RNA.

A growing number of studies in China have found that the deregulation of many microRNAs contributes to the pathogenesis of autoimmune diseases. MicroRNA-130b was down-expressed in kidney tissues from SLE patients, and it was identified to be a novel negative regulator of the type I IFN pathway in renal cells of patients with lupus nephritis. Dysregulation of miR-31 could be an underlying novel molecular mechanism of the IL-2 deficiency in SLE patients since it can enhance IL-2 production during T cell activation. MiR-146a maturation in the type I IFN pathway may lead to uncontrolled excessive inflammation in SLE. The expression of miR-196a-5p was negatively associated with polymyositis (PM), and miR-193b-3p was negatively associated with dermatomyositis (DM) and PM. MiR-210 was also found highly expressed in psoriasis patients. It may play a role in the pathogenesis of psoriasis through STAT6 and LYN inhibition and subsequently, induce Th1/Th17 differentiation.

DNA methylation is another important mechanism in the pathogenesis of autoimmune diseases. Studies have indicated that gene regulatory regions in $CD4^+$ T cells are abnormally regulated by demethylation and methylation which contributes to the development of autoreactivity and overstimulation of autoantibodies [36]. For instance, growth arrest and DNA damage-induced 45α (GADD45α) were proved to conduce to lupus autoimmune reaction through DNA demethylation promotion in SLE $CD4^+$ T cells [37]. The overexpression of JMJD3 may lead to demethylation of H3K27me3 in $CD4^+$ T cells in systemic sclerosis (SSc [38]) patients. The overexpression of CD11a and CD70 in $CD4^+$ T cells from SSc patients may be due to the demethylation of CD11a regulatory elements and the CD70 promoter region. Demethylation of CD40L regulatory elements on the inactive X chromosome also increased the expression of CD40L in $CD4^+$ T cells from female patients with SSc [39].

Several important long non-coding RNAs also have been indicated as critical factors in autoimmune diseases by stabilizing and modulating immune homeostasis [40–43]. For example, Ye et al. found that lncRNA ZFAS1 expression level was increased in synovial tissue from RA patients compared with that in controls and further demonstrated that ZFAS1 promoted the migration and invasion of RA FLS in a miR-27a-dependent manner [44]. Given that T cell play an important role in the pathogenesis of RA, Lu et al. explored ten potential aberrantly expressed lncRNAs in T cells in RA patients and healthy controls and found that LOC100652951 and LOC100506036 were upregulated in RA patients. Besides, the potential role of LOC100652951 and LOC100506036 in RA was further studied. The expression level of LOC100652951 in RA T cells was decreased with the treatment of biologic agents, which indicates that LOC100652951 may be involved in the production of cytokines. Meantime, inhibiting LOC100506036 expression in RA T cells by siRNA could lead to the down-regulated sphingomyelin phosphodiesterase 1 (SMPD1) and nuclear factor of activated T cells (NFAT) which could contribute to the inflammatory responses [45]. In conclusion, lncRNAs affect the development of autoimmune diseases via regulating the expression of disease-related proteins [46].

Overall, a massive effort was made in the last few decades to identify the genetic basis of autoimmune diseases; however, the strongest component of genetic basis still remains the MHC. Further studies are needed to explore the functional variants, particularly across the loci that link to gene expression regulation and the involvement of epigenetic modifications. Moreover, more research is required to focus on epigenetic variation, which builds an essential bridge in understanding gene-environment interactions that lead to autoimmune diseases.

17.3.2 Environmental Factors of Autoimmune Diseases

It has long been widely accepted that environmental factors play crucial roles in developing chronic autoimmune diseases [47]. Defining critical pathogenic environmental risk factors that may trigger the progression of autoimmune disease remains a hot research focus. Chinese researchers have made great effort to identify possible environmental pathogenic factors for autoimmune diseases in the past three decades. Despite identifying specific environmental factors being very important for understanding individual susceptibility, few identified factors have played a clear role in the development of autoimmune diseases. Up to now, the environmental risk factors that may be associated with the onset of autoimmune diseases mainly include cigarette smoking, infectious processes, silica solvents, air pollution, pharmaceutical agents, etc. [47, 48].

17.3.2.1 Cigarette Smoking

Cigarette smoking has been found related to an increased risk of developing RA susceptibility in European populations, but this result has not been replicated in Han populations [49]. Numerous studies have examined the association between smoking and SLE risk. A recent meta-analysis study showed that the association between smoking and SLE risk was significant in Europe (OR = 1.57, 95% CI = 1.18–2.09) and East Asia (OR = 2.24, 95% CI = 1.62–3.09). In contrast, a significant boundary difference for SLE risk was observed in North America (OR = 1.37, 95% CI = 0.97–1.92 [50]). Based on a meta-analysis including 20,626 cases from case-control and cohort studies, results suggested a strong association between cigarette smoking and MS susceptibility (OR = 1.57, 95% CI = 1.50–1.64). However, among these studies included in this meta-analysis, the Chinese Han population was not included [51]. Thus, long-term, prospective, population-based cohort studies are needed to explore the relationship between smoking and autoimmune diseases (e.g., RA, MS) in Chinese population.

Mechanistic evidence exists implicating smoking in autoimmune disease pathogenesis. Cigarette smoke contains a series of toxic components such as tars, free radicals, nicotine, carbon monoxide, polycyclic aromatic hydrocarbons, and so on. It may trigger oxidative stress and direct damage to endogenous proteins and DNA, thus resulting in genetic mutations and gene activation, which may be involved in the progression of autoimmune diseases. In addition, it can upregulate the expression of CD95 on B and CD4 T cells, which may lead to subsequent production of proinflammatory cytokines and autoimmunity [52].

17.3.2.2 Infectious Processes

Bacteria and virus infections are major important environmental factors that may be involved in the development of autoimmune diseases. Among them, Epstein-Barr virus (EBV) is particularly interesting. EBV infection has been suggested as a causal factor for SLE. The first positive correlation between EBV infection and SLE was reported in 1971 in the *Lancet* journal [53]. Since then, many researchers have investigated the possibility of this link from various perspectives. Two studies conducted in mainland China explored the relationship among EBV infection, SLE, and other autoimmune diseases and reported that EBV infection was found to be associated with RA and SLE [54]. Moreover, in the meta-analysis of 33 case-control studies of EBV and SLE, Zhao-Xia Li et al. reported [55] that seroprevalence of EBV VCA-IgG, EBNA IgA, and EA antibody (IgG, IgA, IgM) were significantly higher in SLE patients than controls. Epstein-Barr nuclear antigen-1 (EBNA-1) has a high degree of homology with some proteins that cause an autoimmune humoral response; this molecular mimicry may play essential roles in the induction of antibodies by EBV infection in SLE patients [56]. However, even then, interpretation may be fraught with difficulties. Large prospective studies are needed to identify the correlation between SLE and EBV infection before we can draw a causal relationship between the two.

17.3.2.3 Silica and Silicate

Exposure to occupational respirable silica dust (e.g., the crystalline form of quartz) is an established environmental risk factor for the development of RA, SLE, and other systemic autoimmune diseases [47]. Initial hypotheses linking silicosis dust exposure to autoimmune diseases were ground on hundred case reports and small occupationally based case series. Larger clinic-based case series, occupational cohort, registry-linkage, and case-control studies have also been conducted, many of them published since 1995. In recent years, large population-based cohort studies have conducted to confirm these findings. Unfortunately, no large-scale study has explored the relationship between occupational silicosis exposure and autoimmune diseases in China. Experimental studies suggest that ingested crystalline silica may act as an immune adjuvant which induces oxidative stress and apoptosis; stimulates the release of intracellular antigen, the transcription of proinflammatory cytokines, and T cell responses; and decreases the number of regulatory T cells. Considering the long existence of silica and silicate as natural elements in the environment, with a variety of potential human exposures, further study of their effects on autoimmune disease is warranted.

17.3.2.4 Air Pollution

In recent years, growing attention has been paid to the relationship between air pollution and the development of autoimmune diseases. Exposure to air pollutants has been hypothesized to be linked to the development of systemic autoimmune diseases. However, most studies examining this association were conducted in North America and Europe, where air pollutants concentrations are relatively low. In recent years, Chinese researchers have done a lot of work to provide new insight into the health effects of extreme air pollution in middle-income and low-income countries. For instance, a longitudinal and nationwide study in Taiwan was conducted to evaluate the effect of air pollution exposure on the risk of RA. The study showed that participants exposed to Q4 levels of $PM_{2.5}$ and NO_2 concentration had the highest prevalence of RA compared to those exposed to the Q_1, Q_2, and Q_3 levels [57]. The study of C-N Zhao et al. showed that exposure to a short-term high level of $PM_{2.5}$, NO_2, and SO_2 was positively associated with the rate of SLE hospitalization and the risk of SLE relapse [58]. Jung CR et al. speculated that long-term exposure to traffic-related air pollutants (NO_2 and CO) and $PM_{2.5}$ were significantly associated with the risk of SLE [59].

Air pollution exposure may influence autoimmunity by increasing the production of proinflammatory cytokines, inducing T cell imbalance, oxidative stress, and methylation changes. Noteworthy, the aryl hydrocarbon receptor (AHR) pathway has recently been recognized as involved in the development of autoimmune diseases. AHR is a ligand-activated transcription factor that responds to toxicants present in PM surface. PM contains high-affinity AHR ligands, which can modulate T cell differentiation and effector functions and regulate autoimmunity. To date, the mechanisms linking air pollution to autoimmune diseases have not been fully clarified. Thus further studies are needed to confirm and expand the potential effects of air pollutants on diseases [60]. Owing to the widespread of the air pollution exposure, the potential public health impact is substantial if the causal relationship between air pollution exposure and autoimmune disease is confirmed.

17.3.2.5 Other Environmental Factors

Epidemiologic evidence also supports the association between ultraviolet light (UV) radiation, vitamin D, psychosocial stressors, alcohol consumption, sex steroid hormones, and drugs with increased risk of autoimmune diseases. Although studies have indicated that UV exposure may exacerbate pre-existing SLE, it remains unclear whether UV exposure plays an essential role in developing SLE. UV light exposure is also the main source of vitamin D production. Further studies to strengthen our understanding of the relationship between UV radiation and SLE pathogenesis are needed. In addition, animal studies showed that dietary exposures can induce epigenetic changes and autoimmunity. A high intake of certain antioxidants, including fish, olive oil, and vegetables, may play a protective role in preventing the development of autoimmune disease. Sex steroid hormones, including estradiol, estriol, progesterone, and prolactin, have multiple impacts on the regulation of immunocompetence. The serum levels of sex steroid hormones were demonstrated significantly higher in SLE patients than those in healthy women [61].

17.4 Summary and Perspectives

Overall, although epidemiological data are accumulating in China, the current literature remains challenging due to the lack of national-based epidemiology studies, the difficulty of accurately measuring risk factors and confounders, and the relative rarity of the disease. Ranging from genetic and environmental studies, a multitude of risk factors have been identified in the development of ADs. As a crossroad between environment and genetics, epigenetic modifications will provide more research orientations for further understanding the pathogenesis of ADs.

Autoimmune diseases share many common features, common susceptibility genes, and epigenetic alterations, which can treat and prevent multiple ADs with the same therapeutic strategy. With the rapid development of basic and clinical studies, the survival period of patients has been prolonged; thus, further studies should pay more attention to improving the quality of life of patients, which also lays a foundation for tertiary prevention.

References

1. Damoiseaux JG, Tervaert JW. The definition of autoimmune disease: are Koch's postulates applicable? Neth J Med. 2002;60:266–8.
2. Michet CJ, McKenna CH, Elveback LR, Kaslow RA, Kurland LT. Epidemiology of systemic lupus erythematosus and other connective tissue diseases in Rochester, Minnesota, 1950 through 1979. Mayo Clin Proc. 1985;60:105–13.
3. Flower C, Hennis AJ, Hambleton IR, Nicholson GD, Liang MH. Systemic lupus erythematosus in an African Caribbean population: incidence, clinical manifestations, and survival in the Barbados National Lupus Registry. Arthritis Care Res (Hoboken). 2012;64:1151–8.
4. Jiang B, Zhang YC, Xu XF, Mei HP, Wang G, Ding F, Ding ZB. A prevalence study of rheumatic diseases in eastern coastline of Shandong province. Acta Acad Med Shandong (Chinese). 2001;39:210–1.
5. Huang M, Chen S, Lu G, Wang W, Jiang S, Zhang L, Jin W, Yu J, Xu S, Cai Y. Epidemiological survey on systemic lupus erythematosus. Chin J Intern Med (Chinese). 1985;24:451–3.
6. Xu D, Li B, Chen H, Ruan Z, Zeng Y, Yang X. Epidemiological study of systemic lupus erythematosus in Guangzhou area. Chin J Dermatol (Chinese). 1992;25:50–2.
7. Zou YF, Feng CC, Zhu JM, Tao JH, Chen GM, Ye QL, Cen H, Leng RX, Pan FM, Pan HF, Li R, Fan YG, Wang B, Li XP, Zhang FY, Ye DQ. Prevalence of systemic lupus erythematosus and risk factors in rural areas of Anhui Province. Rheumatol Int. 2014;34:347–56.
8. Mok CC, To CH, Ho LY, Yu KL. Incidence and mortality of systemic lupus erythematosus in a southern Chinese population, 2000–2006. J Rheumatol. 2008;35:1978–82.
9. Chiu YM, Lai CH. Nationwide population-based epidemiologic study of systemic lupus erythematosus in Taiwan. Lupus. 2010;19:1250–5.
10. Zhang Q, Liu Q, Lin C, Baima Y, Li H, Gong H, Lin J. The prevalence of rheumatoid arthritis in middle-aged and elderly people living in Naqu City, Tibet, autonomous region of China. J Orthop Surg Res. 2020;15:338.
11. Zeng XG, Chen B, Zeng F, Hou CZ, He Q, Huang L, Wu JW, Chen QQ. Study on the prevalence rate of rheumatoid arthritis in Zhuang nationality population from Nanning, Guangxi. Zhonghua Liu Xing Bing Xue Za Zhi. 2007;28:1127–9.
12. Yang Z, Wang K, Li T, Sun W, Li Y, Chang YF, Dorman JS, LaPorte RE. Childhood diabetes in China. Enormous variation by place and ethnic group. Diabetes Care. 1998;21:525–9.
13. Zhao Z, Sun C, Wang C, Li P, Wang W, Ye J, Gu X, Wang X, Shen S, Zhi D, Lu Z, Ye R, Cheng R, Xi L, Li X, Zheng Z, Zhang M, Luo F. Rapidly rising incidence of childhood type 1 diabetes in Chinese population: epidemiology in Shanghai during 1997–2011. Acta Diabetol. 2014;51:947–53.
14. Wu HB, Zhong JM, Hu RY, Wang H, Gong WW, Pan J, Fei FR, Wang M, Guo LH, Yang L, Yu M. Rapidly rising incidence of type 1 diabetes in children and adolescents aged 0-19 years in Zhejiang, China, 2007 to 2013. Diabet Med. 2016;33:1339–46.
15. Zhang H, Xia W, Yu Q, Wang B, Chen S, Wang Z, Love EJ. Increasing incidence of type 1 diabetes in children aged 0-14 years in Harbin, China (1990–2000). Prim Care Diabetes. 2008;2:121–6.
16. Tang X, Yan X, Zhou H, Yang X, Niu X, Liu J, Ji Q, Ji L, Li X, Zhou Z. Prevalence and identification of type 1 diabetes in Chinese adults with newly diagnosed diabetes. Diabetes Metab Syndr Obes. 2019;12:1527–41.
17. Cheng Q, Miao L, Zhang J, Ding SJ, Liu ZG, Wang X, Sun XJ, Zhao ZX, Song YJ, Ding XY, Guo ZL, Yang Y, Chen SD, Jiang GX, Fredrikson S. A population-based survey of multiple sclerosis in Shanghai, China. Neurology. 2007;68:1495–500.
18. Lau KK, Wong WW, Sheng B, Yu IT, Fung BH, Li HL, Ma KF, Wong LK, Li PC. The clinical course of multiple sclerosis patients in Hong Kong. J Neurol Sci. 2008;268:78–82.
19. Yu YL, Woo E, Hawkins BR, Ho HC, Huang CY. Multiple sclerosis amongst Chinese in Hong Kong. Brain. 1989;112(Pt 6):1445–67.
20. Lai CH, Tseng HF. Population-based epidemiological study of neurological diseases in Taiwan: I. Creutzfeldt-Jakob disease and multiple sclerosis. Neuroepidemiology. 2009;33:247–53.
21. Liu X, Cui Y, Han J. Estimating epidemiological data of multiple sclerosis using hospitalized data in Shandong Province, China. Orphanet J Rare Dis. 2016;11:73.
22. Hung TP, Landsborough D, Hsi MS. Multiple sclerosis amongst Chinese in Taiwan. J Neurol Sci. 1976;27:459–84.
23. Tsai CP, Yuan CL, Yu HY, Chen C, Guo YC, Shan DE. Multiple sclerosis in Taiwan. J Chin Med Assoc. 2004;67:500–5.

24. Cheng XJ, Cheng Q, Xu LZ, Zhao HQ, Zhao Z, Wang W, Jiang GX, Fredrikson S. Evaluation of multiple sclerosis diagnostic criteria in Suzhou, China--risk of under-diagnosis in a low prevalence area. Acta Neurol Scand. 2010;121:24–9.
25. Liu Y, Duan Y, Yu C, Qin W, Chen H, Dong H, Ye J, Butzkueven H, Li K. Clinical isolated syndrome: a 3-year follow-up study in China. Clin Neurol Neurosurg. 2011;113:658–60.
26. Vyse TJ, Todd JA. Genetic analysis of autoimmune disease. Cell. 1996;85:311–8.
27. Seldin MF, Amos CI, Ward R, Gregersen PK. The genetics revolution and the assault on rheumatoid arthritis. Arthritis Rheum. 1999;42:1071–9.
28. Sadovnick AD, Armstrong H, Rice GP, Bulman D, Hashimoto L, Paty DW, Hashimoto SA, Warren S, Hader W, Murray TJ, Et A. A population-based study of multiple sclerosis in twins: update. Ann Neurol. 1993;33:281–5.
29. Ebers GC, Sadovnick AD, Risch NJ. A genetic basis for familial aggregation in multiple sclerosis. Canadian collaborative study group. Nature. 1995;377:150–1.
30. Han JW, Zheng HF, Cui Y, Sun LD, Ye DQ, Hu Z, Xu JH, Cai ZM, Huang W, Zhao GP, Xie HF, Fang H, Lu QJ, Xu JH, Li XP, Pan YF, Deng DQ, Zeng FQ, Ye ZZ, Zhang XY, Wang QW, Hao F, Ma L, Zuo XB, Zhou FS, Du WH, Cheng YL, Yang JQ, Shen SK, Li J, Sheng YJ, Zuo XX, Zhu WF, Gao F, Zhang PL, Guo Q, Li B, Gao M, Xiao FL, Quan C, Zhang C, Zhang Z, Zhu KJ, Li Y, Hu DY, Lu WS, Huang JL, Liu SX, Li H, Ren YQ, Wang ZX, Yang CJ, Wang PG, Zhou WM, Lv YM, Zhang AP, Zhang SQ, Lin D, Li Y, Low HQ, Shen M, Zhai ZF, Wang Y, Zhang FY, Yang S, Liu JJ, Zhang XJ. Genome-wide association study in a Chinese Han population identifies nine new susceptibility loci for systemic lupus erythematosus. Nat Genet. 2009;41:1234–7.
31. Yang W, Shen N, Ye DQ, Liu Q, Zhang Y, Qian XX, Hirankarn N, Ying D, Pan HF, Mok CC, Chan TM, Wong RW, Lee KW, Mok MY, Wong SN, Leung AM, Li XP, Avihingsanon Y, Wong CM, Lee TL, Ho MH, Lee PP, Chang YK, Li PH, Li RJ, Zhang L, Wong WH, Ng IO, Lau CS, Sham PC, Lau YL. Genome-wide association study in Asian populations identifies variants in ETS1 and WDFY4 associated with systemic lupus erythematosus. PLoS Genet. 2010;6:e1000841.
32. Li Y, Zhang K, Chen H, Sun F, Xu J, Wu Z, Li P, Zhang L, Du Y, Luan H, Li X, Wu L, Li H, Wu H, Li X, Li X, Zhang X, Gong L, Dai L, Sun L, Zuo X, Xu J, Gong H, Li Z, Tong S, Wu M, Li X, Xiao W, Wang G, Zhu P, Shen M, Liu S, Zhao D, Liu W, Wang Y, Huang C, Jiang Q, Liu G, Liu B, Hu S, Zhang W, Zhang Z, You X, Li M, Hao W, Zhao C, Leng X, Bi L, Wang Y, Zhang F, Shi Q, Qi W, Zhang X, Jia Y, Su J, Li Q, Hou Y, Wu Q, Xu D, Zheng W, Zhang M, Wang Q, Fei Y, Zhang X, Li J, Jiang Y, Tian X, Zhao L, Wang L, Zhou B, Li Y, Zhao Y, Zeng X, Ott J, Wang J, Zhang F. A genome-wide association study in Han Chinese identifies a susceptibility locus for primary Sjogren's syndrome at 7q11.23. Nat Genet. 2013;45:1361–5.
33. Zhao J, Ma J, Deng Y, Kelly JA, Kim K, Bang SY, Lee HS, Li QZ, Wakeland EK, Qiu R, Liu M, Guo J, Li Z, Tan W, Rasmussen A, Lessard CJ, Sivils KL, Hahn BH, Grossman JM, Kamen DL, Gilkeson GS, Bae SC, Gaffney PM, Shen N, Tsao BP. A missense variant in NCF1 is associated with susceptibility to multiple autoimmune diseases. Nat Genet. 2017;49:433–7.
34. Shen N, Fu Q, Deng Y, Qian X, Zhao J, Kaufman KM, Wu YL, Yu CY, Tang Y, Chen JY, Yang W, Wong M, Kawasaki A, Tsuchiya N, Sumida T, Kawaguchi Y, Howe HS, Mok MY, Bang SY, Liu FL, Chang DM, Takasaki Y, Hashimoto H, Harley JB, Guthridge JM, Grossman JM, Cantor RM, Song YW, Bae SC, Chen S, Hahn BH, Lau YL, Tsao BP. Sex-specific association of X-linked toll-like receptor 7 (TLR7) with male systemic lupus erythematosus. Proc Natl Acad Sci U S A. 2010;107:15838–43.
35. Fu Q, Zhao J, Qian X, Wong JL, Kaufman KM, Yu CY, Mok MY, Harley JB, Guthridge JM, Song YW, Cho SK, Bae SC, Grossman JM, Hahn BH, Arnett FC, Shen N, Tsao BP. Association of a functional IRF7 variant with systemic lupus erythematosus. Arthritis Rheum. 2011;63:749–54.
36. Zhao M, Zhou Y, Zhu B, Wan M, Jiang T, Tan Q, Liu Y, Jiang J, Luo S, Tan Y, Wu H, Renauer P, Del MAGM, Castillo PM, Ortega CR, Fernandez-Roldan C, Raya E, Faria R, Carvalho C, Alarcon-Riquelme ME, Xiang Z, Chen J, Li F, Ling G, Zhao H, Liao X, Lin Y, Sawalha AH, Lu Q. IFI44L promoter methylation as a blood biomarker for systemic lupus erythematosus. Ann Rheum Dis. 2016;75:1998–2006.
37. Zhao M, Tan Y, Peng Q, Huang C, Guo Y, Liang G, Zhu B, Huang Y, Liu A, Wang Z, Li M, Gao X, Wu R, Wu H, Long H, Lu Q. IL-6/STAT3 pathway induced deficiency of RFX1 contributes to Th17-dependent autoimmune diseases via epigenetic regulation. Nat Commun. 2018;9:583.
38. Wang Q, Xiao Y, Shi Y, Luo Y, Li Y, Zhao M, Lu Q, Xiao R. Overexpression of JMJD3 may contribute to demethylation of H3K27me3 in CD4+ T cells from patients with systemic sclerosis. Clin Immunol. 2015;161:396–9.
39. Lian X, Xiao R, Hu X, Kanekura T, Jiang H, Li Y, Wang Y, Yang Y, Zhao M, Lu Q. DNA demethylation of CD40l in CD4+ T cells from women with systemic sclerosis: a possible explanation for female susceptibility. Arthritis Rheum. 2012;64:2338–45.
40. Pan W, Zhu S, Dai D, Liu Z, Li D, Li B, Gagliani N, Zheng Y, Tang Y, Weirauch MT, Chen X, Zhu W, Wang Y, Chen B, Qian Y, Chen Y, Fang J, Herbst R, Richman L, Jallal B, Harley JB, Flavell RA, Yao Y, Shen N. MiR-125a targets effector programs to stabilize Treg-mediated immune homeostasis. Nat Commun. 2015;6:7096.
41. Wu L, Qin Y, Xia S, Dai M, Han X, Wu Y, Zhang X, Ma J, Wang Y, Tang Y, Liu Z, Zhu W, Jallal B, Yao Y, Qu B, Shen N. Identification of cyclin-dependent

kinase 1 as a novel regulator of type I interferon signaling in systemic lupus erythematosus. Arthritis Rheumatol. 2016;68:1222–32.
42. Han X, Wang Y, Zhang X, Qin Y, Qu B, Wu L, Ma J, Zhou Z, Qian J, Dai M, Tang Y, Chan EK, Harley JB, Zhou S, Shen N. MicroRNA-130b ameliorates murine lupus nephritis through targeting the type I interferon pathway on renal mesangial cells. Arthritis Rheumatol. 2016;68:2232–43.
43. Wang J, Dai M, Cui Y, Hou G, Deng J, Gao X, Liao Z, Liu Y, Meng Y, Wu L, Yao C, Wang Y, Qian J, Guo Q, Ding H, Qu B, Shen N. Association of Abnormal Elevations in IFIT3 with overactive cyclic GMP-AMP synthase/stimulator of interferon genes signaling in human systemic lupus erythematosus monocytes. Arthritis Rheumatol. 2018;70:2036–45.
44. Ye Y, Gao X, Yang N. LncRNA ZFAS1 promotes cell migration and invasion of fibroblast-like synoviocytes by suppression of miR-27a in rheumatoid arthritis. Hum Cell. 2018;31:14–21.
45. Lu MC, Yu HC, Yu CL, Huang HB, Koo M, Tung CH, Lai NS. Increased expression of long noncoding RNAs LOC100652951 and LOC100506036 in T cells from patients with rheumatoid arthritis facilitates the inflammatory responses. Immunol Res. 2016;64:576–83.
46. Gao Y, Li S, Zhang Z, Yu X, Zheng J. The role of Long non-coding RNAs in the pathogenesis of RA, SLE, and SS. Front Med (Lausanne). 2018;5:193.
47. Dooley MA, Hogan SL. Environmental epidemiology and risk factors for autoimmune disease. Curr Opin Rheumatol. 2003;15:99–103.
48. Xia Y, Xie Z, Huang G, Zhou Z. Incidence and trend of type 1 diabetes and the underlying environmental determinants. Diabetes Metab Res Rev. 2019;35:e3075.
49. Yin J, He D, Jiang L, Cheng F, Guo Q, Huang S, Zeng X, Liu Y, Brown MA, Xu H. Influence of cigarette smoking on rheumatoid arthritis risk in the Han Chinese population. Front Med (Lausanne). 2017;4:76.
50. Jiang F, Li S, Jia C. Smoking and the risk of systemic lupus erythematosus: an updated systematic review and cumulative meta-analysis. Clin Rheumatol. 2015;34:1885–92.
51. Zhang P, Wang R, Li Z, Wang Y, Gao C, Lv X, Song Y, Li B. The risk of smoking on multiple sclerosis: a meta-analysis based on 20,626 cases from case-control and cohort studies. PeerJ. 2016;4:e1797.
52. Arnson Y, Shoenfeld Y, Amital H. Effects of tobacco smoke on immunity, inflammation and autoimmunity. J Autoimmun. 2010;34:J258–65.
53. Evans AS, Rothfield NF, Niederman JC. Raised antibody titres to E.B. virus in systemic lupus erythematosus. Lancet. 1971;1:167–8.
54. Zhang X, Li B, Liu Y, Jiang M. Clinical study on antibodies against EBV in sera of patients with rheumatoid arthritis. Zhongguo Yi Xue Ke Xue Yuan Xue Bao. 1999;21:8–12.
55. Li ZX, Zeng S, Wu HX, Zhou Y. The risk of systemic lupus erythematosus associated with Epstein-Barr virus infection: a systematic review and meta-analysis. Clin Exp Med. 2019;19:23–36.
56. Harley JB, Chen X, Pujato M, Miller D, Maddox A, Forney C, Magnusen AF, Lynch A, Chetal K, Yukawa M, Barski A, Salomonis N, Kaufman KM, Kottyan LC, Weirauch MT. Transcription factors operate across disease loci, with EBNA2 implicated in autoimmunity. Nat Genet. 2018;50:699–707.
57. Chang KH, Hsu CC, Muo CH, Hsu CY, Liu HC, Kao CH, Chen CY, Chang MY, Hsu YC. Air pollution exposure increases the risk of rheumatoid arthritis: a longitudinal and nationwide study. Environ Int. 2016;94:495–9.
58. Zhao CN, Mei YJ, Wu GC, Mao YM, Wu Q, Dan YL, Pan HF. Effect of air pollution on hospital admissions for systemic lupus erythematosus in Bengbu, China: a time series study. Lupus. 2019;28:1541–8.
59. Jung CR, Chung WT, Chen WT, Lee RY, Hwang BF. Long-term exposure to traffic-related air pollution and systemic lupus erythematosus in Taiwan: a cohort study. Sci Total Environ. 2019;668:342–9.
60. O'Driscoll CA, Owens LA, Gallo ME, Hoffmann EJ, Afrazi A, Han M, Fechner JH, Schauer JJ, Bradfield CA, Mezrich JD. Differential effects of diesel exhaust particles on T cell differentiation and autoimmune disease. Part Fibre Toxicol. 2018;15:35.
61. Jiang JF, Liu YH, Zhang CX. Sex hormones in female patients with systemic lupus erythematosus. Zhong Nan Da Xue Xue Bao Yi Xue Ban. 2005;30:315–7.

18 Advance in Large-Scale Prospective Cohort Studies of Chinese Adults

Jun Lv, Yuanjie Pang, and Liming Li

Abstract

A cohort study is one of the fundamental study designs in observational epidemiology and plays an irreplaceable role in the etiological research of disease. With the deepening of research on the etiology of complex diseases, increased investment in scientific research, and the development of modern information technology, an increasing number of large-scale population-based prospective cohorts have been established around the world. In China, prospective cohort studies are characterized by the more recent establishment, the limited number, the small scale, the lack of long-term and stable funding, and the short follow-up. This chapter reviews large-scale cohort studies and their applications, with a special emphasis on cohort studies in China. We will review the significance of large-scale cohort studies and research progress abroad, as well as the history, current status, and characteristics of prospective cohort studies in China. Challenges of cohort studies in the era of "multi-omics" will be discussed. We will also review the current situations of large cohorts in China including the basic information and research progress of the China Kadoorie Biobank (CKB), which is one of the few large prospective cohorts worldwide with a biobank. The CKB study has laid the evidence base for environmental and lifestyle factors and diseases (e.g., hemorrhagic stroke) unique to the Chinese population.

Keywords

Cohort study · Chinese · China Kadoorie Biobank

J. Lv · Y. Pang · L. Li (✉)
Department of Epidemiology & Biostatistics, School of Public Health, Peking University, Beijing, China

Peking University Center for Public Health and Epidemic Preparedness & Response, Beijing, China
e-mail: lmlee@bjmu.edu.cn

18.1 Significance of Large-Scale Cohort Studies and Research Progress Abroad

18.1.1 Scientific Value and Public Health Significance of Large-Scale Cohort Studies

The cohort study is a fundamental design in observational studies. In order to test hypotheses of etiological factors, a cohort study can be used to examine the health effects of potentially harmful or protective factors. Population-based cohort studies can be used to investigate the relationships between multiple exposures and health outcomes, and the results are readily generalizable to the larger population, making cohort studies superior to randomized controlled trials. In addition, cohort studies have the following features

D.-Q. Ye (ed.), *Progress in China Epidemiology*, https://doi.org/10.1007/978-981-19-2199-5_18

superior to other observational study designs: (1) a clear temporal relationship between the exposure and the outcome; (2) less affected by several types of biases; and (3) a higher level of evidence for causal inference. Cohort studies are uniquely positioned to examine the following types of exposures and health outcomes: (1) outcomes with a long pre-clinical period; (2) outcomes with a high risk of mortality or a short clinical course; (3) exposures with a long latency period; (4) exposures that are likely to vary because of changes in health status, treatment, and lifestyles at the individual level; (4) exposures that are subject to recall bias (particularly compared with case-control studies); and (5) multiple outcomes that share common exposures. Overall speaking, the design of cohort studies is indispensable in etiological research [1, 2].

One limitation of traditional cohort studies is the unsuitability to investigate diseases with a low incidence rate, which requires a large number of participants and poses considerable difficulty to the conduct of study. Thanks to the growing understanding of etiologies of complex diseases, the recent decade has witnessed research progress in epidemiology, from the assessment of a single environmental or genetic risk factor to the complex interactions of gene-gene and gene-environment. The requirement for sample size is increasing even for diseases that are not considered to be rare. Similarly, the objective of precision medicine is to utilize key characteristics and "multi-omics" biomarkers to differentiate between individuals with varying risks of diseases [3–5], thereby identifying effective measures of disease prevention and treatment. This objective requires an even larger sample size. It is estimated that a sample size of at least 500 thousand is necessary to power the studies of environmental, genetic risk factors, and their interactions on complex diseases such as myocardial infarction, type 2 diabetes, and cancer. Nowadays, population-based studies enrolling larger than 200 thousand individuals are common because of the following reasons: (1) the indispensable role of cohort studies in etiological research; (2) the raised profile of and investment in research by governments and funding organizations; and (3) the development of electronic questionnaires, computerized data entry systems, and comprehensive IT systems for study conduct and database management [6–8].

18.1.2 Current Status and Future Perspectives of Adult Cohort Studies in Western Countries

The Framingham Heart Study (FHS) is one of the most classic prospective cohort studies in modern history, which started in 1948 and had three phases of recruitment (i.e., 1948–, 1971–, and 2020–) [9]. The FHS has established major risk factors for coronary heart disease, stroke, and other chronic diseases. The FHS sparkled a revolution in preventive medicine and has transformed the understanding of disease origin.

Since the 1970s, several high-income countries in Europe and North America have set up population-based cohort studies with long-term follow-ups. The scale of these cohorts was often moderate, and most only collected biological samples from a limited subset of participants. Until now, these cohorts have been followed up for over 20 years, yielding a great deal of impactful evidence on the relationships between multiple exposures (mainly lifestyles and environmental) and major chronic diseases. The early focus of diseases was mainly cardiovascular disease, type 2 diabetes, and cancer that were more common among middle-aged adults. With ongoing follow-ups, the participants of these cohorts are aging, which offers unique opportunities to examine neuro-degenerative and aging-related diseases that are most common among older adults [10].

Since the 1990s, cohort studies have gained considerable attention because of their role in etiological research. Population-based cohort studies spanning a broad range of aims have emerged globally. The *International Journal of Epidemiology* has published over 200 cohort profiles since 2005. The scale is growing for these newly established cohort studies, with 4 cohorts over 500 thousand participants. These studies are the European Prospective Investigation into

Cancer and Nutrition (involving participants from 10 European countries) [11], the National Institute of Health-American Association of Retired Persons Study (NIH-AARP, US) [12], the Million Women Study (UK) [13], and the UK Biobank (UKB) [14]. The Precision Medicine Initiative was started in 2015 to establish a population-based cohort of one million Americans [15]. The enrolment started in May 2017, and by October 2020 359,000 participants had been recruited with 229,000 electronic health records and 277,000 biological samples. There are other types of population-based cohort studies, the enrolment of which was through the country- or region-level census, military records, death registries, hospital records, and medical insurances. This approach amplifies the magnitude of sample size of cohort studies and facilitates the collection of socio-demographic information and health outcomes but lacks individual-level lifestyle factors and environmental exposures. Examples of such studies are the Swiss National Cohort (6.8 million) [16], Scottish Health and Ethnicity Linkage Study (465 million) [17], and Danish Conscription Database (DCD, 728 thousand) [18].

In the recent decade, population-based cohort studies have built into study design the collection and long-term storage of biological samples, which has been made possible because of the rapid development in life sciences and informatics. Until now, UKB and EPIC have established biobanks of the largest scale, with 498 thousand blood and urine samples (UKB) and 388 thousand blood samples (EPIC) [11, 14]. These population-based cohort studies integrate multi-omics biomarkers including genomics, epigenetics, proteomics, and metabolomics and combine multi-omics with the exposome in traditional epidemiology, thereby improving the understanding of mechanisms underlying the origin and development of diseases [3]. This is defined as "systems epidemiology," a discipline originating from the marriage of traditional epidemiology and modern multi-omics technologies of high throughput [19].

In terms of assessing the macro-exposome, traditional cohort studies rely on self-reported data because of the constraints of funding and technologies. In recent years, the rapid advance in smartphones, Internet, and wearable devices has provided unique opportunities for the collection of individual-level data in biomedical research and has broadened the range of data to physical activity, sleep, physiological measures, social activities, and environmental exposures with much higher precision and greater details [20, 21]. Compared with traditional epidemiology, the collection and integration of these new data have enriched the exposures and outcomes under investigation, lowered the cost of data collection, and improved the efficiency of single research. The UKB started to monitor daily physical activity, sitting behaviors, and sleeping patterns of the participants and has collected over eight million hours of behavioral data [8]. The data collection is still ongoing.

The establishment of large-scale population-based prospective studies is still quite recent and these studies are nurturing. In recent years, researchers from the global communities have built consortia involving individual cohort studies of relatively small-scale but long periods of follow-up, in order to answer urgent research questions. These consortia have the strengths of increased statistical power and high external validity. Together with large-scale population-based cohort studies, these consortia have the unique strengths to investigate disease with a low incidence rate.

18.2 History, Current Status, and Challenges of Adult Cohort Studies in China

In China, prospective cohort studies are characterized by the more recent establishment, the limited number, the small scale, the lack of long-term and stable funding, and the short follow-up. Since the 1980s, several prospective studies have been established in the following disease areas: (1) cancer, Breast Cancer Self-Examination Trial Cohort of Shanghai textile workers, Linxian General Population Trial, and prospective cohort study of drinking water and colorectal cancer in

Zhejiang Province; (2) cardiovascular disease, China National Hypertension Survey Epidemiology Follow-up Study (CHEFS), Prospective Cohort Study of Cardiovascular Diseases in Multiple Provinces, and cohort study of cerebrovascular diseases of middle-aged and older adults in Jiangxi Province; and (3) occupational exposures, occupational cohorts of benzene exposure and cancer [10]. For the majority of these cohorts, the follow-ups are finished.

More prospective cohort studies have been established in China in the recent decade, with an increasingly larger scale and a broader range of research aims. Table 18.1 shows prospective cohort studies that are either ongoing or under recruitment. These prospective cohort studies are characterized by the wide geographic coverage, recruitment of participants from various socio-demographic backgrounds, and inclusion of at-risk and high-risk individuals. Importantly, these cohort studies have generated local evidence to understand the etiology of non-communicable diseases (NCDs) in the Chinese population. Since the implementation of "Key Specialized Projects of Precision Medicine" as part of the National R&D plan in 2016, million-scale population-based cohort studies have been planned in China. With the China Kadoorie Biobank (CKB) as the model, the plan is to establish several regional cohorts (Beijing-Tianjin-Hebei, Central, East, South, Northwest, Southwest, and Northeast), disease-oriented cohorts (coronary heart disease, stroke, respiratory diseases, metabolic diseases, breast cancer, etc.), and aging cohorts.

Overall, population-based prospective cohort studies in China are still in their infancy with the following key features: (1) the limited number; (2) the short period of follow-up; and (3) the limited research output of high-quality etiological evidence. A vast amount of funding and resources are warranted to maintain the long-term follow-up and measurement of biological samples, both for existing cohorts and newly established ones. Despite the development of modern technology, multi-omics have yet to achieve high throughput and low costs. The sample size of multi-omics studies is still limited by the costs. Nonetheless, the major strengths of Chinese cohort studies compared with cohort studies in Western populations are the diverse patterns of diseases and risk factors (environmental, lifestyle, and genetic factors), which can generate evidence on disease etiology that is readily generalizable to the Chinese population. This evidence base informs disease prevention strategies.

18.3 China Kadoorie Biobank

In 2004, the China Center for Disease Control and Prevention (China CDC) initiated the CKB (formerly known as the Kadoorie Study of Chronic Disease in China, KSCDC) in collaboration with the University of Oxford. The institution changed from the China CDC to the Chinese Academy of Medical Sciences in phase II of CKB and then changed to Peking University recently. The principal investigators (PIs) were Professor Liming Li (China PI), Professor Sir Richard Peto (UK PI), and Professor Zhengming Chen (UK PI). The CKB project is one of the limited numbers of large-scale prospective cohort studies with biobanks. The primary aims of the study are (1) to survey the distributions of major chronic diseases and associated risk factors; (2) to store biological samples and follow-up individuals for at least 20 years; (3) to examine the incidence and mortality of major chronic diseases; and (4) to explore the complex interplay between genes and environmental factors and between different genes on the development and progression of common chronic diseases and relevant phenotypes [25, 33].

18.3.1 Recruitment of Participants and Baseline Survey

18.3.1.1 Field Investigations and Study Participants

The study took place in ten geographically defined regions (five urban and five rural, Table 18.2). These regions were chosen with consideration of the following factors: levels of economic development, population stability, local disease patterns, exposure to certain risk factors,

Table 18.1 Characteristics of large-scale population-based cohort studies in China

Cohort, regions	Baseline	Sample size	Demographics	Institutions	Principal investigator(s)
The Shanghai Women's Health Study					
Shanghai	1996–2000	74,942	Female, 40–70 years	Shanghai Cancer Institute, Vanderbilt University Medical Center, US. National Cancer Institute	Wei Zheng [22]
The Shanghai Men's Health Study					
Shanghai	2002–2006	61,480	Male, 40–74 years	Shanghai Cancer Institute, Vanderbilt University Medical Center, US National Cancer Institute	Jianmin Yuan, Xiao-ou Shu, Gong Yang [23]
The Guangzhou Biobank Cohort Study					
Guangzhou	2003–2008	30,430	≥50 years, members of the Guangzhou Health and Happiness Association for the Respectable Elders (GHHARE)	Guangzhou No. 12 Hospital, the University of Hong Kong, University of Birmingham	Chaoqiang Jiang, Daqing Lin, Jiaqiang Zheng [24]
The China Kadoorie Biobank					
10 provinces across China	2004–2008	512,891	30–79 years	Peking University, Chinese Academy of Medical Sciences, University of Oxford	Liming Li, Richard Peto, Zhengming Chen [25]
The Taizhou Longitudinal Study					
Taizhou, Jiangsu Province	2007–	200,000	30–80 years	Fudan University, Fudan University Taizhou Institute of Health Sciences	Li Jin [26]
The Dongfeng-Tongji cohort study					
Shiyan, Hubei Province	2008–2010	27,009	≥50 years, retired workers	Tongji Medical College, Huazhong University of Science & Technology	Tangchun Wu [27]
The Shanghai Changfeng Study					
Shanghai	2009–2012	6595	≥45 years	Zhongshan Hospital, Fudan University	Xin Gao [28]
Risk Evaluation of cAncers in Chinese diabeTic Individuals: a lONgitudinal Study (REACTION)					
20–25 communities across China	2011–2012	259,657	Phase 1: 200–250 K Phase 2: 30–40 K Type 2 diabetes, 20–30 K prediabetes, 30–40 K normal glucose regulation (all ≥40 years)	Shanghai Jiao Tong University School of Medicine	Guang Ning [29]
The China Health and Retirement Longitudinal Study					
150 counties/districts and 450 villages/resident committees across China	2011–2012	17,708	≥45	National School of Development (China Center for Economic Research), Peking University	Yaohui Zhao [30]

(continued)

Table 18.1 (continued)

Cohort, regions	Baseline	Sample size	Demographics	Institutions	Principal investigator(s)
The Kailuan cohort study					
Tangshan, Hebei Province	2006–2007	101,510	Working and retired employees from the Kailuan Corporation	Tiantan Hospital, Capital Medical University	Yongjun Wang [31]
The China-PAR Project (Prediction of ASCVD Risk in China)					
15 provinces across China	1992–2008	127,840	≥18 years	Fuwai Hospital, Chinese Academy of Medical Sciences	Dongfeng Gu [32]

Table 18.2 Names of the ten regions in CKB

Urban/rural	Regions
5 urban areas	Licang, Qingdao, Shandong Province Nangang, Harbin, Heilongjiang Province Meilan, Haikou, Hainan Province Wuzhong, Suzhou, Jiangsu Province Liubei, Liuzhou, Guangxi
5 rural areas	Pengzhou, Chengdu, Sichuan Province Maiji, Tianshui, Gansu Province Huixian, Henan Province Tongxiang, Zhejiang Province Liuyang, Hunan Province

quality of death and disease registries, availability and quality of incidence data, convenience of courier service for shipment of biological samples, Internet connectivity, as well as local commitment and capacity.

The inclusion criteria were individuals (1) who were aged 35–74 (born between 1930 and 1970); (2) who were permanent residents of the selected areas; (3) who were able to communicate without severe disabilities; (4) who were willing to participate and sign informed consent; and (5) whose reports of disease and death registration were managed by the local health department. The exclusion criteria were as follows: individuals (1) who were migrant or temporary residents and (2) who were in troops and affiliated agencies in the selected areas (including retirees). To encourage participation, individuals attending the baseline survey who were slightly outside the age range (35–74 years) were also recruited [25].

The administrative units were rural villages or urban residential committees. Extensive publicity campaigns were conducted in all participating communities. Potentially eligible participants in each administrative unit were identified through official residential records. Invitation letters were delivered door-to-door by local community leaders or health workers, and appointments were made for volunteers who agreed to participate in the study. All participants were asked to bring their unique national identity (ID) cards to the assessment center set up in the local community (often in urban residential committees/rural villages, schools, etc.). The target daily recruitment rate was 70–80 participants per region. In addition to meeting the established sample size (i.e., 50,000 people in each area), the recruitment of participants also ensured the balance of age and gender. However, it did not deliberately require the representativeness of the sample population and the overall response rate [25].

18.3.1.2 Baseline Survey

Table 18.3 shows a summary of questionnaire data collected in the baseline survey.

For each participant, a 10-ml random blood sample was collected, with no specific requirement of fasting prior to blood collection. On-site measurements of blood glucose and hepatitis B surface antigen (HBsAg) were done shortly after blood samples were collected. Participants with glucose levels ≥7.8 mmol/L and <11.1 mmol/L were invited to return for a fasting plasma glucose (FPG) test the next day. The samples were then kept in a portable, insulated cool box with ice packs (to maintain their temperature at 4 °C) for up to several hours before being taken to the local study laboratory for immediate processing. After centrifuging and aliquoting, the four cryovials (including one DNA-containing buffy coat) from each blood sample were stored in a – 40 °C freezer, before being couriered on dry ice to the central blood repository in Beijing for storage at –80 °C [25].

Table 18.3 Questionnaire data collected in the CKB project

Questionnaire
(1) Demographics
(2) Socio-economic status: education, occupation, marital status, family members, income, health insurance, and income
(3) Health-related behaviors: tea drinking, alcohol drinking, tobacco smoking, dietary habits, supplements, and physical activity
(4) Passive exposures: food shortage, passive smoking, and household air pollution
(5) Personal and family history: self-rated health, history of major illnesses, medications, blood transfusion, and medical history of first-degree relatives
(6) Female reproductive history: menarche, menopause, history of pregnancy and breastfeeding, oral contraceptive, and surgery history of uterus, ovarian, and breast
(7) Mental health: self-rated satisfaction, major life events, sleeping, chronic pains, anxiety/phobia, depression module (CIDI-A), and anxiety module (CIDI-B)
Physical examinations
(1) Standing and sitting height
(2) Waist and hip circumference
(3) Body weight, bio-impedance, body fat percentage, etc.
(4) Blood pressure, resting heart rate, etc.
(5) Forced expiratory volume in 1 second, forced vital capacity, etc.
(6) Lung carbon monoxide content, lung carbon monoxide hemoglobin ratio, etc.

Between June 2004 and July 2008, a total of 515,681 participants attended the baseline survey. Finally, 512,891 participants were eligible who provided informed consent, had complete information from the baseline survey, and were aged 30–79 years. 41% of the participants were men, 55.9% were from rural areas, and the mean age was 52 years [25].

18.3.2 Follow-Up

The long-term follow-up of the CKB project involves the following: (1) one focusing on the exposures, which are periodical resurveys of 5% of randomly chosen surviving participants every 4–5 years, and (2) one focusing on the surveillance of health outcomes of all cohort participants.

18.3.2.1 Resurveys

Two resurveys have been undertaken in CKB so far. The first resurvey started in 2008 shortly following the completion of the baseline survey. It involved 5% of randomly chosen surviving participants and used administrative unit (i.e., rural village or urban residential committee) as the primary sampling unit (excluding those where the baseline survey was finished within less than 12 months). Apart from several additional questions (e.g., recent hospitalization), the data collection and survey procedures were much the same as in the baseline survey. The first resurvey recruited about 20,000 participants [25].

The second resurvey started in 2014, with all administrative units selected for the first resurvey plus 2–3 additional sites per region. The total number of participants recruited for the second resurvey was around 25,000. In addition to questions included in the baseline survey and first resurvey, the second resurvey included additional questions on dietary patterns, occupational exposures, and chronic obstructive pulmonary disease (COPD), as well as physical and imaging measures including hand grip, electrocardiogram (ECG), lower limb blood pressure, bone mineral density, pulse wave velocity, and carotid ultrasound. Blood lipids and urine tests were also conducted on-site [25].

The third resurvey started in August 2020, with all administrative units selected for the second resurvey plus 1–2 additional sites per region. The target is to recruit 25,000 participants. According to the aging status of the cohort participants and hot topics, this resurvey added questions and measurements including eye examinations (intraocular pressure and fundus imaging), liver ultrasound, e-cigarettes, and aging-related questions and implemented stricter quality control.

18.3.2.2 Follow-Up for Disease Outcomes

Long-term follow-up for all cohort participants started 6 months after the baseline survey, including routine surveillance and active surveillance. The former was established on the existing systems of death and disease registries in local health departments, in close contact with public security, civil affairs (funeral), social security, hospitals, and community medical service centers at all levels. The latter was based on the contact with community delegates (e.g., staff of the residential committees or village doctors) and ascertainment of incident events of participants. The two approaches were complementary, ensuring a dynamic follow-up of the demographics, all-cause mortality, incidence of major chronic diseases, migration, and loss of follow-up of all participants [25].

There are three types of surveillance with relevant information collected [25].

Death surveillance: all-cause mortality. All ten study regions are part of China's Disease Surveillance Points (DSP) system. The vital status of study participants is being monitored regularly through official residential records and death certificates reported to the regional CDC, where office of each regional coordinating center is based. Any deaths occurring among participants are coded (using the 10th International Classification of Diseases, ICD-10) by trained staff "blinded" to baseline information. Causes of death from the official death certificates are being supplemented, if necessary, by review of medical records (which are usually available). For any additional deaths not identified through routine procedures, the causes will be sought by reviewing hospital records or by conducting a verbal autopsy using a validated instrument.

Routine surveillance: mainly five major categories of chronic diseases including ischemic heart disease (IHD), cerebrovascular disease, chronic respiratory disease, diabetes, and cancer. Information about major diseases was collected through linkages with disease registries established in each of ten study regions.

Migration and loss to follow-up: by review of residential records and/or by visits to local communities. Participants who move within the administrative unit are not considered to be lost to follow-up and the new contact information is updated. Permanent loss to follow-up refers to the following situations: (1) participants move out of the administrative unit and the current address cannot be ascertained; (2) of those whose current addresses are available, long-term follow-up cannot be tracked (i.e., moving to another city). To help minimize the underreporting of deaths and to identify participants who have moved permanently out of the study area, active confirmation of vital status is also being carried out annually by review of residential records and/or by visits to local communities.

Based on the initial linkages done in all regions, personal information was matched to the health insurance (HI) databases for most of the participants in 2011 using the unique national ID. In 2014, more than 97% of participants from urban and rural regions were successfully matched to the HI databases. By linkages with the HI databases, the project regularly collects hospitalization information for matched members and can systematically characterize all hospitalization events that occurred during a specific period of follow-up. Through hospitalization information provided by the medical insurance system (e.g., name of hospital, data and numbers of hospitalization), the original medical notes can be collected for those with newly developed major chronic diseases, in order to obtain complete information on clinical characteristics and diagnosis. Information collected through the HI databases has become a crucial and effective approach along with routine monitoring of diseases and death surveillance [25].

By December 31, 2017 (in the analytical database after data cleaning and quality control), the mean follow-up of CKB participants was 10.8 years, with the maximum being 13.5 years, and the total person-years were 551,996. 5302 (1%) participants had lost to follow-up. 49,372 participants had died, and the incident cases were 54,892 for IHD, 60,828 for stroke, 31,067 for cancer, and 21,632 for COPD.

18.3.2.3 Outcome Validation and Adjudication

In 2011, the CKB project initiated outcome adjudication of major diseases with the following aims: (1) to assess the accuracy of diagnosis and phenotyping of reported conditions; (2) to compare the accuracy across regions and hospitals; and (3) to strengthen the quality control of disease surveillance. The focus was to assess the validity of the diagnosis and reporting of diseases, thereby ensuring the accuracy of cases and collecting relevant information. At present, ongoing outcome adjudication covers four major diseases including cancer, stroke, IHD, and respiratory diseases. The basis of outcome adjudication is the collection of medical notes, and the focus is the diagnosis and sub-phenotyping of diseases. The outcome adjudication has become a key and routine piece of work and will include more diseases.

18.3.3 Biological Sample Bank

As one of the world's leading biobanks in terms of storage, the biological sample bank of the CKB stores all samples from the baseline survey and two resurveys of more than 510,000 participants. The current inventory includes more than 17,000 boxes of biological samples, about 4500 boxes of DNA samples, and more than 11,000 boxes of biological samples stored off-site. The total scale of biological sample storage has reached more than 33,000 boxes.

The system of quality and safety management of the CKB sample bank has been perfecting. Since its establishment, the sample bank has been deployed in strict accordance with the standards of sample storage space, temperature, power supply, network, alarm, monitoring, and other standards. It records and monitors the temperature changes of each sample storage device in real time and has developed an emergency response plan. The sample bank ensures that the safety of sample storage is always within a reasonable and controllable range, thereby achieving safe sample storage and quality control. The project has developed an automated process of electronic management of sample storage. Through a series of computer programs and software systems such as sample collection, sub-packaging, transshipment tracking, receiving, positioning, and storage, all samples of the project are fully monitored, thereby minimizing manual operation and errors.

18.4 Research Output of the China Kadoorie Biobank

Population-based cohort studies in Western countries have generated solid evidence on risk factors for major NCDs [6]. However, such evidence may not be generalizable to the Chinese population because of the diverse patterns of risk factors and diseases [34]. As is the case in other low- and middle-income countries (LMICs), there are several health-related conditions unique to the Chinese population. For example, rural areas are greatly affected by indoor air pollutions as a result of using solid fuels for heating and cooking [35]. In the past 5 years, large-scale population-based cohort studies in China, including the CKB, have generated reliable, local evidence that is readily generalizable [34]. Such evidence is crucial to causal inference and can inform guidelines and strategies for the prevention of NCDs in other LMICs.

18.4.1 Hemorrhagic Stroke

Stroke is one of the leading causes of premature death and permanent disability, with approximately three-quarters of deaths (~65 million) occurring in LMICs including China [36]. In recent decades, the age-standardized incidence and mortality rates of stroke have been declining in high-income countries (HICs), but such a declining trend is not seen in many LMICs [36]. In 2013, there were more than three million incident stroke cases and about two million mortality cases in China, with a larger proportion of hemorrhagic stroke (HS) compared with the Western population [37]. Previous studies in Western countries have reported several risk factors for ischemic stroke (IS), including hypertension, diabetes, dyslipidemia, obesity, smoking, alcohol drinking, and physical inactivity [38]. However, there is limited evidence on risk factors for HS. Because of the different etiologies between IS and HS, investigating risk factors for the latter is informative for primary prevention of the disease and serves as the evidence base for understanding disease etiology and developing prevention strategies.

As shown by the CKB study, IS and HS share several risk factors in Chinese adults, including fresh fruit consumption, alcohol, and obesity, while there are some differences in the prognosis and specific risk factors (e.g., dyslipidemia). These findings suggest that targeted prevention strategies should be implemented for different stroke subtypes.

18.4.1.1 Fruits

Despite the high consumption of vegetables in China, the consumption of fruits remains low. In China, fruits are often consumed raw as snacks, which is different from the consumption of both fresh and processed fruits in Western populations. The CKB study reports that higher consumption of fresh fruits is associated with lower risks of both IS and HS [39]. Compared with those who never or rarely consumed fresh fruits, those who consumed daily had lower levels of systolic blood pressure (SBP) and blood glucose; they had a 25% lower risk of IS and a 36% lower risk of HS. There was a dose-response relationship between fresh fruit consumption and these outcomes. In addition, no differences were observed in the protective associations in subgroups by age, sex, and regions.

18.4.1.2 Alcohol Drinking

Studies in Western countries have reported a U-shaped association between alcohol and risk of CVD, suggesting that moderate alcohol intake (about 100 grams per week, g/week) is protective for CVD [38]. However, observational epidemiological studies suffer from reverse causality and residual confounding, meaning that the observed protective associations do not necessarily reflect causality. The health effects of moderate alcohol intake can be examined using genetic tools, namely, Mendelian randomization [40]. In CKB, self-reported alcohol intake shows a U-shaped association with incident stroke in men, including IS and HS [41]. Compared with men who never or rarely drank, those who consumed 100 g/week had the lowest risk of incident stroke. However, such a protective effect is not supported by the genetic evidence. In men, alcohol consumption predicted by genotypes and regions showed a linear, positive association with stroke, with a stronger effect on HS than IS.

18.4.1.3 Adiposity

The CKB study shows a positive association between body mass index (BMI) and incident stroke, with a stronger association for IS than HS [42]. Each 5 kg/m^2 higher BMI was associated with a 30% higher risk of IS and a 11% higher risk of HS. After adjusting for SBP, the positive association attenuated for IS, with each 5 kg/m^2 BMI associated with a 5% higher risk; the positive association of BMI with HS was reversed, with each 5 units higher BMI associated with a 27% lower risk. If the association between BMI and stroke is causal, 16.5% of IS and 6.7% of HS are attributable to a BMI greater than 23 kg/m^2.

18.4.1.4 Blood Lipids

The CKB study demonstrates that the associations of blood lipids with stroke risk differ by disease subtypes [43]. There was a positive association of low-density lipoprotein cholesterol (LDL-C) with IS and an inverse association with HS, while there was an inverse association of high-density lipoprotein cholesterol (HDL-C) with IS and no association with HS. Each 1 mmol/l lower plasma LDL-C (often achievable through statin) was associated with a 15% lower risk of IS but a 15% higher risk of HS. These observational associations have been confirmed by Mendelian randomization in the same population.

18.4.1.5 Lifestyles

The CKB study reports that a healthy lifestyle is associated with lower risk of stroke mortality [44]. A healthy lifestyle is defined as non-smoking, moderate alcohol intake, total physical activity greater than the median, a healthy diet (i.e., high in fruits and vegetables and low in red meat), a BMI between 18.5–27.9 kg/m^2, and a low waist circumference (<90 cm in men and <85 cm in women). Compared with those without any healthy lifestyle factors, those with 1–5 healthy lifestyle factors had a graded lower risk of IS death, ranging from 20% to 79%; for HS death, the corresponding risk reduction ranged from 31% to 63%. If assuming a cause-and-effect association, about 48% of IS deaths and 41% of HS deaths are attributable to non-adherence to the healthy lifestyle.

18.4.1.6 Prognosis

Despite the improvement in diagnosis and treatment of stroke, little is known about the prognosis of stroke in LIMCs including China. The CKB study has investigated both short- and long-term prognosis of stroke including major pathophysiological subtypes [45]. In 480 thousand CKB participants without CVD at baseline, there were 45,732 cases of incident stroke over a median of 9 years of follow-up. The mean age of these cases was 59.3 years and 54% were women. The commonest subtype was IS (80%), followed by intracerebral hemorrhage (16%), subarachnoid hemorrhage (2%), and unspecified type (2%). 28-day mortality was highest for intracerebral hemorrhage (47%) and lowest for IS (3%), while it was 19% for subarachnoid hemorrhage and 24% for unspecified type. Of those who survived stroke at 28 days, 41% developed recurrent stroke within 5 years, with 44% for intracerebral hemorrhage and 41% for IS. 5-year mortality was 17%, with 28% for intracerebral hemorrhage and 16% for IS. After the first IS, 91% of recurrent events were IS; after the first intracerebral hemorrhage, 56% recurrent events were intracerebral hemorrhage and 41% were IS. Overall, the recurrence and mortality rates are high after 5 years of diagnosis. The study findings highlight the need to improve secondary prevention of stroke in China to reduce these risks.

18.4.2 Household Air Pollutions

Around 3 billion people worldwide use solid fuels to cook and heat their homes [35]. These fuels generate smoke which contains a high level of fine particles (mainly PM2.5) and other harmful chemicals, particularly in houses without adequate ventilation [46, 47]. It is estimated that worldwide about 2.5 million deaths are attributable to household air pollution (HAP) [46, 47]. Despite the rapid urbanization in China, around one in three people still rely on solid fuels for domestic usage. Therefore, HAP poses significant health threats to the Chinese population, but there is limited evidence on the health impact of HAP. In China, the health impact of outdoor air pollution is believed to be substantial, but HAP is often ignored. The latter may have greater health consequences.

18.4.2.1 Cardiovascular Diseases

The CKB study shows that using wood or coal for cooking and heating is associated with higher risk of deaths from CHD and stroke [48]. Among 270 thousand participants from 5 rural areas in China, long-term usage of solid fuels for cooking and heating was associated with CVD mortality. Compared with participants who used gas or electricity ("clean fuels"), those who used solid fuels for cooking had a 20% higher risk of CVD mortality, and those who used solid fuels for heating had a 29% higher risk. There was a positive association between the duration of solid fuel use and mortality.

The study also shows that switching from solid to clean fuels for cooking was associated with a 17% lower risk of CVD death and for heating was associated with a 43% lower risk. Importantly, participants who cooked on stoves using solid fuels but had proper ventilation had an 11% lower risk, compared with those whose homes were not properly ventilated. These findings suggest that even if people may have been using solid fuels for a long time, there are still clear health benefits in switching to cleaner fuels. Installing ventilation facilities will be a cheaper alternative for those who cannot afford to switch fuels. Although it cannot be established whether burning coal and wood causes death, irrespective of this, China and other LMICs should encourage people to switch to cleaner domestic fuels and to prioritize policies and practices to allow a swift, widespread, and sustainable switch.

In contrast to rural areas, people from urban areas rarely burn solid fuels for heating and mainly use them for cooking. An analysis of 220 thousand CKB participants from 5 urban areas shows that using solid fuels for cooking is associated with higher mortality risk and cessation of solid fuel use cuts excess mortality risks within 5 years [49]. Ventilation use also lowers mortality risk. Compared with persistent clean fuel users, persistent solid fuel users had a 19% higher risk of all-cause mortality, with the excess risk being 24% and 43% for CVD and respiratory diseases, respectively. The excess risk of all-cause and cardiopulmonary mortality fell by more than 60% in 5 years after cessation of solid fuel use. Ventilation use was associated with a 22% lower risk of all-cause mortality. For both policymakers and the public, it is of paramount importance to promote the transition from solid fuels to clean fuels and the efficient ventilation to reduce the adverse health effects of HAP.

18.4.2.2 Respiratory Diseases

Apart from CVD, HAP has been shown to be associated with respiratory diseases [47]. The CKB study shows that in Chinese adults, using solid fuels for cooking is associated with higher risk of incidence and mortality of major respiratory diseases [50]. Among never smokers, using solid fuels was associated with a 36% higher risk of major respiratory diseases, compared with using clean fuels; switching from solid to clean fuels was associated with a 14% lower risk of the diseases. Among solid fuel users, using wood and coal was each associated with a 22% and 29% higher risk of major respiratory diseases, respectively, and the excess risk for long-term solid fuel users (≥40 years) was 54%. Compared with those without ventilation, the excess risk was 22% and 29% for wood and coal, respectively.

Among respiratory diseases, COPD is a major cause of illness in China [36]. Using solid fuels might be associated with the risk of COPD, but there is limited evidence from prospective studies [51]. According to CKB findings, using solid fuels for cooking and heating is associated with higher risk of COPD. Compared with those who used clean fuels for cooking, those who used coal and wood had a 6% and 14% higher risk of COPD, respectively; the corresponding excess risk was 16% and 21% for those who used coal and wood for heating, respectively. The associations between using solid fuels for cooking and COPD were only observed in women and never smokers. The risk of COPD increased with longer duration of solid fuel use.

18.4.2.3 Other Chronic Diseases

Apart from cardio-pulmonary diseases, the CKB study reports that HAP is associated with mortality of chronic liver disease (CLD) [52]. In Chinese adults, smoking and long-term use of solid fuels for cooking independently increase the risk of CLD mortality, and the excess risk is low among those who stopped smoking and using solid fuels. Long-term solid fuel use for cooking and smoking was associated with a 26% and 28% higher risk of CLD mortality, respectively. Compared with never-smoking clean fuel users, never-smoking solid fuel users had a 41% higher risk of CLD mortality, and the excess risk was 55% for regular-smoking clean fuel users and 71% for regular-smoking solid fuel users. There was no excess risk among those who had switched from solid to clean fuels and ex-regular smokers who stopped because of choice other than pre-existing illnesses. Currently, investigators in CKB study are assessing the associations of HAP with eye diseases as well as with novel biomarkers measured by the multi-omics platform to explore potential mechanisms.

References

1. Zhan S. Epidemiology. 8th ed. Beijing: People's Medical Publishing House; 2017.
2. Rothman KJ. Modern Epidemiology. 3rd ed. Philadelphia: Wolters Kluwer Health/Lippincott Williams & Wilkins; 2008.
3. Manzoni C, Kia DA, Vandrovcova J, et al. Genome, transcriptome and proteome: the rise of omics data and their integration in biomedical sciences. Brief Bioinform. 2018;19(2):286–302.
4. Johnson CH, Ivanisevic J, Siuzdak G. Metabolomics: beyond biomarkers and towards mechanisms. Nat Rev Mol Cell Biol. 2016;17(7):451–9.
5. Schubert OT, Rost HL, Collins BC, et al. Quantitative proteomics: challenges and opportunities in basic and applied research. Nat Protoc. 2017;12(7):1289–94.

6. Chen Z, Emberson J, Collins R. Strategic need for large prospective studies in different populations. JAMA. 2019;323(4):309–10.
7. O'Donnell CJ. Opportunities, challenges and expectations management for translating biobank research to precision medicine. Eur J Epidemiol. 2020;35(1):1–4.
8. Glynn P, Greenland P. Contributions of the UK biobank high impact papers in the era of precision medicine. Eur J Epidemiol. 2020;35(1):5–10.
9. Dawber TR, Moore FE, Mann GV. Coronary heart disease in the Framingham study. Am J Public Health Nations Health. 1957;47(4 Pt 2):4–24.
10. Li L, Lv J. Large prospective cohort studies: a review and update. Chin J Epidemiol. 2015;36:1187–9.
11. Riboli E, Hunt KJ, Slimani N, et al. European prospective investigation into cancer and nutrition (EPIC): study populations and data collection. Public Health Nutr. 2002;5(6B):1113–24.
12. Schatzkin A, Subar AF, Thompson FE, et al. Design and serendipity in establishing a large cohort with wide dietary intake distributions: the National Institutes of Health-American Association of Retired Persons Diet and Health Study. Am J Epidemiol. 2001;154(12):1119–25.
13. Green J, Reeves GK, Floud S, et al. Cohort profile: the million women study. Int J Epidemiol. 2019;48(1):28–9.
14. Sudlow C, Gallacher J, Allen N, et al. UK biobank: an open access resource for identifying the causes of a wide range of complex diseases of middle and old age. PLoS Med. 2015;12(3):e1001779.
15. All of Us Research Program I, Denny JC, Rutter JL, et al. The "all of us" research program. N Engl J Med. 2019;381(7):668–76.
16. Bopp M, Spoerri A, Zwahlen M, et al. Cohort profile: the Swiss National Cohort--a longitudinal study of 6.8 million people. Int J Epidemiol. 2009;38(2):379–84.
17. Bhopal R, Fischbacher C, Povey C, et al. Cohort profile: Scottish health and ethnicity linkage study of 4.65 million people exploring ethnic variations in disease in Scotland. Int J Epidemiol. 2011;40(5):1168–75.
18. Christensen GT, Molbo D, Angquist LH, et al. Cohort profile: the Danish conscription database(DCD): a cohort of 728,160 men born from 1939 through 1959. Int J Epidemiol. 2015;44(2):432–40.
19. Huang T, Li L. Systems epidemiology. Chin J Epidemiol. 2017;39(5):694–9.
20. Onnela JP. Opportunities and challenges in the collection and analysis of digital phenotyping data. Neuropsychopharmacology. 2021;46(1):45–54.
21. Mathews SC, McShea MJ, Hanley CL, Ravitz A, Labrique AB, Cohen AB. Digital health: a path to validation. NPJ Digit Med. 2019;2:38.
22. Zheng W, Chow WH, Yang G, et al. The Shanghai Women's health study: rationale, study design, and baseline characteristics. Am J Epidemiol. 2005;162(11):1123–31.
23. Shu XO, Li H, Yang G, et al. Cohort profile: the Shanghai Men's health study. Int J Epidemiol. 2015;44(3):810–8.
24. Jiang C, Thomas GN, Lam TH, et al. Cohort profile: the Guangzhou biobank cohort study, a Guangzhou-Hong Kong-Birmingham collaboration. Int J Epidemiol. 2006;35(4):844–52.
25. Chen Z, Chen J, Collins R, et al. China Kadoorie biobank of 0.5 million people: survey methods, baseline characteristics and long-term follow-up. Int J Epidemiol. 2011;40(6):1652–66.
26. Wang X, Lu M, Qian J, et al. Rationales, design and recruitment of the Taizhou longitudinal study. BMC Public Health. 2009;9:223.
27. Wang F, Zhu J, Yao P, et al. Cohort profile: the Dongfeng-Tongji cohort study of retired workers. Int J Epidemiol. 2013;42(3):731–40.
28. Gao X, Hofman A, Hu Y, et al. The Shanghai Changfeng study: a community-based prospective cohort study of chronic diseases among middle-aged and elderly: objectives and design. Eur J Epidemiol. 2010;25(12):885–93.
29. Ning G, Reaction Study G. Risk evaluation of cAncers in Chinese diabeTic individuals: a lONgitudinal (REACTION) study. J Diabetes. 2012;4(2):172–3.
30. Zhao Y, Hu Y, Smith JP, Strauss J, Yang G. Cohort profile: the China health and retirement longitudinal study (CHARLS). Int J Epidemiol. 2014;43(1):61–8.
31. Wang A, Liu X, Guo X, et al. Resting heart rate and risk of hypertension: results of the Kailuan cohort study. J Hypertens. 2014;32(8):1600–5.
32. Yang X, Li J, Hu D, et al. Predicting the 10-year risks of atherosclerotic cardiovascular disease in Chinese population: the China-PAR project (prediction for ASCVD risk in China). Circulation. 2016;134(19):1430–40.
33. Chen Z, Lee L, Chen J, et al. Cohort profile: the Kadoorie study of chronic disease in China (KSCDC). Int J Epidemiol. 2005;34(6):1243–9.
34. Pang Y, Lyu J, Yu C, Guo Y, Lee L. Risk factors for cardiovascular disease in Chinese: recent progress and implications. Global Health J. 2020;4(3):65–71.
35. International Energy Agency. World energy outlook 2016. Paris: International Energy Agency; 2016.
36. Zhou M, Wang H, Zhu J, et al. Cause-specific mortality for 240 causes in China during 1990-2013: a systematic subnational analysis for the global burden of disease study 2013. Lancet. 2016;387(10015):251–72.
37. Wang W, Jiang B, Sun H, et al. Prevalence, incidence, and mortality of stroke in China: results from a Nationwide population-based survey of 480 687 adults. Circulation. 2017;135(8):759–71.
38. Benjamin EJ, Muntner P, Alonso A, et al. Heart disease and stroke Statistics-2019 update: a report from the American Heart Association. Circulation. 2019;139(10):56–528.
39. Du H, Li L, Bennett D, et al. Fresh fruit consumption and major cardiovascular disease in China. N Engl J Med. 2016;374(14):1332–43.
40. Holmes MV, Ala-Korpela M, Smith GD. Mendelian randomization in cardiometabolic disease: challenges in evaluating causality. Nat Rev Cardiol. 2017;14(10):577–90.

41. Millwood IY, Walters RG, Mei XW, et al. Conventional and genetic evidence on alcohol and vascular disease aetiology: a prospective study of 500 000 men and women in China. Lancet. 2019;393(10183):1831–42.
42. Chen Z, Iona A, Parish S, et al. Adiposity and risk of ischaemic and haemorrhagic stroke in 0.5 million Chinese men and women: a prospective cohort study. Lancet Glob Health. 2018;6(6):630–40.
43. Sun L, Clarke R, Bennett D, et al. Causal associations of blood lipids with risk of ischemic stroke and intracerebral hemorrhage in Chinese adults. Nat Med. 2019;25(4):569–74.
44. Zhu N, Yu C, Guo Y, et al. Adherence to a healthy lifestyle and all-cause and cause-specific mortality in Chinese adults: a 10-year prospective study of 0.5 million people. Int J Behav Nutr Phys Act. 2019;16(1):98.
45. Chen Y, Wright N, Guo Y, et al. Mortality and recurrent vascular events after first incident stroke: a 9-year community-based study of 0.5 million Chinese adults. Lancet Glob Health. 2020;8(4):580–90.
46. Fatmi Z, Coggon D. Coronary heart disease and household air pollution from use of solid fuel: a systematic review. Br Med Bull. 2016;118(1):91–109.
47. Gordon SB, Bruce NG, Grigg J, et al. Respiratory risks from household air pollution in low and middle income countries. Lancet Respir Med. 2014;2(10):823–60.
48. Yu K, Qiu G, Chan KH, et al. Association of Solid Fuel use with Risk of cardiovascular and all-cause mortality in rural China. JAMA. 2018;319(13):1351–61.
49. Yu K, Lv J, Qiu G, et al. Cooking fuels and risk of all-cause and cardiopulmonary mortality in urban China: a prospective cohort study. Lancet Glob Health. 2020;8(3):430–9.
50. Chan KH, Kurmi OP, Bennett DA, et al. Solid fuel use and risks of respiratory diseases. A cohort study of 280,000 Chinese never-smokers. Am J Respir Crit Care Med. 2019;199(3):352–61.
51. Li J, Qin C, Lv J, et al. Solid fuel use and incident COPD in Chinese adults: findings from the China Kadoorie biobank. Environ Health Perspect. 2019;127(5):57008.
52. Chan KH, Bennett DA, Kurmi OP, et al. Solid fuels for cooking and tobacco use and risk of major chronic liver disease mortality: a prospective cohort study of 0.5 million Chinese adults. Int J Epidemiol. 2020;49(1):45–55.

Some Random Reflections on Evidence-Based Medicine, Precision Medicine, and Big Data Research

19

Jin-Ling Tang and Li-Ming Li

Abstract

Evidence-based medicine remains the best model for medical practice. However, evidence is not decisions; decisions must also consider current resources available and values of people. Evidence shows that the majority of those treated with blood pressure-lowering, cholesterol-lowering, glucose-lowering, and anti-cancer drugs, for example, do not benefit from preventing severe complications such as cardiovascular and death events. This implies that diagnosis and treatment in modern medicine are often imprecise. It has thus become a dream to find out those few who can respond to treatment. Precision medicine has thus come into being. Precision medicine is however not a new idea and cannot rely solely on gene sequencing as initially proposed. Neither is the large, multi-factorial cohort a new concept; it has been used widely in epidemiological research since the 1940s. In fact, medicine has never stopped since its very beginning the search for more precise diagnostic and therapeutic methods and already made achievements at every level of our understanding of the world, such as vaccines, blood transfusion, imaging, and cataract surgery. Genetic biotechnology is not the only path to precision but merely a new method. Most genes are found only weakly associated with diseases and are thus unlikely able to bring about great improvement in diagnostic and therapeutic precision. The traditional multi-factorial approach by embracing big data and incorporating genetic factors is probably the most realistic way ahead for precision medicine. However, big data boasts of possession of the total population and large sample size and claims correlation can displace causation. These are misleading concepts. Science has never observed the totality in order to draw a valid conclusion; a very large sample size is required only when the effect to detect is small and clinically less meaningful; declining causation is equivalent to declining the long-established scientific principles and methods in epidemiology and giving up the assurance for validity in scientific research, which will inevitably lead to use of futile interventions. Thus, in proving the effectiveness of intervention, analyses of real-word big data cannot displace the role of

J.-L. Tang (✉)
Shenzhen Institute of Advanced Technology,
The Chinese Academy of Sciences, Shenzhen, China

The Chinese University of Hong Kong,
Hong Kong, China
e-mail: jltang@cuhk.edu.hk

L.-M. Li
Department of Epidemiology and Biostatistics,
School of Public Health, Peking University,
Beijing, China

D.-Q. Ye (ed.), *Progress in China Epidemiology*, https://doi.org/10.1007/978-981-19-2199-5_19

randomized controlled trials. We expressed these doubts and critiques merely hoping to find out the true potentials of precision medicine and big data.

Keywords

Evidence-based medicine · Precision medicine · Big data · Real-world research Epidemiological methods

19.1 Reasons and Emotions in EBM

Evidence-based medicine (EBM) calls for medical practice to be based on the best available evidence from applied (rather than basic) research [1, 2]. Without EBM's urging, medical research will probably remain as research; without EBM's feedback, medical research will probably lose its orientation; without EBM's shield, medicine will probably be brazenly used for non-medical interests. However, while affirming the importance of evidence in medical decision-making, it must be stressed that evidence itself is not decisions. Current resources, needs of patients, and values of people should also be taken into account in decision-making.

Evidence is reasons. For convenience, in this article I call needs, values, and other personal factors involved in decision-making emotions. Reasons are objective facts obtained from scientific research (e.g., a drug is proved effective) that supports a choice but emotions are personal feelings about the choice. Emotions and reasons are both indispensable factors in medical decision-making. At the beginning of evidence-based medicine in the 1990s, the importance of evidence for medical decision-making was not sufficiently recognized; it was right to overemphasize it. However, in the era when evidence and guidelines are considered by many to have "kidnapped" medical practice, it is important to reiterate the importance of other factors in decision-making, although many medical guidelines and practices have yet to be based on scientific evidence.

The scientific proof that a drug is effective is reason. Reason is neutral, stable, and universal and shows effective options for decision-making. There is no doubt that evidence should permeate into every decision. When evidence exists, ignoring evidence is unwise and irresponsible. However, many misunderstandings and misuse of evidence-based medicine are due to equating evidence with action and overemphasizing the role of evidence in making choices. Human can make atomic bombs, but it does not mean that they should be used to kill. Otherwise it is neglect of emotions in decision-making. The role of evidence in decision-making is to provide the truth. The moment evidence is clearly presented, its role in decision-making is then completed. Evidence cannot tell us whether or not we should do it; it's people who make that decision.

Given that a medicine is effective, whether or not taking it depends on emotions. The long-term propensity of emotions is the values of people. Values determine people's likes or dislikes, their needs, their judgment on the importance of things, and their preferences on using resources (such as manpower, materials, time, and money). People have different values; emotions thus vary from person to person. But there are no right or wrong distinctions among them. Facing neutral and objective evidence, people often make different choices. Distortion of EBM is often due to ignorance or overemphasis of emotions. Ignoring evidence is overemphasizing emotions; equating evidence to decision is ignoring people's emotions. Antihypertensive drugs can prevent about 3 events of myocardial infarction or stroke within 5 years in every 100 treated. The cost is relatively low and side effects are few and minor. Targeted anti-cancer drugs can prolong survival for several months and are expensive. To treat or not to treat? There is no absolutely right or wrong answers. The right answer depends on emotions and varies from person to person.

In fact, evidence is not completely emotionless. Take treatments as an example, why are some treatments developed instead of others? Why are some treatments evaluated instead of others? Why are some outcomes used instead of others? Why are the evaluations carried out in these patients instead of others? In fact, every step of scientific efforts toward the truth is more or less affected by the values of scientists. Even the most fundamental issue of medicine – what is disease – is not entirely determined by the truth, but also has a component of human "feelings." Where should the diagnostic cut-off points of hypertension, hyperlipidemia, and diabetes be placed? What is the minimum size of tumors that should be diagnosed as cancer? There are no absolutely objective standards [3, 4]. So disease is not a black and white entity free of human negotiations. There is always a subjective element in the definition of disease [5, 6].

Due to variations in people's needs, values, and feelings, most of the "rigid" international guidelines or consensus on whether or not to intervene are debatable. The appropriate or reasonable treatment is the one that is safe, effective, and affordable, the patient is willing to accept, and is performed by a competent doctor in the right place and at the right time. The "reasonable" treatment is defined by both "reasons" and "emotions." Contrary to the guidelines, the reasonable treatment is bound to vary from person to person and can only be an individualized decision due to changeable emotions.

We emphasize reasonable treatments because there are many unreasonable conducts. Why do such unreasonable conducts still exist even if decisions are evidence-based? It is because the role of "emotion" in scientific exploration and evidence interpretation and application is overlooked or misused. As there can be invested interests behind unreasonable medical conducts, the original doctrine of medicine should be upheld: the patient first. Only in this way will medicine not go astray.

Moreover, some said that evidence-based medicine denied intuition, experiences, and assumptions, equated randomized controlled trial (RCT) and meta-analysis or clinical research to evidence-based medicine, equated statistical significance to clinical significance, relied too much on statistics, and used evidence to force doctors to do what they shouldn't do. These criticisms are mostly a result from misunderstanding of evidence-based medicine [7]. Some others complained that there was a lack of humanities in evidence-based medicine, and RCTs and guidelines were driven by commercial interests which have led to over-diagnosis and over-treatment. For example, some expensive anti-cancer drugs are over-hyped but have little effect in prolonging survival. These problems are mostly the result of misuse of evidence-based medicine [8, 9]. Misunderstanding and misuse of evidence-based medicine are not the problems of evidence-based medicine itself, but the problems of its users. It was also noted that patients in RCTs do not represent all patients, and the average results obtained in studies do not apply to all patients. RCTs and meta-analyses surely have their own problems. There may be biased, misleading, and even forged results in clinical studies. These problems reflect the limitations of modern medicine and medical research as a whole and adverse human factors that exist in any human activities. There are yet no solutions better than that provided by evidence-based medicine [10, 11].

19.2 Precision Medicine Cannot Reply Only on New Technologies

Since the middle of the twentieth century, chronic diseases have become the major burden of disease and cause of deaths, but prevention and treatment of chronic diseases are far less precise and effective than antibiotics and vaccines for infectious diseases. For example, research evidence shows that in 100 patients taking antihypertensive drugs for 5 years, only 3 can avoid coronary heart disease or stroke due to treatment, suggesting the treatment does not benefit the remaining 97 patients. A treatment that is effective only in 3% of the treated is appallingly imprecise. The precision of treatments for cancer, hyperlipidemia, and diabetes are similar. Finding the handful of patients who can respond to treatment has become the dream of modern medicine; precision medicine was thus proposed. If the above discussion on EBM is about individualizing treatment according to the value people give to the treatment, precision medicine is about individualizing treatment according to people's biological responses to treatment.

Discovery of the double helix structure of DNA, the human genetic materials, is the greatest breakthrough in biomedicine in the twentieth century. The discovery has cracked the secret codes of human heredity. Through DNA sequencing, genes that predispose people to disease can be found and prevention can be made more precise. It can also help identify genes that are related to people's response to a treatment and thus make treatment more precise. Since the birth of polymerase chain reaction (PCR) in the 1980s, gene-related research has become the hottest spot in biomedical research, which foreshadows infinite prospects for conquering cancers and cardiovascular diseases [12]. We have allocated our limited biomedical research resources hugely to this field [13, 14].

The original vision of precision medicine is to find patients sensitive to prevention and treatment through the latest gene sequencing technology, thus improving the precision of prevention and treatment and enhancing effectiveness [15–18]. However, many doubted from the very beginning that genomic technologies could independently and successfully solve the problem of precision medicine [15–19]. Therefore, other new technologies were also incorporated into the tool kits of precision medicine, such as proteomics, metabolomics, and gut microbiota. It is then anticipatable to further include traditional factors and old technologies we have long been using to predict the effectiveness of prevention and treatment. These factors include age, sex, family history, disease subtypes, physical, pathological, physiological, biochemical, immune and imaging features, and so on. Therefore, while many are still seriously pondering what precision medicine is, the United States, which first proposed the concept of precision medicine, changed the name of its flagship precision medicine project from "The Precision Medicine Initiative Cohort Program" to "All of Us Research Program" [20]. This precision medicine project has changed from initially a genomic project to essentially a typical epidemiological cohort study, in which genomic characteristics are only one of the many characteristics which are to be measured and studied. Among all the factors, it is still unknown whether genomic factors can outperform the others on the road to precision.

In fact, apart from including new measurements, precision medicine is not a new concept but an old wine in a new bottle. Moving toward precision of diagnosis and treatment is the eternal pursuit of medicine as it is the ultimate goal of medical progress and the representative feature of every major progress in medicine. However, precision medicine is by no means only that at the genetic level, nor can it be arrived only after genetic measurements are made possible. For example, since the middle of the nineteenth century, discovery of microorganisms and emergence of microbiological methods had made diagnosis and treatment of infectious diseases revolutionarily more precise. Imaging technologies such as X-ray are another revolution in precision medicine by detecting, locating, and treating diseases.

In a broad sense, recognition of specific symptoms and signs of disease; invention of thermometers, stethoscopes, X-rays, ultrasound, CT, endoscopes, and microscopes; and examinations via physiological, biochemical, pathological, microbiological, and immunological equipment are all steps toward precision in medicine. With these theories and innovations, diagnosis and treatment of many diseases have now been made highly precise. Precise prevention and treatment of infectious diseases are good examples. Other examples include blood transfusion owing to identification of blood groups and location of disease and surgery owing to imaging technologies. Precision in medicine has in fact been made at every level of our perception of the world. For example, CT location of fracture is precision at the gross anatomical level, endoscopic location of lesions is precision at the organ level, microscopic typing of cancer is precision at the cellular level, immunological determination of bacterial infection is precision at the molecular level, and genetic diagnosis is precision at the gene level.

These achievements in precision are mostly on diagnosis and prognosis, but precision in diagnosis and prognosis is not the ultimate goal of precision medicine. The ultimate goal of precision medicine is precise prevention and treatment [21]. Whether precision in diagnosis and prognosis brought about by genetic testing (or any other new technologies at present and in the future) can lead to more precise prevention and treatment is a question that must be answered. In predicting effect of prevention and treatment, genetic examination may eventually surprise us again. However, at present, targeted therapies for cancer, supposedly a landmark achievement of precision medicine, can at most prolong survival for only a few months [8, 9], nowhere near the precision in prevention and treatment achieved as a result of discovery of organisms and X-ray. There will certainly be new miracles in medicine, but are we too optimistic about genetic diagnosis and should we put all eggs in one basket? The subsequent concessions, adjustments, and "sourcing" of precision medicine are exactly responses to these concerns and doubts.

The flagship project of precision medicine in the United States is now essentially a large cohort study (PMI 2016) [20], which include many other factors in addition to the new genetic measurements. In search for the causes of chronic diseases, large-scale cohort studies were invented and launched in the middle of the twentieth century. As the archetype of cohort studies, the British Doctors Study with 40,000 doctors involved revealed the relationship between smoking and lung cancer [22], and the 73-year Framingham Heart Study revealed the major risk factors of cardiovascular diseases [23]. In 2004, China carried out a chronic disease cohort study (China Kadoorie Biobank Study) with 500,000 people enrolled and biological and genetic specimens collected [24, 25]. Findings of these studies have made prevention of lung cancer and cardiovascular diseases more precise. Large randomized controlled clinical trials designed evaluating treatment efficacy are in essence similar to the concept of large cohort studies. Therefore, cohort study of precision medicine is not a new idea either. They are just including more and more people and taking more and more measurements.

Why are more people required for research? An important rule of medical research is that the smaller the effect is, the larger the study (i.e., sample size) is required. For example, cataract surgery can let patients to see again immediately and completely, and thus operation of a few patients is sufficient to prove the effect. However, thousands of people will be needed with years of follow-up to demonstrate the effect of antihypertensive drugs in preventing coronary heart disease, stroke, or death [26]. An effect of this size cannot be a surprise in any case, let alone precision of the treatment. Therefore, a paradox arises: the effect of intervention must be extremely small if it requires to study a million of people to prove and the intervention cannot be precise as most people it treats will not respond [27].

The size of the effect of a risk factor on the occurrence of disease can be estimated by the relative risk. In the United Kingdom, the relative risk of smoking on lung cancer is about 15. This means that 93% of lung cancer cases are attributable to smoking. If eliminating smoking, 93% of lung cancer in smokers can be prevented. Even so, many still have doubts about and ignore the harms of smoking. In view of this, we must think about the question – what is the value of a gene with a relative risk below 1.5 in preventing a disease? Not to mention the complexity, difficulty, and possible negative consequences of interventions on genes.

However, people's expectations of genes far outweigh their recognition of the importance of quitting smoking. Due to our own limits, we sometimes turn to gods. The more incredible a thing is, the more likely it is to be deified, despite the fact that common sense is more likely to be right. For this reason, sometimes we may collectively become blind. The DNA strand that contains the codes of each and every one of us is so magical that we cannot help but deify it.

Does this DNA chain that controls our lifeblood really control our fate, including sickness, recovery, and longevity? There is a paradox about fate: when the fate is predicted, it changes. This is a bit like Schrodinger's cat in quantum mechanics. When we know that we will be rich in the future, we may get relaxed and the fortune may not come; when we know that we will be bad off in the future, we may work hard so our fate will change. If genes determine that we are bound to live a long life, why don't we get ravenous and overeat? If this DNA chain really determines our fate, why can't it control its own fate and why does it need to hide itself in the body for protection? What a fate this physical body of ours will possibly come to pass in this ever-changing world? We doubt that the DNA strand can truly tell.

A person is greater than the sum of the basic elements that make him, so reductionism is not the only strategy that can win out. If the genetic path is only one of many paths possible to precision medicine, there are reasons that the cost of putting all the eggs in one basket is too high. First, even though precision medicine has a promising future, whether it can precisely guide treatment must ultimately be verified in population studies. Second, it is often unnecessary to make interventions precise at the individual level because there exists commonalities among individuals. Third, it may only be a theoretical premise to be precise for everyone [28] because it cannot be verified through repetition unless the effect is extremely large. Fourth, if it can be precise at the subgroup level, the randomized controlled trial is still the most reliable method to verify whether a genetic marker can effectively predict effectiveness in a subgroup. For example, a typical example is to randomly assign patients of KRAS wild-type colon cancer to the treatment and control groups and similarly allocate KRAS mutant patients and then perform subgroup analyses to compare the therapeutic effect (i.e., interactions) of a targeted cancer drug in KRAS wild-type patients with that in mutant patients [21, 29–31]. This is exactly the way we generate scientific evidence to inform evidence-based decision-making. In this sense, there is no conflict between EBM and precision medicine.

Thus, precision medicine and evidence-based medicine are complementary but not substitutive; evidence from precision medicine research can make EBM practice more precise. It is unrealistic to consider that evidence-based medicine is probabilistic and imprecise and thus will eventually be replaced by precision medicine. Historical experiences show that interventions that are 100% effective are only unusual cases.

Finally, precision medicine is not necessarily the best model for medical practice. Public health measures are mostly built on the recognition of equal benefits to all, such as sewage discharge, water supply, disinfection, and other measures to prevent infectious diseases. They can benefit all and have good fairness. In fact, individuality and commonality, or particularity and generality, are two different sides of the same issue. Even interventions for individuals, such interventions as antibiotics and vaccines that are designed based on commonalities rather than individualities, are often the most effective. Wherever individualized treatment is emphasized, it is often the case in which the commonalities and fundamental mechanisms of the matter have not been found. As a result, we try various methods with a hope that some may work in some occasions.

19.3 Big Data: Statistical Precision Versus Scientific Credibility

Computers and the Internet have brought unprecedented convenience to the storage, processing, and analysis of data. The mass of routinely collected data have brought great convenience to scientific research. The arrival of the era of big data has provided unprecedented new opportunities for generating evidence for medical practice and the development of precision medicine. Due to the scarcity of resources, scientific studies are usually conduced with a limited size of samples. When the sample size is large enough, a general conclusion can be precisely drawn from the samples. It is claimed that sample size can be ignored in big data research because they have data of the entire population [32]. The possibility of studying the whole population seems the most prominent advantage of big data research.

However, representing the whole population is only a false promise. Representativeness of a study is an abstract concept referring to the limited population relative to the sampling population and depending on the sampling method. If the whole population is referred to the sum of all relevant individuals in the world, say hypertensive patients, no database can possibly represent the whole population. Patients in a hospital cannot represent all the patients in a city; patients in all the hospitals in a city cannot represent all the patients in the country; all patients in a country cannot represent all patients in the world; and all patients in the world at present cannot represent all patients in the world in the future. Therefore, the whole population of a database is relative and finite and so is its representativeness. Therefore, it is thus not guaranteed a conclusion based on the observation of the so-called whole population can be generalized to other populations without an error. In addition, the so-called broad representativeness often leads to serious practical errors. For example, if a drug is effective in a 5% subgroup of patients, the best studies are those on patients who represent only these 5% of patients instead of all relevant patients. Extending studied patients beyond the 5% seems to broaden the representativeness, but the consequence is that the drug will be mistakenly recommended according to the trial result to many in whom the drug is ineffective. In this case, the broader the representativeness a study is intended, the greater the error will be, and the farther away will the use of the drug be from precision medicine.

In fact, studies and inferences about the whole population so far are all based on samples, and there is no need to study the whole population. We have never observed all the men and women in the world before we can tell the difference between them. It is also impossible for us to observe all men and women in the world because we cannot observe those who have passed away or those who have not yet been born. If we really have to wait till we can observe all the people in the whole, we will have to wait forever and never come to a conclusion. Similarly, to know the taste of Maotai, a famous Chinese liquor, we don't have to drink all the Maotai in the world. We can only study the samples and it is sufficient to study samples.

It is also argued that in big data research correlation is enough so we can ignore causation because big data covers the whole population [32]. For medicine, this is a more dangerous signal. First, representativeness and causality are different concepts and so good representativeness does not lead to good evidence on causality. Second, causality is fundamentally important in medicine. For example, we say smoking can cause lung cancer, because there is causality between them. By the same token, we say antihypertensive drugs can reduce the risk of cardiovascular diseases. By the nature of causality, we then know quitting smoking can prevent cancer and taking antihypertensive drugs can prevent cardiovascular diseases. Smokers often carry lighters, which are also associated with lung cancer. However, smokers cannot expect to prevent cancer by throwing away their lighters because there is no causality between them.

Identifying the causality between cause and disease and between treatment and effect is an important part of medical research. We have developed a set of theories and methods for studying causation in human populations [33–35], which are largely about control of biases and confounding, making discovered correlations more likely to be real causations and eventually making sure changing the causes will prevent and cure diseases [36]. If medical interventions are based on associations rather than causations, they will not be guaranteed to be effective [36, 37].

Denying the difference between association and causation is tantamount to denying the scientific principles of epidemiological research established in the past century, such as control of confounding in observational studies and randomization and blinding in clinical trials. Large sample size can only reduce random errors and improve the precision of results but cannot make up for deficiencies in study design, cannot control biases, and cannot improve the validity of findings.

The relationship between validity and precision is similar to that between the power of a tool and the number of times it is repeatedly used. For example, if we liken the randomized controlled trial to a microscope, the cohort study is the human eye. If we cannot see bacteria under the microscope, it is unarguable that we cannot see bacteria with naked eyes. If it is false to say that bacteria can be seen with naked eyes, the false statement will not become true regardless of how many people (the sample size) repeatedly saying so. Internal validity is the prerequisite for external extrapolation. The statement that correlation is enough is a sheer disregard of the long-established theories and methods of medical research.

It is precisely because of excessive attention to sample size, disregard for causality, and limited understanding of scientific principles of population studies that it is proposed to evaluate medical interventions by using real-world observational studies based on big data and believe that they can replace randomized controlled trials and become final confirmation of treatment effects. However, the fundamental difference between real-world studies (whether based on big data or not) and randomized controlled trials is not sample size or the degree of restriction on PICOS (population, intervention, comparator, outcome, and setting) and other factors. If necessary, randomized controlled trials can also include a large sample size and be conducted in the real-world setting [38, 39]. The essential difference between the two, in fact, lies in the capability of control for biases and confounding, which is in essence the difference between observation and experiment. They are at different levels of scientific validity [40–42]. In other words, conclusions drawn from randomized controlled trials are much more credible than real-world observational studies. Therefore, given the importance of interventions in medicine and the validity of findings for research, real-world observational studies cannot displace experimental randomized controlled trials in evaluating medical interventions.

In addition, for those medical questions that can ethically be studied through only observational studies, real-world big data studies are no difference from specially organized ones and even superior to the latter in some aspects. Those questions cover in fact most issues related to medical practice other than interventions, such as causes, diagnosis, prognosis, rare chronic side effects, prevalence and incidence (if the data cover all members in a defined population), and economic evaluation of medical interventions. Even with regard to treatment effects, big data has a great potential in generating research hypotheses and preliminary results on new uses of drugs and can also be used to support the development of pragmatic randomized trials. In research on causes and prognoses, big data can provide numerous, unprecedented new risk factors, greatly broadening the spectrum of potential risk factors and further expanding the possibilities of prevention. For medical and health management, big data provide an unprecedented opportunity to be explored. Having said all those, it is also worth noting that the accuracy, precision, and completeness of data and the consistency of the same measurement in different time periods and/or different institutions may be one of the major obstacles restricting the use of big data at present.

Last but not least, the sample size and even methodological quality is not the key factor that determines the significance of a study. The significance of a study primarily lies in the significance of the research question addressed. Each of us faces mountains of data every day, just like walking into a big forest; trees cannot tell what they can do but it requires people to ask questions.

19.4 Conclusions

Evidence-based medicine emphasizes both reasons and emotions and is still the best model for medical practice today. However, most drugs are effective only in a fraction of patients. It has become a big challenge to modern medicine to find the handful of patients who respond to treatment. However, scientific breakthroughs require time and accumulation. Their occurrence is often accidental rather a result of planned activities. For example, invention of the microscope, control of puerperal fever, control of cholera, discovery of microorganisms as a cause of disease, discovery of antibiotics and vaccines, and so on, each took hundreds of years and often transpired with a play of luck.

It took thousands of years or even longer for human beings to conquer infectious diseases. Perhaps we have become too impatient facing the problem of chronic diseases which became prevalent less than a hundred years ago. Using the latest biomedical technologies to make the treatment more precise is the purpose of precision medicine, but it is not just around the corner. In fact, individualized treatment for every patient is only a theoretical possibility. Currently the successful and precise interventions (such as antibiotics and vaccines) are not individually specific ones, but the same approach for all by targeting at the commonalities of the problem. Moreover, factors that determine health go far beyond genes and medical interventions. Thus precision medicine cannot be the only way out. Big data does offer a new path for medical research. However, it will be a serious retrogression for medical research if we simply think that a large sample size and correlation are all that is needed without making efforts to prove causality. This thinking mistakes random error as bias, confuses statistical significance with scientific validity, and denies the well-established principles and methods of population research in medicine.

However, in the field of science, we should always have an open mind, because scientific breakthroughs are often not predictable. Those who laugh at others may eventually be laughed at and those who wish to predict the future may badly be mistaken. Lord Kelvin, former President of the Royal Society of England, once said heavier than air flying machines were impossible. Einstein also once proclaimed there was not the slightest indication that nuclear energy would ever be obtainable. More than 100 years ago, who was possibly sure that Semmelweis' investigation on puerperal fever would open the door for effective control of infectious diseases? Science always takes us with surprise. Through doubting and criticizing, we only hope this article can stimulate more discussions and studies that will eventually realize the great potentials of precision medicine and big data research.

References

1. Sackett DL, Rosenberg WMC, Gray JAM, et al. Evidence based medicine: what it is and what it isn't [J]. BMJ. 1996;312:71.
2. Tang JL, Glasziou P. Essentials in evidence-based medicine [M]. 2nd ed. Beijing: Peking University Medical Press; 2016.
3. Tang JL. Chapter 6: an example of evidence-based decision making: the evidence and logic behind the strategies for prevention of cardiovascular disease [G]. In: Tang JL, Glasziou P, editors. Essentials in evidence-based medicine. 2nd ed. Beijing: Peking University Medical Press; 2016. p. 72–84.
4. Tang JL. Chapter 30: progress in medicine and definition of disease [G]. In: Tang JL, Glasziou P, editors. Essentials in evidence-based medicine. 2nd ed. Beijing: Peking University Medical Press; 2016. p. 339–53.
5. Doust J, Vandvik PO, Qaseem A, et al. Guidance for modifying the definition of diseases: a checklist [J]. JAMA Intern Med. 2017;177(7):1020–5.
6. Yang ZY, FAN H, Tang JL. Correspondence to "Guidance for modifying the definition of diseases: a checklist" [J]. JAMA Intern Med. 2017;177(7):1020–5. (in press)
7. Medlive-Cardiology. Personal opinions on evidence-based medicine [EB/OL]. 2017(Sep-12)(2014). http://mp.weixin.qq.com/s/6p0M77-Yh0L_wleEfwLDhQ.
8. Kim C, Prasad V. Cancer drugs approved on the basis of a surrogate end point and subsequent overall survival: an analysis of 5 years of US Food and Drug Administration approvals [J]. JAMA Intern Med. 2015;175(12):1992–4.
9. Rupp T, Zuckerman D. Quality of life, overall survival, and costs of cancer drugs approved based on surrogate endpoints [J]. JAMA Intern Med. 2017;177(2):276–7.
10. Greenhalgh T, Howick J, Maskrey N, et al. Evidence based medicine: a movement in crisis? [J]. BMJ. 2014;348:g3725.
11. Ioannidis JPA. Evidence-based medicine has been hijacked: a report to David Sackett [J]. J Clin Epidemiol. 2016;73:82–6.
12. Collins FS. Exceptional opportunities in medical science: a view from the National Institutes of Health [J]. JAMA. 2015;313(2):131–2.
13. Chalmers I, Glasziou P. Avoidable waste in the production and reporting of research evidence [J]. Obstet Gynecol. 2009;114(6):1341–5.
14. Macleod MR, Michie S, Roberts I, et al. Biomedical research: increasing value, reducing waste [J]. Lancet. 2014;383(9912):101–4.
15. Coote JH, Joyner MJ. Is precision medicine the route to a healthy world? [J]. Lancet. 2015;386(9978):1617.
16. Lu YF, Goldstein DB, Angrist M, et al. Personalized medicine and human genetic diversity [J]. Cold Spring Harb Perspect Med. 2014;4(9):a008581.
17. Rubin R. Precision medicine: the future or simply politics? [J]. JAMA. 2015;313(11):1089–91.
18. Tonelli MR, Shirts BH, et al. Knowledge for precision medicine [J]. JAMA, Oxford University Press, Oxford, England. 2017;12(3):248–56.
19. Collins FS, Varmus H. A new initiative on precision medicine [J]. N Engl J Med. 2015;372(9):793–5.
20. Precision Medicine Initiative. Cohort program announces new name: the all of US research program National Institute of health [EB/OL]. All of US research program, Maryland, USA: National Institute of Health, 2016, 2017(Sep-12)(2016). https://www.nih.gov/AllofUs-research-program/pmi-cohort-

program-announces-new-name-all-us-research-program.
21. Hunter DJ. Uncertainty in the era of precision medicine [J]. N Engl J Med. 2016;375(8):711–3.
22. Doll R, Peto R, Wheatley K, et al. Mortality in relation to smoking: 40 years' observations on male British doctors [J]. BMJ. 1994;309(6959):901–11.
23. Mahmood SS, Levy D, Vasan RS, et al. The Framingham heart study and the epidemiology of cardiovascular disease: a historical perspective [J]. Lancet. 2014;383(9921):999–1008.
24. Du H, Li L, Bennett D, et al. Fresh fruit consumption and major cardiovascular disease in China [J]. N Engl J Med. 2016;374(14):1332–43.
25. Chen Z, Chen J, Collins R, et al. China Kadoorie biobank of 0.5 million people: survey methods, baseline characteristics and long-term follow-up [J]. Int J Epidemiol. 2011;40(6):1652–66.
26. Sutcliffe P, Connock M, Gurung T, et al. Aspirin for prophylactic use in the primary prevention of cardiovascular disease and cancer: a systematic review and overview of reviews [J]. Health Technol Assess. 2013;17(43):1–253.
27. Tang JL, Yang ZY, Mao C. The use and pitfalls of large randomized controlled trials [J]. Chin J Epidemiol. 2017;38(10):1299–304. [in press]
28. Ogino S, Lochhead P, Chan AT, et al. Molecular pathological epidemiology of epigenetics: emerging integrative science to analyze environment, host, and disease [J]. Mod Pathol. 2013;26(4):465–84.
29. Fisher DJ, Copas AJ, Tierney JF, et al. A critical review of methods for the assessment of patient-level interactions in individual participant data meta-analysis of randomized trials, and guidance for practitioners [J]. J Clin Epidemiol. 2011;64(9):949–67.
30. Dahabreh IJ, Terasawa T, Castaldi PJ, et al. Systematic review: anti-epidermal growth factor receptor treatment effect modification by KRAS mutations in advanced colorectal cancer [J]. Ann Intern Med. 2011;154(1):37–49.
31. Yang ZY. Predictive biomarkers of the efficacy of epidermal growth factor receptor tyrosine kinase inhibitors in treating advanced non-small cell lung cancer: A systematic review of randomized controlled trials [D]. School of Public Health and Primary Care, Hong Kong, China: The Chinese University of Hong Kong, 2014, Doctor.
32. Schönberger VM, Cukier K. Big data: a revolution that will transform how we live, work and think [M]. Boston: Houghton Mifflin Harcourt; 2013.
33. Rothman KJ. Modern epidemiology [M]. Boston: Little, Brown and Company; 1986.
34. Feinstein AR. Clinical epidemiology: the architecture of clinical research [M]. Philadelphia, PA: W.B. Saunders; 1985.
35. Tang JL, Han XR. Chapter 2: epidemiology—methods for producing evidence [G]. In: Tang JL, Glasziou P, editors. Essentials in evidence-based medicine. 2nd ed. Beijing: Peking University Medical Press; 2016. p. 19–33.
36. Tang JL. Chapter 5: causes, causal models and causal inference [G]. In: Li LM, editor. Epidemiology, vol. 1. 3rd ed. Beijing: People's Medical Publishing House; 2015.
37. Khoury MJ, Ioannidis JP. Medicine big data meets public health [J]. Science. 2014;346(6213):1054–5.
38. Ware JH, Hamel MB. Pragmatic trials--guides to better patient care? [J]. N Engl J Med. 2011;364(18):1685–7.
39. Ford I, Norrie J. Pragmatic trials [J]. N Engl J Med. 2016;375:454–63.
40. Hill AB. Observation and experiment [J]. N Engl J Med. 1953;248(24):995–1001.
41. Tang JL, Yang ZY. Observation versus experiment and efficacy versus effectiveness [J]. Chin J Epidemiol. 2014;35(3):221–7.
42. Sherman RE, Anderson SA, Dal Pan GJ, et al. Real-world evidence - what is it and what can it tell us? [J]. N Engl J Med. 2016;375(23):2293–7.

20 Research Progress in Biomedical Big Data

Bo Wang and Liming Li

Abstract

Currently, the value in biomedical big data has been ascending. Notable sources of biomedical big data include medical claims data, electronic medical records, public health data, medical research data, medical market and costs data, individual behavior and mentality data, human genetics and omics data, social demography data, environmental and geographic information data, and health network and media data. Biomedical big data can be applied to conduct omics studies and association studies among different omics, quickly search for biomarkers and develop new drugs, rapidly screen unknown pathogens and find suspicious agents, carry out the real-time implementation of biological monitoring and public health surveillance, prevent and control of emerging infectious diseases, understand the changing spectrum of diseases in the population, evaluate the efficacy and safety of drugs and vaccines in real world, conduct precise health management, and allow more powerful work on data mining. Meanwhile, biomedical big data does face challenges, including standardization and normalization of data collection, merging of current data islands, computer management of massive data, efficient use of data for research and practice, and lack of talents with the comprehensive expertise in both biomedicine and information technology. Biomedical big data will change the pattern of medical practice and improve the quality of healthcare services.

Keywords

Biomedicine · Big data · China · Application

20.1 Introduction

We have entered the era of big data. The research results of International Data Corporation showed that the amount of data generated globally in 2011 was as high as 1.82 ZB (1 ZB = 2^{70} B) [1]. The United Nations released a white paper in May 2012, entitled *Big data for development: challenges and opportunities*, pointing out that big data is a historic opportunity for the United Nations and governments. People can now use abundant data resources to carry out unprecedented real-time analyses of the social economy to help the government better respond to social and economic operations [2].

B. Wang
Department of Epidemiology and EBM, Meinian Public Health Institute, Peking University Health Science Center, Beijing, China

L. Li (✉)
Department of Epidemiology and Biostatistics, School of Public Health, Peking University, Beijing, China
e-mail: lmlee@bjmu.edu.cn

D.-Q. Ye (ed.), *Progress in China Epidemiology*, https://doi.org/10.1007/978-981-19-2199-5_20

20.1.1 Definition and Characteristics of Big Data

Big data refers to a dataset that is too large and complex to be captured, managed, stored, retrieved, shared, transmitted, and analyzed with conventional software tools within a certain period of time. Big data has the characteristics of "4Vs" [3]. The amount (volume) of data is large, often above the PB level (1PB = 2^{50} B). There are many different data types (variety), including structured data, semi-structured data, and unstructured data from many data sources. The speed of generation and update (velocity) is fast, such as real-time data stream, with high timeliness requirements. Big data may have great scientific merit (value). Although the utilization density is low, it often contains new knowledge or has important predictive value.

The main characteristics of big data that are different from traditional data sets include distributed storage and complexity [4]. Big data is not necessarily stored in a fixed database but is generally distributed in different places in the network space. Big data mainly consists of semi-structured or unstructured data with high complexity. Traditional data sets, which are mostly small amounts of pure data, are used to carry out hypothesis-driven, advanced model-based analysis and explore causal relationship. Big data, on the other hand, which is usually data-driven, predominantly employ uncleaned large data sets to conduct data-driven analysis and explore correlation relationship within a relatively loose analysis framework.

20.1.2 Development Status of Big Data in China and Abroad

Big data science continues to grow. Driven by the technical demands of big data application, data science research and talent training have attracted the attention of all countries. Many universities in Europe and the US have set up data science research institutions and opened data science courses [5]. There are also increasing forums, conferences, and journals about big data science. In April 2012, researchers from the UK, the USA, Germany, Finland, and Australia launched Global Big Data Week, to encourage governments to formulate strategic big data measures. In 2008, *Nature* published a special issue *Big Data*, which introduced the challenges brought by massive data. In 2011, *Science* published a special issue on data processing, *Dealing with Data*, which discussed the challenges posed by data deluge, and pointed out that if these data can be organized and used more effectively, there will be more opportunities to exert the important role of science and technology in promoting social development. In 2012, *ERCIM News*, the official journal of the European Research Consortium for Informatics and Mathematics, published a special issue *Big Data*, which discussed data management in the era of big data, and innovative technologies for data-intensive research, and introduced research activities and innovative progress made by European research institutions. As an international authoritative academic institution in the field of data science, the Committee on Data for Science and Technology (CODATA) set up a big data session in its 2012 academic conference.

The Chinese government and research institutions also pay great attention to big data. The application of big data in health and medicine is a national priority for China [6]. In December 2012, National Development and Reform Commission listed the development of data analysis software and relevant service in a special guide. In 2013, the Ministry of Science and Technology included big data in the 973 Basic Research Plan. Department of Management Sciences, Department of Information Sciences and Department of Mathematical and Physical Sciences listed big data in the 2013 National Natural Fund Guide. In August 2015, the State Council issued *Action Plan for Promoting the Development of Big Data*, to comprehensively promote the development and application of big data in China and accelerate the construction of a data powerhouse [7]. In June 2016, the General Office of the State Council issued *Guiding Opinions of the General Office of the State Council on Promoting and Regulating the*

Application and Development of Big Data in Health and Medical Care [8], blowing the horn of development and application of healthcare big data in China. The *Guiding Opinions* proposed that healthcare big data is an important strategic resource, and its development will bring about profound changes in healthcare patterns and help improve the efficiency and quality of healthcare services. Chinese Academy of Sciences, Fudan University, Peking University, and Shandong University have successively established specialized institutions for data science research. Since 2018, Peking University, the University of Chinese Academy of Sciences, Nanjing University had set up the National Institutes of Health Data Science. Theory and application of big data were also specially discussed in Xiangshan Science Conference and Shuangqing Forum, held by the Ministry of Science and Technology and National Natural Science Foundation of China.

20.2 Sources and Application of Biomedical Big Data

Biomedical big data comes from a wide range of sources. Currently, global research hotspots in biomedical big data mainly focus on interaction networks of protein and other biomacromolecules, application in drug databases and electronic health records, application of genome sequence data in disease prediction, data mining of drug bioinformatics, systems biology and systems medicine, etc. [9].

20.2.1 Major Sources of Biomedical Big Data

The following factors promote the emergence of big data in the biomedical field. The first is the integrity of life and the complexity of diseases. For example, chronic diseases that pose a serious threat to human health are mostly complicated diseases with complex genetic and molecular mechanisms and are influenced by genes, environment, and their interactions. The etiological studies of these diseases will generate a large amount of data [10]. The second factor is the development of high-throughput technology and the reduction of genome sequencing costs. High-throughput sequencing technology enables simultaneous sequencing of millions of DNA molecules, making it possible to perform a detailed and complete analysis of the transcriptome and genome of a species [11]. With the completion of the Human Genome Project and the rapid development of computing power, the cost of genome sequencing has been greatly reduced, which will contribute to the generation of massive sequencing data [12]. The last but not the least factor is the rapid development of hospital informatization and the IT industry. The human body itself is an important source of biomedical big data. With the quick development of hospital informatization and IT industry, more and more human body data can be stored and utilized. For example, X-ray, 3D MRI, mammography, and 3D CT scans include 30M, 150M, 120M, and 1G of data, respectively. By 2015, an average hospital in the USA needs to manage 665T of data [13].

Biomedical big data covers a wide range of fields related to human health, including medical claims data, electronic medical records, public health data, medical research data, medical market and cost data, individual behavior and mentality data, human genetics and omics data, social demography data, environmental and geographic information data, and health network and media data [14]. Table 20.1 lists the main sources of biomedical big data.

20.2.2 Application of Biomedical Big Data

Biomedical big data can be applied in the following areas [15]. First, the conduct of systems biomedical research to better understand etiologies of diseases, involving exposure omics of environment and lifestyles, genomics, epigenomics, transcriptomics, proteomics, metabolomics, metagenomics, and phenotypic omics of individual health and diseases. The integration of

Table 20.1 The main sources of biomedical big data

Sources	Detailed types
Clinical data	Electronic medical records, medical imaging, medical device monitoring, etc.
Public health data	Disease and death registration, public health surveillance, food sales, nutrition labeling, etc.
Medical research data	Clinical trials, observational studies, real-world studies, drug development, medical equipment development, etc.
Medical market and cost data	Medical service expenses, medical equipment sales records, pharmacy sales records, medical insurance, etc.
Individual behavior and mentality data	Real-time video, individual behavior, fitness records, physical activity records, absence records, sensors, etc.
Human genetics and omics data	Genomics, transcriptomics, proteomics, metabolomics, etc.
Social demography data	Gender, age, marital status, economic income, etc.
Environmental and geographic information data	Geographical location, administrative area, meteorological conditions, pollution, leisure places, crime, traffic, etc.
Health network and media data	Health websites, search engines, communication operators, microblog, WeChat, forums, instant messaging, etc.

big data of various omics, will not only provide comprehensive and new understanding for the development of prevention and treatment occurrence of diseases, but also facilitate the practice of personalized medicine, which means more accurate prediction of risk and prognosis, and more targeted prevention and treatment measures [12, 16]. Second, rapid identification of biomarkers and drug development. Using the omics data of patient population, it is possible to quickly identify biomarkers related to disease occurrence, prognosis or treatment effect [17]. In drug development, big data can provide an in-depth understanding of the etiology and pathogenesis of diseases, so as to help detect biological targets and develop drugs. Meanwhile, drug screening process will be sped up by making full use of massive omics data, research data of existing drugs, and a high-throughput drug screening strategy [12]. Third, quick detection for unknown pathogens and identification of suspected pathogens. Through collecting samples, sequencing, and comparing to sequences of known pathogens, it can be determined whether a known or an emerging pathogen (and the closest known relatives) causes an outbreak, so as to infer its origin and routes of transmission, guide drug screening, treatment and prevention [18]. Fourth, real-time implementation of biological monitoring and public health surveillance. Public health surveillance includes surveillance of infectious diseases, surveillance of chronic non-communicable diseases and related risk factors, and health-related surveillance (such as birth defects, food safety hazards, etc.). In addition, it is also possible to conduct epidemic surveillance through a nationwide electronic medical record database [19], and predict the epidemic of certain infectious diseases by monitoring social media or frequently retrieved entries [20]. For example, influenza early warning based on big data analysis has become the focus of research [21]. Google Trends has been used to predict the outbreak of influenza before hospital emergencies increased in certain areas, by finding the peaks of search terms such as "flu symptoms" and "flu treatment" [22, 23]. Fifth, prevention and control of emerging infectious diseases. Big data can also be used for contact identification and tracing for emerging infectious diseases [24]. In the prevention and control of COVID-19 in China, big data technology has played an important role in contact tracking, early warning, resource allocation and production recovery, by using location and travel data, medical and health data, news media data, government data, online consumption data, data collected by intelligent equipment, and epidemic prevention data [25]. Sixth, investigation of the changes in the disease burden. This could help develop new disease prevention strategies. The Global Burden of Disease Study is an example of applying big data [26], which applies a wide range of and a huge amount of data. Nearly 4700 parallel computers completed automated and standardized calculations of data mining analysis. The findings relevant to China demonstrated that compared with 1990, the disease spectrum of Chinese residents has undergone major changes in 2017. The burden of infectious diseases, malnutrition, and maternal diseases has been greatly reduced, while the burden of non-communicable diseases has increased substantially. Stroke and ischemic heart disease, instead of respiratory tract infection and neonatal diseases, have become the main cause of disease burden [27]. Seventh, the conduct of precise health management. Real-time and continuous monitoring of individual physical signs (heart rate, pulse rate, respiratory rate, body temperature, heat consumption, blood pressure, blood sugar, blood oxygen, body fat content, etc.) through wearable devices will help formulate timely health advice, so as to provide precise health management [14, 28, 29]. Finally, implementation of more powerful data mining. The tasks of data mining include association analysis, cluster analysis, classification analysis, anomaly analysis, etc. Big data mining can increase the degree of power and the ability to find weak correlation, thus contributing to the discovery of new knowledge and insights [19]. In recent years, medical claims data and electronic medical records have been used to analyze epidemiological characteristics of major and rare diseases, to investigate the etiology and prognosis of non-communicable diseases, to evaluate the efficacy and safety of drugs and vaccines in the real world, and to compare relative efficacy of different treatments.

20.3 Biomedical Big Data Initiatives and Actions

In recent years, big data initiatives and actions relevant to biomedical field have been carried out both in China and abroad, such as *Big Data Research and Development Initiative*, *Data to Knowledge to Action*, *Global Pulse*, *National Population Health Data Sharing Platform*, etc.

20.3.1 Big Data Research and Development Initiative

In March 2012, the US government launched *Big Data Research and Development Initiative* [30, 31], which was dedicated to improving the ability to extract knowledge and ideas from big data and to serve energy, health, finance, information technology, and other fields. In the biomedical field, data research was solicited by NSF and NIH to advance the core scientific and technological means of managing, analyzing, visualizing, and extracting useful information from large and diverse data sets, with particular interests in imaging, molecular, cellular, electrophysiological, behavioral, epidemiological, clinical and other data sets related to health and disease. NSF also provided $1.4 million to support a focused research group of statisticians and biologists to determine protein structures and biological pathways. The International 1000 Genomes Project aimed to establish the world's largest set of data on human genetic variation.

20.3.2 Data to Knowledge to Action

In November 2013, *Data to Knowledge to Action* was released by the US as the second phase of *Big Data Research and Development Initiative* [32]. OSTP's *Predicting the Next Pandemic Initiative* aimed to establish a consortium consisting of government departments and agencies, NGOs, academic institutions, industry partners and others, to enhance multi-sector collaboration and the use of big data to predict pandemics before they occur. NIH's *Big Data to Knowledge (BD2K) Initiative* aimed to develop new approaches, standards, methods, tools, software, and competencies necessary for biomedical scientists to capitalize on the big data being generated by the research community, and enhance access to available biomedical data through technologies, approaches, and policies that enable and facilitate widespread data sharing, discoverability, management, duration, and meaningful re-use. This initiative formed The Cancer Genome Atlas (TCGA), the Cardiovascular Research Network (CVRN) and other outputs [33]. TCGA aimed to map genetic changes in more than 20 cancers using large-scale genomic data sets. CVRN built a large cohort of more than 34,000 patients with atrial fibrillation by collaborating with health care providers and accessing electronic medical records. Using this large cohort, researchers developed and validated new stroke risk scoring tools for patients with atrial fibrillation, and improved stroke prevention strategies in patients with atrial fibrillation. American Society of Clinical Oncology launched the CancerLinQ™, as a virtual clinical trial, to obtain anonymized, vast amounts of information available online about treatment outcomes and quality of life from many cancer patients, so as to improve the quality of care for cancer patients.

20.3.3 Global Pulse

Global Pulse, initiated by the United Nations in 2009, aimed to promote awareness of the opportunities brought by big data, build public-private data sharing partnerships, develop efficient analysis tools and methods, so as to drive the application of data mining and real-time analysis in the UN system, and track and monitor the impact of global regional social and economic crisis in a more timely manner [34]. In biomedical field, this project used big data to predict disease outbreaks, and utilized digital early warning signals to guide aid programs.

20.3.4 National Population Health Data Sharing Platform

The platform, launched in 2003, aimed at assembling national population health data resources in basic medicine, clinical medicine, public health, traditional Chinese medicine, pharmacy, population, and reproductive health [35]. These data sources were mainly generated by science and technology programs. As of 2012, the platform had integrated data resources totaling 2.1TB, including 265 shared data sets. At present, the main function of the platform is to provide databases according to user needs, including Chinese physiological constants database, liver tumor database, eye disease database, infectious disease monitoring database, chemical composition database for Chinese herb, adverse drug reaction database, drug target database, and population and reproductive health survey database.

20.3.5 Big Data-Driven Management and Decision-Making Research

This major research plan, initiated by the National Natural Science Foundation of China in 2015, aimed to explore theory paradigm, data governance, value analysis and discovery, and analysis methods and technology, relevant to big data-driven management and decision-making [36]. In biomedical field, *Study on Harmonization Platform for Big Data of Population Health* was initiated, to explore theoretical mechanisms, data integration and sharing, data technology development and visualization for biomedical big data in China, so as to serve population health.

20.3.6 National Pilot Program for Healthcare Big Data Centers and Industrial Parks

This program, announced by National Health and Family Planning Commission in 2016, aimed to establish more regional and national centers and industrial parks focusing on big data in health and medicine to make more meaningful use of these data [37]. Fujian, Jiangsu, Fuzhou, Xiamen, Nanjing, and Changzhou were designated as the first batch of pilot provinces and cities, so as to promote and standardize the application and development of healthcare big data. The following data sets were integrated in these pilot provinces and cities: medical claims data, public health surveillance data, birth and death registries, and electronic medical records from hospitals.

20.3.7 Yichang Big Data Platform for Health Management

Yichang city locates in the southwest of Hubei province, China. Since 2014, Yichang has initiated the construction of *Big Data Platform for Health Management* [38]. This platform integrates population health information, including demography, medical services, health examination, public health surveillance, intelligent health monitoring, disease prevention and control, food safety, environmental health, geographic information in this city, so as to develop health interventions and explore the new pattern of life-cycle health management.

20.3.8 Regional Health Big Data Platform in Yinzhou District

Yinzhou, a district of Ningbo in Zhejiang province, locates 230 km south of Shanghai, China. This platform assembles multiple epidemiological surveys; electronic health records for chronic disease management; and health administrative, clinical, laboratory, drug and electronic medical record databases [39]. In addition, planned immunization, maternal and child healthcare, and public health surveillance have been integrated to realize collaboration and information sharing between public health and other sectors. Currently, Yinzhou district is promoting the combination of the regional health big data platform and artificial intelligence to promote population health and provide residents with personalized, precision health management services.

20.4 Major Problems and Trends of Biomedical Big Data

As an emerging field, biomedical big data is forming a new interdisciplinary direction and has obvious development advantages. Meanwhile, we should also be aware of the inherent flaws of big data, as well as the problems facing the development of biomedical big data in China.

20.4.1 Advantages and Flaws of Biomedical Big Data

From an epidemiological perspective, biomedical big data has unique advantages [5]. Big data can solve the problem of sample size in epidemiological studies, and large sample size can improve the accuracy of results and reduce the random/sampling error. Objective collection methods can help reduce information bias. The collection of big data is usually more objective, and it can record individual behaviors throughout the whole course. Information bias may be reduced compared to traditional epidemiological studies, which often collect information by recalling certain behaviors. Big data also provides unprecedented new risk factors for etiologic studies, and largely widens the range of available prevention measures [40].

As an emerging field, big data is also accompanied by some controversies [41, 42]. First, since data is always increasing, is it necessary to distinguish big data from traditional data? Second, it has been suspected that big data may be a kind of commercial propaganda in more sense. Third, the types of variables in big data increase and become more complex, correspondingly the probability of false-positive results will also increase. Fourth, bigger data does not necessarily mean better data, the representativeness and purity of the data must be considered. Finally, is it ethical to use data from the population without informing the individuals? These controversies must be addressed in the future development of big data.

Although biomedical big data has received much attention, we must realize that it also has some inherent flaws [40, 43]. First, it is still an observational study in nature, and it is difficult to avoid the shortcomings of observational studies, such as confounding bias. Without the increase of data sources and the diversification of data types, the mere increase in data volume can only improve the power and precision, and cannot affect the validity of results. Second, big data research is often a secondary application of data, which is not collected by the researchers personally, hence the quality of data is particularly noteworthy. A small amount of missing or inaccuracy may not affect the application of big data, however, a large amount of data inaccuracy or missing may lead to false discoveries. Third, big data may not be suitable for causal inference. The advantage of big data lies in finding associations, but it cannot indicate whether these associations are meaningful. The prediction based on data integration and correlation analysis is the core of big data. Fourth, Big data is essentially data-driven analysis without a predefined hypothesis, which makes data mining and multiple comparisons prone to false-positive results (that is, caused by chance), so as to produce false correlation and ecological fallacy. Finally, compared with probability random sampling, there may be selection bias in big data as collection methods often cover individuals with certain characteristics (such as medical insurance patients and people using wearable devices).

20.4.2 Main Problems Faced by Biomedical Big Data

The main problems faced by biomedical big data include the following [24, 44, 45]. First, how to realize the standardization of biomedical data? Data standardization is the prerequisite for data sharing. Only standardized data can be effectively integrated, so as to give full play to the value of big data [46]. Second, how to break data islands and achieve biomedical data sharing. It should be avoided that data can only be used by a few people or institutions, and data sharing is a prerequisite for the application of biomedical big data. Many public funding agencies have required that data from the funded research must be shared within a certain range [47]. Take electronic medical records as an example. China has more than 300 commercial providers of hospital information systems with various technical structures and data standards [6]. Such incompatibility has impeded the adoption of individual electronic health records in China. Third, how to store and manage biomedical big data? Data in biomedical field is extremely huge and is generated and updated faster. Its storage method affects not only the efficiency of data analysis but also the cost of data storage [3]. Fourth, how to realize efficient use of biomedical big data? China has accumulated a huge amount of biomedical data, and the utilization of the data also depends on the development of big data technology to a certain extent [48]. Fifth, how to perform analysis, integration, and mining of biomedical big data. In particular, the processing of semi-structured and unstructured data (such as electrocardiogram and medical imaging) and the processing of streaming data (real-time video, sensor data and medical device monitoring data) are important challenges for biomedical big data analysis [49]. Finally, there is a lack of interdisciplinary talents in biomedicine and information science. This dilemma needs to be solved by promoting the education of interdisciplinary disciplines of computer science and biomedicine [3, 26].

20.4.3 Trends of Biomedical Big Data

The trend of biomedical big data in the future has been raised [50, 51]. First, from "concept" to "value," big data will become the basis of smart health. Biomedical big data will be able to generate new knowledge, change medical practice with information and ultimately improve human health and public health [17]. Second, biomedical big data will contribute to the generation, integration, and transformation of scientific evidence. For example, large amounts of health data can be integrated, to obtain more reliable evidence [14]. In addition, virtual clinical trials can be carried out to produce evidence through real-time network data [33]. Third, there is a huge risk of privacy leakage while mining massive data. Data security and privacy protection have received increasing attention. Relevant policies and legislation need to be strengthened urgently, and corresponding technological development will play an important role [14]. Fourth, big data-oriented population cohort study has become a hot spot. The mega cohort studies are characterized by large sample size (hundreds of thousands of participants), prospective follow-up (even for decades), multidisciplinary cooperation, addressing both multiple diseases and multiple risk factors, sharing in biological specimens and data resources. After a long-term follow-up, such studies can produce a large number of population data [52]. Fifth, closely relating to information images and statistical graphics, visualization of biomedical big data will communicate the information contained in big data more clearly and effectively [19, 53]. Sixth, personalized health management based on biomedical big data is becoming increasingly popular. Real-time sensors (wearable devices) can be used to conduct real-time and continuous health monitoring and assessment, providing real-time health guidance for individuals [48]. With the development of individualized medicine based on biomedical big data, individualized prevention, diagnosis, and treatment will be realized [17]. Big data in biomedicine has become a strategic industry. Many countries have made big data a national strategy, and the industrialization of biomedical big data has begun to emerge.

Human has entered the age of big data. Big data science, as an emerging interdisciplinary field spanning information science, social science, network science, systems science, biomedicine, psychology, economics, and many other fields, is gradually taking shape and has become a hot spot of scientific research. There is a huge amount of data in the field of biomedicine, and how to share, regulate, manage and utilize is the key. Meanwhile, the cultivation of biomedical big data professionals needs to be solved urgently. Biomedical big data will change the pattern of medical practice, improve the quality of healthcare services, and ultimately contribute to the medical goals of individualized treatment and prevention.

References

1. Mayer-Schönberger V, Cukier K. Big data: a revolution that will transform how we live, work, and think. Boston: Houghton Mifflin Harcourt; 2013.
2. UN Global Pulse. Big data for development: challenges and opportunities. 2012 [cited 9 Dec 2020]. Available from: http://www.unglobalpulse.org/sites/default/files/BigDataforDevelopment-GlobalPulseMay2012.pdf.
3. Li G, Cheng X. Research status and scientific thinking of big data. Bull Chin Acad Sci. 2012;27(6):647–57.
4. Jee K, Kim GH. Potentiality of big data in the medical sector: focus on how to reshape the healthcare system. Healthc Inform Res. 2013;19(2):79–85.
5. Wang B, Lv J, Li L. Big data in biomedicine: status quo and perspective. Chin J Epidemiol. 2014;35(6):617–20.
6. Zhang L, Wang H, Li Q, et al. Big data and medical research in China. BMJ. 2018;360:j5910.
7. The State Council of China. Action outline for promoting the development of big data. 2015 [cited 9 Dec 2020]. Available from: http://www.gov.cn/zhengce/content/2015-09/05/content_10137.htm.
8. The General Office of the State Council of China. Guiding opinions of the General Office of the State Council on Promoting and Regulating the Application and Development of Big Data in Health and Medical Care. 2016 [cited 9 Dec 2020]. Available from: http://www.gov.cn/zhengce/content/2016-06/24/content_5085091.htm
9. Li C, Zhang W. Clustering analysis of research hotspots of the big data and health management. Chin Hosp Manag. 2016;10:63–5.
10. Hu Y. Population based etiological research on complex diseases. J Peking Univ (Health Sci). 2007;39(2):113–5.
11. Wang X, Yang Z, Wang M, et al. High-throughput sequencing technology and its application. China Biotechnol. 2012;32(1):109–14.
12. Costa FF. Big data in biomedicine. Drug Discov Today. 2014;19(4):433–40.
13. Zarrouk M. Delivering excellence in patient care with ready access to clinical data. 2012. [cited 28 July 2016]. Available from: http://www.netapp.com/us/media/wp-7169.pdf.
14. Groves P, Kayyali B, Knott D, et al. The big data revolution in healthcare: accelerating value and innovation. New York: McKinsey Global Institute; 2013.
15. Mooney SJ, Pejaver V. Big data in public health: terminology, machine learning, and privacy. Annu Rev Public Health. 2018;39:95–112.
16. Murdoch TB, Detsky AS. The inevitable application of big data to health care. JAMA. 2013;309(13):1351–2.
17. Chawla NV, Davis DA. Bringing big data to personalized healthcare: a patient-centered framework. J Gen Intern Med. 2013;28(Suppl 3):S660–5.
18. Yang R. Preventive medicine research in the era of big data: digital preventive medicine. Chin J Prev Med. 2014;48(3):1–4.
19. Gao H, Xiao L, Xu D, et al. Medical data mining platform based on cloud computing. J Med Inform. 2013;34(5):7–12.
20. Chunara R, Andrews JR, Brownstein JS. Social and news media enable estimation of epidemiological patterns early in the 2010 Haitian cholera outbreak. Am J Trop Med Hyg. 2012;86(1):39–45.
21. Fu Z, Bao C, Li Z, et al. Progress of research regarding the influenza early warning system, based on "Big Data". Chin J Epidemiol. 2020;41(6):975–80.
22. Dugas AF, Jalalpour M, Gel Y, et al. Influenza forecasting with Google Flu Trends. PLoS One. 2013;8(2):e56176.
23. Carneiro HA, Mylonakis E. Google trends: a web-based tool for real-time surveillance of disease outbreaks. Clin Infect Dis. 2009;49(10):1557–64.

24. Song J, Hu Y. Medical big data and precision medicine: prospects of epidemiology. Chin J Epidemiol. 2016;37(8):1164–8.
25. Wu J, Wang J, Nicholas S, et al. Application of big data technology for COVID-19 prevention and control in china: lessons and recommendations. J Med Internet Res. 2020;22(10):e21980.
26. Yu S, Xiao G. Research on global burden of disease-big data analysis application examples. J Med Inform. 2013;34(9):12–6.
27. Zhou M, Wang H, Zeng X, et al. Mortality, morbidity, and risk factors in China and its provinces, 1990-2017: a systematic analysis for the Global Burden of Disease Study 2017. Lancet. 2019;394(10204):1145–58.
28. Xu D, Yang H. The application of big data on healthcare personalized service. Chin J Health Inform Manag. 2013;10(4):301–4.
29. Zhou G, Xin Y, Zhang Y, et al. Study on big data's application in medical and health field. Chin J Health Inform Manag. 2013;10(4):296–300.
30. Office of Science and Technology Policy, Executive Office of the President of the United States. Obama Administration unveils "Big Data" Initiative: announces $200 million in new R&D investments 2015. [cited 9 Dec 2020]. Available from: https://obamawhitehouse.archives.gov/the-press-office/2015/11/19/release-obama-administration-unveils-big-data-initiative-announces-200.
31. Siva N. 1000 Genomes project. Nat Biotechnol. 2008;26(3):256.
32. Executive Office of the President of the United States. Fact sheet: data to knowledge to action 2015. [cited 9 Dec 2020]. Available from: https://obamawhitehouse.archives.gov/the-press-office/2015/11/19/fact-sheet-data-knowledge-action
33. Magid DJ, Gurwitz JH, Rumsfeld JS, et al. Creating a research data network for cardiovascular disease: the CVRN. Expert Rev Cardiovasc Ther. 2008;6(8):1043–5.
34. UN Global Pulse. 2009. [cited 9 Dec 2020]. Available from: http://www.unglobalpulse.org
35. Jiang J, Zhao H, Liu R. Discussion on the information organization of the scientific data sharing platform-take the National Scientific Data Sharing Platform for Population and Health as an example. J Inform Resour Manag. 2012;4:52–6.
36. National Natural Science Foundation of China. Major research plan "big data driven management and decision-making research": 2020 Annual Project Guide 2020. 2020. [cited 15 Dec 2020]. Available from: http://www.nsfc.gov.cn/publish/portal0/tab568/info79030.htm
37. National Health and Family Planning Commission of the PRC. China to build health care big data centers, industrial parks. 2016. [cited 15 Dec 2020]. Available from: http://en.nhc.gov.cn/2016-10/24/c_70573.htm
38. Liu J, Zhang P, Xu C, et al. Construction and use of big data for health management. Chin J Epidemiol. 2019;40(2):227–30.
39. Lin H, Tang X, Shen P, et al. Using big data to improve cardiovascular care and outcomes in China: a protocol for the CHinese Electronic health Records Research in Yinzhou (CHERRY) Study. BMJ Open. 2018;8(2):e019698.
40. Tang J, Li L. Some reflections on evidence-based medicine, precision medicine, and big data-based research. Chin J Epidemiol. 2018;39(1):1–7.
41. Chiolero A. Big data in epidemiology: too big to fail? Epidemiology. 2013;24(6):938–9.
42. Fan W, Bifet A. Mining big data: current status, and forecast to the future. SIGKDD Explor. 2012;14(2):1–5.
43. Khoury MJ, Ioannidis JP. Medicine. Big data meets public health. Science (New York, NY). 2014;346(6213):1054–5.
44. Willems SM, Abeln S, Feenstra KA, et al. The potential use of big data in oncology. Oral Oncol. 2019;98:8–12.
45. Pastorino R, De Vito C, Migliara G, et al. Benefits and challenges of Big Data in healthcare: an overview of the European initiatives. Eur J Public Health. 2019;29(Suppl_3):23–7.
46. Lynch C. Big data: how do your data grow? Nature. 2008;455(7209):28–9.
47. National Institutes of Health Office of Extramural Research. NIH sharing policies and related guidance on NIH-funded research resources. 2018 [cited 10 Dec 2020]. Available from: https://grants.nih.gov/policy/sharing.htm.
48. Trifonova OP, Il'in VA, Kolker EV, et al. Big data in biology and medicine: based on material from a joint workshop with representatives of the international Data-Enabled Life Science Alliance, July 4, 2013, Moscow, Russia. Acta Naturae. 2013;5(3):13–6.
49. Green DE, Rapp EJ. Can big data lead us to big savings? Radiographics. 2013;33(3):859–60.
50. China Computer Federation. Trends of big data in 2014. Commun CCF. 2014;10(1):32–6.
51. Shilo S, Rossman H, Segal E. Axes of a revolution: challenges and promises of big data in healthcare. Nat Med. 2020;26(1):29–38.
52. Xiong W, Lv J, Guo Y, et al. Overview on the practice and characteristics of large prospective cohort studies. Chin J Epidemiol. 2014;35(1):93–6.
53. Callebaut W. Scientific perspectivism: a philosopher of science's response to the challenge of big data biology. Stud Hist Philos Biol Biomed Sci. 2012;43(1):69–80.

21 Cultural Epidemiology in China

Dong-Qing Ye, Yan-Mei Mao, Jun Wu, Xin-Yu Fang, and Bao-Zhu Li

Abstract

Culture affects health by influencing individual behaviors and habits, and plays an important role in the occurrence and development of diseases. However, the extent of culture's influence on identified diseases remains uncertain, and further studies in medical anthropology and epidemiology are needed. It is undeniable that the relationship between culture and epidemiology has received more and more attention in recent years. As an interdisciplinary research field, cultural epidemiology is of great significance in the formulation of international health policies. There are many notable examples of cultural and epidemiological integration around the world with good results, especially in China. This review provides a brief summary of progress in cultural epidemiology, particularly in China, to provide clues for disease prevention and control.

Keywords

Cultural epidemiology · Patriotic health campaign · The Healthy China Strategy · China

21.1 Introduction

Anthropology is the study of human beings with biological and social attributes [1]. Epidemiology is the study and analysis of the patterns, causes, and effects of health and disease conditions in populations. Epidemiology is the analysis of problems affecting health and disease from a population perspective. It starts with the various distribution phenomena of the population and looks for the various related factors affecting health and disease, including physical, biological, social, cultural, and behavioral factors [2]. Since the Renaissance, biomedicine has been developing, gradually forming a biomedical model based on experimental medicine and pathology. It has a solid biological science foundation and huge technical resources, and has made amazing achievements in elucidating the mechanism of disease and designing new treatments. Biomedicine has always been a great driving force to promote the development of medicine. However, the biomedical model cannot explain and solve the influence of psychological and social factors on diseases. Due to the social

D.-Q. Ye (✉) · Y.-M. Mao · J. Wu · X.-Y. Fang · B.-Z. Li
Department of Epidemiology and Biostatistics, School of Public Health, Anhui Medical University, Hefei, China
e-mail: ydq@ahmu.edu.cn

D.-Q. Ye (ed.), *Progress in China Epidemiology*, https://doi.org/10.1007/978-981-19-2199-5_21

progress, the development of science and technology and the change of the disease spectrum, the biomedical model has not been able to fully adapt to the development of modern medicine. Biopsychosocial medical model arose at the historic moment and is accepted by more and more people. In 1977, Engel, a professor of psychiatry and internal medicine at the University of Rochester in New York, proposed that the biomedical model should be replaced by the biological psychosocial medical model. Biopsychosocial medical model's understanding of human's attributes rises from biological natural person to social economic person, and the occurrence and change of diseases deepen from biological level to psychological and social level [3]. Biopsychosocial medical model not only attaches importance to human's biological living state, but also attaches more importance to human's social living state. It comprehends human life, health, and disease from the perspective of biology and society, and seeks for the mechanism of disease phenomena, diagnosis and treatment methods. Anthropology and epidemiology are both subjects of human study, and share common and specific research methods. Therefore, there is inevitable crossover between them, and the cases of cooperation between anthropology and epidemiology are common at home and abroad. While the value of interdisciplinary collaboration between epidemiology and anthropology is widely recognized and hotly debated, effective international health policies and multicultural health programs require such collaboration. The EMIC framework for cultural studies of illness was developed in response to such needs, and a cultural epidemiology emerged from that framework as an interdisciplinary field of research on locally valid representations of illness and their distributions in cultural context [4]. Culture is a set of shared understandings of beliefs, values, norms, and social practices that influence the behavior of a relatively large group. Cultural differences can be manifested through daily behavior, which is relatively external and dominant. Cultural factors have an important influence on human psychology and society. Sociocultural contexts strongly influence the measurement of diseases such as epilepsy, cholera, Titanic mortality, breastfeeding, and adolescent smoking. How to communicate with different audiences and intervene to improve health and prevent disease is the goal of practitioners in the field of cultural epidemiology [5]. In specific disease prevention and control projects, it is beneficial to analyze the influence of relevant cultural factors on the occurrence and development of diseases, so as to find prevention and intervention measures suitable for the cultural logic of specific regions or populations, which will greatly help to analyze and solve public health problems.

21.2 The Intersection of Anthropology and Epidemiology Is an Interdisciplinary Collaboration in Health and Disease Research

Over the past two decades, there has been increasing attention to the possible contribution of the social sciences to the epidemiological study of health and disease patterns. This growing interest is largely due to the rise of chronic noncommunicable diseases, which were a major cause of morbidity and mortality in western populations in the twentieth century. There are many kinds of noninfectious diseases, mainly including malignant tumors, cerebrovascular diseases, hypertension, other types of heart disease, coronary heart disease, etc. The rise of industrialization has made chronic noncommunicable diseases more severe in developing countries. In 2003, the economic burden of chronic noncommunicable diseases in China was 858.054 billion RMB, accounting for 71.45% of the total economic burden of all diseases and 7.31% of GDP [6]. The economic burden of chronic noncommunicable diseases is enormous, and its increasing speed is higher than that of GDP, which makes a dominating contribution to the economic burden of all diseases in China [6]. In general, chronic noncommunicable diseases are strongly influenced by lifestyle variables, which are themselves strongly influenced by social and cultural forces. Understanding the impact of behavioral factors on hypertension requires understanding the social and cultural factors that contribute to obesity, a sedentary lifestyle, non-compliance with blood pressure medications (or other prescription regimens), and stress. Similarly, it is increasingly recognized that consideration of human behavior and its social and cultural determinants is important for understanding the distribution and control of infectious diseases. Related to the expansion of epidemiological interest into the field of behavior is the development of etiological models that focus on the psychological, biological, and sociocultural characteristics of the host rather than just exposure to specific pathogens or even behavioral risks. Since the 1970s and 1980s, the mainstream medical model has gradually developed from the "biomedical model" to the "biopsychosocial model." The biopsychosocial model is a broad view that attributes disease outcome to the intricate, variable interaction of biological factors (genetic, biochemical, etc.), psychological factors (mood, personality, behavior, etc.), and social factors (cultural, familial, socioeconomic, medical, etc.). The basic principle of this model is that a person must be treated as a whole rather than an isolated organ, and that the biological, psychological and social aspects of a person's life must be included in the consideration of disease. The biopsychosocial medical model of human-centered diagnosis links science with humanism, using every possible means to enable clinicians, patients, and their families to work together to manage disease more effectively [3, 7]. In addition to biological factors, diseases and health are also influenced and restricted by complex external environment, among which psychological and social factors play an important role. For example, the psychological stress brought by some emergencies can interfere or weaken the immune system of the human body through nerve and endocrine regulation, and increase the susceptibility of the body to various diseases. It is now widely accepted that disease and health are the result of the interaction of biological, psychological, and social factors. The biopsychosocial medical model is also widely recognized and plays a role in many diseases, such as psychosocial disorders and chronic diseases [8]. However, cultural factors play a crucial role in explaining certain psychiatric symptoms and can guide treatment [9]. For example, as more and more immigrants come to the USA, many of whom require treatment for mental illness, clinicians must recognize the need to take cultural factors into account when treating these patients [10]. In the USA, the health care system has increasingly focused on addressing the social and cultural determinants of health.

During this period, advances in statistical and computational techniques made it easy to test multivariate causal models, thus encouraging the measurement of the influence of social and cultural factors on disease occurrence [11, 12]. Multilevel regression modeling at two levels is emphasized because of its prevalence in psychosomatic medicine research [13]. The scale of social dominance orientation (SDO), used to measure the degree of preference for inequality among social groups, is a predictive measure of social and political attitudes toward stigmatized outgroups, and the effect of SDO on discrimination is mediated by prejudice [14]. Regression analysis is also a routine analysis method that can be used to analyze the influencing factors of disease, such as sociocultural, gender, age, and ethnicity [15–17]. In general, advances in statistical and computational techniques have allowed the role of culture in disease to be quantitatively calculated, which has promoted the development of cultural epidemiology. The development of cultural epidemiology suggests that we should take more comprehensive measures to prevent and control diseases. For example, it seems that there is a lack of a health-based approach of human papillomavirus (HPV) diseases. Due to the weakness of cultural management in society, this may be a major problem and requires the involvement and intervention of all policy makers, health planners, authorities, professors, elites, and clergy to control this major cultural health problem [18].

21.3 Cultural Epidemiology

In the late 1950s, anthropologists and epidemiologists began collaborating. At that time, many epidemiology textbooks believed that social environment was an important causative factor for both infectious and chronic diseases. At the same time, the literature of medical anthropology began to discuss epidemiology, and the two disciplines crossed. The ecological research methods in epidemiology investigate diseases from different levels and significantly add to the content of social and environmental aspects. The environment of public health concern is not only the physical and spatial environment, but also the immaterial network such as culture, the social relations that profoundly affect the human state [5]. Culture is the social behavior and norm in human society, and also a central concept of anthropology. It covers all kinds of phenomena in human society that are transmitted through social learning. Some aspects of human behavior, such as language, social practices (e.g., kinship and marriage), expressive forms (e.g., art, music, dance, ritual, and religion), and technologies (e.g., tool usage, cooking, shelter, and clothing) are said to be cultural universals, found in all human societies. The concept of material culture includes the material manifestations of culture, such as technology, architecture and art, and the non-material aspects of culture, such as the principles of social organization (including the practice of political organization and social institutions), mythology, philosophy, literature (written and oral), science. The concept of cultural epidemiology focuses on the role of health-related behaviors, of which culture is a difficult concept to grasp, with rich connotations including beliefs, customs, etc. Health behavior theory is a commonly used theory in the field of public health, which usually attributes problems to or is related to individual behaviors or omissions. This framework suggests that poor health results from individuals' inability or unwillingness to pay attention to prevention information or recommended therapeutic actions [19]. Diseases can cross borders, and as communication between countries has increased, epidemiologists have become increasingly concerned with transnational disease patterns. When epidemiologists work in different countries or between different groups within the same country, they inevitably have to deal with cultural differences. Many people believe that culture can be used as an explanatory variable to a large extent to predict and explain observed behaviors and diseases.

It has been proved in a variety of diseases that culture influences human health by influencing people's behavior and mental spirit. Research in western cultures demonstrates that practitioners form negatively biased impressions associated with patient masking. Cultural systems, such as cultural racism, undergird the social conditions that shape racial inequities in health, including social and health policy decision-making, governance, practice, and public reception [20]. In the USA, it is important to consider specific cultural mediators in the development of weight loss interventions among overweight and obese Hispanics [21]. Heritage diets and culturally appropriate dietary advice may help combat chronic diseases [22]. Health literacy is an important factor in improving patient compliance, cancer screening, and chronic disease management. Cultural beliefs around health and illness contribute to an individual's ability to understand and act on the directives of health care providers [23]. Culture-bound syndromes are a syndrome associated with cultural background and is often unique to ethnic or regional populations. Culture influences how people perceive symptoms, interpret them, and where they seek help [24]. The prevalence of different types of hallucinations in schizophrenia is the result of the interaction of multiple factors, including cultural patterns and clinical parameters, and culture seems to play a decisive role [25]. The food-sharing culture of northeastern Thailand makes social relationships among villagers through food-sharing as a risk factor that plays an important role in liver fluke infection and transmission [26]. One study found that caregivers' beliefs concerning dementia and the concept of family harmony as evidenced through the practice of filial piety are permeating cultural values, which together affect the attitudes toward research and help-seeking behaviors (i.e., seeking information on diagnosis and using formal services). The intersection of culture and dementia has been identified to include dementia awareness, care, and family roles [27]. These cultural beliefs impinge on key elements of the caregiving process, including caregivers' appraisal of stress, coping strategies, and informal and formal support [27, 28]. Ethnocultural factors also influence the natural history of Parkinson's disease [29]. Cultural background, including the beliefs the patient holds, whether religious or more broadly spiritual, can influence a patient's response to illness [30]. We can easily find a high prevalence of diseases of the digestive system and cervical spine among people who work in long-term sitting positions, such as drivers [31]. It is a culture-related disease. The standard of human body aesthetics and its influence on health are common in many countries. Historically, waist girdling in Europe has been linked to a range of health problems, including muscle wasting and liver damage. In Chinese history, the practice of foot binding, which is the result of the beauty of small feet, has caused many women's feet to suffer from impaired development and even fatal infections. The development of modern medicine to achieve breast augmentation technology has also brought about a number of health consequences. Esthetics and people's esthetic ideas are constantly changing and cosmetic surgery is extremely popular today. Culture influences human health through a series of processes, such as the behavior of people and the attitude and way of seeking medical treatment. Cultural history influences the way in which medical knowledge is formed, maintained, and changed.

21.3.1 An Important Case of the Integrated Application of Anthropology and Epidemiology in Foreign History

Emergent infectious diseases often have a great impact on social culture, and the disease culture phenomenon formed in the process also deserves special attention. Therefore, the plague or the Black Death, a typical disease event that took place in the Middle Ages in Europe, has been continuously studied and presented in different ways, including literature. For example, the description of plague in the Decameron by Italian writer Boccaccio makes us find that literature actually records those major diseases or plagues in the historical process in its unique way, and the influence of diseases on human society and collective mind cannot be underestimated. The human organism is a life form that needs to constantly adapt to the natural conditions. In the long process of evolution, groups in various regions must constantly adapt and make use of the surrounding conditions, and thus accumulate the experiences and patterns of their daily life. The foundation of folk culture is actually related to this. Diseases will not only affect people's lives, but also the large-scale infectious diseases because of their huge impact, and the human society interwoven into a complex phenomenon of a disease culture. Some of the basic concepts we have today, such as public health, life expectancy, and safety of drinking water and food, are actually social consensus that has evolved in the fight against mass disease. Therefore, the importance of disease culture relates to contemporary development models, social governance, community awareness, and international cooperation. For example, the traumatic memories of the Black Death brought to human society in the Middle Ages in Europe led to a sharp decline in the population of Europe. But the cataclysm also led to a heightened understanding of man's destiny, which was essential to the Renaissance. The Renaissance, a large-scale ideological and cultural movement, always revolves around the spirit of humanism. Due to the impact of the European plague or the Black Death on human cognition, many writers, playwrights, and painters since the Renaissance not only describe the huge plague in different ways in their works, but also use the plague as a kind of metaphor to reflect the inner world of the characters. These historical traces of disease not only left questions to be considered and solved in the field of medicine and sociology, but also triggered the study of humanities, including culture and literature. While the epidemic of the Great Plague had a huge impact on human beings, it also made people start to think about the potential problems in daily life and social structure, including getting rid of the bad habits of eating wild animals, and starting to organize the construction of the protection system. Therefore, since modern times, the concept of public health has been introduced all over the world. Disease is about all regions and groups, about development patterns and lifestyles, about ideas that are linked to scientific inquiry and cultural ideas. As Mr. Hu Shi once pointed out, every new development cannot be isolated, it must have other cultural background and it must be the product of that cultural background [32].

Epilepsy is a brain disorder caused by periodic abnormal electrical activity in the brain. It may be characterized by convulsions in certain limbs, sudden feelings and thoughts, or convulsions throughout the body [33]. The incidence of epilepsy in industrialized countries is about 50 cases per 100,000 people per year, with a prevalence rate of about 5 to 6 per 1000. Epilepsy is a disease that has traditionally been enveloped in magical beliefs, and these beliefs take many forms around the world. Throughout history, man has struggled to find explanations for diseases. It is perhaps not surprising that there has been a widespread struggle to understand, treat, and prevent the disease, since epilepsy has many strange and frightening symptoms. According to Scandinavian folk belief, epilepsy is caused by hidden people or magic. The popular treatment was to drink the blood of the criminals and eat the ashes of the charred clothes of the captured. In Norway and Sweden, epilepsy has for many centuries been considered a strange and mysterious disease. The explanations of its causes have been many and imaginative. One being that epilepsy was caused by the hidden people inhabiting the woods and the mountains. To avoid the disease, these hidden people should not be annoyed [34]. Epilepsy is a disease closely related to culture, which is greatly influenced by traditional culture and belief. Epilepsy remains one of the most common neurological disorders in the world, but seems to be widely misunderstood, especially in low-income countries. Patients with epilepsy (PWE) may face considerable stigma in society. Misconceptions about epilepsy are common in rural areas of sub-Saharan Africa. Understanding misconceptions is a critical stage in developing culturally appropriate intervention programs to improve medical compliance, quality of life and reduce stigma. Awareness-raising campaigns are needed among both urban and rural populations to reduce misunderstanding and combat stigma [35].

The influence of culture in epilepsy lies in whether and how the condition is brought to the attention of epidemiologists, and in its effect on morbidity, prevalence, causes, and consequences. Culture helps us understand incidence and prevalence in epidemiological studies of epilepsy. Cultural epidemiological methods have shown that the various local meanings and control strategies of epilepsy influence the number and severity of cases of interest to epidemiologists, so understanding the cultural meanings can help determine the number of cases and the severity of the epidemic. Olmsted County, Minnesota, USA, has been the focus of epilepsy epidemiology research since the middle of the 1950s. A study centered around understanding doctors' and patients' perceptions of epilepsy, its effects and treatment has revealed a gap between what people know about epilepsy from their doctors and what they want to know about their own epilepsy. Different people have different perceptions of epilepsy. The accepted causes of epilepsy at the time included emotional stress and supernatural forces, and biological mechanisms were not generally considered to be the cause of the disease. Residents, doctors, and social workers had very different interpretations of epilepsy, and their perceptions of this disorder determined the course of treatment. For example, patients attributing the cause to neuroticism or supernatural forces may take antispasmodic pills and drink tea to relieve tension, or visit a witch doctor for treatment. And the cultural aversion to epilepsy may affect doctors' diagnosis. And that can have an impact on things like prevalence that epidemiologists look at. The problem of selection bias in epidemiology is also the problem of selection bias that has previously occurred when cases in specialized medical centers were used to represent cases in the general community. Extrapolating from the clinic to the community is not a description of what is actually happening in the population. This may exaggerate or decrease the incidence of epilepsy in the population, which is known as selection bias. From the epidemiological study of epilepsy, the measurement tool itself can affect the actual condition of the disease. Epidemiology is a report-based observational discipline, and when the reporting standards are inconsistent, the results are not the same. Standards and methods for district cultural impact reporting. Seizures are the criteria for diagnosis, and these need to be reported by the patient or by eyewitnesses. Cultural differences can lead to inconsistent results in reports. The occurrence and prevalence of epilepsy are influenced by many factors, including natural factors, social factors and cultural factors. Epilepsy is a disease greatly influenced by cultural factors. A more comprehensive and symptomatic treatment of causes and treatment combining anthropological and sociological methods is more culturally symptomatic.

Neurasthenia is a disease which consists of increased fatigue or bodily weakness and exhaustion plus pantalgia, dizziness, headache, and other symptoms relevant to autonomic nerve dysfunction. There are plenty of studies investigating the history of diagnostic criteria of neurasthenia, which is influenced by diverse cultural (or social) environment [36]. Explanatory models of Neurasthenia Spectrum Disorders (NSDs) highlighted social distress, "tensions," and both general and clinic-specific physical, psychological, and cultural ideas. Findings indicate the importance of social contexts and cultural meaning in explanatory models of neurasthenia, as well as the potential clinical relevance of the construct of Neurasthenia Spectrum Disorder [37]. Depression is the most common depression disorder, with significant and persistent low mood as the main clinical feature. It is the main type of mood disorder and the mortality rate of depression increases year by year and the racial difference is obvious [38]. There are significant ethnic differences in the prevalence, symptoms, developmental mechanisms, patient cognition, and treatment of major depressive disorder (MDD) [39]. Culture may shape aspects of the autobiographical life structure in MDD [40]. Most gender differences in MDD patients in one study are not consistent with findings of Western studies suggesting that gender differences in MDD may be determined by both biological and sociocultural differences among ethnically different patient populations [41]. For instance, the prevalence of lifetime MDD in East Asia was less than 3%, versus 16% in the USA; however, according to a World Health Organization report, the suicide rate in Korea is the highest (31.2/100,000 population and one out of five in MDD patients) among developed countries, which is in contrast to the findings of other prevalence studies, suggesting hidden underlying mental health problems, including MDD [42]. The remarkably low prevalence rates of depression in the Asian population may arise from study methodologies, cultural backgrounds in thinking about emotional distress and MDD symptoms, fear of being stigmatized by addressing mental disorders, or the protective effects of family and social support. According to a recent large epidemiological study in Korea, only 10% of subjects with clinical depression were found to receive any form of treatment for depression, which is lower than in western countries. Interestingly, there are different descriptions of depressive symptoms in Asian and Western countries: Asian MDD patients show more irritability, anxiety, and irritability, lower positive emotions, and physical symptoms are common, while Western patients show more emotional symptoms than physical symptoms. Treatment compliance also varies widely by race and ethnicity [43]. Thus, ethno-cultural modifications in the evaluation and treatment of MDD should also be considered to reflect their cultural diversity maximally. All in all, neurasthenia and depression are culturally influenced disorders. Neurasthenia and depression are concepts of diseases originating from the West, which had a long history of development in the West before they were introduced into Chinese society. However, there are serious cultural differences between neurasthenia and depression in different cultural backgrounds of China and the West from the perspectives of cardiology, somatization and changes in clinical diagnostic criteria. Chinese and western cultures have different views on body and disease. Western philosophy pursues the tradition of subject-object dichotomy, emphasizing the spiritual self over the physical self, which leads to the strict distinction between physical diseases and mental diseases in medicine. It is under the influence of this dualistic view of mind and body that the change in the concept of neurasthenia and depression has resulted in a shift from emphasizing somatic symptoms to emphasizing psychological symptoms. In contrast, traditional Chinese medicine and culture view the body and mind as a unified whole that is interconnected with each other and connected with the social environment. In ancient Chinese philosophy and medical tradition, the mind-body monism of the unity of form and spirit and the use of form and quality occupy a dominant position. As a result, TCM does not distinguish between physical diseases and mental diseases, and tends to use the principle of syndrome differentiation for treatment in terms of treatment methods and means. Both in the West and in China, the concepts of neuropathy and depression are controversial both theoretically and clinically. Western disease classification caters to western notions of personality that emphasize individualism and independence, while Asian cultures emphasize interdependence, interconnectedness, and collectivism. When western diagnostic criteria are applied to Asian cultures, the culture may encounter some adaptive problems [44]. With the increasing trend of migration worldwide, the cultural characteristics of depression have become increasingly important in clinical practice. The good news is that people have recognized that depression presents differently in different cultures, and efforts are being made to develop depression assessment tools sensitive enough to capture these changes [45, 46].

21.4 The Integration of Culture and Epidemiology in Disease Prevention and Control in China

China is a big country with a history of 5000 years and rich cultural deposits. In China, culture and epidemiology are closely intertwined. We summarized the progress of cultural epidemiology in China based on the development history of modern and contemporary Chinese history.

21.4.1 Patriotic Health Campaign

The patriotic health campaign is a great initiative and successful practice of public health in New China. In general, the patriotic health movement is a movement that combines the health movement with patriotism, which needs the participation of the whole society and benefits the whole society [47]. It started around 1950, when the new China was just founded and there were many things to be done. At that time, the Chinese people's health and hygiene level was very low, due to the long war, economic backwardness and the prevalence of various diseases and other reasons. Shortly after the founding of the People's Republic of China, the vast rural areas suffered from a severe shortage of medical resources, rampant infectious and endemic diseases and poor health. For example, plague spread to more than 500 counties in 20 provinces (autonomous regions); 11 million schistosomiasis patients, endemic area of more than 2 million square kilometers. More than 30 million filariasis patients; The prevalence of tuberculosis is as high as 4%. The total number of leprosy patients is nearly half a million [48]. China's 1981 Economic Yearbook showed that in 1949, the annual per capita income in China was only 69.29 yuan, the annual per capita grain was only 209 kilograms, and the average life expectancy was 35 years [49]. Controlling the spread of the disease and ensuring the health of the people has become an urgent problem for China. Therefore, the Communist Party of China (CPC) linked health work with patriotic awareness, leading the people of the country to launch a vigorous patriotic health campaign. In the 1950s, the

Chinese government started a social movement called the Patriotic Health Campaign headed by the Patriotic Health Campaign Committee (PHCC) at both the national and provincial/city level. As part of the campaign, the government declared war on "the four demons-the fly, the mosquito, the mouse and the sparrow." People had been instructed to clean their homes, schools and workplaces daily and to conduct personal hygiene. The sanitary conditions in the countryside had also been greatly improved. The incidence of smallpox, cholera, dysentery, and other infectious diseases had been greatly reduced due to the cut-off of vectors and transmission routes. The number of medical institutions and medical and health professionals had also been greatly improved. Under the leadership of the CPC Central Committee and governments at all levels, the active participation of the general public had effectively reduced the density of mosquitoes, flies, rats, and cockroaches, and significantly reduced the occurrence and prevalence of plague, malaria, Japanese encephalitis, and other diseases. Many urban and rural areas had been cleared of a large number of garbage and filth, and have taken on a new look. On April 3, 1978, the CPC Central Committee and the State Council decided to re-establish the Central Committee for Patriotic Health Campaign, and issued the Circular on Insisting on Carrying out the Patriotic Health Campaign, which fully resumed the patriotic health campaign. We have launched a series of efforts to eliminate the "four pests," promote the "five stresses four beauties and three loves," build clean cities and towns, and revolutionize toilets, and achieved remarkable results. The CPC Central Committee and the State Council had always attached great importance to the patriotic health campaign, and the reports of the 16th, 17th, and 18th National Congress of the CPC all put forward the idea of "carrying out the patriotic health campaign." In the report of the 19th National Congress of the Communist Party of China, patriotic health has been strengthened. Chairman Xi Jinping proposed to "adhere to prevention first, carry out in-depth patriotic health campaigns, advocate healthy and civilized lifestyles, and prevent and control major diseases" [47, 50].

Schistosomiasis has always been a serious endemic disease in Chinese history. It causes severe physical, social and economic disability and, together with other major parasitic diseases, severely reduces the productive capacity of developing countries. Schistosomiasis has been prevalent and rampant in China for more than 2000 years. In the early days of P.R.C., the disease spread throughout 350 counties (cities) in 12 provinces (cities), including Jiangsu, Zhejiang, Hunan, Hubei, Anhui, Jiangxi, Sichuan, Yunnan, Guangdong, Guangxi, Fujian, and Shanghai, affecting more than 10 million people and threatening more than 100 million lives [51]. The type, distribution, and intensity of schistosomiasis varies in different regions. The distribution of schistosomiasis is closely related to occupation, local water distribution, and living habits [52]. In the 1950s and 1960s, the Chinese central government and the National PHCC declared that snails were responsible for the transmission of schistosomiasis. Therefore, in the schistosomiasis epidemic areas, massive campaigns were implemented to eliminate snails with poisonous drugs provided by the government. Diseases Control in China issued the "criteria for control and elimination of schistosomiasis in China." Health education programs were also being developed with an emphasis on behavioral change through the dissemination of scientific knowledge and skills training. Subsequently, in areas where schistosomiasis was highly prevalent, almost all villagers were aware of the risks and obtained the knowledge and skills to implement the required preventive measures, but they had no incentive to change their traditional lifestyles and rely mainly on government efforts to control the problem [53, 54]. It has been 70 years to implement schistosomiasis control in China, which can be divided into five stages including the initiating preparedness, mass-based campaign, achievement consolidation, mass drug administration, control of infection source. The second national health conference in 1952 determined the four principles of health work, namely, facing workers, peasants, and soldiers, giving priority to prevention, uniting traditional Chinese and western medicine, and combining health work with mass movements. In 1953, the State

Council pointed out that schistosomiasis prevention and control institutions should be established in every province, city, and county. From the mid-1950s to the mid-1980s, the strategy of schistosomiasis prevention and control in China focused on controlling the spread of schistosomiasis by means of population chemotherapy, drug extermination, environmental improvement, and clean water supply. Subsequently, simultaneous chemotherapy for both human and animal, combined with health education and continuous extermination of snails in susceptible areas resulted in effective control of schistosomiasis in endemic areas. In accordance with the principle of "taking measures in accordance with local conditions, providing classified guidance and joint prevention and control" and in conjunction with the construction of a new socialist countryside, all epidemic areas nationwide have actively implemented a comprehensive prevention and control strategy focusing on the control of infectious sources [55, 56]. The number of schistosomiasis patients had dropped from 9.49 million in the early years of the founding of P.R.C. (1957) to 30,000 in 2018, a remarkable achievement thanks to the leadership of the Party and government, comprehensive management, scientific prevention and treatment, and professional teams [57]. These achievements not only demonstrate the success of disease control, but also represent a particularly successful social practice with unique cultural attributes. Although rich experiences are being reported on schistosomiasis prevention and control, it is necessary to sublimate the experience to the cultural level, as cultural and spiritual values historically far outweigh the value of achievement. Culture is crucial in the fight against schistosomiasis. The effective prevention and control work is not only based on the strong patriotic culture of the Chinese people, but also has formed a more specific schistosomiasis control culture Narrowly speaking, the culture of schistosomiasis control is the spiritual culture that is jointly created and nurtured by schistosomiasis control workers since the founding of P.R.C. The spiritual features of Chinese schistosomiasis control culture are characterized by the patriotism and care about the people, the matter-to-fact attitude, the pioneering and enterprising spirit, and the spirit of sacrifice and dedication [58]. One study has also pointed out that the meaning of "China's culture for schistosomiasis control," i.e., people-first, government-oriented, science-respected, collective wisdom and efforts, and diversity-embracing. China has successfully integrated culture into schistosomiasis control and achieved good results.

Plague is a deadly and rapidly spreading infectious disease caused by the bacterium Yersinia pestis, which killed more than a third of the Europe's population, or 25 million people, in the fourteenth century [59]. It has killed millions of people throughout human history and continues to cause sporadic outbreaks nowadays. In the autumn of 1910, a virulent infectious disease broke out in northeast China. The epidemic spread rapidly with a high fatality rate, killing tens of thousands in a few months. Japan and Russia, on the grounds of health and epidemic prevention, are ready to seize the control of the three northeastern provinces. The disease was unknown at the time. Chinese doctor Wu Liande dissected a patient's corpse and isolated the plague pathogen for observation and culture, confirming that the pathogen of the epidemic was Yersinia pestis. Based on epidemiological data and bacteriological tests, Wu Liande first suggested that the epidemic was an extremely dangerous form of pneumonic plague, which could be transmitted from person to person in droplets. Therefore, he encouraged people to wear masks and advocated isolating plague patients and restricting the movement of people as the priority. The Chinese government appointed Wu Liande as commander in chief of the health and epidemic prevention campaign. Prevention and control measures had been taken to control the source of infection, cutoff transmission routes and protect vulnerable groups, including establishing plague hospitals, centrally treating infected people, isolating epidemic areas, strictly disinfecting houses and clothing, controlling traffic, restricting population movement, promoting the use of simple masks, and vaccinating and injecting Pest serum. However, due to the high number of deaths, the cold weather and the difficulty of burial, a large number of dead bodies were exposed to the ground. Wu Liande advocated cremation of plague victims, which was not in keeping with traditional Chinese culture and met resistance. As the implementation of cremation is contrary to the traditional Chinese funeral and burial system, it was necessary to have the courage to break through the obstacles of traditional customs. Finally, under the threat of the spread of the epidemic, the Qing government approved the centralized cremation [60]. Under the leadership of Wu Liande, the plague epidemic in China, which had shocked the world, was brought under control. Experience with plague prevention shows that epidemic control is a key factor in safeguarding national sovereignty. The major epidemic crisis in northeast China has helped cement the conceptual link between the physical health of the individual and the political health of the country. Since then, China's public health began to modernize. Human plague was basically under control by the end of 1950s, but China persisted in carrying out patriotic health campaigns and taking measures to prevent and control plague, such as rodent eradication and uprooting, which made the plague epidemic basically stable. By the end of the 1970s, a nationwide investigation of plague foci was basically completed. In 1981, the Ministry of Health established the National Plague Surveillance Program to conduct systematic surveillance of plague throughout the country. In 1989, the Law of P.R.C. on the Prevention and Treatment of Infectious Diseases officially listed plague as a Class A infectious disease and brought it under legal management. Since then, laws and regulations on plague management and prevention continued to emerge.

Cholera is a severe diarrheal disease that spreads rapidly, affecting millions of people and killing tens of thousands each year. The disease is caused by O1 and is characterized by watery diarrhea, which can be fatal if not treated properly. Cholera had not been reported in South America from the late 1800s until 1991, when it was introduced in Peru, wreaking havoc in one of the biggest epidemics reported to date [61]. Up to 1961, there were six cholera pandemics in China. In the Qing Dynasty, there were four cholera pandemics with two types. Compared with the world cholera pandemic years, it can be seen that almost every time when the world cholera pandemic occurred, there would be strong or weak cholera epidemic in China, which showed the characteristics of China's organism and its sensitivity to the world situation [62]. Cholera is one of a series of infectious diseases affected by climate, geography, and other natural environments. The occurrence of cholera is closely related to the local natural and cultural environment, thus cholera is integrated with water, sanitation, and hygiene activities [63]. Since the implementation of the patriotic health campaign, China has made remarkable progress in environmental and personal hygiene, and the incidence of cholera was kept at a relatively low level. From 1977 to 1986, cholera was prevalent in China, and the number of reported cases, regional distribution, and incidence scale increased significantly. The number of cholera cases in 1980 was as high as 40,611. The cholera epidemic in China has been kept at a relatively low level since 2002, when the epidemic was brought under control. However, local outbreaks occurred occasionally, mainly caused by food-borne infections, especially those caused by *Vibrio cholerae* contaminated by aquatic products. The occurrence of food-borne cholera is closely related to local food culture and natural environment. In 2009, for example, a cholera outbreak in Sichuan, China, was caused by eating soft-shelled turtles [64]. Vibrio cholerae is easy to be detected in seafood and aquatic products. To control and prevent Vibrio cholerae, it is necessary to supervise the sanitary condition of aquatic products [65]. Vibrio cholerae is more likely to be detected in the aquatic products of coastal cities, such as Guangdong and Zhejiang, and because people in coastal cities tend to eat and drink aquatic products, the risk of cholera outbreaks is higher in these areas than in other provinces [66, 67]. Cholera is one of the "Class A infectious diseases" that shall be subject to compulsory management according to the Law of P.R.C. on the Prevention and Treatment of Infectious Diseases, and also one of the international quarantine infectious diseases that must be subject to health quarantine according to the International Health Regulations. Since 1995, the Ministry of Health of China has formulated and issued numerous cholera prevention and control programs and manuals, and set up a number of state-level monitoring stations to carry out monitoring. China adheres to the basic principle of prevention first, and takes comprehensive preventive measures mainly to cut off transmission routes. Specific measures include establishing and improving all levels and various types of diarrhea disease clinics to detect cholera-infected patients in time, and conducting inspection, quarantine and epidemiological investigation promptly to find out the source of infection. Leading institutions for disease prevention at all levels should be improved, and a rigorous network of epidemic reporting and monitoring should be established.

Smallpox (variola) is a virulent infectious disease caused by Smallpox virus. It is characterized by strong infectivity and high lethality. The Chinese people's struggle against smallpox lasted for thousands of years, and it was not until 1961 that smallpox was completely eradicated [68]. Smallpox was first recorded in Chinese history as far back as the Jin Dynasty, and then spread in mainland China as a result of war. In China, the Kangxi Emperor, known as the greatest emperor in history, was also plagued by smallpox. Therefore, when Kangxi became the emperor, he attached great importance to the prevention and treatment of smallpox. Ancient Chinese medical scientists made a long study on the prevention and control of smallpox and achieved good results. As early as in the Northern Song Dynasty, China had invented the method of pox inoculation, which was of great significance in reducing the harm of smallpox and was also an important contribution of the Chinese nation to preventive medicine in the world [69]. Later, human pox inoculation was spread from China to the West. On this basis, E. Jenner invented vaccinia inoculation and introduced it to China. The human pox inoculation method invented in China and the cowpox inoculation method invented in the West played an important role in the eradication of smallpox and became the forerunner of artificial immunity against severe infectious diseases. In the early days of New China, smallpox was still one of the highest mortality acute infectious diseases in China. In order to combat smallpox, China promulgated a number of laws to carry out the planned work of universal vaccinia. The law stipulates that all residents of the People's Republic of China, regardless of nationality, must be vaccinated with vaccinia. With the successful implementation of the nationwide vaccination policy, the vaccination rate of Chinese residents has risen sharply. The patriotic health campaign eliminated the vectors of various infectious diseases on a large scale, improved the environmental health, established a health system, publicized and popularized the knowledge of health and epidemic prevention, and laid a good social foundation for the eradication of smallpox. The number of smallpox cases dropped dramatically. Between 1952 and 1958, the number of smallpox cases in China dropped from more than 100,000 to more than 300 [70]. Smallpox is the first human eradication of an infectious disease, is the only disease to be eliminated.

Health is not only the absence of disease and weakness, but also refers to the perfect state of physical, psychological, and social adaptability [71]. With the change of times, a series of patriotic health campaigns have been carried out, such as building civilized cities, improving water and toilets in rural areas, health education, food safety, and tobacco control. Although the patriotic health campaign has different contents in different times, it shows strong medical humanistic care and Chinese cultural heritage. In a word, patriotic health movement is a great invention and successful practice in the history of human health development.

21.4.2 The Healthy China Strategy

In October 2016, the CPC Central Committee and the State Council jointly released an outline for the Healthy China 2030 initiative, specifying the targets and programs of action. "Healthy China 2030" is comprised of 29 chapters that cover five areas such as public health services, environment management, the medical industry, and food and drug safety. On October 18, 2017, Chairman Xi Jinping pointed out in his report to the 19th National Congress of the CPC that we should implement a healthy China strategy [72]. People's health is an important symbol of a prosperous nation and a strong and prosperous country. It is very important to improve the national health policy and provide people with full range of full-cycle health services [73]. The report of the 19th National Congress of the Communist Party of China further proposed to implement the strategy of healthy China, marking that the Party and the government have raised the health of the people to the height of bearing on the overall modernization drive, and officially established the healthy China strategy as a national strategy [74]. Due to industrialization, urbanization, aging population, and the changing disease spectrum, ecological environment and lifestyle, China faces the health problems of both developing and developed countries. Health culture is an important part of socialist culture. It is one of the important tasks of social construction to maintain and protect people's health in an all-round and full cycle. The state's emphasis on people's health is inseparable from the CPC purpose of serving the people wholeheartedly. Moreover, health is the foundation of social productivity, and also the cornerstone and symbol of national prosperity and rejuvenation. Since then, China has implemented the Healthy China strategy in various aspects and achieved remarkable results.

Under the Healthy China strategy, the city's infrastructure and sanitation environment have been greatly improved [75]. China has also stepped up tobacco control efforts to reduce smoking rates [76]. In China, the national basic public health service project is a basic public health service for key groups such as the elderly, women and children, for key diseases such as chronic diseases and infectious diseases, and to meet people's basic health needs such as vaccination and health education. It is a major measure to implement the Healthy China strategy. The level and capacity of community-level services in China have been greatly improved, health benefits are emerging, equal access to services has been achieved, and the gap between regions, urban and rural areas, and between different groups of people is narrowing [77]. The coverage of basic public health services in China is expanding, the quality and quantity of services are improving, and the provision and management of basic public health services are becoming more standardized. China is constantly increasing its research and development efforts in traditional Chinese medicine (TCM), so that TCM can make greater contributions to human health [78, 79]. An important part of the Healthy China strategy is to put prevention first, carry out intensive patriotic health campaigns, advocate healthy and civilized lifestyles, and prevent and control major diseases. Lifestyle is an important modifiable factor in the occurrence of cancer, and the cultural impact on the pursuit of health in the lifestyle of Chinese cancer survivors remains largely unexplored. Chinese cultural beliefs concerning the nature of food, TCM, minimizing social disturbances, and collaborative control influenced their lifestyle.

Since 1978, the lifestyle, dietary structure, consumption and entertainment mode, working mode, economic relationship, and interpersonal relationship communication mode of the social population in China have been constantly changing. As a result, the disease spectrum and medical model have also changed accordingly. By the end of the 1970s, China had basically completed the transformation of the disease spectrum, and the main cause of death of the population had changed from acute infectious diseases to chronic diseases, completing the transformation from the biomedical model to the modern medical model. China's first health revolution, which focused on the control of infectious diseases, has yet to be completed, while the second health revolution, which focused on the control of chronic diseases, has arrived ahead of schedule. Chronic diseases have become a major threat to people's health, and the prevention and treatment of central cerebrovascular diseases and malignant tumors is the focus of the second health revolution. In recent years, chronic diseases, such as malignant tumor, cerebrovascular disease, cardiovascular disease and respiratory disease, have become serious threats to the life and health of urban and rural residents in China [80]. Obesity and diabetes have also become major public health problems that endanger people's health [81, 82]. Chronic diseases are strongly influenced by lifestyle. China actively promotes health education activities to prevent chronic diseases. In 2007, the National Healthy Lifestyle Initiative was launched to spread health knowledge and promote the formation of healthy behaviors among the population [83]. Since the national healthy lifestyle campaign was launched in 2007, local governments have actively participated in it. By the end of December 2015, 2507 counties (districts) in China had launched the campaign, accounting for 80.9 percent of the country's total [84]. In carrying out healthy lifestyle publicity activities, all places pay attention to the combination of traditional culture, so that publicity is easy to understand, easy to accept. For example, Danzhou Tune is an intangible cultural heritage project of Hainan Province. Danzhou Health Bureau and the Culture and Sports Bureau have worked together to turn the core message of a healthy lifestyle into a folk song feature film for performance among the people. In addition to combining with traditional culture, local propaganda has kept pace with The Times and made full use of microblog, WeChat and other new media to carry out propaganda.

China is one of the countries with severe endemic diseases. There are about 70 kinds of endemic diseases, mainly including IDD, endemic fluorosis, endemic arsenicosis, Kashin-Beck disease and Keshan disease. There were 30 provinces and Xinjiang Production and Construction Corps in China where iodine deficiency disease was prevalent to varying degrees [85]. Endemic disease control agencies have also changed over the decades as epidemics have changed. On March 6, 1960, the CPC Central Committee approved the establishment of the Leading Group for the Prevention and Control of Local Diseases in Northern China. The Party committees of 13 provinces, autonomous regions and municipalities directly under the Central Government in northern China also established leading groups for the prevention and control of endemic diseases, mainly responsible for the prevention and control of Keshan disease and Kashin-Beck disease. In 1973, the control mission of ground nail disease was added. In 1977, the prevention and control of endemic fluorosis was added. In 1981, the Leading Group for Endemic Diseases Prevention and Control in the Northern Region of the CPC Central Committee was renamed the Leading Group for Endemic Diseases Prevention and Control of the CPC Central Committee, and its scope of work was expanded to 28 provinces, autonomous regions and municipalities directly under the Central Government, and 17 ministries and commissions. In 1986, the Central Leading Group for Prevention and Control of Endemic Diseases was abolished, and the Ministry of Health established the Bureau for Prevention and Control of Endemic Diseases to take charge of the leading work of prevention and control of endemic diseases nationwide. In 1998, the National Office for the Prevention and Control of Endemic Diseases was abolished and its responsibilities were transferred to the Department of Disease Control (in 2006 the name was changed to the Bureau for Disease Control and Prevention of the Ministry of Health). Through the joint efforts of local and national prevention and control workers at all levels for decades, the prevention and control of endemic diseases has achieved remarkable results. The effective control and elimination of endemic diseases in China benefits from the superior socialist system [86]. In 2016, the Outline of the "Healthy China 2030" Plan proposed to strengthen public health services covering the whole people, maintain the control and elimination of key endemic diseases, so that endemic diseases will no longer become a major problem endangering people's health. Accordingly, in March 2017, the National Health and Family Planning Commission, the National Development and Reform Commission and the Ministry of Finance jointly issued the National Endemic Disease Prevention and Control Plan during the 13th Five-Year Plan Period, which set the targets for the prevention and control of seven endemic diseases, including eliminating iodine deficiency and basically eliminating Keshan disease by 2020. In a word, under the Healthy China strategy, the Chinese government and local governments have taken various measures tailored to local conditions to combat endemic diseases, thus ensuring the health of the Chinese people. The prevalence of these endemic diseases is not only related to the local natural environment but also related to the local cultural environment, including diet and living habits. In the 1970s, iodine deficiency diseases were prevalent to varying degrees in most areas of China, threatening about 720 million people. Since 1994, China has gradually implemented nationwide measures to prevent and control salt iodization, and the incidence of iodine deficiency diseases has dropped significantly. Moreover, the iodine nutrition status of the population has been monitored in all regions, and the iodine supplement strategy has been adjusted in time according to the monitoring results [87]. Epidemiologic data has implicated *T. venenata* as a probable cause of clusters of sudden unexplained death (SUD) in northwestern Yunnan Province. This phenomenon is related to the local good consumption of wild mushrooms. The government warns the villagers about the precautions of eating wild mushrooms, which can effectively reduce the incidence of USD [88]. The prevalence of both cystic echinococcosis and alveolar echinococcosis (AE and CE) is 1.66% in Tibet, China, and an estimated 50 million people in western China are at risk of contracting the disease. Poor sanitary conditions, the Buddhist doctrine of allowing old livestock to die a natural death, and the unrestricted disposal of the animal's internal organs after slaughter may account for the high prevalence of human CE here. Some studies suggest that it is necessary to shorten the treatment time of this disease and adopt special methods adapted to local culture to improve the healthy quality of life in Tibetan communities [89, 90]. These measures are based on the understanding of local customs and food culture and other characteristics of the formulation. Culture plays an important role in the prevention and control of endemic diseases.

21.5 Conclusion

Although the intersection of anthropology and epidemiology has only been taken seriously in recent years, the influence of culture on disease has a long history. It is an inevitable trend to attach importance to cultural factors in the study of the development of diseases. Combined with the social and cultural background of the population, targeted public health prevention and control measures and epidemiological studies have a more significant effect on disease prevention and control.

References

1. Marjetka J. The partnership of public health and anthropology. Coll Antropol. 2016;40(2):151.
2. Frérot M, Lefebvre A, Aho S, Callier P, Astruc K, Aho Glélé LS. What is epidemiology? Changing definitions of epidemiology 1978-2017. PLoS One. 2018;13(12):e0208442.
3. Papadimitriou G. The "biopsychosocial model": 40 years of application in psychiatry. Psychiatriki. 2017;28(2):107–10.
4. Weiss MG. Cultural epidemiology: an introduction and overview. Anthropol Med. 2001;8(1):5–29.
5. Trostle JA. Epidemiology and culture. Cambridge: Cambridge University Press; 2004.
6. Hu JP, Rao KQ, Qian JC, Wu J. The study of economic burden of chronic non-communicable diseases in China. Chin J Prev Control Chron Dis. 2007;03:189–93.
7. Toppelberg CO. Biopsychosocial model. Am J Psychiatry. 1997;154(9):1328–9.
8. Wade DT, Halligan PW. The biopsychosocial model of illness: a model whose time has come. Clin Rehabil. 2017;31(8):995–1004.
9. Burkett GL. Culture, illness, and the biopsychosocial model. Fam Med. 1991;23(4):287–91.
10. Roy D, Jayaram G, Vassila A, Keach S, Rao V. Depression after traumatic brain injury: a biopsychosocial cultural perspective. Asian J Psychiatr. 2015;13:56–61.
11. Janes CR, Stall R, Gifford SM. Anthropology and epidemiology: interdisciplinary approaches to the study of health and disease. Dordrecht: Springer; 1986.
12. Joseph N, Watson NN, Wang Z, Case AD, Hunter CD. Rules of engagement: predictors of Black Caribbean immigrants' engagement with African

American culture. Cultur Divers Ethnic Minor Psychol. 2013;19(4):414–23.
13. Myers ND, Brincks AM, Ames AJ, Prado GJ, Penedo FJ, Benedict C. Multilevel modeling in psychosomatic medicine research. Psychosom Med. 2012;74(9):925–36.
14. Michinov N, Dambrun M, Guimond S, Méot A. Social dominance orientation, prejudice, and discrimination: a new computer-based method for studying discriminatory behaviors. Behav Res Methods. 2005;37(1):91–8.
15. Kyung-Sook W, SangSoo S, Sangjin S, Young-Jeon S. Marital status integration and suicide: a meta-analysis and meta-regression. Soc Sci Med. 2018;197:116–26.
16. Stolz E, Fux B, Mayerl H, Rásky É, Freidl W. Passive suicide ideation among older adults in Europe: a multilevel regression analysis of individual and societal determinants in 12 countries (SHARE). J Gerontol B Psychol Sci Soc Sci. 2016;71(5):947–58.
17. Wang W, Lau Y, Chow A, Thompson DR, He HG. Health-related quality of life and social support among Chinese patients with coronary heart disease in mainland China. Eur J Cardiovasc Nurs. 2014;13(1):48–54.
18. Soltanizadeh N, Ameri Shahrabi M, Masjedi MR, Ainy E, Kavousy E, Hashemi SM. Health culture and presenting a paradigmatic model focusing on human papillomavirus disease. J Family Reprod Health. 2020;14(2):116–23.
19. Airhihenbuwa CO, Ford CL, Iwelunmor JI. Why culture matters in health interventions: lessons from HIV/AIDS stigma and NCDs. Health Educ Behav. 2014;41(1):78–84.
20. Cogburn CD. Culture, race, and health: implications for racial inequities and population health. Milbank Q. 2019;97(3):736–61.
21. Lindberg NM, Stevens VJ, Halperin RO. Weight-loss interventions for Hispanic populations: the role of culture. J Obes. 2013;2013:542736.
22. Kuehn BM. Heritage diets and culturally appropriate dietary advice may help combat chronic diseases. JAMA. 2019;322(23):2271–3.
23. Shaw SJ, Huebner C, Armin J, Orzech K, Orzech K, Vivian J. The role of culture in health literacy and chronic disease screening and management. J Immigr Minor Health. 2009;11(6):460–7.
24. Ventriglio A, Ayonrinde O, Bhugra D. Relevance of culture-bound syndromes in the 21st century. Psychiatry Clin Neurosci. 2016;70(1):3–6.
25. Bauer SM, Schanda H, Karakula H, Olajossy-Hilkesberger L, Rudaleviciene P, Okribelashvili N, Chaudhry HR, Idemudia SE, Gscheider S, Ritter K, T. S. Culture and the prevalence of hallucinations in schizophrenia. Compr Psychiatry. 2011;52(3):319–25.
26. Phimpraphai W, Tangkawattana S, Kasemsuwan S, Sripa B. Social influence in liver fluke transmission: application of social network analysis of food sharing in Thai Isaan culture. Adv Parasitol. 2018;101:97–124.
27. Brooke J, Cronin C, Stiell M, Ojo O. The intersection of culture in the provision of dementia care: a systematic review. J Clin Nurs. 2018;27(null):3241–53.
28. Sun F, Ong R, Burnette D. The influence of ethnicity and culture on dementia caregiving: a review of empirical studies on Chinese Americans. Am J Alzheimers Dis Other Dement. 2012;27(1):13–22.
29. Sauerbier A, Aris A, Lim EW, Bhattacharya K, Ray Chaudhuri K. Impact of ethnicity on the natural history of Parkinson disease. Med J Aust. 2018;208(9):410–4.
30. Speck P. Culture and spirituality: essential components of palliative care. Postgrad Med J. 2016;92(1088):341–5.
31. Murray KE, Buul A, Aden R, Cavanaugh AM, Kidane L, Hussein M, Eastman A, Checkoway H. Occupational health risks and intervention strategies for US taxi drivers. Health Promot Int. 2019;34(2):323–32.
32. Wang XL. Disease culture and literary representation—the case of black death in medieval Europe. J Sichuan Univ (Philos Soc Sci Ed). 2020;03:27–33.
33. Gulcebi MI, Bartolini E, Lee O, Lisgaras CP, Onat F, Mifsud J, Striano P, Vezzani A, Hildebrand MS, Jimenez-Jimenez D, Junck L, Lewis-Smith D, Scheffer IE, Thijs RD, Zuberi SM, Blenkinsop S, Fowler HJ, Foley A, Epilepsy Climate Change Consortium, Sisodiya SM. Climate change and epilepsy: insights from clinical and basic science studies. Epilepsy Behav. 2021;116:107791.
34. Tuft M, Nakken KO, Kverndokk K. Traditional folk beliefs on epilepsy in Norway and Sweden. Epilepsy Behav. 2017;71:104–7.
35. Mbelesso P, Luna J, Yangatimbi E, Mboukou C, Preux PM. Sociocultural representations of epilepsy in the Central African Republic: a door-to-door survey. Seizure. 2019;67:23–6.
36. Lee MH, Kim Y, Cho SH. Review on diagnostic criteria of neurasthenia: suggesting pathway of culture-bound diseases. J Pharmacopuncture. 2017;20(4):230–4.
37. Paralikar V, Agashe M, Sarmukaddam S, Deshpande S, Goyal V, Weiss MG. Cultural epidemiology of neurasthenia spectrum disorders in four general hospital outpatient clinics of urban Pune, India. Transcult Psychiatry. 2011;48(3):257–83.
38. Das-Munshi J, Chang CK, Schofield P, Stewart R, Prince MJ. Depression and cause-specific mortality in an ethnically diverse cohort from the UK: 8-year prospective study. Psychol Med. 2019;49(10):1639–51.
39. Weissman MM, Bland RC, Canino GJ, Faravelli C, Greenwald S, Hwu HG, Joyce PR, Karam EG, Lee CK, Lellouch J, Lépine JP, Newman SC, Rubio-Stipec M, Wells JE, Wickramaratne PJ, Wittchen H, Yeh EK. Cross-national epidemiology of major depression and bipolar disorder. JAMA. 1996;276(4):293–9.
40. Jobson L, Miskon N, Dalgleish T, Hitchcock C, Hill E, Golden AM, Zulkefly NS, Mukhtar F. Impact of culture on autobiographical life structure in depression. Br J Clin Psychol. 2018;57(3):382–96.
41. Xiang YT, Wang G, Guo T, Hu C, Ungvari GS, Kilbourne AM, Lai KY, Wong SY, Si TM, Zheng QW,

Chen DF, Fang YR, Lu Z, Yang HC, Hu J, Chen ZY, Huang Y, Sun J, Wang XP, Li HC, Zhang JB, Chiu HF. Gender differences in demographic and clinical features and prescribing patterns of psychotropic medications in patients with major depressive disorder in China. Compr Psychiatry. 2013;54(8):1198–202.
42. Kessler RC, Berglund P, Demler O, Jin R, Koretz D, Merikangas KR, Rush AJ, Walters EE, Wang PS, Replication NCS. The epidemiology of major depressive disorder: results from the National Comorbidity Survey Replication (NCS-R). JAMA. 2003;289(23):3095–105.
43. Han C, Pae CU. Do we need to consider ethnocultural variation in the use of atypical antipsychotics for Asian patients with major depressive disorder? CNS Drugs. 2013;27:S47–51.
44. Xing XH. Cultural differences in the development of concepts of neurasthenia and depression. Electron J Clin Med Lit. 2018;5(71):195.
45. Widiana HS, Simpson K, Manderson L. Cultural expressions of depression and the development of the Indonesian depression checklist. Transcult Psychiatry. 2018;55(3):339–60.
46. Atkins R, Gage G, Kelly TA, Joseph PV, Johnson S, Ojo K, Williams W. Exploring expressions of depression in black single mothers. Issues Ment Health Nurs. 2018;39(11):935–45.
47. Mao YM, Wu J, Pan HF, Fan YG, Ye DQ. The patriotic health movement is a great pioneering work of public health in new China and an important support for an all-round well-off. Chin J Dis Control Prev. 2020;24(10):1120–3.
48. Wang L, Wang Z, Ma Q, Fang G, Yang J. The development and reform of public health in China from 1949 to 2019. Glob Health. 2019;15(1):45.
49. China NBoSo. China statistical yearbook 1981. Beijing: China Statistics Press; 1982.
50. Zhang SN, Liu ZB, Gu ZW. Disease control and prevention in China in the 20th century and prospects for the new millennium. Environ Health Prev Med. 2002;7(3):132–7.
51. Li YS, Cai KP. Epidemiological trends and challenges of schistosomiasis in China. Chin J Epidemiol. 2004;07:7–8.
52. Dai SM, Xu ZM, Zhang LJ, Xu J, Lv S. Analysis of schistosomiasis cases report in National Notifiable Disease Report System in China, 2015-2017. Chin J Schistosomiasis Control. 2019;31(2):121–5.
53. Wang RT. Critical health literacy: a case study from China in schistosomiasis control. Health Promot Int. 2000;null(3):269-274(266).
54. Guan Z, Dai SM, Zhou J, Ren XB, Qin ZQ, Li YL, Lv S, Li SZ, Zhou XN, Xu J. Assessment of knowledge, attitude and practices and the analysis of risk factors regarding schistosomiasis among fishermen and boatmen in the Dongting Lake Basin, the People's Republic of China. Parasit Vectors. 2020;13(1):273.
55. Yang Y, Zhou YB, Pan X, Song XX, Jiang Q. Comparative analysis of epidemiological situation and strategies to control schistosomiasis between China and African countries. Zhongguo Xue Xi Chong Bing Fang Zhi Za Zhi. 2015;27(03):328–31.
56. Zhou XN, Xu J, Lv S, Li SZ. Progress of the national programme and achievements of scientific researches on schistosomiasis elimination in China. Chin J Dis Control Prev. 2019;23(07):749–53.
57. Lv S, Xu J, Cao CL, Zhang LJ, Li SZ, Zhou XN. China fighting against schistosomiasis for 70 years: progress and experience. Chin J Parasitol Parasit Dis. 2019;37(05):514–9.
58. Deng WC, Li YS, Cheng XH, Ren GH, He HB, Zhou YB, Zhang YY, Hu BJ, Liu HQ, Lu SK, Li SM, XN. Z. Implications, spiritual characteristics and practical significance of Chinese schistosomiasis control culture. Zhongguo Xue Xi Chong Bing Fang Zhi Za Zhi. 2020;32(3):222–4.
59. Glatter KA, Finkelman P. History of the plague: an ancient pandemic for the age of COVID-19. Am J Med. 2021;134(2):176–81.
60. Mao YM, Wu J, Pan HF, Ye DQ. Practice with erudition patriotism with sincerity: in memory of Wu Lien Teh: a plague fighter and pioneer of public health in China. Chin J Dis Control Prev. 2019;23(08):1021–4.
61. Balasubramanian D, Murcia S, Ogbunugafor CB, Gavilan R, Almagro-Moreno S. Cholera dynamics: lessons from an epidemic. J Med Microbiol. 2021;70(2):undefined.
62. Dan L. Seeing the number of Chinese cholera popularity from Fang Zhi - a modern significance of the first big popularity of cholera. J Chin Hist Geogr. 2017;32(01):146–58.
63. Pezzoli L. Oral cholera vaccine working group of the global task force on cholera control. Global oral cholera vaccine use, 2013-2018. Vaccine. 2020;2020:A132–40.
64. Tang XF, Liu LG, Ma HL, Zhu BP, Hao CX, Wu XY, Fei N, Zhu XP, Zhang LJ. Outbreak of cholera associated with consumption of soft-shelled turtles, Sichuan province, China, 2009. Zhonghua Liu Xing Bing Xue Za Zhi. 2009;31(9):1050–2.
65. Zhang J, Chang ZR, Zhong HJ, Wang DC, Xu J, Kan B, Ran L, Wang ZJ. Investigation on status of pollution of vibrio cholera in seafood and aquatic products in 12 provinces of China in 2005. Zhonghua Yu Fang Yi Xue Za Zhi. 2007;41(3):208–11.
66. Deng XL, Li BS, Tan HL, Sun LM, Ke BZ, Ke CW, Wang DC, Kan B, Zhong HJ. The etiologic characteristics of Vibrio cholerae in Guangdong province in 2007. Zhonghua Liu Xing Bing Xue Za Zhi. 2008;29(7):696–9.
67. Lü HK, Chen EF, Xie SY, Chai CL, Wei YD, Mo ST, Ye JL, Luo Y. Investigation on vibrio cholera carried in aquatic products of littoral areas, Zhejiang Province. Zhonghua Yu Fang Yi Xue Za Zhi. 2006;40(5):336–8.
68. Duggan AT, Perdomo MF, Piombino-Mascali D, Marciniak S, Poinar D, Emery MV, Buchmann JP, Duchêne S, Jankauskas R, Humphreys M, Golding GB, Southon J, Devault A, Rouillard JM, Sahl JW, Dutour O, Hedman K, Sajantila A, Smith GL, Holmes EC, Poinar HN. 17 century Variola virus

reveals the recent history of smallpox. Curr Biol. 2016;26(24):3407–12.
69. Xu WM, Wang CC, Jiang LJ, Hu JQ, Gu DL. Enlightenment of the invention and spread of Chinese variolation art on the prevention and treatment of severe infectious diseases with traditional Chinese medicine. Modernization of traditional Chinese medicine and Materia Medica-world. Sci Technol. 2021;23(06):2141–5.
70. Liu DC, Li J. Vaccination campaign in the early of new China. Contemp China Hist Stud. 2016;23(06):69–79.
71. Leonardi F. The definition of health: towards new perspectives. Int J Health Serv. 2018;48(4):735–48.
72. Key terms to understand reform and opening up. Beijing Rev. 2019;62(10):44.
73. Han XP, Sun XJ. Fully implement the healthy China strategy. Frontline. 2018;12:54–7.
74. Tan X, Wu Q, Shao H. Global commitments and China's endeavors to promote health and achieve sustainable development goals. J Health Popul Nutr. 2018;37(1):8.
75. Yue D, Ruan S, Xu J, Zhu W, Zhang L, Cheng G, Meng Q. Impact of the China healthy cities initiative on urban environment. J Urban Health. 2017;94(2):149–57.
76. Goodchild M, Zheng R. Tobacco control and healthy China 2030. Tob Control. 2019;28(4):409–13.
77. Liu ZY, Xiao Y, Zhao K, Liu AZ. Implementation progress and effect of National Essential Public Health Services Program in China. Chin J Public Health. 2019;35(06):657–64.
78. Xiao XH. Study and thought on the safety of traditional Chinese medicines under healthy China strategy. Zhongguo Zhong Yao Za Zhi. 2018;43(5):857–60.
79. Xiao X. Development of traditional Chinese medicine: new era and new strategy. Zhongguo Zhong Yao Za Zhi. 2019;44(18):3837–41.
80. Li R, Cheng X, Schwebel DC, Yang Y, Ning P, Cheng P, Hu G. Disability-adjusted life years associated with population ageing in China, 1990-2017. BMC Geriatr. 2021;21(1):369.
81. Wang LM, Chen ZH, Zhang M, Zhao ZP, Huang ZJ, Zhang X, Li C, Guan YQ, Wang X, Wang ZH, Zhou MG. Study of the prevalence and disease burden of chronic disease in the elderly in China. Zhonghua Liu Xing Bing Xue Za Zhi. 2019;40(3):277–83.
82. Hua J, Zhang L, Gao D, Huang Y, Ning P, Cheng P, Li Y, Hu G. Prevalence of overweight and obesity among people aged 18 years and over between 2013 and 2018 in Hunan, China. Int J Environ Res Public Health. 2020;17(11):4048.
83. Li Y, Wang JL, Zhang XC, Wu J, Liang XF. Retrospect and prospect of healthy lifestyle for all, 2007–2015. Chin J Health Educ. 2016;32(12):1143–5.
84. Zhang M, Wang LM. Epidemic status and prevention strategies of chronic noncommunicable diseases in China. Chin J Front Med Sci. 2016;8(12):1–6.
85. Sun DJ, Gao YH, Liu H. Achievements and prospects of endemic disease prevention and control in China in past 70 years. Chin J Public Health. 2019;35(07):793–6.
86. Sun DJ, Gao YH, Liu H. Effective control and even elimination of endemic diseases in China benefits from the superior socialist system. Chin J Dis Control Prev. 2019;23(07):745–748, 753.
87. Shao J, Zhou L, Yang JB, Gao DL. Research progress of iodine deficiency disease in China. Jiangsu J Prev Med. 2014;25(01):46–8.
88. Shi GQ, Huang WL, Zhang J, Zhao H, Shen T, Fontaine RE, Yang L, Zhao S, Lu BL, Wang YB, Ma L, Li ZX, Gao Y, Yang ZL, Zeng G. Clusters of sudden unexplained death associated with the mushroom, Trogia venenata, in rural Yunnan Province, China. PLoS One. 2012;7(5):e35894.
89. Shan X, Chen Y, Liu K, Zhang S, Yu J, Yin J, Kaji L, Song R, Wang Y, Wang Y, Qing Y, Li S, Yang Z, Zhang H. Health-related quality of life (HRQoL) associated with echinococcosis patients in Tibetan communities in Shiqu County, China: a case-control study. Qual Life Res. 2020;29(6):1559–65.
90. Yang YR, McManus DP, Huang Y, Heath DD. Echinococcus granulosus infection and options for control of cystic echinococcosis in Tibetan communities of Western Sichuan Province, China. PLoS Negl Trop Dis. 2009;3(4):e426.

22 Progress and Perspective of Transmission Dynamics Models in Prevention and Control of Infectious Diseases

Yongyue Wei, Jinxing Guan, Yang Zhao, and Feng Chen

Abstract

The current respiratory infectious disease has expanded over the world, posing a serious threat to people's physical and mental health, as well as their lives. Science and technology immediately united to fight against such deadly infectious disease in the past 100 years. Mathematical models have proved invaluable to understand and help control infectious disease epidemics. By simplifying real world phenomena, these models describe, analyze, and predict disease transmission patterns, producing tractable solutions in the face of quickly changing situations. In this Chapter, we firstly summarized the history and development of the mathematical models in infectious diseases. Afterwards, the specific transmission dynamics models with different model structures used in fitting and forecasting the situation of the current respiratory infectious disease were introduced, aiming different analytical objectives including but not limited to parameter estimation, trend prediction and early warning, prevention and control measures effectiveness evaluation, and transmission uncertainty exploration. Summary in values of transmission dynamics models is followed to illustrate their contribution in understanding and combating infectious disease outbreaks. Despite their utility, however, mathematical models are facing several important challenges which, if ignored, would result in biased estimation of the crucial epidemiological parameters, bad fitting of the data, or misinterpretation of the results. In conclusion, mathematical modeling should be one of the most valuable tools to reflect such huge uncertainties or, on the other hand, warn of the worst situation. An appreciation of models' shortcomings not only clarifies why they cannot do but helps anticipate what they can.

Keywords

COVID-19 pandemic · Transmission dynamics model · SEIR

22.1 Preface

Infectious diseases are diseases caused by pathogenic agents or microorganisms and able to spread person-to-person, animal-to-animal, or animal-to-person. The history of mankind is the history of fighting infectious diseases. In the long history, infectious diseases constructed a grave

Y. Wei · J. Guan · Y. Zhao · F. Chen (✉)
Department of Biostatistics, School of Public Health, Nanjing Medical University, Nanjing, China
e-mail: fengchen@njmu.edu.cn

D.-Q. Ye (ed.), *Progress in China Epidemiology*, https://doi.org/10.1007/978-981-19-2199-5_22

danger to people's lives and well-being; smallpox, plague, cholera, influenza, and so on have brought huge disasters to mankind.

Since the twentieth century, with the invention of vaccines and antibiotics, humans have achieved brilliant success in conquering infectious diseases, eradicating or eliminating smallpox, leprosy, poliomyelitis, diphtheria, whooping cough, tetanus, measles, etc., which have been raging for thousands of years. However, with the development of international trade, the increase of international travel and the changes of environment, some infectious diseases that had been eliminated or controlled (such as venereal tuberculosis, etc.) started to spread again. As a result of environmental pollution and ecological changes, many pathogens mutated and rapidly spread, and virus of a variety of zoonotic infectious diseases mutated rapidly and accelerated transmission to humans, resulting in the uninterruptedly, as well as powerful occurrence of new infectious diseases. In addition, infectious diseases spread faster with the rapid development of traffic, long-distance, and cross-regional communication [1]. In this situation, the researches on prevention and control measures of the pathogenesis and transmission of emerging infectious diseases are timely and long-term effects. The infectious disease epidemiology studies mainly include the following aspects: the etiology of infectious disease, the occurrence and transmission of infectious diseases in a population; the natural and social factors that affect the transmission of infectious disease; preventions and control measures to block the transmission route and protect the susceptible population; and the effectiveness of preventive and control strategies.

Describing and analyzing the changing laws of the amount in the transmission of infectious disease is a key method in transmission dynamics study. Based on the characteristic of infectious disease, such as the occurrence, transmission mechanism, biological factors and social influence, mathematical models could be established. Through qualitative, quantitative analysis and numerical simulation of these models, exploring epidemic laws, predicting the future trend, analyzing the source and the key point of epidemic could be conducted to deeper the understanding of diseases and better prevent and control the transmission.

22.2 Development of Transmission Dynamics Model

It is a huge challenge to predict the epidemic trend of an emerging infectious disease timely, accurately, and reliably. Epidemiologists, statisticians, and public health decision-makers must deal with the uncertainty of poor data quality, limited understanding of diseases, rapid changes in the social environment, and the impact of various interventions.

The earliest mathematical model in infectious disease could be traced back to the eighteenth century. Daniel Bernoulli developed a smallpox model in 1760 to assess the effectivity of variolation of healthy people with the smallpox virus, and, in 1766, he revealed the necessity of smallpox vaccination, which could extend the median life span by 14 years [2]. In the twentieth century, the development of mathematical models in infectious disease had reached a climax. A discrete time model [3] to realize the recurrence of measles epidemics, built by Hamer in 1906, is possibly the first to assume that the product of the susceptible and infective densities determines the incidence. Four years later, Rose formulated differential equation models to study the transmission dynamic of malaria between mosquito and human [4]. The results showed that if the number of mosquitoes was reduced below a critical value, the epidemic of malaria would be controlled. In 1927, Kermack and McKendrick [5] proposed the well-known SIR (susceptible, infectious, and recovered) model, also called KM model, to study the epidemic regularity of bubonic plague in London from 1665 to 1666 and the plague in 1906. The basic SIR model only considers the ideal situation of the three groups of people, that is to say, the susceptible (S), the infectious (I) and the recovered (R) (Fig. 22.1).

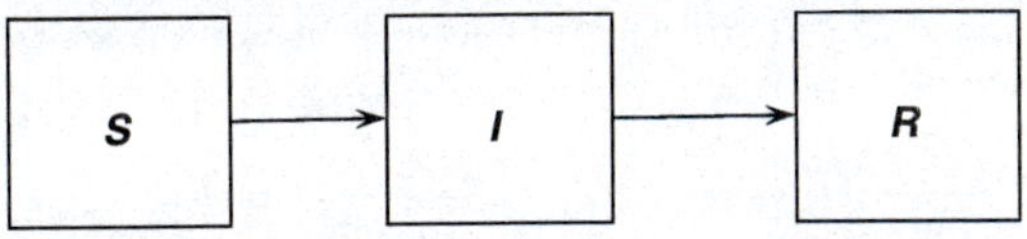

Fig. 22.1 Diagram of SIR transmission dynamics model

The ordinary differential equations of SIR model were as follows:

$$\begin{cases} \frac{dS(t)}{dt} = -\beta I(t)S(t)/N \\ \frac{dI(t)}{dt} = \beta I(t)S(t)/N - \gamma I(t) \\ \frac{dR(t)}{dt} = \gamma I(t) \\ N = S(t) + I(t) + R(t) \end{cases} . \quad (22.1)$$

The basic assumptions of the above model are as follows: (1) People are classified into three groups: susceptible (*S*), infected (*I*), and recovered (*R*); (2) The total population is *N*. *S*(*t*), *I*(*t*), and *R*(*t*) represent the total size of people in category *S*, *I*, or *R* at time *t* respectively, $S(t) + I(t) + R(t) = N$; (3) The number of people infected by a patient in a unit time is relative to the number of healthy people at the time, and the proportional coefficient is β, which is called the transmission rate; (4) It is assumed that the proportion of patients who are cured every day and have immunity to the disease, indicating that they would no longer enter the compartment *S* and are removed, in all infected patients is γ (the cure rate).

Whereafter, in 1932 they proposed SIS (susceptible, infectious, susceptible) model [5]. Based on the two models, they obtained the epidemic threshold theory to identify whether a disease will spread, laying the foundation for the study of transmission dynamics model. With the emergence and development of computers in the mid-twentieth century, mathematical epidemiology seems to have grown exponentially (the first edition of Bailey's book [6], published in 1957, represents a significant milestone). Thus, a wide range of models in different infectious diseases has now been developed, mathematically analyzed, and widely used in infectious diseases.

For the past few years, transmission dynamics model had extremely rapid development. Transmission dynamics model was extended to involve aspects such as the incubation period of the disease (with or without infectiousness), quarantine, stage of infection, immunity (including loss of immunity) of susceptible and infected individuals, age structure, birth, natural death, population migration, immunity of prognostic individuals, vertical transmission, spatial spread, disease vectors and other conditions and have been used in human diseases such as measles, rubella, chickenpox, whooping cough, diphtheria, smallpox, malaria, onchocerciasis, filariasis, rabies, gonorrhea, herpes, syphilis, and HIV/AIDS [2].

In December 2019, the novel respiratory viral infections attacked the world, and soon became the public health emergency worldwide [7]. Up to March 3, 2021, such infectious disease has caused over 114 million confirmed cases and 2.5 million deaths. Scholars and professionals worldwide have proposed a large number of transmission dynamics models to study the laws and trends of the epidemic and evaluate the effect of quarantine and prevention and control measures to provide reference for decision-making departments. Applying the transmission dynamics models correctly can effectively help the prevention and control of emerging infectious diseases.

22.3 Transmission Dynamics Modeling in the Respiratory Infectious Disease

SEIR model was the most used model in the respiratory infectious disease studies. The conventional SEIR model included four compartments (Fig. 22.2): susceptible (*S*), exposed (*E*), infectious (*I*), removed (*R*). Once a susceptible individual exposed to an infected individual effectively, then the transmission happens. The

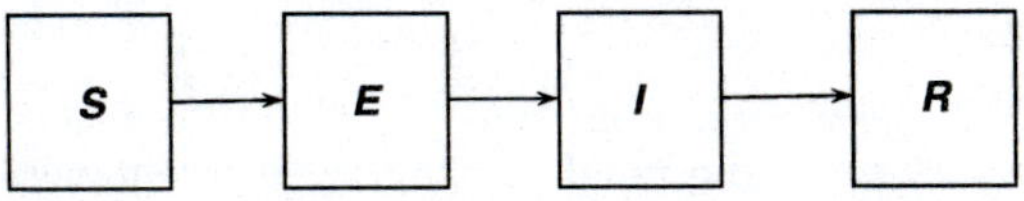

Fig. 22.2 Diagram of SEIR transmission dynamics model

susceptibles enter into the incubation period (class E), during which they are infected while in absent of symptoms. The incubation period is defined as the period from initial exposure to the onset of symptoms.

Dynamics of these compartments across time (t) are described by the following set of ordinary differential equations:

$$\begin{cases} \frac{dS(t)}{dt} = -\beta I(t)S(t)/N \\ \frac{dE(t)}{dt} = \beta I(t)S(t)/N - \alpha E(t) \\ \frac{dI(t)}{dt} = \alpha E(t) - \gamma I(t) \\ \frac{dR(t)}{dt} = \gamma I(t) \\ N = S(t) + E(t) + I(t) + R(t) \end{cases} \quad (22.2)$$

in which β is the transmission rate for infections (defined as the number of people that a case can infect per day); α is equal to 1 divided by the incubation period; the reciprocal of infectious period is γ; and the entire population is denoted by N.

A key parameter in transmission dynamics models is the basic reproductive number (R_0), which is defined as the average number of secondary infections produced when one infected individual is introduced into a host population where everyone is susceptible [2]. An infection can get started in a fully susceptible population if and only $R_0 > 1$. If $R_0 < 1$, the infectious disease will not spread. R_0 of SEIR model is calculated by the following equation:

$$R_0 = \frac{\beta}{\gamma}. \quad (22.3)$$

22.3.1 Model Instances Fitting the Current Respiratory Infectious Disease Dynamics in China

With increasing knowledge of the current respiratory virus and rapidly changing interventions, simple SIR/SEIR mode could not properly describe epidemiologic characteristics and biologic features. Previous studies had developed a series of models with different extensions. Models could be divided into three types: compartment extension, parameter extension, and metapopulation extension. In this section, we will introduce essential structures of different extension models and in next section, we will illustrate the application of these models (Table 22.1).

Table 22.1 Extensions of the transmission dynamics model

Type of extension	Extending
Compartment extension	Asymptomatic
	Unascertained
	Presymptomatic
	Disease severity stage
	Hospitalized
	Quarantine
Parameter extension	Effect indicator for control measures
	Time-varying transmission rate
	Relative transmission rate of E/A vs. I
	Population flow
Population-stratified model	Age structure
	Geographical unit

22.3.1.1 SEIR Model with Extended Compartments

To achieve different purposes and better describe the epidemic, studies extended the SIR/SEIR model with various compartments. Compartment extension included the following parts: presymptomatic individuals, asymptomatic individuals, unascertained individuals, disease severity stage, hospitalized process, quarantine, and so on.

Previous studies had revealed the infectiousness of asymptomatic [8–10] and presymptomatic [11] cases. Thus, to better depict the epidemic picture, some studies developed modified SEIR/SIR model with an additional compartment representing asymptomatic cases (A), abbreviated to

SEIAR, or presymptomatic cases (P), abbreviated to SEPIR (Fig. 22.3).

In SEIAR model, infected individuals in incubation period would enter the infected compartment at proportion σ and others, who have no symptoms till recovery, would enter the asymptomatic compartment.

Using SEIARD model, SEIAR model with additional death compartment, incorporating mobility data in Wuhan before January 30, 2020, Li et al. estimated that the ratio of asymptomatic to symptomatic infections and simulated scenarios where Wuhan travel restrictions were delayed by 3, 5, and 7 days, respectively [12].

Similar to SEIAR model, another model extended SEIR model with an additional compartment of unascertained cases (U) owing to mild, limited, or lack of symptoms, to explore how many cases were unascertained possibly on account of deficient nucleic testing capacity (Fig. 22.4).

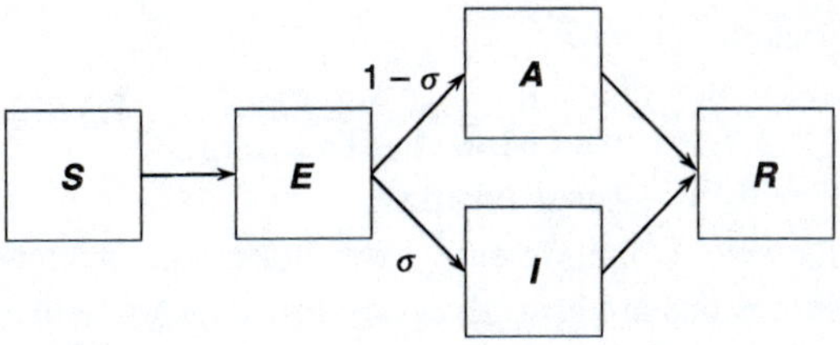

Fig. 22.3 Diagram of SEAIR model

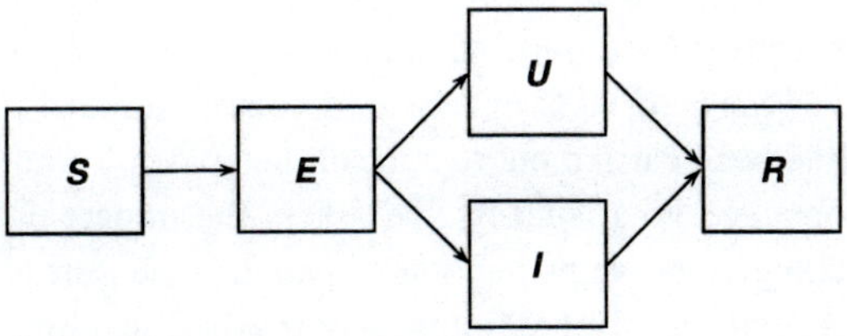

Fig. 22.4 Diagram of SEIRU model

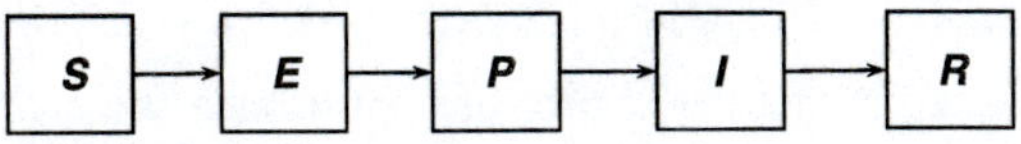

Fig. 22.5 Diagram of SEPIR model

In SEPIR model, the infected individuals in incubation period are divided into two compartments: exposed compartment (E), exposed but without infectiousness, and presymptomatic compartment, exposed and with infectiousness (Fig. 22.5).

These two categories of infection, A and P, have separate rates of transmission compared with infection with symptoms, I. β, the transmission rate due to infected and symptomatic individuals; and $\mu\beta$, the transmission rate due to asymptomatic individuals and presymptomatic individuals, which is β by a factor μ. The related transmission factor, μ, will be discussed in next section.

Another extension of compartment is disease severity stage. The infection, I in SEIR model, is divided into three compartments due to disease severity: infected individuals with mild symptoms (I_{mild}), infected individuals with severe symptoms (I_{severe}) and infected individuals with critical symptoms (I_{critical}) (Fig. 22.6).

The rapidly increasing number of infections would cause heavy burden to health care system. To quantize the burden of health care system, a series of models considering the hospitalized, ICU patients and so on had been constructed. In these models, the exposed individuals would

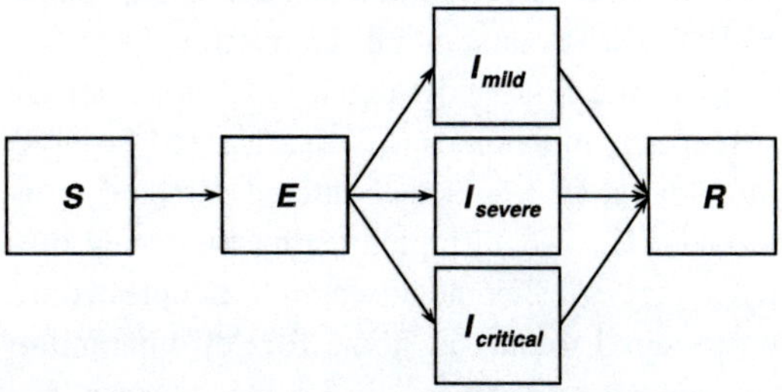

Fig. 22.6 Diagram of SEIR model with severity compartments

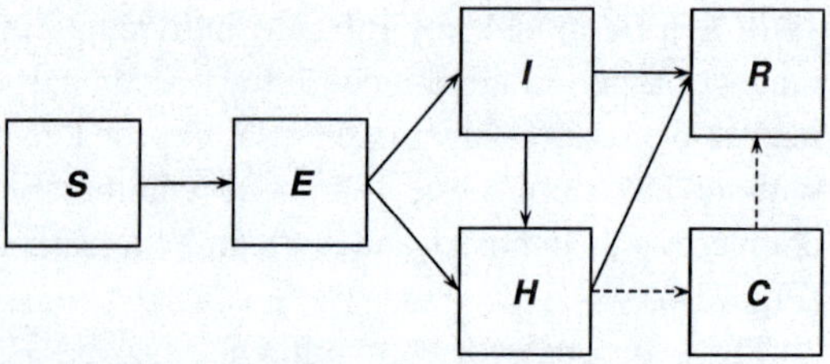

Fig. 22.7 Diagram of SEIRHC model

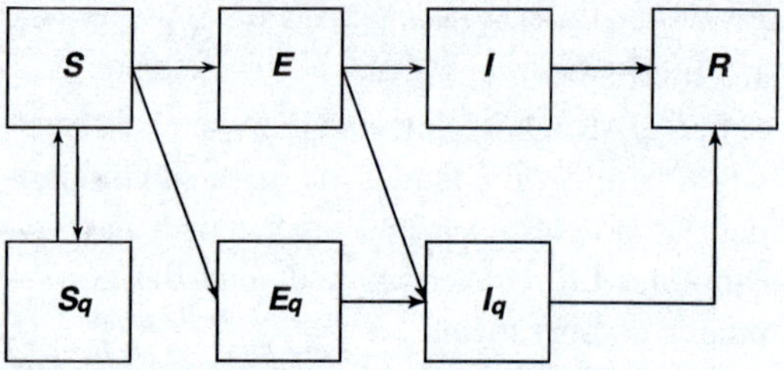

Fig. 22.8 Diagram of SEIR^{+Q} model with severity compartments

enter compartment H if they have symptoms and need emerging health care, even to be sent to intensive care unit (ICU), they would enter compartment H, while others, with no/mild symptom, would enter compartment I and recover naturally (Fig. 22.7).

By SEIR model incorporating hospitalized and ICU patients, hospitalized data up to May 3, 2020, a platform for short-term forecasting was constructed in Switzerland and predicted that the need for ICU beds could be 761 (95% CI 541–1164) by May 6, 2020 [13].

At the beginning of epidemic, the number of infections would have an exponential increase without any intervention and control measures. To flatten the epidemic curve, plenty of nonpharmaceutical interventions (NPIs), especially social distance strategies, had been implemented. Considering the implementation of quarantine strategies, models with quarantine compartments were constructed. Modified SEIR models, named SEIR^{+Q}, with quarantine compartments often contain the following extensions: quarantined susceptible individuals (S_q), quarantined exposed individuals (E_q), and quarantined infected individuals (I_q). When implementing the social distance strategies, some susceptible people would be required to stay at home for self-quarantine and enter compartment S_q. Besides, susceptible individuals who had contacted with infections and being tracked would be quarantined, E_q, and then become symptomatic, I_q, while some are not quarantined, E (Fig. 22.8).

Using SEIR^{+Q} model, Wei et al. estimated that nearly 40% of the total infections was unconfirmed and predicted that on May 31, the daily new cases in Wuhan would reduce to 0. Besides, comprehensive interventions and control measures implemented in Wuhan had reduced 19,951 cases by March 30 [14].

To achieve different purposes considering different factors, there are also models similar to SEIR^{+Q} developed. For instance, to study the effect of kinds of wearing masks, researchers extended SEIR model with a series of compartments representing individuals with face masks, S_u, E_u, and I_u. Furthermore, to explore the possible impact of vaccination, models are extended with a compartment, S_v similar to S_q, representing individuals vaccinated. With different assumptions, these models could explore the possible epidemic trend in the future.

22.3.1.2 SEIR Model with Specific Parameters

Except compartment extensions, parameter extensions are also necessary to characterize the epidemic in the modeling studies. In this section, we will introduce four types of parameter extensions: effect indicator for control measures, time-varying transmission rate, relative transmission rate of compartment E/A compared with compartment I and population flow.

Plenty of interventions and control strategies had been carried out to control the epidemic and obtained great success. To assess the impact of comprehensive prevention and control measures, an indicator for control measures was added into the equations.

$$\frac{dS}{dt} = -w\beta IS / N \tag{22.4}$$

w represents the impact of control measures on transmission rate. For example, Wei et al. developed SEIR model with an additional w parameter and incorporating onset data before June 11 in Beijing, which estimated that comprehensive control measures taken in Beijing for preventing the second outbreak had reduced 95% transmission ($w = 0.95$) and avoided 99% infections [15].

Similarly, considering the impact of other indicators, such as meteorological factors and the increase of health consciousness, on transmission, other studies set transmission rate as a continuous time-varying variable or a discrete variable.

$$\frac{dS}{dt} = -\beta(t) IS/N. \quad (22.5)$$

Considering the effect of environmental temperature on transmission, Shi et al. constructed a modified SEIR model to estimate a time-varying parameter for transmission rate [$\beta(t)$] [16].

As mentioned in last section, infected individuals in incubation period had been proved infectious, and studies extended SEIR model with compartment *A*/*P*. These studies, considering the transmission of the exposed (*E*), the presymptomatic (*P*) or the asymptomatic (*A*), added a transmissibility factor in Eq. (22.6), the ratio of the transmission rate of infections to that of asymptomatic cases/presymptomatic cases/incubation population. In SEIR model, the transmission from *S* to *I* was described by the following equation:

$$\frac{dS}{dt} = -\beta(I + \varepsilon E) S/N. \quad (22.6)$$

For instance, assuming different contact rate, Hou et al. used SEIR model setting 7 days as the incubation period and $\varepsilon = 0.5$ to investigate possible effect of quarantine and isolation interventions on disease transmission [17].

In SEIR model with the additional compartment of asymptomatic individuals, the transmission was described by the following equation:

$$\frac{dS}{dt} = -\beta(I + \varepsilon E + \varepsilon A) S/N. \quad (22.7)$$

If a presymptomatic compartment was added, compartment *E* was assumed not infectious, and the transmission was shown as follows:

$$\frac{dS}{dt} = -\beta(I + \varepsilon P + \varepsilon A) S/N, \quad (22.8)$$

where ε represent the relative transmissibility factor, and often set as 0.55, according to previous studies [18, 19].

Due to inflow and outflow population, the total population in the modeling system is changing. Thus, a series of studies incorporated population movement or migration data in the model. SEIR Models considering population flow are described by the following equations:

$$\begin{cases} \dfrac{dS(t)}{dt} = -\beta I(t) S(t)/N + S_{\text{in}}(t) - S_{\text{out}}(t) \\ \dfrac{dE(t)}{dt} = \beta I(t) S(t)/N - \alpha E(t) + E_{\text{in}}(t) - E_{\text{out}}(t) \\ \dfrac{dI(t)}{dt} = \alpha E(t) - \gamma I(t) \\ \dfrac{dR(t)}{dt} = \gamma I(t) \\ N = S(t) + E(t) + I(t) + R(t) + S_{\text{in}}(t) - S_{\text{out}}(t) + E_{\text{in}}(t) - E_{\text{out}}(t) \end{cases}, \quad (22.9)$$

where $S_{\text{in}}(t)$ and $E_{\text{in}}(t)$ represent the inflow susceptible individuals and exposed individuals, while $S_{\text{out}}(t)$ and $E_{\text{out}}(t)$ represent the outflow individuals. In this model, we assume that the infected and symptomatic individuals, *I*, would be isolated once they become symptomatic and could not migrate.

Yang et al. developed a similar SEIR model incorporating confirmed data before February 9,

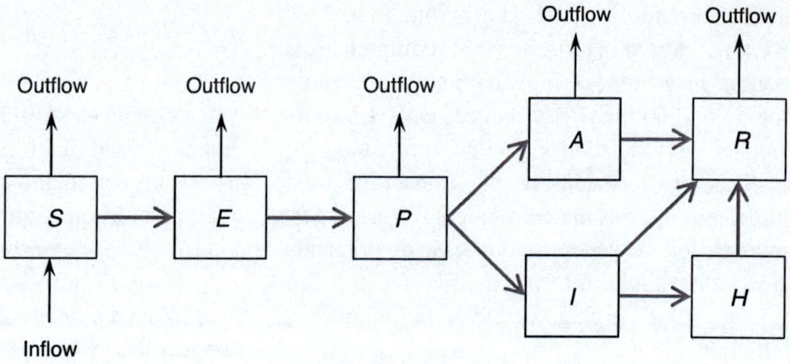

Fig. 22.9 Diagram of SAPHIRE model

2020, population flow, and setting 7 days as the incubation period, which predicted 42,792 (62,031 actually) individuals would be infected in Hubei province as of February 20 and, by late April, cumulated infections would reach 59,578 (68,128 actually) [20].

22.3.1.3 Mathematical Model with Stratified Populations

In the recent pandemic, individuals are not unmovable but could move from one place to another, enhancing the spread of the virus all over the world. Although simple compartment model, SIR/SEIR model and their extensions, can be applied in small communities or cities, but it is not suitable at large spatial scales and cannot account for population heterogeneity and interaction between metapopulations via mixing/commuting [21]. As a result, metapopulation models were formulated, which divide the population into smaller groups depending on the geographic location or age structure. Here, we introduce a type of metapopulation model divided by geographic location. The ordinary differential equations of this metapopulation model were shown as follows:

$$\begin{cases} \dfrac{dS_i(t)}{dt} = -\beta I_i(t) S_i(t)/N_i(t) + \sum\limits_{j=1,i\neq j}^{n} M_{ji}(t)\dfrac{S_j(t)}{N_j(t)-I_j(t)} - \sum\limits_{j=1,i\neq j}^{n} M_{ij}(t)\dfrac{S_i(t)}{N_i(t)-I_i(t)} \\ \dfrac{dE_i(t)}{dt} = \beta I_i(t) S_i(t)/N_i(t) - \alpha E_i(t) + \sum\limits_{j=1,i\neq j}^{n} M_{ji}(t)\dfrac{E_j(t)}{N_j(t)-I_j(t)} - \sum\limits_{j=1,i\neq j}^{n} M_{ij}\dfrac{E_i(t)}{N_i(t)-I_i(t)} \\ \dfrac{dI_i(t)}{dt} = \alpha E_i(t) - \gamma I_i(t) \\ \dfrac{dR_i(t)}{dt} = \gamma I_i(t) + \sum\limits_{j=1,i\neq j}^{n} M_{ji}(t)\dfrac{R_j(t)}{N_j(t)-I_j(t)} - \sum\limits_{j=1,i\neq j}^{n} M_{ij}(t)\dfrac{R_i(t)}{N_i(t)-I_i(t)} \\ N_i(t) = S_i(t) + E_i(t) + I_i(t) + R_i(t) + \sum\limits_{j=1,i\neq j}^{n} M_{ji}(t) - \sum\limits_{j=1,i\neq j}^{n} M_{ij} \end{cases} \quad (22.10)$$

For notational convenience, the compartments are now labelled by a subscript, i.e., $S_i(t)$, $E_i(t)$, $I_i(t)$, and $R_i(t)$, to denote the number of individuals belonging to the respective compartments of city i at time t. $M_{ji}(t)$ represents the number of individuals moving from city j to i at time t and vice versa. In this model, we assume the infected individuals with symptoms are isolated.

In actual modeling, the above extensions are not singly used, and studies often developed combinations of different extensions to better describe the epidemic. For this purpose, Hao et al. reconstructed the full transmission dynamics of the recent pandemic in Wuhan, named SAPHIRE model, incorporating compartments for presymptomatic infections, unascertained infections--asymptomatic or mildly symptomatic individuals, and hospitalized individuals transmission for the presymptomatic and the unascertained (22.8), and population flow, a combination of five above extensions (Fig. 22.9) [19].

The ordinary differential equations of SAPHIRE model are as follows:

$$\begin{cases} \frac{dS}{dt} = n - \frac{\beta S(\alpha P + \alpha A + I)}{N} - \frac{nS}{N} \\ \frac{dE}{dt} = \frac{\beta S(\alpha P + \alpha A + I)}{N} - \frac{E}{D_e} - \frac{nE}{N} \\ \frac{dP}{dt} = \frac{E}{D_e} - \frac{P}{D_P} - \frac{nP}{N} \\ \frac{dA}{dt} = \frac{(1-r)P}{D_P} - \frac{A}{D_I} - \frac{nA}{N} \\ \frac{dI}{dt} = \frac{rP}{D_P} - \frac{I}{D_I} - \frac{I}{D_q} \\ \frac{dH}{dt} = \frac{I}{D_q} - \frac{H}{D_H} \\ \frac{dR}{dt} = \frac{A+I}{D_I} + \frac{H}{D_H} - \frac{nR}{N} \end{cases}, \quad (22.11)$$

where β is the transmission rate for ascertained cases; α is the ratio of the transmission rate of unascertained cases to that of ascertained cases, set as 0.55; r is ascertainment rate; D_e is the latent period, set as 2.9 days; D_p is the presymptomatic infectious period, assumed as 2.3 days; D_i is the symptomatic infectious period, set as 2.9 days; D_q is the duration from illness onset to isolation; and D_h is the isolation period in hospital, set as 30 days.

According to Hao's study, the basic reproductive number (R_0) is 3.54 (95%CI: 3.40–3.67), much higher than that of SARS and MERS, and 87% of the infections in Wuhan before March 8, 2020, were unascertained (individuals who are asymptomatic or mildly symptomatic may be included.). Besides, the multipronged control policies taken in Wuhan had decreased the effective reproductive number (R_t) to 0.28 (95%CI: 0.23–0.33) and reduced 96% total infections as of March 8, 2020.

In this section, we listed several types of extending transmission dynamics models and gave a brief introduction for each extension. Nobody knows for sure which model is the best, and it depends on what you want to achieve through modeling.

22.3.2 Objectives of Transmission Dynamics Models

Being aware of the early transmission dynamics and judging the impact of control measures play a vital role in preventing the epidemic [22]. Transmission dynamics models, which can allow people to make more accurate predictions, determine and evaluate control strategies due to acquiring a better knowledge of transmission mechanisms and the most influential factors in COVID-19 spread, had been widely used and obtained great success [2]. In this section, we will illustrate the application of transmission dynamics model for the current respiratory infections from four aspects by examples: epidemiological parameter estimation, trend prediction, prevention and control measures evaluation and exploring possibility.

22.3.2.1 Epidemiological Parameters Estimation

At the beginning of the epidemic, our knowledge of this virus and the epidemic is limited. In this period, main purpose of the models is exploring the epidemiological characteristics and estimating relative parameters.

Published on January 31, 2020, Wu et al. used SEIR model incorporating limited actual data before Jan 25, 2020, population flow, and a set of empirical/theoretical parameters, which estimated 75,815 individuals that had been infected in Greater Wuhan as of Jan 25, 2020, and warned that cities including Chongqing, Beijing, Shanghai, Guangzhou, and Shenzhen had imported hundreds of infections from Wuhan before Wuhan lockdown [23]. The ordinary differential equations are as follows:

$$\begin{cases} \frac{dS(t)}{dt} = -\frac{S(t)}{N}\left(\frac{R_0}{D_I} I(t) + z(t)\right) + L_{I,W} + L_{C,W}(t) - \left(\frac{L_{W,I}}{N} + \frac{L_{W,C}(t)}{N}\right) S(t) \\ \frac{dE(t)}{dt} = \frac{S(t)}{N}\left(\frac{R_0}{D_I} I(t) + z(t)\right) - \frac{E(t)}{D_E} - \left(\frac{L_{W,I}}{N} + \frac{L_{W,C}(t)}{N}\right) E(t) \\ \frac{dI(t)}{dt} = \frac{E(t)}{D_E} - \frac{I(t)}{D_I} - \left(\frac{L_{W,I}}{N} + \frac{L_{W,C}(t)}{N}\right) I(t) \end{cases}, \quad (22.12)$$

where $S(t)$, $E(t)$, $I(t)$, and $R(t)$ were the number of susceptible, latent, infectious, and removed individuals at time t; D_E and D_I were the mean latent (assumed to be the same as incubation of SARS-CoV and MERS-CoV, 6 days [24]) and infectious period (equal to the serial interval minus the mean latent period,8.4 days − 6 days = 2.4 days [24]); $L_{W,I}$ is the daily average number of international outbound air passengers from Wuhan, while $L_{I,W}$ is that of international inbound air passengers; $L_{W,C}$ is the daily number of all domestic outbound travelers from Wuhan and $L_{C,W}$ is that of all domestic inbound travelers; R_0 was the basic reproductive number; $z(t)$ was the zoonotic force of infection equal to 86 cases per day in the baseline scenario before market closure on Jan 1, 2020, and equal to 0 thereafter. In this study, R_0 was estimated as 2.68 (95% CI: 2.47–2.86) by Markov Chain Monte Carlo (MCMC) methods with Gibbs sampling and non-informative flat prior.

Besides, in the early dynamics, the infectiousness of asymptomatic or mild symptomatic cases had been proved [25–27] but the contagiousness and proportion of these infections in China and how they would contribute to the spread remains unclear. Thus, Li et al. simulated the spatiotemporal dynamics of infections among 375 Chinese cities by a metapopulation model, using the data from one of the world's largest social media and technology businesses named Tencent [18], with the following equations:

$$\begin{cases} \frac{dS_i}{dt} = -\frac{\beta I_i^r S_i}{N_i} - \frac{\mu\beta I_i^u S_i}{N_i} + \theta \sum_{j=1, i\neq j}^{n} M_{ij} \frac{S_j}{N_j - I_j^r} - \theta \sum_{j=1, i\neq j}^{n} M_{ji} \frac{S_i}{N_i - I_i^r} \\ \frac{dE_i}{dt} = \frac{\beta I_i^r S_i}{N_i} + \frac{\mu\beta I_i^u S_i}{N_i} - \frac{E_i}{Z} + \theta \sum_{j=1, i\neq j}^{n} M_{ij} \frac{E_j}{N_j - I_j^r} - \theta \sum_{j=1, i\neq j}^{n} M_{ji} \frac{E_i}{N_i - I_i^r} \\ \frac{dI_i^r}{dt} = \alpha \frac{E_i}{Z} - \frac{I_i^r}{D} \\ \frac{dI_i^u}{dt} = (1-\alpha)\frac{E_i}{Z} - \frac{I_i^u}{D} + \theta \sum_{j=1, i\neq j}^{n} M_{ij} \frac{I_j^u}{N_j - I_j^r} - \theta \sum_{j=1, i\neq j}^{n} M_{ji} \frac{I_i^u}{N_i - I_i^r} \\ N_i = N_i + \theta \sum_{j=1, i\neq j}^{n} M_{ij} - \theta \sum_{j=1, i\neq j}^{n} M_{ji} \end{cases}, \quad (22.13)$$

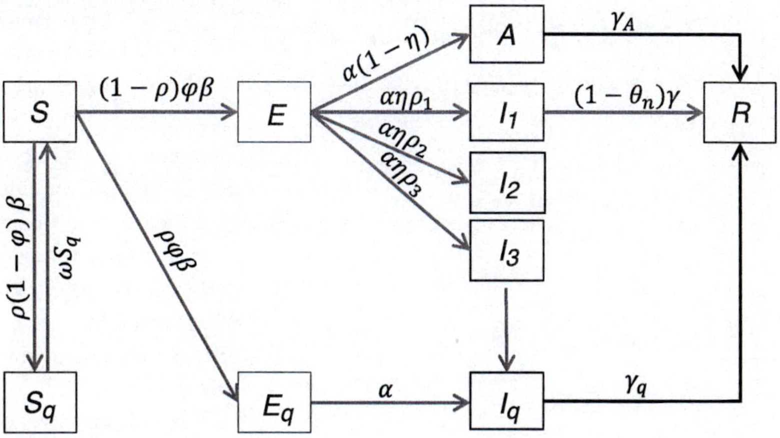

Fig. 22.10 Diagram of SEIR^{+CAQ} model

where S_i, E_i, I_i^r, I_i^u and N_i are the susceptible, exposed, documented infected, undocumented infected and total population in city i. In this model, patients with symptoms severe enough to be confirmed are defined as documented infected individuals, I_i^r, whereas other infected persons are defined as undocumented infected individuals, I_i^u. β represents the transmission rate due to documented infected individuals. The relative transmission rate due to undocumented individuals is reduced by a factor μ. In addition, α is the fraction of documented infections, Z is the average latency period and D is the average duration of infection. The effective reproduction number (R_e) is calculated as $R_e = \alpha\beta D + (1 - \alpha)\mu\beta D$. M_{ij} represents the daily number of people traveling from city j to city i, and θ, greater than 1, reflect underreporting of human movement. Individuals in the compartment I_i^r are assumed do not move between cities.

This model is a combination of unascertained extension, relative transmission rate extension and metapopulation we mentioned above. According to this study, R_e, equivalent to the basic reproductive number, R_0, at the beginning of the epidemic, is 2.38 (95%CI: 2.03–2.77) and undocumented infections, source of 79% of the documented cases, had 55% transmission rate compared with documented infections (95% CI: 46–62%). Besides, the median estimates for the latency and infectious periods are 3.69 and 3.47 days, respectively, and only 14% (95% CI: 10–18%) of total infections in China were reported during 10–23 January, 2020. These findings contribute to explain the rapid spread of the current pandemic around the world.

Except above two, transmission dynamics models are also widely used to estimate the doubling time of infections, reporting rate, mortality and explore the possibility of new outbreaks in a city.

22.3.2.2 Dynamic Trend Prediction

With the increasing knowledge and more data, transmission dynamics models could be refined to fit the data to forecast epidemic trends in the future, such as the peak time and size, hospitalization needs, the number of deaths, and so on. Trend prediction is one of the main objectives of dynamic models, providing reference for the prevention and control measures [28]. Here, we will illustrate the application of dynamic model in prediction through a case of complex model.

Wei et al. [28] modeled the cumulated confirmed cases in three divided regions, Wuhan, Hubei except Wuhan and China except Hubei, up to February 12 by SEIR^{+CAQ} (SEIR with Infected severity stages, Asymptomatic infected and Quarantined individuals) (Fig. 22.10). The ordinary differential equations are as follow:

$$\begin{cases} \frac{dS}{dt} = -(1-\rho)\beta\varphi(\varepsilon E+I+A)S - \rho\beta(1-\varphi) \\ (\varepsilon E+I+A)S - \rho\beta\varphi(\varepsilon E+I+A)S + \omega S_q \\ \frac{dE}{dt} = (1-\rho)\beta\varphi(\varepsilon E+I+A)S - \alpha E \\ \frac{dA}{dt} = \alpha(1-\eta)E - \gamma_A A \\ \frac{dI_1}{dt} = \alpha\eta\rho_1 E - \gamma I_1 \\ \frac{dI_2}{dt} = \alpha\eta\rho_2 E - \gamma I_2 \\ \frac{dI_3}{dt} = \alpha\eta\rho_3 E - \gamma I_3 \\ \frac{dR}{dt} = \gamma_A A + (1-\theta_1)\gamma I_1 + (1-\theta_2)\gamma I_2 + \\ (1-\theta_3)\gamma I_3 \\ \frac{dS_q}{dt} = \rho\beta\varphi(\varepsilon E+I+A)S - \omega S_q \\ \frac{dE_q}{dt} = \rho\beta(1-\varphi)(\varepsilon E+I+A)S - \alpha E_q \\ \frac{dI_q}{dt} = \alpha E_q + \theta_1\gamma I_1 + \theta_2\gamma I_2 + \theta_3\gamma I_3 - \gamma_q I_q \\ 1 = \rho_1 + \rho_2 + \rho_3 \\ I = I_1 + I_2 + I_3 \end{cases} , \quad (22.14)$$

where A represents the asymptomatic infections; I_1, I_2, I_3 are, respectively, the infections with mild symptom, severe symptom and critical symptom; S_q, E_q, I_q are susceptible individuals, exposed individuals and infected individuals who are quarantined; ρ represents quarantine rate; $1/\omega$ is the quarantine period; φ is the proportion of susceptible individuals contact with infections and will become infected; ε represents the relative transmission rate mentioned above; $1 - \eta$ is the proportion of asymptomatic infections; ρ_1, ρ_2, ρ_3 are the proportions of mild, severe, and critical infections; γ, γ_A, γ_q are reciprocals of treatment periods; θ_1, θ_2, θ_3 are quarantine rate of mild, severe, and critical infections.

The results showed that the pandemic in China except Hubei and Hubei except Wuhan had reached the peak on February 1 or February 2 and the peak time of Wuhan was February 9. The study predicted that under the current strength of prevention and control, there would be 80,417 (79,215 in actual) confirmed cases in China up to February 29.

22.3.2.3 Effectiveness Evaluation for Prevention and Control Measures

A series of public health (nonpharmaceutical) interventions could be applied to control the epidemic but how the interventions strategies influence the transmission should be investigated. The main purpose of transmission dynamics model is to assess the poorly understood efficacy of non-pharmaceutical interventions, such as travel restrictions, social measures, in preventing the spread of infection.

The Wuhan travel ban, which looks to be the absolute maximum attempted cordon sanitaire in human history, enacted on January 23, 2020, forbade every transportation in and out of Wuhan city, in attempt to prevent further spread. Later, Level 1 response was implemented all over China [29]. To evaluate the effect of transmission control measures at early pandemic in China, Tian et al. [30] added a parameter of control effect into SEIR model and considered the imported cases from Wuhan (Eq. (15)). Based on Tian's study, R_0 in Wuhan before January 23 was 3.15 (95%CI: 3.04 ~ 3.26) and the implementation of Wuhan travel ban and the national emergency response had reduced 3% ~ 69% transmission in provinces except Hubei and avoided 96% cases (nearly 450,000) outside Wuhan up to February 19.

$$\begin{cases} \frac{dS_i}{dt} = -\frac{C_{\text{Segment}}\beta I_i S_i}{N_i} \\ \frac{dE_i}{dt} = \frac{C_{\text{Segment}}\beta I_i S_i}{N_i} - \delta E_i + \lambda_i \\ \frac{dI_i}{dt} = \delta E_i - \gamma I_i \\ \frac{dR_i}{dt} = \gamma I_i \end{cases} . \quad (22.15)$$

The role of control measures at different stages of the outbreak are captured by estimated parameter C (range 0–1), which reduces transmission and R_e proportionally as a multiplicand of β.

In modeling studies, the effect of interventions is reflected in the following aspects: the reduction of parameters related to transmission, such as contact rate, transmission rate and R_e or R_t, a parameter representing the effect of control measures (such as C_{Segment} mentioned above), the avoided cumulated cases and the averted hospitalizations. Evaluating the effect of containment strategies could help decision-makers develop better measures to control the transmission. By quantifying the effect of interventions, the possible trend after implementing control measures which had not been introduced can be better simulated. Thus, choosing the optimal combinations of control measures become achievable.

22.3.2.4 Exploration of Dynamic Uncertainty

Transmission dynamics models based on the SIR/SEIR structure, which imitate the mode of transmission, can be used to simulate future transmission scenarios through a series of hypotheses about transmission, disease and immunity parameters. The disease-specific parameters driving it in transmission dynamics models can be modified based on knowledge of the underlying transmission process to test how the pandemic would vary if different assumptions about the disease and nonpharmaceutical interventions were used [31]. With in-depth knowledge of characteristics of infectious disease and the influence of interventions estimated by models, simulating the future trend becomes logical and believable.

Assuming different effects and implementing time of control measures, the theoretical trend of epidemic could be simulated. Zhong et al. used an extending SEIR model incorporating population flow with different assumptions of implementing time of strict quarantine measures in Hubei. They found that the scale of the outbreak in mainland China would quadruple owing to implementation being delayed by 5 days [20].

Serious control tactics must strike a compromise between the following competing risks: the risks of mortality and health system collapse, against economic risks and attendant hardships (and health consequences). Transmission dynamics model could be used to explore long-term intervention strategies. In May, 2020, prevention and control of the novel respiratory infectious disease in Canada had achieved initial success. If it is possible, to relax some distancing measure and resume economic activities becomes a new consideration. Thus, Tang et al. [32] simulated de-escalation of control measures in Ontario, Canada and explored the possibility of reopening. The less social distance strategies maintained, the more exposed contacts (maybe unrealistically high) should be effectively traced and isolated to keep $R_t < 1$.

Before the introduction of vaccine, how vaccine would influence the dynamics of the epidemic in the future was unknown. In this situation, Saad-Roy et al. [33] developed a modified model (Fig. 22.11) for a variety of immunization scenes to simulate the future trend with and without vaccines. The ordinary differential equations of Saad-Roy's model are as follows:

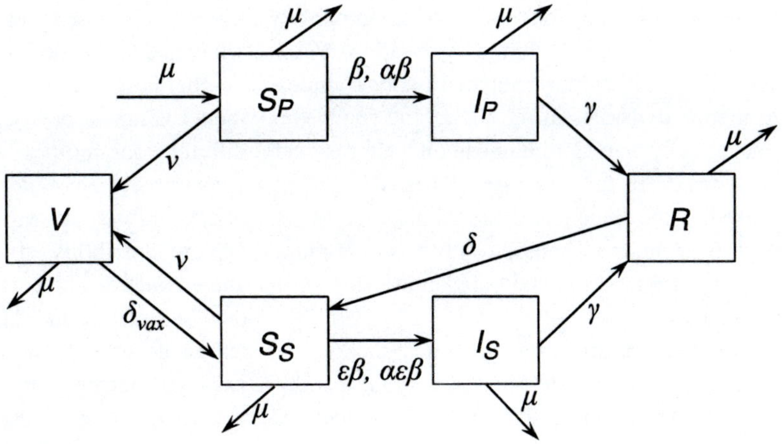

Fig. 22.11 Modified model flowchart that incorporates a vaccinated class V and reinfection classes

$$\begin{cases} \dfrac{dS_P}{dt} = \mu - \beta(t)S_P(I_P + \alpha I_S) - \mu S_P - s_{\text{vax}}\nu S_P \\ \dfrac{dI_P}{dt} = \beta(t)S_P(I_P + \alpha I_S) - (\gamma + \mu)I_P \\ \dfrac{dR}{dt} = \gamma(I_P + I_S) - \delta R - \mu R \\ \dfrac{dS_S}{dt} = \delta R + \delta_{\text{vax}}V - \varepsilon\beta(t)S_S(I_P + \alpha I_S) - \mu S_S - s_{\text{vax}}\nu S_S \\ \dfrac{dI_S}{dt} = \varepsilon\beta(t)S_S(I_P + \alpha I_S) - (\gamma + \mu)I_S \\ \dfrac{dV}{dt} = s_{\text{vax}}\nu(S_P + S_S) - (\delta_{\text{vax}} + \mu)V \end{cases} \quad (22.16)$$

In this model, six compartments are included: fully susceptible, S_P; partially immune, S_S; and fully immune, R; vaccinated, V; primary infected, I_P; secondary infected, I_S. α and ε represent varying degrees of transmission of secondary infections and susceptibility of S_s relative to primary infections. ν is a constant fraction representing the fully and partially susceptible populations are vaccinated each week (thus entering the vaccinated class V). $1/\delta_{\text{vax}}$ represents vaccinal immunity duration. Full immunity from natural infection is assumed to wane at rate δ, while immunity from vaccine wane at rate δ_{vax}. The birth rate μ is assumed to be equal to the death rate. s_{vax} is a binary variable representing vaccination is introduced or not.

By assuming different values of susceptibility to secondary infections, ε, natural immunity duration, $1/\delta$, vaccinal immunity duration, $1/\delta_{\text{vax}}$, and so on, this model simulated likely complex pandemic dynamics in the future and found the substantially varied immunization patterns and the burdens of critically severe cases might be caused by the change of the potential vaccine, as well as immune responses to primary infection, ranging from sustained epidemics to near elimination.

Besides, transmission dynamics model, by simulating the possible scenarios, could also be used to explore the start time of an epidemic, optimal vaccination strategy, the feasibility of a new control strategy, and help understand how small changes in interventions would affect the future dynamics. The core value of transmission dynamics model is exploring different possibilities under various assumptions, which could increase our knowledge of the wide range of conditions that might happen at some time in the future or some location, even in an alternative reality, and thereby enrich the scope of our understanding.

22.4 Values of Transmission Dynamics Models

As stated in 1976 by the British statistician George Box, all models are wrong, but some are useful. It is sometimes important to understand what models can do what they cannot [34].

The core value of transmission dynamics model is not to precisely predict but to explore different possibilities. At the beginning of the epidemic, when almost nothing of the novel pathogen was known, models could help to explore possibility of epidemiological features and estimate relative parameters, helpful to predict the situation and shed light on virologic studies. Later, with the increasing knowledge of the pathogen, mathematical models could be modified to fit the data and then predict the future trend of epidemic. Predictions are valuable even if they are inaccurate. Any deviation of the actual data and the predicted data would provide quick and valuable evidence that the current interventions are very likely effective. After the implementation of comprehensive prevention and control measures, compartment models could also assist to quantitatively assess the efficacy of these control countermeasures and, further, explore the appropriate control strategies. At the end of the pandemic, the model could be used to explore the probability of resurgence. As mentioned above, transmission dynamics model was used to explore epidemic trends with different assumptions before the first vaccine is developed.

Transmission dynamics model should be one of the tools to reflect uncertainties or warn of the worst situation. Sometimes it is not the complex models but the deceptively simple models that are most effective for understanding a system's large-scale behavior, although it may not be precise enough. When the epidemic had been controlled, models can be used to simulate what would happen if current interventions were lifted and provide references and warnings. The purpose of modeling is not to long-term prediction but to near forecast, not to exact predicting but to early warning. What we know and what we assume is a double-edged sword. For one thing, models are limited by them, but if we use properly and absorb them, we will be guided to get over the hump.

22.5 Challenges of Transmission Dynamics Models

It is a huge challenge to predict the epidemic trend of an emerging infectious disease timely, accurately, and reliably. Epidemiologists, statisticians, and public health decision-makers must deal with the uncertainty of poor data quality, limited understanding of diseases, rapid changes in the social environment, and the impact of various interventions.

Without enough understanding of the virus, models would be wrong. At the beginning of epidemic, crucial epidemiological characteristics of the pathogen remain largely unclear. Thus, the model could only be constructed by borrowing the information from similar respiratory infections. Besides, some models ignored the incubation period [35, 36]—an interval between virus infection and developing symptoms, or set the length of incubation period as 2–3 days in reference of SARS, which is underestimated. Furthermore, the infectiousness of asymptomatic cases and patients in incubation period was not considered in early modeling, contradictory to the facts. The structure of transmission dynamics model is highly depending on our comprehension of the virus, and without fully knowledge of the pathogen, the models would be inappropriate.

Without accurate data, models would be wrong. In the studies on the recent pandemic, the most commonly used data was the number of confirmed cases. However, at the early epidemic, nucleic testing capacity was insufficient, resulting in a considerable delay from the individual suffering virus-induced symptoms to laboratory-confirmed virus infection. Even in Beijing, the capital of China, there were also a 2-day delay from infection to be confirmed in 2021 (Fig. 22.12). Thus, models fitting the pandemic using confirmed cases data, which could not reflect the actual epidemic trend, would obtain biased crucial epidemiological parameters and delayed turning point, and should be interpreted with caution.

All the predictions, especially long-term predictions, are inaccurate as a result of rapidly changing interventions and human behaviors, the rapid evolvement of the virus, the dynamic capacity of diagnosis and treatments and the knowledge of the pathogen. In the absence of fully understanding of virus and data accurate enough, trying to pin down details in a model and making precise prediction, possibly leading to overfitting, are futile and meaningless. If there is a 50% uncertainty due to other aspects or assumptions, refining a model by 10% is nonsense. If a model could not properly depict the true dynamics, what is the point of high precision and complexity of this model?

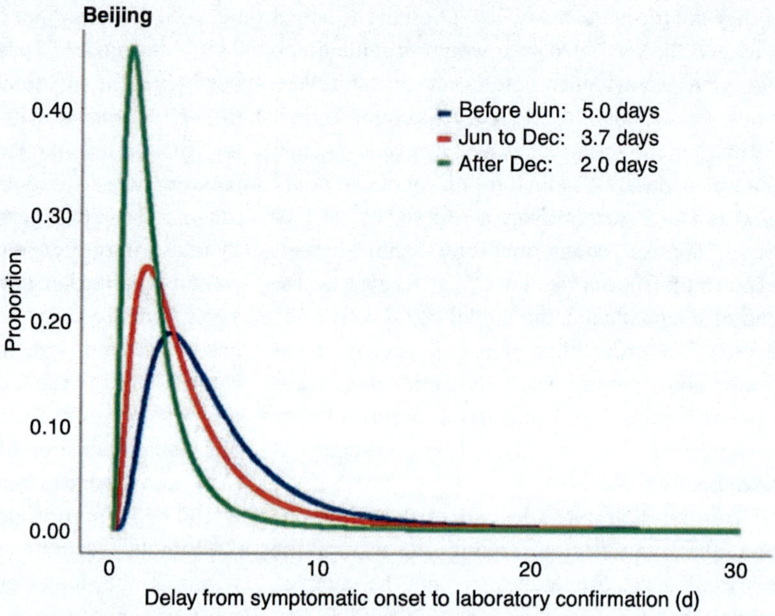

Fig. 22.12 Delay from symptomatic onset to laboratory confirmation in Beijing

In addition, when estimating the effect of control measures, transmission dynamics model could not tell us the impact of each given intervention. What we can obtain from transmission dynamics model is how the comprehensive interventions had reduced the transmission and infections. Further, the effect of interventions is often defined as the difference between the epidemic in the real world and the epidemic had no interventions performed, may be contrary to the fact.

References

1. Martens P. How will climate change affect human health? Am Sci. 1999;87(6):534–41.
2. Ma S, Xia Y. Mathematical understanding of infectious disease dynamics, vol. 16. Singapore: World Scientific; 2009. p. 229.
3. Hamer WH. Epidemic disease in England. Lancet. 2021;1:733–9.
4. Ross R. The prevention of malaria. J Am Med Assoc. 1911;LVII:1715–6.
5. Kermack WO, McKendrick AG. Contributions to the mathematical theory of epidemics--I. 1927. Bull Math Biol. 1991;53(1–2):33–55.
6. Bailey NTJ. The mathematical theory of infectious diseases. 2nd ed. New York: Hafner Press; 1975.
7. Wirawan IMA, Januraga PP. Forecasting COVID-19 transmission and healthcare capacity in Bali, Indonesia. J Prev Med Public Health. 2020;53(3):158–63.
8. Mizumoto K, et al. Estimating the asymptomatic proportion of coronavirus disease 2019 (COVID-19) cases on board the diamond princess cruise ship, Yokohama, Japan, 2020. Euro Surveill. 2020;25(10):2000180.
9. Bai Y, et al. Presumed asymptomatic carrier transmission of COVID-19. JAMA. 2020;323(14):1406–7.
10. Sutton D, et al. Universal screening for SARS-CoV-2 in women admitted for delivery. N Engl J Med. 2020;382(22):2163–4.
11. He X, et al. Temporal dynamics in viral shedding and transmissibility of COVID-19. Nat Med. 2020;26(5):672–5.
12. Li Y, et al. Effect of travel restrictions of Wuhan City against COVID-19: a modified SEIR model analysis. Disaster Med Public Health Prep. 2021;16:1–7.
13. Zhao C, et al. icumonitoring.ch: a platform for short-term forecasting of intensive care unit occupancy during the COVID-19 epidemic in Switzerland. Swiss Med Wkly. 2020;150:w20277.
14. Wei Y, et al. Implementation of clinical diagnostic criteria and universal symptom survey contributed to lower magnitude and faster resolution of the COVID-19 epidemic in Wuhan. Engineering (Beijing). 2020;6(10):1141–6.
15. Wei YY, et al. Inference of start time of resurgent COVID-19 epidemic in Beijing with SEIR dynamics model and evaluation of control measure effect. Zhonghua Liu Xing Bing Xue Za Zhi. 2020;41(11):1772–6.
16. Shi P, et al. Impact of temperature on the dynamics of the COVID-19 outbreak in China. Sci Total Environ. 2020;728:138890.

17. Hou C, et al. The effectiveness of quarantine of Wuhan city against the Corona virus disease 2019 (COVID-19): a well-mixed SEIR model analysis. J Med Virol. 2020;92(7):841–8.
18. Li R, et al. Substantial undocumented infection facilitates the rapid dissemination of novel coronavirus (SARS-CoV-2). Science. 2020;368(6490):489–93.
19. Hao X, et al. Reconstruction of the full transmission dynamics of COVID-19 in Wuhan. Nature. 2020;584(7821):420–4.
20. Yang Z, et al. Modified SEIR and AI prediction of the epidemics trend of COVID-19 in China under public health interventions. J Thorac Dis. 2020;12(3):165–74.
21. Belik V, Geisel T, Brockmann D. Natural human mobility patterns and spatial spread of infectious diseases. Phys Rev X. 2011;1:01101.
22. Yousefpour A, Jahanshahi H, Bekiros S. Optimal policies for control of the novel coronavirus disease (COVID-19) outbreak. Chaos Solitons Fractals. 2020;136:109883.
23. Wu JT, Leung K, Leung GM. Nowcasting and forecasting the potential domestic and international spread of the 2019-nCoV outbreak originating in Wuhan, China: a modelling study. Lancet. 2020;395(10225):689–97.
24. Lipsitch M, et al. Transmission dynamics and control of severe acute respiratory syndrome. Science. 2003;300(5627):1966–70.
25. Chan JF, et al. A familial cluster of pneumonia associated with the 2019 novel coronavirus indicating person-to-person transmission: a study of a family cluster. Lancet. 2020;395(10223):514–23.
26. Munster VJ, et al. A novel coronavirus emerging in China - key questions for impact assessment. N Engl J Med. 2020;382(8):692–4.
27. Du Z, et al. Risk for transportation of coronavirus disease from Wuhan to other cities in China. Emerg Infect Dis. 2020;26(5):1049–52.
28. Wei YY, et al. Fitting and forecasting the trend of COVID-19 by SEIR^{+CAQ} dynamic model. Zhonghua Liu Xing Bing Xue Za Zhi. 2020;41(4):470–5.
29. China Daily. Tibet activates highest-level public health alert. 29 January 2020. Available from http://www.chinadaily.com.cn/a/202001/29/WS5e318a36a3101282172739c1.html.
30. Tian H, et al. An investigation of transmission control measures during the first 50 days of the COVID-19 epidemic in China. Science. 2020;368(6491):638–42.
31. Holmdahl I, Buckee C. Wrong but useful - what Covid-19 epidemiologic models can and cannot tell us. N Engl J Med. 2020;383(4):303–5.
32. Tang B, et al. De-escalation by reversing the escalation with a stronger synergistic package of contact tracing, quarantine, isolation and personal protection: feasibility of preventing a COVID-19 rebound in Ontario, Canada, as a case study. Biology (Basel). 2020;9(5):100.
33. Saad-Roy CM, et al. Immune life history, vaccination, and the dynamics of SARS-CoV-2 over the next 5 years. Science. 2020;370(6518):811–8.
34. Siegenfeld AF, Taleb NN, Bar-Yam Y. Opinion: what models can and cannot tell us about COVID-19. Proc Natl Acad Sci U S A. 2020;117(28):16092–5.
35. Wu JT, et al. Estimating clinical severity of COVID-19 from the transmission dynamics in Wuhan, China. Nat Med. 2020;26(4):506–10.
36. Dehning J, et al. Inferring change points in the spread of COVID-19 reveals the effectiveness of interventions. Science. 2020;369(6500):eabb9789.

23 Propensity Score and Mendelian Randomization for Control of Confounding

Tong Wang, Xue Gao, and Qian Gao

Abstract

Confounding factors are inevitable in real-world study. In order to obtain effective research conclusions, it is essential to reasonably consider the influence of the confounding factors and eliminate the bias. The propensity score (PS) and Mendelian randomization (MR) methods are widely used to control for the confounding effects in real-world studies. PS utilizes methodologies such as matching, stratification, weighting, and regression adjustment to improve the comparability of the distributions of the potential confounders between groups, thereby weakening or balancing the influence of measurable confounding factors on effect estimation and expecting to achieve a mimic-randomization; MR relies on the natural, random assortment of genetic variants during meiosis and uses genetic variants as instrumental variables to simulate the randomization in a population, thereby controlling for the confounding effects, especially for the unknown and unmeasurable confounding factors in the effect estimation. These two methods are distinctive in research design, model assumptions, analysis procedures, and the interpretation of the estimation results, and they each have their statistical advantages and limitations in obtaining valid effect estimates. In this chapter, the authors briefly introduce the recent research progress and findings of the methodology aspects in terms of the PS and MR models in China. The main content includes formulating the theoretical background of the two methods on basic principles and model construction, methodological research progress, limitations and issues that should be aware of, and illustrating the application of the two methods in real-world study through some examples.

Keywords

Real-world study · Propensity score · Mendelian randomization · Confounding bias

In epidemiological studies, the control of potential confounders is a frequently encountered problem that must be properly addressed. Generally, methods such as restriction, matching, and randomization can be used in the study design phase and multivariate analysis in the data analysis phase to control their potential confounding effects; however, these methods have certain conditions in application. For example, multivariate analysis requires, theoretically, all

T. Wang (✉) · X. Gao · Q. Gao
Department of Health Statistics, School of Public Health, Shanxi Medical University, Taiyuan, Shanxi, China
e-mail: tongwang@sxmu.edu.cn

D.-Q. Ye (ed.), *Progress in China Epidemiology*, https://doi.org/10.1007/978-981-19-2199-5_23

the confounding variables should be measured. Restriction and matching are used for known confounding factors, and the number of matching variables should be limited. On the other hand, a randomized controlled trial (RCT) can effectively control for confounding effects and thus is the gold standard for evaluating causal effects, but these types of studies are difficult to implement in many cases owing to issues of ethics, participant compliance, study duration, and funding constraints. Additionally, the strict inclusion and exclusion criteria in RCTs result in participants probably differing from the real-world populations. Thus, the findings of RCTs should be further validated in the real-world study. In public health, potentially modifiable intervention factors like lifestyle and body weight cannot be randomized per se, and the causal relationship between such factors and health outcomes cannot be verified in RCTs. Real-world studies often have non-RCT designs, and propensity score and Mendelian randomization are commonly used to control for confounding and estimate the causal effects between the risk factors of interest and health outcomes, depending on whether confounding factors are measured. The first section of this chapter will introduce these two commonly-used methods for controlling confounding and give examples of their application. The second section of this chapter presents a review of advances in these methods in China, and the third section identifies issues that need attention in their application.

23.1 Introduction to Propensity Score and Mendelian Randomization Methods

Confounders must usually satisfy the following three criteria: having an association with the risk factor of interest, having an association with the outcome variable given the risk factor of interest, and not being an intermediate variable in the causal pathway from the risk factor to the outcome. The presence of confounders would distort the actual causal association between the risk factor and the outcome [1]. If known confounders are measured, their effects can be controlled with the help of propensity scores. If unknown or unmeasured confounders are present, Mendelian randomization based on instrumental variables is commonly used to estimate causality between phenotype and disease.

23.1.1 Propensity Score

The propensity score, first proposed by Rosenbaum and Rubin (1983) based on a counterfactual framework, is a function of multiple covariates and the conditional probability of the ith individual being assigned to a treatment group based on the known values of the covariates ($\boldsymbol{X}_i$) [2, 3]:

$$e(X) = P(G = 1|\mathbf{X})$$

where G denotes the group or treatment or exposure factor and $G = 1$ means that the individual is in the treatment group and $G = 0$ means the individual in the control group; $\boldsymbol{X}$ is the covariate vector $\boldsymbol{X} = (x_1, x_2, \ldots, x_m)$. If the propensity score is calculated using traditional logistic regression, i.e., a logistic regression model with group G as the dependent variable and the factors to be controlled as the independent variables:

$$\text{logit}\left[P(G = 1|\mathbf{X})\right] = \alpha + \beta_1 x_1 + \cdots + \beta_m x_m$$

The propensity score for each individual can be estimated by substituting the values of the covariates taken for each individual into the model as follows:

$$PS = P(G = 1|X) = \frac{e^{\alpha + \beta_1 x_1 + \cdots + \beta_m x_m}}{1 + e^{\alpha + \beta_1 x_1 + \cdots + \beta_m x_m}}$$

Therefore, the propensity score is an estimate of the probability of an individual receiving the treatment ($G = 1$) given the covariates $\boldsymbol{X}$.

The propensity score itself does not control for confounding but improves the balance between the comparison groups through matching, regression adjustment, stratification, or weighting. This balances the distribution of the covariates between treatment and achieves a randomization-like effect, also known as post hoc randomization. The propensity score matching method involves matching study participants with the same or similar propensity score values in different groups to theoretically equalize the distribution of covariates between the groups and then estimating the between-group effects based on the successfully matched participants. Propensity score adjustment is a regression model constructed to estimate between-group effects using the outcome variable as the response variable, the grouping variable as the independent variable, and the propensity score value as a new covariate. The propensity score value can also be used as a stratification variable, and participants are divided according to the propensity score values for stratified analysis. When there is a sufficient sample size within the strata, the analysis can be performed directly on individual strata or the effects of each stratum can be weighted and averaged. Propensity score inverse probability weighting (IPW) is similar to the traditional standardization method in which each study participant is assigned a corresponding weight based on the propensity score value, thus constructing a pseudo-population in which the distribution of covariates does not differ between groups, thereby eliminating the effect of confounding factors.

Example 23.1

Job burnout is a psychological syndrome, which is a reflection of long-term emotional and interpersonal stressors at work. Situational aspects and individual aspects are factors that may influence the experience of job burnout. One such factor could be sleep status. For this reason, we examine the relationship between sleep quality and job burnout on Chinese coal mine staff with propensity score method [4].

Step 1: Study Sample

3832 subjects were selected from a coal mine group located in Shanxi Province in China. Job burnout was evaluated by the Chinese version of Maslach Burnout Inventory-General Survey, and a widely accepted and applied standard was utilized to distinguish the clinical burnout from non-burnout individuals, i.e., either score > 2.20 on the exhaustion dimension or score > 2.00 on the cynicism dimension was diagnosed as experiencing clinically job burnout. Sleep quality was assessed with a self-administered questionnaire including eight items, and higher scores of the sum of these eight items represented more sleep complaints. Subjects with summation of the eight items higher than 0 represented sleep complainers who had a poorer sleep quality.

First of all, we calculated the standardized difference for each covariate to check the balance of covariates between exposure and control groups.

Bigger values of standardized difference predicted severer imbalance, and a value bigger than 0.1 indicated statistically significant imbalance of the covariate distributions. Age, sex, marital status, educational level, current smoker, and current drinker are included as demographic covariates, and work type, work seniority, workplace, monthly income, condition of work shifts, and occupational injury are included as working-related covariates.

As displayed in Table 23.1, before weighting the sample, substantial differences were observed between two groups on most of the covariates. Robust weighting approaches are therefore needed to limit the extent of confounding bias.

Step 2: Estimate the Propensity Score (PS) and Weight the Sample

We estimated the PS and weighted the subjects using the propensity score. Firstly we estimated the PS with the generalized boosted model (GBM), which exhibited robust properties and low prediction error among various PS estimation methods. Then we weighted the sample with the IPW using PS. To assess whether resulting propensity score weights had removed the imbalance between the exposure and control groups, we calculated the standardized difference to check the balancing performance after weighting the sample.

As displayed in Table 23.2, after weighting the subjects with inverse probability using the propensity scores, differences between two groups diminished substantially. The absolute of standardized difference for all the covariates were less

Table 23.1 Study sample characteristics

	Total (n = 3433)	Good sleep quality (n = 1327)	Poorer sleep quality (n = 2106)	d^{a}
Age (year) (mean ± SD)	41.03 ± 8.64	40.10 ± 8.67	41.62 ± 8.57	−0.176
Male sex (%)	84.6	81.7	86.40	−0.130
Marital status (%)				
Married	93.6	93.1	94.0	−0.036
Unmarried	4.8	6.0	4.0	0.081
Others	1.6	1.0	2.0	−0.103
Bachelor degree/above (%)	12.9	13.7	12.3	0.042
Current smoking (%)	57.8	53.4	60.5	−0.146
Alcohol consumption (%)	41.4	35.6	45.1	−0.194
Manual labor (%)	74.1	73.9	74.3	−0.011
Work seniority (year) (%)				
1–3	12.6	15.1	11.1	0.114
4–10	23.9	25.8	22.7	0.069
11–15	16.5	16.4	16.5	−0.003
≥16	47.0	42.7	49.7	−0.142
Underground workers (%)	55.9	52.6	58.0	−0.109
Monthly income (%)				
≤4000	24.8	22.1	26.4	−0.105
4000–6000	42.7	41.4	43.5	−0.042
6000–8000	22.5	25.4	20.8	0.107
≥8000	10.0	11.1	9.3	0.056
Work shifts (%)	48.3	39.5	53.8	−0.287
Occupational injury (%)	9.8	8.3	10.7	−0.082

Abbreviations: *SD* standard deviation

[a]Standardized difference in the original sample, $d = \frac{\left(\overline{x}_{\text{treatment}} - \overline{x}_{\text{control}}\right)}{\sqrt{\frac{s^2_{\text{treatment}} + s^2_{\text{control}}}{2}}}$ for continuous covariates; $d = \frac{\left(\hat{p}_{\text{treatment}} - \hat{p}_{\text{control}}\right)}{\sqrt{\frac{\hat{p}_{\text{treatment}}\left(1-\hat{p}_{\text{treatment}}\right)+\hat{p}_{\text{control}}\left(1-\hat{p}_{\text{control}}\right)}{2}}}$ for dichotomous covariates

Refer from: Gao X, Ma KL, Wang H, Gao Q, Lei LJ, Wang T (2019) Association of sleep quality with job burnout among Chinese coal mine staff: a propensity score weighting analysis. Sci Rep 9 (1):8737. doi:10.1038/s41598-019-45329-2

Table 23.2 Inverse probability weighted sample characteristics

	Good sleep quality	Poorer sleep quality	d^a
Age (mean ± SD)	40.97 ± 8.51	41.09 ± 8.59	−0.014
Male sex (%)	84.4	84.6	−0.006
Marital status (%)			
Married	94.3	93.9	0.016
Unmarried	4.5	4.5	0.003
Others	1.2	1.6	−0.041
Bachelor degree/above (%)	12.7	13.0	−0.010
Current smoking (%)	57.2	58.0	−0.017
Alcohol consumption (%)	40.8	41.8	−0.020
Manual labor (%)	74.9	74.1	0.019
Work seniority (year) (%)			
1–3	12.6	12.0	0.016
4–10	24.4	24.2	0.004
11–15	16.5	16.3	0.004
≥16	46.6	47.4	−0.017
Underground workers (%)	55.8	56.5	−0.014
Monthly income (%)			
≤4000	24.3	25.0	−0.016
4000–6000	42.1	42.4	−0.007
6000–8000	23.7	22.5	0.027
≥8000	10.0	10.0	−0.003
Work shifts (%)	47.4	48.7	−0.026
Occupational injury (%)	9.3	9.9	−0.018

Abbreviations: *SD* standard deviation

[a]Standardized difference in the weighted sample, $d = \frac{\left(\bar{x}^{w}_{\text{treatment}} - \bar{x}^{w}_{\text{treatment}}\right)}{\sqrt{\frac{s^2_{w,\text{treatment}} + s^2_{w,\text{control}}}{2}}}$ for continuous covariates; $d = \frac{\left(\hat{p}^{w}_{\text{treatment}} - \hat{p}^{w}_{\text{control}}\right)}{\sqrt{\frac{\hat{p}^{w}_{\text{treatment}}\left(1-\hat{p}^{w}_{\text{treatment}}\right)+\hat{p}^{w}_{\text{control}}\left(1-\hat{p}^{w}_{\text{control}}\right)}{2}}}$ for dichotomous covariates

Refer from: Gao X, Ma KL, Wang H, Gao Q, Lei LJ, Wang T (2019) Association of sleep quality with job burnout among Chinese coal mine staff: a propensity score weighting analysis. Sci Rep 9 (1):8737. doi:10.1038/s41598-019-45329-2

than 0.05. There was no longer any statistical difference between the two groups after weighting of the sample, thus validating the good balance of subjects after executing the weighting process.

Step 3: Estimate the Relationship of Exposure with Outcome

The next step was to estimate the association of sleep quality and job burnout with the weighted sample. We examined the association between sleep quality and the binary outcome with the logistic model. Using the generalized boosted PS weighting regression model, we identified that in comparison with poorer sleepers, good sleepers were significantly associated with lower risk of job burnout (Table 23.3).

23.1.2 Mendelian Randomization

Mendelian randomization is a statistical causal inference model that uses genetic variations as instrumental variables. Mendelian randomization was firstly proposed by Katan in exploring the hypothesis that low serum cholesterol levels directly increase cancer risk, and this method has been widely used in medical research in recent years [5]. Mendelian randomization uses the random assortment of genetic variants during gamete formation to simulate the random distribution of a population: whether an individual carries a genetic variant at birth that affects a particular phenotype is random, and genetic variation is

Table 23.3 The model examining the association of sleep quality with job burnout

	GBM-based PS weighting model			
	OR	SE	*p* value	95%CI
Sleep quality	0.70	0.08	6.02e-06	(0.60,0.82)

Abbreviations: *GBM* generalized boosted model, *SE* standard error, *CI* confidence interval, *OR* odds ratio

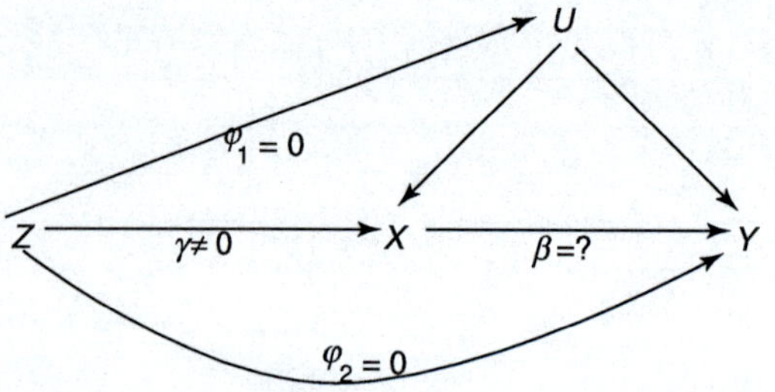

Fig. 23.1 Core assumptions for instrumental variables. *Z* Instrumental variable, *X* exposure, *Y* outcome, *U* confounding

usually uncorrelated with acquired environmental confounders. Thus, differences in an outcome between those who carry the variant and those who do not can be attributed to variation in exposure factors, thus excluding the effects of confounding factors [6]. The main advantage of the Mendelian randomization model using genetic variation as instrumental variables over the traditional instrumental variable models is that genetic variation is randomly segregated and combined during gamete formation, independent of the social environment, lifestyle, and other phenotypes, which ensures that confounding factors are balanced across different subgroups of genetic variation, to theoretically avoid the influence of confounding factors. However, genetic variation precedes the occurrence and changes in environmental exposure, confounding, and disease outcome, and the exposure variation explained by genetic variation as a proxy variable for exposure also precedes outcome, thus excluding the problem of reverse causation [7].

To serve as a valid instrumental variable, genetic variation must satisfy the following core assumptions (Fig. 23.1):

1. Association assumption: genetic variant *Z* is associated with exposure *X* ($\gamma \neq 0$).
2. Independence assumption: genetic variant *Z* is independent of confounder *U* that affects the "exposure–outcome" relationship ($\varphi_1 = 0$).
3. Exclusive assumption: genetic variant *Z* affects outcome *Y* only through exposure factor *X* ($\varphi_2 = 0$).

According to the type of sample data, Mendelian randomization models can be divided into one-sample Mendelian randomization and two-sample Mendelian randomization.

Two-sample Mendelian randomization allows investigators to use summary-level data for analysis, and its application is more common owing to its more convenient data acquisition. Summary-level data are summary statistics (including association estimates, standard errors, and significance *P* values) of the association between genetic variants and phenotypes (or disease outcomes). Assuming that there are *j* mutually independent instrumental variables ($G_1,\ldots,G_j$) that meet the core assumptions, estimates of the association of the *j*th genetic variant G_j with the exposure and the outcome are denoted as $\widehat{\beta}_{X_j}$ and $\widehat{\beta}_{Y_j}$, respectively. The causal effect of exposure on outcome are estimated using the inverse variance weighting (IVW) method, which is based on the idea that the Wald estimates corresponding to each genetic variant are first calculated separately:

$$\hat{\theta}_{R_j} = \frac{\widehat{\beta}_{Y_j}}{\widehat{\beta}_{X_j}}$$

The inverse of the variance of the Wald estimates are then used as the weight to integrate the proportional estimates for each genetic variant, and the integrated IVW estimates are used as the final estimates of the causal effect of exposure on outcome:

$$\widehat{\beta}_{\text{IVW}} = \frac{\sum_{j=1}^{J} \hat{\theta}_{R_j} \sigma_{R_j}^{-2}}{\sum_{j=1}^{J} \sigma_{R_j}^{-2}} = \frac{\sum_{j=1}^{J} \widehat{\beta}_{X_j} \widehat{\beta}_{Y_j} \sigma_{Y_j}^{-2}}{\sum_{j=1}^{J} \widehat{\beta}_{X_j}^{2} \sigma_{Y_j}^{-2}}$$

Table 23.4 shows the meaning of symbols involved in the estimate of causal effect using IVW method.

Table 23.4 The meaning of symbols involved in the estimate of causal effect using IVW method

Symbols	Meaning
G_j	The jth genetic variant
$\widehat{\beta}_{X_j}$	The association between the G_j with the exposure
$\widehat{\beta}_{Y_j}$	The association between the G_j with the outcome
$\widehat{\beta}_{\mathrm{IVW}}$	The estimate of causal effect using IVW method
$\widehat{\theta}_{R_j}$	The Wald estimates of casual effect corresponding to the G_j
$\sigma_{R_j}^{-2}$	The inverse of the variance for the $\widehat{\theta}_{R_j}$ corresponding to the G_j
$\sigma_{Y_j}^{-2}$	The inverse of the variance for the $\widehat{\beta}_{Y_j}$ corresponding to the G_j

Refer from: Burgess S, Butterworth A, Thompson SG (2013) Mendelian randomization analysis with multiple genetic variants using summarized data. Genet Epidemiol 37 (7):658–665. doi:10.1002/gepi.21758

The advantage of using summary-level data for analysis is that summary-level data are often derived from the results of genome-wide association studies (GWAS) of large samples, ensuring higher confidence in the causal effect estimates while improving the precision of the study results. However, further subgroup-specific analyses cannot be performed based on summary data alone, and it is more difficult to adjust variables according to research needs.

Example 23.2

Type 2 diabetes mellitus (T2DM) is a chronic condition which describes a group of metabolic disorders characterized by insulin resistance, and it leads a heavy health burden of disability and mortality. Previous research put forward the link between insomnia and T2DM; however, little is known about the underlying causality. Herein, we utilized the two-sample summary data-based MR framework to investigate the causal relation between insomnia and T2DM [8].

Step 1: Select the Study Sample

We acquire the summary-level data for insomnia from the largest available meta-analysis of GWAS, which contains unrelated European descent individuals from UK Biobank and 23andMe. The two-sample MR may develop biased estimates when using the study sample that have significant overlap between the exposure and outcome GWAS. Thus, we excluded the GWASs involving UKB or 23andMe as the T2DM sample. Furthermore, to reduce the potential confounding bias due to population stratification, we chose the European-descent adults as the T2DM cohort. According to the above criteria, summary statistics of T2DM was selected from the largest GWAS which was conducted by the DIAbetes Genetics Replication And Meta-analysis (DIAGRAM) consortium.

The data can be found at GWAS Catalog (https://www.ebi.ac.uk/gwas/) and DIAGRAM (http://diagram-consortium.org/index.html). The form of the summary statistics can be seen in Table 23.5.

Step 2: Select the Genetic Instruments

The independent lead single-nucleotide polymorphisms (SNPs) that are genome-wide significantly ($P < 5 \times 10^{-8}$, $r^2 < 0.1$) associated with insomnia were included as preliminary instruments. Then we extracted the T2DM summary statistics according to the SNP ID of the preliminary instruments and matched the associations of the selected instruments with insomnia and T2DM (some of results can be seen in Table 23.6).

To further ensure the independence of the SNP instruments, we excluded the SNPs from the instrument variable set that were in linkage disequilibrium (LD) using the clumping algorithm (r^2 threshold = 0.01 and window size = 1 Mb).

Step 3: Estimate the Causality of Exposure with Outcome

Lastly, we examined the causal relationship of insomnia on T2DM with the inverse-variance

Table 23.5 GWAS summary data for insomnia (sectional)

SNP	beta.exposure	se.exposure	a1	a2	eaf	pval.exposure
rs113851554	0.206	0.014	T	G	0.051	1.56E-51
rs62149809	0.148	0.025	A	G	0.986	5.71E-09
rs1064939	0.130	0.020	A	T	0.978	2.16E-10
rs79204944	0.079	0.014	A	G	0.045	4.24E-08
rs72899452	0.074	0.012	T	C	0.065	1.00E-09
rs55972276	0.073	0.009	A	C	0.137	4.19E-17
rs77641763	0.071	0.009	T	C	0.122	6.53E-15
rs138014720	0.070	0.013	A	T	0.941	3.46E-08
rs2286729	0.070	0.011	A	G	0.086	5.37E-11
rs118166957	0.068	0.008	T	C	0.159	1.95E-16
rs11650304	0.067	0.012	C	G	0.931	1.23E-08
rs62158170	0.066	0.007	A	G	0.786	1.20E-19
rs62264767	0.065	0.008	A	C	0.853	1.63E-14
rs7168238	0.064	0.011	C	G	0.074	1.80E-08
rs699844	0.060	0.011	A	G	0.920	4.11E-08
rs7566062	0.059	0.007	T	C	0.225	1.37E-16
rs28611339	0.058	0.009	T	G	0.128	8.46E-11

beta.exposure, beta estimate for the association of SNP with exposure; se.exposure, standard error of the beta.exposure; a1, effect allele; a2, reference allele; eaf, effect allele frequency; pvalue.exposure, two-sided P-value from the meta-analysis for exposure

Table 23.6 SNP instruments for causal effect of insomnia on T2DM (sectional)

SNP	beta.exposure	se.exposure	pval.exposure	beta.outcome	se.outcome	pval.outcome
rs1015438	0.078	0.008	2.51E-14	0.0046	0.016	0.77
rs1031654	−0.051	0.007	3.88E-12	−0.032	0.015	0.031
rs1038093	0.039	0.006	2.47E-10	0.011	0.013	0.37
rs10502966	−0.039	0.006	8.54E-11	0.0083	0.012	0.49
rs1064213	−0.037	0.006	6.41E-10	0.015	0.012	0.2
rs1064939	0.130	0.02	2.16E-10	0.097	0.046	0.035
rs10756571	0.036	0.006	1.80E-08	0.015	0.013	0.25
rs10761240	−0.043	0.006	2.12E-12	−0.015	0.012	0.21
rs10800992	0.042	0.006	3.84E-12	−0.0084	0.012	0.49
rs10825503	0.033	0.006	1.43E-08	−5.00E-04	0.012	0.97
rs10865954	0.078	0.006	1.92E-11	0.0057	0.013	0.65

beta.exposure, beta estimate for the association of SNP with exposure; se.exposure, standard error of the beta.exposure; pvalue.exposure, two-sided *P*-value from the meta-analysis for exposure; beta.outcome, beta estimate for the association of SNP with outcome; se.outcome, standard error of the beta.outcome; pvalue.outcome, two-sided *P*-value from the meta-analysis for outcome

Refer from: Gao X, Sun H, Zhang Y, Liu L, Wang J, Wang T (2020) Investigating Causal Relations Between Sleep-Related Traits and Risk of Type 2 Diabetes Mellitus: A Mendelian Randomization Study. Front Genet 11:607865. doi10.3389/fgene.2020.607865

weighted (IVW) estimates, simple weighted median (SME), weighted median estimates (WME), and MR-Egger estimates.

With the three MR models, we all found significant adverse effect of insomnia on the risk of T2DM (Table 23.7).

Table 23.7 MR causal relationship of insomnia with T2DM

Methods	OR	*p* value	95%CI
IVW	1.14	2.03e-07	(1.08, 1.19)
SME	1.13	5.56E-04	(1.06, 1.22)
WME	1.14	3.48E-04	(1.06, 1.22)
MR-Egger	1.25	2.44E-02	(1.03, 1.52)

23.2 Progress in Propensity Score and Mendelian Randomization Methodology and Application in China

23.2.1 Progress Regarding Propensity Score

The propensity score method is conducted in two main steps: first, a treatment model is constructed to estimate the propensity score values; second, the propensity score values are applied to construct an outcome model to estimate the treatment effects. However, the traditional propensity score method does not take into account the influence of the uncertainty of the propensity score on the treatment effect and does not utilize a priori information in estimating the treatment effect. Therefore, some researchers have proposed introducing the idea of Bayesian statistics into the propensity score, including the intermediate Bayesian propensity score method proposed by An (2010) [9] and the two-step Bayesian propensity score method proposed by Kaplan and Chen (2012) [10]. However, the theoretical study and practical application of both methods are only applicable to dichotomous variables. In view of this, Wu (2014) [11] extended the Bayesian propensity score method to the case where the treatment factors contained multiple categories and constructed two new models: the intermediate Bayesian generalized propensity score method and the two-step Bayesian generalized propensity score method, which also considered both unordered multi-categorical variables and ordered multi-categorical variables. The simulation results show that when the treatment factor is unordered multi-categorical, the Bayesian method can obtain results that are closer to the true value of the treatment effect than the general method when the prior precision is zero. When the treatment effect estimates obtained by the general method are biased, the Bayesian method estimates can greatly reduce the bias. When the treatment factor is ordered multi-categorical, the researchers recommend the intermediate Bayesian generalized propensity score method based on higher prior precisions when applying regression or weighting methods or the two-step Bayesian generalized propensity score method for regression or stratification based on an outcome model with a prior precision of zero. However, which of the two Bayesian generalized propensity score methods is superior is not defined. Additionally, that study used either logistic regression models or cumulative logit models for estimating propensity score values in the first step and considered only the main effects of the covariates.

In practice, there are a large amount of large-scale data with multi-level hierarchical structure, and the treatment factors are mostly unordered multi-categorical and ordered multi-categorical. Yu (2016) [12] proposed applying the estimation of propensity score using a boosting algorithm to multi-level data and constructed multi-level propensity score models with treatment factors of unordered multi-categorical and ordered categorical data (mainly taking tri-categorical as an example). The simulation results show that the accuracy and precision of different multi-level propensity score models for estimating the treatment effects vary greatly under different data structures, and each has its own conditions of applicability. The boosting algorithm is superior in estimating multi-level propensity score models, but it is not applicable in all cases and should be chosen according to the different settings of the data.

The traditional propensity score matching (PSM) method uses point estimates of propensity score without considering the effect of sampling error. Some researchers have proposed using confidence intervals of propensity scores for matching, called propensity score interval matching (PSIM). PSIM can significantly improve the matching rate when the sample size is small but may lead to poorer balance of covariates between groups after matching. Guo (2019) [13] proposed using of the global optimal matching algorithm constructed according to the basic idea of the assignment problem in the integer programming problem to optimize PSIM and constructed the global optimal PSIM algorithm. The algorithm focuses on minimizing the sum of propensity score distances or maximizing the sum of propensity score confidence interval overlaps for all objects that form a match, thereby increasing the matching rate while further balancing the intergroup covariates. Guo (2019) had also extended the matching algorithm from dealing with binary factors to the case of unordered tri-categorical factors. The simulation results show that this matching method estimated treatment effects is with closest confidence interval coverages to nominal level and with smaller standardized differences and higher matching rates. However, the mean squared error of the method for estimating treatment effects is large.

In health economics studies, the propensity score matching differences-in-differences (PSM-DID) model is widely used as a powerful tool in policy analysis. The PSM-DID model was first proposed by Heckman (1997) [14], and it was noted that the propensity score matching model could screen control groups for the DID model. However, when facing the challenge of applying propensity score matching (which is originally applicable to cross-sectional data) to panel data, traditional schemes based on transforming panel data into cross-sectional data and matching phase by phase based on panel data are prone to the problems of self-matching or inconsistency of matched participants before and after policy implementation. Xie et al. (2021) [15] improved the traditional phase-by-phase matching scheme. First, the matching variables were differentiated, and the matching was controlled by a special class of variables (categorical variables that contained a large amount of unobservable information and should be maintained the same in the control group and the treatment group in the actual study) and the propensity score. Second, the matching method was changed from point-to-point matching of propensity score values to overall matching between propensity score value sequences. An example of its application show that the improved PSM-DID model can be used to more effectively identify policy effects when the control group differs significantly from the treatment group and when there are special class variables.

The marginal structural model-based IPW method is an important class of methods that can be used to estimate treatment effects in non-randomized studies. For IPW, the estimation of the inverse probability weights in the first phase is critical and determines whether the final treatment effect estimates are unbiased. In recent years, some researchers have used data-adaptive methods, including many statistical learning algorithms, to estimate inverse probability weights and have achieved good results. However, most current studies are limited to binary treatment factors and single longitudinal survival outcome. In view of this, Guo (2018) [16] used multiple statistical learning algorithms to estimate the inverse probability weights when the treatment factors were continuous variables and time-dependent competitive risk survival outcome and explored truncation of the weights to avoid the influence of extreme weights on the estimation of treatment effects. The simulation results show that (1) CBGPS (covariate balancing generalized propensity score) and non-parametric CBGPS (npCBGPS) are better at balancing covariates for continuous treatment variables; statistical learning algorithms such as boosted CART (classification and regression tree) and RF (random forest) perform better in reducing estimation bias. When using IPW for effect estimation, the distribution of the weight variables should be considered first; if there are many outliers, the weights should be truncated before performing the effect estimation. (2) For time-dependent competitive risk survival data, when using marginal structural cause-specific hazard models for effect estimation, as the treatment assignment mechanism in the actual data is often unknown, the researchers suggest using two methods, boosted CART and RF, instead of traditional logistic regression to construct inverse probability weights, so as to reduce the influence of model misspecification on effect estimation. Unfortunately, Guo (2018) [16] did not consider the problem of variable selection in generalized PS models. These methods may have poor performance when there are high-dimensional covariates because the inclusion of unnecessary covariates into generalized PS models can be detrimental to the accuracy and precision of an estimation. In view of this, Gao et al. (2021) [17] proposed generalized outcome-adaptive LASSO (GOAL) method. The simulation results show that when the outcome model is linear, (1) the GOAL can accurately select covariates needed to achieve an unbiased and statistically efficient estimation; (2) the GOAL provide an estimation with high accuracy and precision; and (3) the GOAL is robust to the generalized PS model misspecification.

Balancing assessment for covariates in the propensity score model is needed before and after propensity score matching, and Flury and Reidwyl (1986) [18] first proposed the standardized difference method to evaluate the balance of covariates for two groups. For data from multiple groups, the maximum value of the standardized differences between any two groups is used as the evaluation index. However, calculation in this method is cumbersome and inconvenient for practical application. Huang (2018) [19] constructed the FQ statistic for evaluating the intergroup balance of tri-categorical covariates using the combined variance and compared it with the hypothesis test method and the standardized difference method. The simulation results show that the standardized difference method and the FQ statistic can better evaluate the balance of the tri-categorical covariates than the hypothesis test method, and they are not affected by the sample size. The distribution of tri-categorical covariates can be considered balanced when the FQ statistic of covariates is less than 0.2. The FQ statistic is more advantageous for application because the calculation steps of the FQ statistic are easier than those of the standardized difference method. However, the researchers only simulated the cases of binary covariates and continuous covariates and did not consider the cases of multi-categorical covariates and non-normally distributed continuous covariates.

In practice, propensity score subgroup analysis can lead to unbalanced covariates within the subgroups owing to inconsistency between the estimated propensity scores of the total sample and the actual values, resulting in biased estimates of subgroup causal effects. However, direct estimation of subgroup propensity scores magnifies the bias-variance tradeoff, i.e., it achieves covariate balance within subgroups while leading to variance inflation. In view of this, Dong (2020) [20] proposed the subgroup balancing propensity score. For each subgroup, to optimize the sample covariates balancing condition, the method adaptively selects either the total sample or the subgroup sample, to estimate the propensity scores of individuals within that subgroup, and develops two versions based on matching and weighting. Additionally, a random search algorithm is designed for estimating subgroup balancing propensity scores when the number of subgroups is large. Simulation results show that this method is effective in improving the performance of estimating subgroup treatment effects using the propensity score method. Researchers have applied this method to the Italian Survey on Household Income and Wealth (SHIW) to estimate the causal effect of debit cards on household consumption across income groups.

Adverse drug events (ADEs) from a spontaneous reporting system (SRS) are the main data source of drug–drug interaction (DDI) studies. However, there are two main problems in detecting DDIs from the SRS: confounding bias and the false-positive rate. Wang et al. (2020) [21] proposed the propensity score-adjusted three-component mixture model (PS-3CMM) based on disproportionality analysis and the three-component mixture model in DPAs (disproportionality analysis). Simulations and example studies show that the PS-3CMM model can adjust the confounding bias of all drug–drug–ADE combinations in the US Food and Drug Administration Adverse Event Reporting System (FAERS) database while estimating the false discovery rate. PS-3CMM performs better than existing methods in detecting true DDIs. Additionally, the model is more sensitive in selecting DDI signals with non-positive individual drug relative ADE risk. The PS-3CMM model has limitations in dealing with highly relevant drugs and does not consider drug regimen and dose information when applied to the FAERS.

23.2.2 Progress in Mendelian Randomization

The validity of instrumental variables that satisfy the core assumptions is necessary for correct estimation in Mendelian randomization models; however, when genetic variants are pleiotropic, use of such genetic variants as instrumental variables violates the core assumptions and is therefore referred to as an invalid instrumental variable. When invalid instrumental variables are included in the model, the use of Mendelian randomization models assuming all instrumental variables being valid for effect estimation will certainly lead to biased effect estimates, as well as an increase in the type I error rate (false-positive rate). Based on this, Zhao et al. (2020) [22] proposed a Bayesian-weighted Mendelian randomization (BWMR) for causal inference. In the BWMR model, the uncertainty of weak effects owing to polygenicity is taken into account, and the bias caused by pleiotropy is detected and resolved by Bayesian weighting. To render the BWMR-based causal inference stable and effective, the researchers also constructed a variational expectation-maximization algorithm. Additionally, an exact closed-form formula was derived to correct the posterior covariance. The simulation results showed that BWMR outperformed existing methods such as the MR-Egger model. In an example study using BWMR to explore the causal relationships between 130 metabolites and 93 complex phenotypes, BWMR revealed new causal relationships between exposure and outcome traits. Xu et al. (2021) [23] proposed the Mendelian randomization approach accounting for correlated and idiosyncratic pleiotropy (MRCIP), which aims to solve the problem of correlation between instrumental variables as well as pleiotropy. The researchers first constructed a random-effects model to represent the pleiotropy in the model simultaneously, and then they used the PRW-EM algorithm, which combines the expectation–maximization (EM) algorithm with extra updating steps for the weights, to estimate the model parameters. The model simultaneously estimates the proportion of correlated pleiotropy in the instrumental variables and performs a likelihood ratio test. The results of the simulation study showed that the MRCIP method outperformed the established methods. Lin et al. (2021) [24] proposed Mendelian randomization with refined instrumental variable from genetic score (MR-RIVER) based on summarized data. Borrowing linkage disequilibrium (LD) information from public database, the researchers adjusted the point effect of each SNP and got the genetic score from the adjusted effect. Then the genetic score was used as an instrumental variable to estimate the causal effect between exposure and outcome. The results showed that the MR-RIVER can improve the performance in statistical power and controlment of type I error, compared with IVW and GSMR, which are MR methods based on summarized data.

Li et al. (2018) [25] discussed the identifiability and estimation of causal effects of continuous treatment on a binary response when the treatment is measured with errors, and there are latent categorical confounders between the treatment and the response. Based on multiple widely used parametric models, they first discussed the identifiability of causal effects and then proposed a method for estimation and inference. The method can exclude the biases owing to latent confounders and measurement error using a single instrumental variable. Based on the identification results, the presence of categorical confounders and the selection of latent confounder levels are given.

The rapid development of modern sequencing technologies and the widespread reporting and application of GWAS have provided a sufficient theoretical basis for screening genetic variation as instrumental variables associated with specific exposure factors in Mendelian randomization analysis. However, the vast majority of genetic variants obtained from GWAS that are significantly associated with exposure do not include a complete understanding of the biological mechanisms of association, resulting in estimates of causal effects obtained from GWAS have no pathway or mechanism-related explanations, as well as difficulties in validating the relationships between identified genetic variants and disease. Transcriptome-wide association studies (TWAS) integrate results from GWAS and gene expression studies and are used to study the gene regulation mechanisms behind diseases, which can better help elucidate causal associations between disease causes. Yuan et al. (2020) [26] proposed the probabilistic Mendelian randomization method, PMR-Egger, for TWAS, which is based on the Mendelian randomization likelihood framework and combines several existing TWAS and Mendelian randomization methods to test for gene-to-trait causality in the presence of horizontal pleiotropy and can be extended to thousands of individuals. In simulations, PMR-Egger has good robustness under various model parameter settings, and type I errors were better controlled in the presence of horizontal pleiotropy; PMR-Egger outperformed existing TWAS and Mendelian randomization methods. The researchers applied the PMR-Egger method to an example study of 39 diseases and complex traits obtained from three GWAS repositories, including UK Biobank; the results also showed that the PMR-Egger method outperformed other existing research methods.

Existing TWAS methods focus on the analysis of one outcome trait at a time and are univariate in nature. However, many complex traits are interrelated and share a common genetic basis. Multivariate analysis of multiple traits can better improve TWAS efficacy. Liu et al. (2021) [27] constructed the multiple outcome probabilistic Mendelian randomization with Egger assumption (moPMR-Egger) model for analyzing multiple outcome traits in TWAS. The moPMR-Egger examines one gene at a time, relies on cis-single-nucleotide polymorphisms (SNPs) with potential linkage disequilibrium as instrumental variables, and jointly tests their causality for multiple traits. A key feature of moPMR-Egger is the ability to test and control for potential horizontal pleiotropy of instrumental variables, thereby maximizing the efficacy and reducing false associations in TWAS. The results of a simulation study showed that moPMR-Egger outperformed existing TWAS methods in terms of causal effect estimation, and it has a lower type I error rate in causal effect estimation and better horizontal pleiotropic effect testing. The researchers also applied moPMR-Egger to analyze 11 traits out of 5 trait categories in UK Biobank. The results showed that moPMR-Egger identified 13.15% more genetic associations than a univariate method with different trait categories and revealed unique regulatory mechanisms of systolic and diastolic blood pressure.

GWAS-based pathway association analysis is a powerful approach for genetic studies of complex human diseases. However, genetic confounding effects of genes associated with environmental exposures can reduce the accuracy of GWAS-based pathway association analysis for target diseases. Fan et al. (2018) [28] proposed the Mendelian randomization-based pathway enrichment analysis (MRPEA) method; based on GWAS summary data, this method was able to correct for genetic confounding effects of environmental exposures. Simulation studies have shown that MRPEA generally outperforms traditional pathway association analysis (TPAA) in a variety of scenarios. The researchers also applied this method to real GWAS summary data on cardiovascular disease and smoking and observed significantly improved performance of MRPEA compared with TPAA; adjustment for environmental exposures was not required during this process.

Mendelian randomization and instrumental variables research methods have not been widely used in the study of survival data. Huang et al. (2020) [29] proposed an instrumental variables analysis method for the survival context, using a semiparametric linear transformation model to transform survival time and survival probability and then perform causal effect estimation. The researchers explored the conditions that could estimate the hazard ratio and effect on the survival probability. For statistical inferences, estimating equations were constructed in the study. The asymptotic properties of the proposed estimators can give an estimation without making parametric assumptions about confounding factors, thus avoiding the difficulty of estimating associations between exposure and outcome due to unknown confounding.

23.3 Issues to Be Considered in the Propensity Score and Mendelian Randomization

Although the propensity score and Mendelian randomization provide non-randomized controlled studies with a means to control for confounding and estimate causal associations, there are corresponding restrict assumptions to be met in their application. Additionally, it should be emphasized that conducting an RCT is still the most reliable method for obtaining causal evidence, and non-randomized controlled studies have a certain gap with respect to RCTs in terms of evidence level. If non-RCTs comply with the Transparent Reporting of Evaluations with Nonrandomized Designs (TREND) guideline, the results of those studies can be used as a complement to evidence-based medicine.

23.3.1 Issues Regarding Propensity Score

Referring to the procedures of a typical propensity score method for data analysis, the following aspects should be noted in its application.

1. Selection of covariates for a propensity score estimation model

   The most commonly used models for propensity score calculation include logistic regression, probit regression, and certain machine learning methods. Regardless of the model used, the probability of each observation entering the treatment group is non-zero. The key covariates should include those affecting treatment and outcome and should incorporate as many measured confounders as possible, provided that the covariates take reliable values. A simulation study found that variables unrelated to treatment factor G but related to outcome variable Y should always be included in the propensity score estimation model, and their inclusion would improve the precision of the estimates without increasing bias [30]. Conversely, including variables that are related to treatment factor G but not to outcome variable Y will reduce the precision of the estimates and increase bias and will result in larger mean squared errors in studies with small sample sizes. Therefore, standard model establishment tools designed to create good predictive models for treatment variable G do not necessarily lead to the optimal propensity score models.
2. Selection of propensity score methods and parameter settings

   The selection of propensity score methods should be carried out in conjunction with the research questions and data characteristics. Usually, the propensity score matching method can be selected when the sample size is large and the minimum sample size requirement can still be met after loss of the sample due to matching; when the sample size is limited, the method that involves all the data, such as the IPW method, should be preferably selected.

   After obtaining the propensity score, the propensity score distribution should be analyzed to examine the overlap assumption, i.e., the common support for the ranges of propensity score values in the treatment group and the control group. If the propensity score value of an individual in the treatment group is significantly higher than the maximum propensity score value of the control group or significantly lower than the minimum propensity score value of the control group, the individual is considered to be removed; however, if the overlapping range of propensity score values is limited, the propensity score method should not be used.
3. Evaluation of the balance

   Whether the covariates achieve balance after propensity score matching is something that must be evaluated, which can be done using the standardized difference method and the graphical method. For example, a standardized difference with an absolute value less than 0.1 can be considered good balance.

4. Sensitivity analysis

   Application of the propensity score method is very flexible, and choosing different matching methods and setting different parameters in the analysis process may lead to different analysis results. Therefore, adequate sensitivity analysis is necessary in the application of the propensity score method and should be considered in advance in the analysis procedure. Usually, the following aspects can be considered in sensitivity analysis of propensity score methods: using different models to calculate propensity score values; matching with different ratios or matching with different methods; and sensitivity analysis with different propensity score methods (e.g., propensity score matching method vs. regression adjustment based on propensity score).

23.3.2 Issues Regarding Mendelian Randomization

Applying instrumental variables that satisfy the core assumptions is a necessary condition for Mendelian randomization models to effectively control for confounding, and when the assumptions are violated, biased estimates will be obtained. For most genetic variants obtained from GWAS that are significantly associated with traits, the biological mechanisms of their association with exposure are unclear, and the use of genetic variants with unclear biological mechanisms as instrumental variables increases the possibility of violating the core assumptions of the instrumental variables. Therefore, the methods used for testing the core assumptions of Mendelian randomization and the related sensitivity analysis are particularly important.

1. Weak instrumental variables

   The strength of an instrumental variable refers to the extent to which the instrumental variable is associated with the exposure. When genetic variation satisfies the three core assumptions but is weakly associated with exposure, it is called a weak instrumental variable. The strength of instrumental variables is generally evaluated using the Cragg–Donald F statistic, and a rule of thumb is that the strength of the instrumental variable's F statistic in Mendelian randomization models is at least 10; when the strength is less than 10, the estimates of causal effects are heavily biased. Additionally, the F statistic corresponds to the significance P value of the "instrumental variable–exposure" association. The genome-wide level of 5×10^{-8} is usually used as a threshold for screening instrumental variables, thus avoiding potentially weak instrumental variable bias [31].

2. Pleiotropy

   Pleiotropy refers to the effect of genetic variation on outcome through pathways other than the specific "instrumental variable–exposure-outcome" pathway (Fig. 23.2). Genetic variants are invalid as instrumental variables in the presence of pleiotropy, and the application of invalid instrumental variables can lead to biased estimates of causal effects.

   For the problem of pleiotropy, the current correction methods can be divided into two main categories: the first category is to first identify and exclude the instrumental variables with pleiotropy and then construct Mendelian randomization models for the remaining instrumental variables without pleiotropy. The other approach is to directly construct Mendelian randomization models based on adjusting for the pleiotropy bias, which allow for the presence of pleiotropy in the instrumental variables; in this case pleiotropic effects are corrected to estimate causal effects. Alternatively, sensitivity analysis can be performed using different pleiotropy cor-

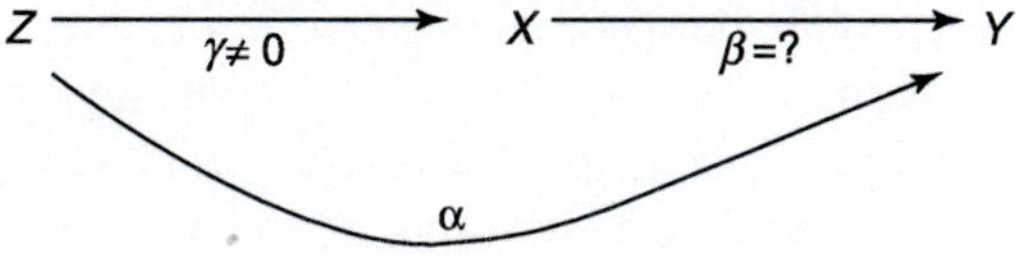

Fig. 23.2 Pleiotropic instrumental variables. Z: instrumental variable; X: exposure; Y: outcome

rection models to assess the robustness of the study results [32].

3. Linkage disequilibrium

   Linkage disequilibrium (LD) describes the correlation between genetic variants, which is usually caused by the proximity of physical locations among genetic variants. Mendelian randomization usually selects mutually independent SNPs as instrumental variables. When LD exists between the selected genetic variants, the correlations between instrumental variables should be incorporated into the Mendelian randomization model, thus correcting for the effect of LD between instrumental variables on the model [24].

4. Population stratification

   Population stratification refers to the heterogeneity of the association between genetic variants and phenotypic traits among subgroups of different races or countries. In two-sample Mendelian randomization studies, this heterogeneity can lead to instrumental variables that fail to achieve randomization for confounders, resulting in spurious associations between genetic variants and exposures, confounders, and outcomes, resulting in biased estimates of causal effects [33]. To avoid population stratification, homogeneous populations are usually selected as the study population when constructing Mendelian randomization models.

5. Statistical power

   The statistical power of Mendelian randomization models for estimating causal effects is related to the proportion of exposure variance explained by all instrumental variables included in the model; when other parameters are consistent, the higher this proportion of explanation, the more representative the instrumental variables are of the exposure variance and the higher the statistical power of its corresponding model. Existing Mendelian randomization models usually select multiple genetic variants as instrumental variables, thus increasing the proportion of instrumental variables explaining the exposure variance and improving the statistical power of the estimates. Sample size is another major factor in determining the statistical power of Mendelian randomization models. Most current studies use the summary statistics of association between genetic variants and traits to establish Mendelian randomization models based on summary-level data, which have higher statistical power than Mendelian randomization models based on individual data as the summary-level data contain larger sample sizes. There are some online calculators that can estimate the power of MR according to the sample size and the proportion of exposure variance explained by all instrumental variables (http://218.2.247.110:9094/#/login).

6. Conclusion extrapolation

   When interpreting the causal effect estimates obtained from the Mendelian randomization model, it should be noted that the exposure variation explained by genetic variations is only one part of the total variation in exposure; therefore, the effect estimates obtained by Mendelian randomization are only the effects of this part of exposure variation on the outcome determined by the instrumental variable, whereas the effects of exposure variation on the outcome owing to other non-genetic factors cannot be obtained using Mendelian randomization models. The complete causal association should be explored in the context of biological mechanisms and the results of further clinical studies or randomized controlled trials [34].

In summary, with small sample sizes, population stratification, LD, gene–environment interactions, canalization and developmental compensation, an unreliable genotype–disease relationship, or low population incidence of the selected genetic variants, the above three core assumptions of the instrumental variable will not be satisfied, resulting in biased results. This is the limitation of the Mendelian randomization method.

Acknowledgments We thank Simin He and Yu Zhang for their help in preparing the manuscript, and support from the National Natural Science Foundation of China (grant numbers: 82073674, 81872715 and 82103949) is acknowledged.

References

1. Velentgas P, Dreyer NA, Nourjah P, Smith SR, Torchia MM. Developing a protocol for observational comparative effectiveness research: a User's guide. Rockville: Agency for Healthcare Research and Quality; 2013.
2. Rosenbaum PR, Rubin DB. The central role of the propensity score in observational studies for causal effects. Biometrika. 1983;70(1):41–55. https://doi.org/10.1093/biomet/70.1.41.
3. Wang YJ, Cai HW, Xia JL, Jiang ZW, Wang L. Propensity score (III) key issues in practice of propensity score. Chin J Epidemiol. 2010;31(7):823–5. https://doi.org/10.3760/cma.j.issn.0254-6450.2010.07.025.
4. Gao X, Ma KL, Wang H, Gao Q, Lei LJ, Wang T. Association of sleep quality with job burnout among Chinese coal mine staff: a propensity score weighting analysis. Sci Rep. 2019;9(1):8737. https://doi.org/10.1038/s41598-019-45329-2.
5. Katan MB. Commentary: Mendelian randomization, 18 years on. Int J Epidemiol. 2004;33(1):10–1. https://doi.org/10.1093/ije/dyh023.
6. Emdin CA, Khera AV, Kathiresan S. Mendelian randomization. Jama. 2017;318(19):1925–6. https://doi.org/10.1001/jama.2017.17219.
7. Smith GD, Lawlor DA, Harbord R, Timpson N, Day I, Ebrahim S. Clustered environments and randomized genes: a fundamental distinction between conventional and genetic epidemiology. PLoS Med. 2007;4(12):e352. https://doi.org/10.1371/journal.pmed.0040352.
8. Gao X, Sun H, Zhang Y, Liu L, Wang J, Wang T. Investigating causal relations between sleep-related traits and risk of type 2 diabetes mellitus: a Mendelian randomization study. Front Genet. 2020;11:607865. https://doi.org/10.3389/fgene.2020.607865.
9. An W. Bayesian propensity score estimators: incorporating uncertainties in propensity scores into causal inference. Sociol Methodol. 2010;40(1):151–89. https://doi.org/10.1111/j.1467-9531.2010.01226.x.
10. Kaplan D, Chen J. A two-step Bayesian approach for propensity score analysis: simulations and case study. Psychometrika. 2012;77(3):581–609. https://doi.org/10.1007/s11336-012-9262-8.
11. Wu M (2014) Statistical modeling and application for multi-treatment Bayesian propensity score analysis. Doctoral, The Second Military Medical University, Shanghai.
12. Yu F (2016) The study and application of multilevel propensity score model of categorical data in the hierarchical structure data. Doctoral, The Second Military Medical University, Shanghai.
13. Guo Y (2019) Research and application in global optimal propensity score interval matching for categorical data. Doctoral, The Second Military Medical University, Shanghai.
14. Heckman JJ, Hidehiko I, Todd PE. Matching as An econometric evaluation estimator: evidence from evaluating a job training Programme. Rev Econ Stud. 1997;64(4):605–54. https://doi.org/10.2307/2971733.
15. Xie SX, Fan PF, Wan YY. Improvement and application of classical PSM-DID model. Stat Res. 2021;38(2):146–60. https://doi.org/10.19343/j.cnki.11-1302/c.2021.02.011.
16. Guo W (2018) Research and application in medical studies of inverse probability weighting based on statistical learning. Doctoral, The Second Military Medical University, Shanghai.
17. Gao Q, Zhang Y, Liang J, Sun H, Wang T. High-dimensional generalized propensity score with application to omics data. Brief Bioinform. 2021; https://doi.org/10.1093/bib/bbab331.
18. Flury BK, Riedwyl H. Standard distance in univariate and multivariate analysis. Am Stat. 1986;40(3):249–51. https://doi.org/10.1080/00031305.1986.10475403.
19. Huang FQ, Xu J, An SL. A research on methods of balance evaluation among the covariates of multiple groups. Chin J Health Stat. 2018;35(2):172–6. https://doi.org/10.3969/j.issn.1002-3674.2018.02.003.
20. Dong J, Zhang JL, Zeng S, Li F. Subgroup balancing propensity score. Stat Methods Med Res. 2020;29(3):659–76. https://doi.org/10.1177/0962280219870836.
21. Wang X, Li L, Wang L, Feng W, Zhang P. Propensity score-adjusted three-component mixture model for drug-drug interaction data mining in FDA adverse event reporting system. Stat Med. 2020;39(7):996–1010. https://doi.org/10.1002/sim.8457.
22. Zhao J, Ming J, Hu X, Chen G, Liu J, Yang C. Bayesian weighted Mendelian randomization for causal inference based on summary statistics. Bioinformatics. 2020;36(5):1501–8. https://doi.org/10.1093/bioinformatics/btz749.
23. Xu S, Fung WK, Liu Z. MRCIP: a robust Mendelian randomization method accounting for correlated and idiosyncratic pleiotropy. Brief Bioinform. 2021; 22(5):bbab019. https://doi.org/10.1093/bib/bbab019.
24. Lin L, Zhang R, Huang H, Zhu Y, Li Y, Dong X, Shen S, Wei L, Chen X, Christiani DC, Wei Y, Chen F. Mendelian randomization with refined instrumental variables from genetic score improves accuracy and reduces bias. Front Genet. 2021;12:618829. https://doi.org/10.3389/fgene.2021.618829.
25. Li W, Jiang Z, Geng Z, Zhou XH. Identification of causal effects with latent confounding and classical additive errors in treatment. Biom J. 2018;60(3):498–515. https://doi.org/10.1002/bimj.201700048.
26. Yuan Z, Zhu H, Zeng P, Yang S, Sun S, Yang C, Liu J, Zhou X. Testing and controlling for horizontal pleiotropy with probabilistic Mendelian randomization in transcriptome-wide association studies. Nat Commun. 2020;11(1):3861. https://doi.org/10.1038/s41467-020-17668-6.
27. Liu L, Zeng P, Xue F, Yuan Z, Zhou X. Multi-trait transcriptome-wide association studies with probabilistic Mendelian randomization. Am J Hum Genet.

2021;108(2):240–56. https://doi.org/10.1016/j.ajhg.2020.12.006.

28. Fan Q, Zhang F, Wang W, Xu J, Hao J, He A, Wen Y, Li P, Liang X, Du Y, Liu L, Wu C, Wang S, Wang X, Ning Y, Guo X. GWAS summary-based pathway analysis correcting for the genetic confounding impact of environmental exposures. Brief Bioinform. 2018;19(5):725–30. https://doi.org/10.1093/bib/bbx025.
29. Huang YT. Mendelian randomization using semiparametric linear transformation models. Stat Med. 2020;39(7):890–905. https://doi.org/10.1002/sim.8449.
30. Patrick AR, Schneeweiss S, Brookhart MA, Glynn RJ, Rothman KJ, Avorn J, Stürmer T. The implications of propensity score variable selection strategies in pharmacoepidemiology: an empirical illustration. Pharmacoepidemiol Drug Saf. 2011;20(6):551–9. https://doi.org/10.1002/pds.2098.
31. Burgess S, Butterworth A, Thompson SG. Mendelian randomization analysis with multiple genetic variants using summarized data. Genet Epidemiol. 2013;37(7):658–65. https://doi.org/10.1002/gepi.21758.
32. Gao X, Wang H, Wang T. Review on correction methods related to the pleiotropic effect in Mendelian randomization. Chin J Epidemiol. 2019;40(3):360–5. https://doi.org/10.3760/cma.j.issn.0254-6450.2019.03.020.
33. Davey Smith G, Hemani G. Mendelian randomization: genetic anchors for causal inference in epidemiological studies. Hum Mol Genet. 2014;23(R1):R89–98. https://doi.org/10.1093/hmg/ddu328.
34. Wang Y, Shen H. Challenges and factors that influencing causal inference and interpretation, based on Mendelian randomization studies. Chin J Epidemiol. 2020;41(8):1231–6. https://doi.org/10.3760/cma.j.cn112338-20200521-00749.

Progress of Air Pollution Epidemiology Research in China

24

Hongbing Xu and Wei Huang

Abstract

Adverse health effects resulting from short- and long-term exposure to air pollution have been confirmed by a large number of epidemiologic studies globally. Meanwhile, air pollution epidemiology research has been under rapid development with significant improvement. Epidemiologic research methodology has also become an important tool to support health risk assessment and evidence-based air quality management. Combining with air pollution exposure and risk assessment, cohort studies have been extensively conducted in North American and European countries to identify the hazardous substances, health risk factors, and pollution sources. Based on the global research findings, the International Agency for Research on Cancer (IARC) classified particulate matter in ambient air as a Group I human carcinogen in 2013, and the World Health Organization (WHO) has updated the Global Air Quality Guidelines in 2021. In recent years, with the rapid social and economic development, the health impact of air pollution has become increasingly prominent, with substantial spatiotemporal differences in the levels and sources of pollution worldwide. In this chapter, we have focused on methodological development and health effects in epidemiologic research of air pollution in China, and findings around the world and potential implications for China.

Keywords

Epidemiology · Air pollution · Exposure assessment · Health effect

24.1 Air Pollution

Air pollution is a common atmospheric phenomenon worldwide, resulting from interactions between anthropogenic activities (e.g., intensive emissions of particulate matter [PM] air pollutants) and specific climatic conditions. Air pollution episodes occurring in atmospheric environment are often known as ambient or outdoor air pollution, whereas episodes occurring in constructed environments (e.g., residences and office buildings) are called indoor air pollution. In this chapter, the terminology regarding air pollution mainly refers to pollutants in ambient air, because indoor air pollution, especially in urban environments, is predominantly originated from outdoor emission sources (e.g., combustion). Extreme air pollution episodes occur when dust or particles suspending in ambient air sharply accumulate in relatively dry conditions, along

H. Xu · W. Huang (✉)
Department of Occupational and Environmental Health, Peking University School of Public Health, Beijing, China
e-mail: whuang@bjmu.edu.cn

D.-Q. Ye (ed.), *Progress in China Epidemiology*, https://doi.org/10.1007/978-981-19-2199-5_24

with complex processes of physical and chemical reactions, including gas-to-particle conversion and aerosol hygroscopic growth. The frequent occurrence of air pollution events characterized as high levels of ambient PM is strengthened when the total emissions exceed the limitation of the atmospheric environmental carrying capacity. Also, ambient air quality can be worsened by specific meteorological conditions, such as static and stable weather. In addition to causing poor air quality and reducing atmospheric visibility, ambient air pollution has been known to be a potential environmental toxicant. The initial epidemiologic research on the health effects of pollutant mixtures was sparked by a few famous episodes of extreme air pollution that occurred in the 1930–1950s, such as the smog events in the Meuse River Valley, Belgium, and London, UK [1, 2]. For instance, dense smog indicative of PM and sulfur dioxide (SO_2) with levels exceeding 1000 μg/m^3 in December 1952 in London resulted in an excess deaths toll of over 4000.

Over the past decades, a growing body of epidemiologic studies has shown strong linkages between air pollution and a wide array of adverse effects, including respiratory diseases, cardiometabolic disorders, adverse birth outcomes, and neurological disorders, in differential real-world scenarios [3]. Under real-world exposure settings, inhaled exposures contaminated with various pollutants, including PM with aerodynamic diameter <10 and 2.5 μm (PM_{10} and $PM_{2.5}$), ultrafine particles (UFPs, with aerodynamic diameter <100 nm), black carbon (BC), nitrogen dioxide (NO_2), nitrogen oxides (NO_x), SO_2, carbon monoxide (CO), and ozone (O_3). Although air pollutants can enter into the human body via multiple routes (e.g., inhalation, ingestion, and skin penetration); however, the amount of internal dose in exposed individuals may be primarily dominated by inhalation routes. Evidence from experimental studies has demonstrated that PM in small-size fractions, such as UFPs, can rapidly reach the systemic circulation [4]. Controlled human exposure studies suggest that inhalation of UFPs is capable of diffusions from the lung to the circulation, consequently accumulating at sites of vascular injury [5, 6]. Among the pollutants, $PM_{2.5}$ is the principal pollutant of health concerns because numerous studies have consistently confirmed that $PM_{2.5}$ poses a greater threat to public health globally. Both the American Heart Association and the European Society of Cardiology have identified $PM_{2.5}$ as an important modifiable risk factor for cardiometabolic diseases. The most recent Global Burden of Disease (GBD) data estimates that 4.6 million premature deaths worldwide are associated with exposure to ambient $PM_{2.5}$, and the largest portion of deaths is attributed to cardiorespiratory diseases [7]. The health burden posed by $PM_{2.5}$ is much higher in heavily polluted regions (e.g., East Asia). Further, the components of PM and gaseous pollutants vary substantially over space and time given. $PM_{2.5}$ represents a heterogeneous mixture with differential species whose components mainly include carbonaceous fractions (e.g., organic carbon [OC] and elemental carbon [EC]), sulfate (SO_4^{2-}), ammonium (NH_4^+), and metals, and with various sources, such as traffic emission and biomass combustion. Thus far, evidence of associations between PM components/sources and adverse health responses remains somewhat limited, and most studies assessed the impacts of PM mass concentrations as the whole exposure metric. From public health standpoints, a better understanding of the risks caused by specific PM components/sources is crucial in setting up control measures for pollutant emissions.

Expedite urbanization has resulted in worsening air quality in China, and ambient air pollutants (particularly $PM_{2.5}$, NO_x, and SO_2) originating from fossil fuel combustion have increased overall in densely populated regions. In January 2013, most Chinese cities experienced persistent heavy air pollution episodes [8]. Based on monitoring data collected in the 190 largest cities in China from January 18, 2013, to December 31, 2013, the variations in hourly ambient $PM_{2.5}$ concentrations revealed that only 6% of the measured time met the guideline values of the World Health Organization interim target-1 (WHO IT-1) at 35 μg/m^3. Additionally, pollutant data showed that the northern and eastern of China were the most polluted area. In recent years, the widespread episodes of photochemical and air pollution events in the city-clusters areas have aroused great attention from the Chinese government, environmental protection departments, scientific research institutions, and the public to the problem of air pollution. In 2012, the Chinese National Ambient Air Quality Standard (NAAQS) was updated for stringent air pollutant regulation, and $PM_{2.5}$ as a new criterion pollutant was added into the revision of the NAAQS. For ambient $PM_{2.5}$, the 24-h mean concentration limited value for Category I places (e.g., natural protection zones) and II places (e.g., residential zones) is 35 $\mu g/m^3$ and 75 $\mu g/m^3$, respectively. Nevertheless, the revised NAAQS on mean $PM_{2.5}$ for 24-h is still far exceeding the updated air quality guideline value of 5 $\mu g/m^3$ recommended by WHO [9]. To date, evidence of air pollution exposure on health status in China is primarily generated based on short-term exposure studies. It should be noted that research on the effect of long-term exposure is still largely sparse, which is essential in setting up evidence-based ultimate objective goals to protect public health. In this context, we aim to provide a comprehensive review regarding the progress of air pollution epidemiology research in China, with an emphasis on exposure assessment methods and pollutants-associated cardiorespiratory effects.

24.2 Progress in Air Pollution Epidemiologic Study Methods

24.2.1 Principals of Exposure Assessment

Since the 1970s, air pollution exposure assessment has become a key step in assessing the associations between air pollutants and human health effects. Indeed, exposure assessment is the basis in environmental epidemiology of air pollution, which provides information on the characteristics of exposed population, exposure concentrations, exposure routes, and the source contribution of different environment factors to air pollution exposure. The primary steps of air pollution exposure assessment include estimating or measuring pollutant concentrations, exposure frequency, and duration of exposure to an agent (e.g., air pollutant) in exposed individuals. The determining factors of exposure assessment include systematically qualitative and quantitative evaluations of toxicant concentrations, individual and population exposures, exposure doses, and biological (or health) effect indicators.

The toxic property of air pollution is largely dependent on the intrinsic nature of pollutants as well as individual exposure levels. For assessment of exposure levels, it is primarily determined by the processes of migration, transport, and transformation of air pollutants, direct personal contact, and body's absorption of biological reactions. In practice, the main procedures of exposure assessment include: (1) exposure prediction: mathematical models are used to estimate pollutants in ambient and individual levels, based on the emission sources of pollutants or their precursors; (2) air monitoring: measurements of ambient pollutants were obtained from the monitoring station located nearby the residential address; (3) microenvironmental monitoring: exposures in each microenvironment are weighted for the mean time spent there and added to estimate total personal exposures; (4) personal monitoring: exposures of the subjects by directly measuring near the breathing zone of the subjects; (5) biological monitoring: internal dose of pollutant exposures by measuring biomarkers indicative of inhaled pollutant or its metabolites.

24.2.1.1 Assessments of Air Pollution Exposure

Measurements or estimations of the pollutant dose received by exposed individuals are essential for determining the health effects of air pollution in environmental epidemiologic studies. Direct assessment methods of exposure concentrations include personal monitoring and biological monitoring, based on obtained individual exposure levels or measured biological biomarkers. Personal active monitors/samplers (e.g., Thermo Scientific DataRAM pDR-1500) are used to measure pollutant concentrations (e.g., $PM_{2.5}$) at the individual levels. The primary advantage of using these instruments is the direct measurements of pollutant concentrations with inhalation exposures occurring during the sampling/monitoring period. Biological biomarkers indicate the part of toxicants or their metabolites detected in exposed individuals, which could be ideal indicators for the internal dose of the human following exposure to exogenous toxicants. Therefore, biomarker concentrations measured in biosamples (e.g., blood and urine) may reflect the effective exposure levels of pollutants more directly than measurements of contact levels. Emerging evidence suggests that special adducts in tissues or body fluids (e.g., DNA adducts and hemoglobin adducts) could be used as a surrogate indicator of the effective dose of air pollution exposure [10]. Biological monitoring may reflect the sum of internal dose via differential exposure routes (e.g., inhalation, digestion, and skin penetration), whereas cannot provide adequate information on the contribution of each route. Further, the ability of DNA and protein adducts to assess the carcinogenesis of environmental factors might be limited, because they primarily reflect shorter time periods of exposure (e.g., 1 month) due to a shorter biological half-life of the proteins. Indirect exposure assessment refers to estimation exposures using the fixed ambient monitoring station and mathematical modeling prediction. Incorporating monitoring concentration data and parameters of an individual's time-activity patterns and questionnaire surveys can significantly improve the validity of estimated exposures. Qualitative and retrospective approaches based on results of questionnaires or diary surveys have become a useful method of exposure assessment for pollutants characterized by specific types of emission sources (e.g., individuals categorized as two groups: exposed/unexposed to asbestos dust).

More recently, mathematical modeling prediction has emerged as an important technique for exposure assessment at both individual and population levels. Land use regression (LUR) model has been developed for exposure estimations of the distribution of regional pollutant concentrations, which is mainly conducted using data of pollutants measured at the fixed monitoring station, land use information, traffic network and flow, population density, meteorology, topography, greening, and other site-specific variables. Existing evidence suggests that pollutant concentrations estimated by the LUR model could explain approximately 60–80% of regional pollutant concentration changes [11]. Also, the LUR model shows a good performance in estimating the spatial distribution of long-term air pollution exposure, whereas the application to the estimation of short-term variations in concentrations of ambient air pollutants has been limited because this approach is inadequate for modeling data with high temporal resolution. Additionally, the satellite remote sensing technique provides a relatively accurate and cost-effective way to model spatiotemporally-resolved concentrations of PM mass and its components by using aerosol optical depth (AOD) in regions where air monitoring stations are largely sparse or not available. Compared with LUR, the primary parameter used in satellite-based exposure prediction is AOD measures, including the spectral eigenvalues of atmospheric scattering, absorption, and radiation. Although the development and application of LUR models and satellite-retrieved AOD products in China are largely limited, numerous exposure prediction models performed in developed countries have successfully applied to estimate concentrations of ambient PM and NO_2 at residential levels to assess the associations with adverse health effects.

24.2.1.2 Determinants of Air Pollution Exposure

The key components of air pollution exposure assessment include contact duration in and evaluations of pollutant concentrations in specific microenvironments (e.g., outdoors and indoors). The sum of individual exposure in each microenvironment is often presented as the integrated exposure, which can be directly or indirectly affected by: (1) factors relevant to the spatial distribution of pollutants and contact rates, including important sources, routes, and pathways of exposure; (2) factors relevant to temporal variations of contaminant concentrations and contact time, such as the duration and periodicity of exposure, the peak exposure, and the frequency and duration of contact; (3) factors relevant to interpersonal variability of dose, such as chemical intake and uptake rate and metabolism.

Exposure duration can be obtained on the basis of rational assumptions or individual information on time-activity patterns and lifestyle characteristics. Exposure concentration refers to a pollutant concentration at a contact boundary, such as human breathing zone. The concentration distribution of air pollutants can be used to estimate exposure levels of pollutants to individuals at a certain time and place. There are several approaches to evaluating pollutant concentrations, including personal monitoring, measurements of pollutants in ambient air and various microenvironments, and model simulations according to the pollutant emission intensity, transportation, and transformation process in the atmosphere. Among the approaches, microenvironmental assessment has the potential to supplement the outdoor fixed monitoring networks to improve the accuracy of estimated pollutant concentrations among exposed individuals. Typical microenvironments consist of living room, office, motor vehicle, public place, or other indoor environments, and they can also be further categorized as time spent in the kitchen and non-cooking time, based on the characteristics of kitchen activities. The major advantage of microenvironment assessment is that pollutant concentrations measured in course of daily activities are pollutants contacted by the human body when exposure occurs.

Model simulation and prediction techniques are also important in deriving data on pollutant concentrations for exposure assessment. According to the nature of pollutants, the commonly used models include those based on the principles of thermodynamics and kinetics. Thermodynamic principle model (e.g., pollutant environmental model) is suitable for pollutants, which are distributed among various environmental media, such as atmosphere, water, and soil, and have a certain lifetime in the environment, such as semi-volatile polycyclic aromatic hydrocarbons. Kinetic principle models, particularly air quality models based on the transport and transformation of PM and gaseous pollutants, focus on pollutants with inhalation as the main exposure route. Exposure assessments based on these models often use emission source data to simulate and predict temporal and spatial distributions of pollutant concentrations, along with parameters of pollutant property, meteorological/environmental factors, time-activity patterns, and indoor/outdoor ratios. It is worth noting that the data derived from model simulations should be validated via the observational measurements determined by monitor services to reduce potential estimation error. The development of more refined air quality assessment modeling techniques is expected to accurately qualify temporal and spatial distributions of pollutant concentrations, and improve the accuracy of exposure assessment. In 2010, the US Environmental Protection Agency proposed a 5-year plan to combine regional- and local-scale air quality models with environmental health studies, which include a three-dimensional chemical transmission model, community multiscale air quality model (CMAQ), and the local air quality dispersion model (AERMOD system).

24.2.2 Uncertainty and Variability in Assessment

Uncertainty and variability in the estimation of air pollution exposure are primarily generated by factors-related exposure parameters. The uncertainty regarding exposure assessment can be divided into three categories as following: (1) scenario uncertainty: uncertainty with regard to the wrong or incomplete information needed to comprehensively assess the exposure and dose; (2) parameter uncertainty: uncertainty with regard to some parameter of sources, including potential errors originating from the processes of measurement and sampling, and use of surrogate data; (3) model uncertainty: uncertainty with regard to the gaps in scientific knowledge required to make predictions based on causal inferences. The sources of uncertainty include descriptive and aggregation errors, as well as errors in insufficient professional judgment and incomplete analysis. Nevertheless, several methods can be used to reduce uncertainty mainly by: (1) using larger sample sizes or time-activity patterns assessed by survey-reported and global positioning system-recorded trips; (2) using rational simulations and analysis tools, such as statistical and sensitivity analyses, improved probabilistic methods based on the Monte Carlo analysis.

Spatial variability can occur regionally or locally. Generally, air pollutants at a regional scale are greatly affected by industrial activities, while pollutant levels at a local scale are affected by individual activities. The microenvironment method, which is usually applied to estimating personal exposures, assesses segments of time and location of exposure and thereby sums over all segments for approximately true exposure through the respiratory tract. Temporal variability is variability over the short- and long-term time duration. Long-term variations include seasonal changes, heating fuel use, and outdoor time, whereas short-term variations include differences in industrial production and personal activities during working days and weekends and differences in activities within a day. Individual variability includes individual and behavioral characteristics, such as age, sex, weight, spatial condition, and activity pattern. These variabilities are associated with other potential individual differences. For example, differences of individual weight are the results of a combination of genetic factors, nutritional conditions, lifestyle, and environmental factors.

24.3 Progress in Effect Estimates of Air Pollution

24.3.1 Short-Term Effects

Although epidemiologic research on air pollution and health in China started late, numerous publications emerging in recent years have demonstrated the short-term effects of air pollution. Short-term effects indicate that variations in air pollutant concentrations over shorter time periods (e.g., several hours to weeks) can prompt the onset or exacerbation of health status (e.g., mortality) and mediate the pathophysiological progression of diseases. Methodologically, epidemiologic study designs used to capture short-term effects of air pollution include population-based time series, case-crossover study, and panel study. Time series and case-crossover studies are the most common ecological methods of environmental science and health, which are designed to evaluate the impact of short-term air pollution on health status, focusing on daily mortality and hospital admission. The associations with temporal change in air pollution exposure are influenced by individual characteristics, such as age, gender, ethnicity, socioeconomic characteristics, smoking, and drinking. Other confounders are the seasons or other periodic patterns or long-term trends, such as time trends, days of the week, holidays, weather, and influenza epidemic.

With the development of individual exposure monitoring technology, the panel study as a prospective study design has been widely conducted in China, which allows to follow a small group (usually a dozen to a few hundred healthy and vulnerable population) of individuals intensively over a short time period and thereby capture the short-term effects of time-varying environmental stressors (e.g., air pollutants) on measured health outcomes. The outcomes tend to be symptoms and measurements of multiple subclinical health outcomes, such as spirometric parameters, vascular functions, blood and urinary biomarker profiles. For example, researchers at Peking University took the opportunity of the 2008 Summer Olympics to follow a panel of healthy adults before, during and after the Olympics, namely the study of Health Effects of Air Pollution Reduction Trial (HEART), and assessed the impacts of air quality interventions at individual exposure levels on a series of health indicators of cardiovascular physiology [12].

Another powerful research method assessing short-term effects of air pollution is the intervention study (epidemiologic experiment) that applies intervention measures to changes in pollutant concentrations and subsequently compares the health indicators between groups before versus after the implementation of interventions to validate the effectiveness of interventions. Because the design of the intervention study can well reduce the impacts of confounding factors, and investigate the effects of the interventions on human health, thus the intervention design is considered as a reasonable method to assess the causality of an observed association. For example, a randomized crossover intervention study of short-term indoor air filtration intervention on cardiopulmonary function in non-smoking elderly with chronic obstructive pulmonary disease (COPD) in Beijing, and a randomized, double-blind crossover trial of indoor air purifier intervention and face mask intervention on cardiopulmonary health in healthy college students in Shanghai [13]. This type of study design is of critical importance to validate the effectiveness of air quality management practices and personal-level interventions.

24.3.1.1 Mortality Risk

Extensive epidemiologic studies conducted in the past decades have revealed linkages between ambient air pollution and mortality. Nevertheless, high-quality evidence on the impact of air pollution on health status is primarily originated from studies conducted in Europe and North America, and few data are available in developing countries. Examples of such studies are the US National Mortality, Morbidity and Air Pollution Studies (NMMAPS) and the project of Air Pollution and Health: A European Approach 2 (APHEA-2). Data from the 20 largest cities and metropolitan areas, obtained from NMMAPS showed a statistically robust association of mortality with per 10μg/m^3 increase in PM_{10} (0.51%, 95% confidence interval [CI]: 0.07–0.93) [14]. The study of APHEA-2 covering 29 European cities has shown that the excess risk of total mortality increased by 0.6% (95% CI: 0.4–0.8) was associated with per 10 μg/m^3 increase in exposure to PM_{10} [15]. To the best of our knowledge, the first multicity time-series study that examined the effects of short-term air pollution exposure on mortality in China was the project of Public Health and Air Pollution in Asia (PAPA), using data from three representative cities: Hong Kong, Shanghai, and Wuhan [16]. In this analysis, effect estimates were firstly determined for individual city, and then combined effects were computed using a random-effects approach. With adjustments for time trend, meteorologic factors, and additional potential covariates (e.g., influenza epidemic), increases of 0.37% (95% CI: 0.21–0.54) for total mortality, 0.44% (95% CI: 0.19–0.68) for cardiovascular mortality, and 0.60% (95% CI: 0.10–1.04) for respiratory mortality were observed in association with per 10 μg/m^3 increase in 2-day moving average (MA) of PM_{10} exposures. Based on data from 1996 to 2008 in 16 Chinese cities, the China Air Pollution and Health Effects Study (CAPES) provided evidence confirming the effects of short-term air pollution exposure on mortality and reported per 10 μg/m^3 increase in exposure to PM_{10} at 2 MA days in relation to elevations of 0.35% (95% CI: 0.18–0.52) for total mortality [17]. For cause-specific analysis, increased risk of cardiovascular and respiratory mortality was 0.56% (95% CI: 0.31–0.81) and 0.44% (95% CI: 0.23–0.64), respectively. Two-pollutant models showed that the associations with PM_{10} exposures remained robust and independent of gaseous pollutant SO_2 or NO_2. Further, a national study including 38 large cities in China (2010–2013) also confirmed the effects of air pollution on mortality, per 10 μg/m^3 increase in PM_{10} at 1 MA day of exposure was associated increased risk of 0.44% (95% CI: 0.30–0.58) for total mortality and 0.62% (95% CI: 0.43–0.81) for cardiorespiratory mortality [18]. Generally, the findings found in the Chinese population are remarkably consistent with those observed in developed countries, supporting that air pollution exposure poses a tremendous threat to global public health.

More recently, considerable research attention has been shifted from large particles (e.g., PM_{10}) to particles in small size fractions (e.g., $PM_{2.5}$ and UFPs), because smaller size-fractioned particles may deposit in lung airways and alveoli deeper, and even translate into the circulation. Ambient $PM_{2.5}$ has been indicated to be the fourth leading risk factor for mortality in China, high levels of $PM_{2.5}$ exposures might be potentially responsible for 1.2 million premature deaths per year [19]. In a meta-analysis of 33 time-series and case-crossover studies performed in the Chinese population until 2012, significant increases in excess risks of premature death were observed in the pooled association estimates of various pollutants, using fixed-effect or random-effect models [20]. The results showed that the magnitude of associations with ambient $PM_{2.5}$ exposures was generally greater than with PM_{10}, indicating that the larger proportion of the health effects caused by PM_{10} could be attributed to $PM_{2.5}$. In specific, increases of 0.32% (95% CI: 0.28–0.35) for total mortality, 0.43% (95% CI: 0.37–0.49) for cardiovascular mortality, and 0.32% (95% CI: 0.23–0.40) for respiratory mortality were significantly associated with per 10 μg/m^3 increase in exposure to PM_{10}. Additionally, per 10 μg/m^3 increase in concentrations of $PM_{2.5}$ corresponded to increased risks of total, respiratory, and cardiovascular, and mortality increased by 0.38% (95% CI: 0.31–0.45), 0.51% (95% CI: 0.30–0.73), and 0.44% (95% CI: 0.33–0.54), respectively. It is notable that the pooled estimates in this study are largely weighed by the findings from more developed areas in China (e.g., Pearl River Delta Region and Yangtze River Delta) due to most of the air pollution epidemiology studies conducted in these cities. The relevant evidence is still sparse to evaluate the effects of air pollution in less developed areas. The updated analysis up to 2016 from the same study groups showed that per 10 μg/m^3 increase in $PM_{2.5}$ was associated with 0.51% (95% CI: 0.38–0.63), 0.62% (95% CI: 0.52–0.73), and 0.75% (95% CI: 0.54–0.95) increases in risks of total, respiratory, cardiovascular mortality, respectively [21]. In a recent meta-analysis of studies until 2018, a short-term increase in concentrations of $PM_{2.5}$ was associated with an elevated risk for total mortality by 0.49% (95% CI: 0.39–0.59) in the Chinese population [22]. Also, the pooled association estimate from study locations with daily $PM_{2.5}$ levels <75 μg/m^3 was larger than those with high levels of exposure (>75 μg/m^3), which extended the existing evidence that the adverse health effects are still detectable at $PM_{2.5}$ concentrations below the current regulatory limit value of the Chinese NAAQS.

Although dozens of studies have shown associations of daily mortality with PM exposures, the effects of temporal variations in pollutant concentrations at a long-term scale on mortality in China remain poorly understood. One important reason is that PM concentrations nationwide have been routinely measured and disclosed only since 2013, thus data on long time-series measurements of ambient $PM_{2.5}$ are largely absent. A recent analysis performed by Wu et al. [23] examined the associations between ambient air pollution and daily mortality in Guangzhou, China, based on a unique 11-year dataset (2006–2016). They found that statistically robust associations of $PM_{2.5}$ with risks of total, cardiovascular, and respiratory mortality existed; per 10 μg/m^3 increase in $PM_{2.5}$ concentrations at 6 MA days of exposure was associated with excess risks of 0.55% (95% CI: 0.24–0.86), 1.15% (95% CI: 0.68–1.62), and 0.78% (95% CI: 0.10–1.46), respectively. This analysis provided population-based evidence on the short-term effects of ambient $PM_{2.5}$ concentrations at a global scale (ranging from 2.7 to 263.8 μg/m^3), but the magnitude of association estimates for $PM_{2.5}$ was not comparable with those found in study locations with a relatively good air quality [24, 25]. A national analysis involving 112 US cities from 1999 to 2005 has shown that increase of 0.98% (95% CI: 0.75–1.22) in total mortality and 0.85% (95% CI: 0.46–1.24) in cardiovascular mortality, as well as 1.68% (95% CI: 1.04–2.33) in respiratory mortality, were observed in association with per 10 μg/m^3 increase in $PM_{2.5}$ exposures [24]. Further, an analysis including Mediterranean metropolitan areas showed that per 10 μg/m^3 increase in $PM_{2.5}$ exposures was associated with significant elevations of 0.32%, 0.54%, and 1.12% for total, cardiovascular, and respiratory mortality, respectively [25]. The differential city-to-city health risks of air pollution might be partially explained by differential characteristics of study population and various component species of pollutant mixtures across locations [26]. To date, coal is still the primary source of energy use in China, accounting for approximately 58% of total energy consumption. Further, the rapid urbanization results in significantly increasing number and use of motor vehicles. Consequently, the current source contribution of air pollution in China is predominantly dominated by a mixed emission type, characterized as coal smoke and motor vehicle emissions. Whereas the principal source of air pollutants in developed world is motor vehicle emissions. A 2014 systematic review and meta-analysis has quantified adverse effects of PM components and revealed that per 1 μg/m^3 increase in $PM_{2.5}$-bound EC (an indicator of traffic-related air pollution) and SO_4^{2-} (an indicator of regional pollution from coal-fired power plants) increased excess risk of total mortality by 1.30% (95% CI: 0.17–2.43) and 0.15% (95% CI: 0.06–0.25), respectively [27]. More research is needed to conduct assessing the difference in health responses observed between typical Asian areas and the western world. Selected studies on associations of short-term ambient PM and gaseous air pollution exposure with mortality in the Chinese population are summarized in Table 24.1.

24.3.1.2 Hospitalization

Hospitalization as a crucial proxy measure of morbidity has been widely used to investigate the health effects following air pollution exposure. Although the daily numbers of hospitalization are often analyzed using statistical approaches in a manner similar to assessing mortality effects; however, hospitalization data has several characteristics that substantially differ from those of mortality-related events, such as disease compositions and demographics. The impacts of ambient air pollution exposure on hospital admissions for respiratory diseases have been assessed in a series of epidemiologic studies in China. Recently, a nationwide time-series study was conducted to examine associations of short-term exposure to air pollutants with cause-specific diseases, based on data of hospital admissions in 252 Chinese cities from 2013 to 2017 [33]. For individual-day lag patterns, the association estimates between $PM_{2.5}$ and diseases of the respiratory system were largely on the current day of exposure and reduced sharply in the extended exposure period. For instance, the risks of hospital admissions for total respiratory diseases increased by 0.34% (95% CI: 0.28–0.39) and 0.17% (95% CI: 0.11–0.22) were associated with per 10 μg/m^3 increase in $PM_{2.5}$ at the current day and previous day of exposure, respectively. In cause-specific analysis, per 10 μg/m^3 increase in

Table 24.1 Summary of selected evidence of the risks of short-term ambient air pollution exposure on mortality in the Chinese population

Author (published year)	Study period	Pollutants	Increases (μg/m^3)	Percent increases in mortality (95% confidence interval)		
				Total	Cardiovascular	Respiratory
Wong et al. (2008) [16]	1996–2004[a]	PM_{10}	10	0.37 (0.21–0.54)	0.44 (0.19–0.68)	0.60 (0.16–1.04)
		SO_2	10	0.98 (0.74–1.23)	1.09 (0.72–1.47)	1.46 (0.84–2.08)
		NO_2	10	1.19 (0.71–1.66)	1.32 (0.79–1.86)	1.63 (0.62–2.64)
Chen et al. (2012) [17, 28, 29]	1996–2008	PM_{10}	10	0.35 (0.18–0.52)	0.44 (0.23–0.64)	0.56 (0.31–0.81)
		SO_2	10	0.75 (0.47–1.02)	0.83 (0.47–1.19)	1.25 (0.78–1.73)
		NO_2	10	1.63 (1.09–2.17)	1.80 (1.00–2.59)	2.52 (1.44–3.59)
Huang et al. (2012) [30]	2004–2008	$PM_{2.5}$	10	0.20 (0.07–0.33)	0.27 (0.08–0.46)	0.19 (−0.20–0.59)
Hou et al. (2011) [31]	2004–2008	PM_{10}	10	0.35 (0.11–0.58)	–	0.32 (−0.42–1.06)
		NO_2	10	2.42 (1.57–3.27)	–	3.71 (1.09–6.40)
		SO_2	10	0.60 (0.16–1.05)	–	1.02 (−0.32–2.38)
Yin et al. (2017) [18]	2010–2013	PM_{10}	10	0.44 (0.30–0.58)	–	–
Wu et al. (2018) [23]	2006–2016	PM_{10}	10	0.44 (0.22–0.65)	0.82 (0.49–1.14)	0.56 (0.09–1.03)
		$PM_{2.5}$	10	0.55 (0.24–0.86)	1.15 (0.68–1.62)	0.78 (0.10–1.46)
Wu et al. (2019) [32]	2006–2016	NO_2	10	1.89 (1.49–2.29)	2.18 (1.59–2.77)	2.29 (1.46–3.12)

[a]This combined analysis using data from three representative China cities: Hong Kong, from 1996 to 2002; Shanghai and Wuhan, both from 2001 to 2004. Abbreviations: PM_{10}, particulate matter (PM) with aerodynamic diameter <10 μm; $PM_{2.5}$, PM with aerodynamic diameter <2.5 μm; SO_2, sulfur dioxide; NO_2, nitrogen dioxide

exposure to $PM_{2.5}$ at the current day was related to increases in hospital admissions of 0.36% (95% CI: 0.28–0.44) for pneumonia, 0.32% (95% CI: 0.18–0.46) for acute bronchitis, and 0.52% (95% CI: 0.40–0.64) for the total number of COPD and bronchiectasis, but no significant effects were observed for asthma (–0.52% [95% CI: –0.36–0.16]). These results add to previous findings that COPD-related diseases might be responsible for the large portion of air pollution-associated adverse effects of respiratory system. The GBD study indicated that COPD was one of the leading causes of premature deaths in 2015, which could account for 3.2 million mortality globally [34]. In China, COPD ranked as the third most common cause of death in 2013, and more than 0.9 million deaths could be explained by COPD-related events [35]. A pooled analysis of the NMMAPS study including 14 US cities reported that the risks of hospital admissions for COPD increased by 1.98% (95% CI: 1.49–2.47), in relation to per 10 μg/m^3 increase in PM_{10} at 2 MA days of exposure [36]. In a 2014 systematic review and meta-analysis of studies conducted in the East Asian region, short-term exposure to PM_{10} and gaseous pollutants (e.g., NO_2 and SO_2) was associated with increased risks for COPD hospitalizations [37]. Per 10 μg/m^3 increase in PM_{10}, NO_2 and SO_2 increased the relative risk (RR) of COPD hospitalizations by 1.0% (RR: 1.010; 95% CI: 1.002–1.018), 1.9% (RR: 1.019; 95% CI: 1.016–1.022), and 0.7% (RR: 1.007; 95% CI: 1.003–1.010), respectively. Nevertheless, population-based studies of gaseous components, especially for CO at differential levels of exposure, have yielded mixed findings. A recent time-series analysis from Beijing, China from 2013 to 2017 was performed to assess the impact of short-term air pollution exposure on acute exacerbation of COPD [38]. Extreme levels of ambient particulate and gaseous pollutants were found during the study period, with daily averaged concentrations of $PM_{2.5}$ ranging from 5.0 to 467.0 μg/m^3 and CO ranging from 0.2 to 7.0 ppm. Results of regression models showed that the risks of hospitalizations for COPD corresponding to per interquartile range (IQR) increase in pollutant concentrations increased by 2.9% (RR: 1.029 [95% CI: 1.023–1.035]) for PM_{10}, 2.8% (RR: 1.028 [95% CI: 1.021–1.034]) for $PM_{2.5}$, 3.6% (RR: 1.036 [95% CI: 1.028–1.044]) for NO_2, 1.9% (RR: 1.019 [95% CI: 1.013–1.024]) for SO_2, and 2.4% (RR: 1.024 [95% CI: 1.018–1.029]) for CO. However, a study conducted in Hong Kong reported that short-term exposure to CO at low levels (ranging from 0.1 to 2.1 ppm) was associated with a reduced risk of hospital admissions for COPD [39]. The potentially protective role of lower CO in ambient air was also found for reduced hospital admissions for respiratory tract infection [40]. These findings suggest that CO under certain circumstances may exert differential effects on the respiratory system, and further studies are warranted to confirm and elucidate underlying mechanisms.

Apart from affecting the respiratory system, exposure to air pollution can also be a trigger of cardiovascular events. There are numerous epidemiologic and clinical studies that have examined associations between short-term variations in air pollution and daily hospital admissions for cardiovascular diseases. Considering the comparatively large sample size and importance, the findings from the National Health Insurance Database for Urban Employees covering 0.28 billion enrollees in 218 Chinese cities were merited to be discussed [41]. Daily averaged concentrations of ambient PM_{10} across all cities were 89 μg/m^3 throughout the study period (2014–2016). For individual-day lag patterns, the largest association estimate occurred on the current day of PM_{10} elevations. For instance, a significant increase of 0.29% (95% CI: 0.23–0.66) in daily hospitalizations was associated with per 10 μg/m^3 increase in exposure to concentrations of ambient PM_{10}, and the effect estimate remained robust after adjusting for gaseous pollutant (CO or SO_2). Additional analyses of this Database, based on health data within the period of 2014–2017, further investigated the impacts of short-term exposure to $PM_{2.5}$ on hospital admissions for cause-specific cardiovascular diseases [42]. Using random-effect models, per 10 μg/m^3 increase in ambient $PM_{2.5}$ at the current day of exposure was related to increases in hospital admissions of 0.26% (95% CI: 0.17–0.35) for cardiovascular disease, 0.29% (95% CI: 0.18–0.40) for ischemic stroke, 0.31% (95% CI: 0.22–0.40) for ischemic heart disease, 0.27% (95% CI: 0.04–0.51) for heart failure, and 0.31% (95% CI: 0.22–0.40) for heart rhythm disturbances. Compared to days with $PM_{2.5}$ concentrations ≤15 μg/m^3, higher $PM_{2.5}$ exposures were associated with significant increases of 1.1% (95% CI: 0.0–2.2) to 3.8% (95% CI: 2.1–5.5) in cardiovascular admissions. In line with mortality effects reported in previous studies [43], exposure-response curve derived from this study revealed that a steeper slope was observed at lower ambient $PM_{2.5}$ concentrations (0–50 μg/m^3), whereas a relatively stable plateau was reached at $PM_{2.5}$ concentrations >250 μg/m^3. Collectively, these findings confirmed the existing evidence that the relationships between ambient air pollution exposure and adverse health effects (e.g., mortality and morbidity) approximately appeared to be non-linear changes.

24.3.1.3 Surrogate Outcomes

Accumulating evidence supports that a variety of pathophysiologic alterations could occur among both healthy and susceptible individuals following air pollution exposure, in a manner predisposing to the onset of cardiorespiratory morbidity and mortality. These subclinical effects of air pollution provide crucial insights into the underlying mechanisms whereby air pollution may acutely prompt biochemical and cellular events that are implicated in the observable outcome associations. In this section, the potential pathways linking air pollution exposure to respiratory and cardiometabolic health are summarized, based on evidence from a series of human studies.

24.3.1.3.1 Pulmonary Pathophysiological Response

Biosamples of exhaled breath condensate (EBC) are reliable approaches for capturing the pathophysiologic alterations in the lower respiratory airways. One prominent hypothesis regarding the mechanisms of air pollution-associated adverse health effects is that inhalation of air pollution, especially for PM air pollution, is capable of triggering oxidative stress responses and subsequent inflammatory cascades in the lung. Nitric oxide (NO) in exhaled air is primarily originated from inducible nitric oxide synthase (NOS2) responsive to up-regulation of inflammation in the airway epithelium [44]. Exhaled NO has been used as a complementary marker in clinical practice to monitor the procession of respiratory diseases. Biomarkers of nitrite and nitrate (or nitrite plus nitrate) measured in EBC are the metabolic oxidative products of NO, which can be produced by activation of NOS2 and reflect the levels of airway oxidative and nitrosative stress [44]. Reactive oxygen species can react with lipids and nucleic acids to form various stable compounds indicative of oxidative stress, such as 8-isoprostane, 8-hydoxydeoxyguanosine [8-OHdG], and malondialdehyde [MDA]) [45]. Further, worsening of airway acidification exerts detrimental effects on several aspects of airway functions, including increased bronchoconstriction and viscosity of the airway mucus, as well as impaired epithelial function [46].

To date, more convincing evidence for pulmonary oxidative stress and inflammation responses attributable to ambient air pollution exposure is primarily derived from studies performed during the 2008 Beijing Olympics. In the HEART study, 125 healthy nonsmoking adults (aged 19–33 years old) were recruited and followed up with six clinical visits from June 2, 2008, to October 30, 2008 [47]. Based on the timelines of pollution control actions, the entire study period was decomposed into three subperiods, namely pre-, during-, and post-Olympics periods. Each participant experienced "high-low-high" levels of exposure corresponding to drastic changes in ambient pollutant concentrations that occurred in three subperiods. Statistically significant elevations of exhaled NO levels were observed in association with IQR increases in concentrations of ambient $PM_{2.5}$ and its major components (OC, EC, and SO_4^{2-}) and gaseous pollutants (NO_2, SO_2, and CO), during the preceding 1–7 days of exposure. Higher pollutant levels were also related to elevations levels of EBC nitrite, nitrate, nitrite plus nitrate, 8-isoprostane, and MDA. Further, an indicator of airway acidification was observed to be reduced in EBC as evidenced by lowering pH. Generally, the strongest associations for exhaled NO, nitrite, nitrate, and nitrite plus nitrate occurred on the current day of exposure, but for MDA and 8-isoprostane occurred during the preceding 3–6 days of exposure, indicating that air pollution could affect the process of NO metabolism faster than lipid peroxidation response. Additionally, 36 schoolchildren (8 asthma patients and 22 healthy individuals) were followed up with five visits during the periods before and during the Olympic Games (June 2007–September 2008) [48]. Significant increases in exhaled NO levels of 16.4% (95% CI: 11.8–21.2) and 18.8% (95% CI: 15.4–22.2) were associated with IQR increases in concentrations of $PM_{2.5}$ and BC at 2 MA days of exposure, respectively. The association estimates for $PM_{2.5}$ and BC exposures were slightly larger in healthy children than in those with diagnosed asthma. In 107 children with asthma residing in Mexico City, Romieu et al. [49] found that MDA levels in EBC could serve as a useful biomarker to capture the effects of $PM_{2.5}$ exposures, and increased MDA levels were associated with reductions in indices of lung function (e.g., forced expiratory volume in 1-s [FEV1]) and elevated secretions of IL-8 in nasal lavage. More recently, a panel of patients with diagnosed COPD residing in Beijing were recruited and followed with two repeated measurements between September 2014 and May 2015, Chen et al. [50] reported a positive association between particles in the size range of 100–200 nm and EBC nitrite plus nitrate. These findings provided preliminary but potentially crucial evidence on how inhaled air pollution may prompt the pathogenesis of respiratory diseases.

24.3.1.3.2 Cardiometabolic Function

A growing body of studies has been conducted to assess the effects of air pollution on cardiometabolic health within several minutes to days of exposure, with focusing on functional intermediate outcomes implicating in the development of cardiometabolic disorders, such as atherosclerosis and thrombosis. Mechanically, the prevailing hypothesis is that inflammatory mediators provoked by inhaled air pollutants (e.g., particles with a high content of pro-oxidative components) can leave the lung and thereby spill over into the circulation, inducing vascular inflammatory responses [51]. Individuals exposed to various ambient air pollutants have signs of activation of the lipid peroxidation process, along with elevated levels of oxidative DNA damage. In Chinese studies, significant elevations of DNA damage levels were detected in blood lymphocytes among traffic policemen versus indoor traffic officers in Shanghai and Guangzhou [52, 53]. In the HEART study, heightened systemic oxidative and inflammatory burdens were observed in association with air pollution exposure [54]. High levels of air pollutants were positively related to indicators reflecting endothelial dysfunction or platelet activation, including adhesive endothelial glycoprotein von Willebrand factor (vWF), soluble CD40 ligand (sCD40L) and soluble CD62P (sCD62P) [55]. Emerging evidence indicates that air pollution-associated heightened thrombogenicity might be a crucial mechanism to partially explain clinical manifestations of acute cardiovascular events [56]. Indeed, thrombotic events caused by platelet activation are well known to underlie the complications of atherosclerotic plaque instability [57]. Recently, a prospective study of Air Pollution and Cardiovascular Dysfunctions in Healthy Adults Living in Beijing (Beijing AIRCHD) has shed novel insight into the potential mechanisms responsible for air pollution-associated acute cardiovascular events. Seventy-three non-smoking young adults were followed up with repeated measurements in 2014–2016, Xu et al. [58] confirmed that exposure to high levels of air pollutants over a few days (e.g., ambient $PM_{2.5}$ ranging from 31 to 236 μg/m^3) could potentiate the prothrombotic reaction and atherosclerotic plaque vulnerability, as evidenced by elevated levels of sCD62P, sCD40L, fibrinogen/fibrin degradation product, matrix metalloproteinases (MMPs), and reductions in levels of prothrombin time and tissue inhibitor of MMPs. Mediation analyses revealed that activations of MMPs could be mediated through heightened systemic inflammation, and these cardiovascular responses could further worsen blood thrombogenicity. In addition, results also revealed the linkages between ambient air pollution exposure and impaired anti-atherosclerotic properties of high-density lipoprotein (HDL), and elevated levels of proatherogenic lipoproteins [59]. Similar findings were also found in individuals residing in North America, despite low levels of $PM_{2.5}$ exposures (ranging from 0.2 to 94.0 μg/m^3) [60, 61].

Additionally, neuropathophysiologic activities and metabolic changes may also act as crucial mechanistic pathways that are likely to explain the elevated risks of air pollution attributed to cardiometabolic disorders (e.g., hypertension and diabetes). Growing evidence has shown that hypertension and diabetes commonly coexist and may share initial pathophysiologic mechanisms, such as autonomic dysfunctions, worsening of insulin resistance, and increased inflammatory potential at the vasculature and adipose tissue [62]. In a clinical study of 62 cardiac rehabilitation patients in Boston, the USA, Zanobetti et al. [63] observed positive associations between ambient $PM_{2.5}$ and arterial blood pressure (BP) levels, and the effects were stronger among individuals with a resting heart rate ≥70 bpm (a proxy for assessment of sympathetic activity). Heart rate variability (HRV) is an essential clinical tool for the evaluation of autonomic nervous system function, and reduction of HRV indices reflects decreasing parasympathetic and increasing sympathetic tone. Numerous studies have shown that exposure to air pollution was related to autonomic dysfunctions, based on HRV indices (e.g., the standard deviation of all normal-to-normal intervals [SDNN]) derived from electrocardiographic (ECG) recordings. For example, in a 2-year longitudinal follow-up of 40 patients with cardiovascular diseases before and during the Beijing Olympics, reductions in SDNN of 3.5–4.7% were found to be significantly associated with IQR increases in $PM_{2.5}$ at prior 1–12-h MAs of exposure [64]. Also, Langrish et al. [65] reported that reducing personal exposure to PM air pollution using a facemask could improve a variety of cardiovascular health outcomes (e.g., HRV indices) among 98 patients with coronary heart diseases living in Beijing. Several studies have indicated that the underlying metabolic abnormalities (e.g., obesity and insulin resistance) observed in patients and healthy individuals confer susceptibility to the adverse cardiometabolic effects of air pollution. Sun et al. [66] reported significant inverse associations of SDNN with UFPs and BC exposures in a panel of elderly participants in Shanghai, China, with stronger associations in individuals with diabetes risk factors, including obesity and impaired glucose tolerance. In the Veterans Administration Normative Aging Study, Baja et al. [67] found that prolongation of ECG-derived QT intervals was associated with exposure to NO_2 and CO, and the associations were stronger among individuals who were obese and with diagnosed diabetes. QT is a reliable index of cardiac ventricular repolarization and has been found to be associated with heightened myocardial vulnerability to life-threatening arrhythmias and acute cardiovascular events [68]. Likely, additional analyses from the Beijing AIRCHD also showed the air pollution attributed to prolonged QT intervals and pro-hypersensitive actions were found in modifications by overweight status [69, 70]. Moreover, Air Pollution and Cardiometabolic Disease (AIRCMD-China) study, 65 nonsmoking adults with metabolic syndrome were followed up with repeated visits in 2012–2013. Brook et al. [71] found that short-term exposure to $PM_{2.5}$ and BC resulted in insulin resistance status and higher levels of BP. Results further showed the adverse impacts of air pollutants on myocardial perfusion and oxygen demand, and the effects could be modified by dyslipidemia (e.g., low levels of HDL cholesterol) [72].

24.3.1.3.3 Epigenetic Changes

As discussed earlier, exposure to air pollution is associated with DNA damage locally and systematically. Emerging evidence suggests that air pollution can also alter epigenetic states such as global and gene-specific DNA methylation [73, 74]. Epigenetic changes, particularly DNA methylation abnormalities, have been implicated in the development and exacerbation of respiratory and cardiovascular diseases associated with ubiquitous environmental exposures (e.g., air pollution) [74]. Among 718 elderly individuals in the Greater Boston area, Baccarelli et al. [75] found rapid reductions in levels of DNA methylation in long interspersed nucleotide element-1 (LINE-1) responsive to ambient $PM_{2.5}$ and BC at prior up to 7 MA days of exposure. Particles in size ranges of 0.007–3 μm at prior 7 MA days of exposure were also found to be negatively associated with DNA methylation in tissue factor (F3), a key player implicating in the blood coagulation cascades and subsequent fibrinogen production [76]. Limited experimental trials have been conducted to assess whether epigenetic changes caused by inhaled pollutants may prompt the pathogenesis of cardiorespiratory diseases. In a randomized controlled study on 16 asthmatic patients, the authors found methylation of cysteinyl leukotriene receptor 1 (CysLTR1) genes in association with lung function among 16 asthmatic patients exposed to traffic-related air pollution [77]. Also, the linkages between particles exposures and impaired lung function could be partially mediated via alterations in methylation and gene expression of CysLTR1. Elevated LTE4 has been demonstrated to recruit immune cells to the airway mucosa, leading to heightened airway inflammatory response [78]. Recently, significant reductions in methylation of Alu and Toll-like receptor-4 (TLR4) were reported in 15 healthy adults exposed to concentrated ambient $PM_{2.5}$ for 2 h, and these epigenetic changes may in turn worsen the pro-hypersensitive action of $PM_{2.5}$ [79]. A panel study performed in Shanghai revealed that reduced CD40LG methylation could serve as a potential mediator responsible for the association of $PM_{2.5}$ exposures with sCD40L elevations [80]. It should be noted that the change in DNA methylation is not an exclusive mechanism that regulates gene expression, and other potential regulatory mechanisms, including activation of transcription factors and chromatin remodeling, may also affect expressions of protein-coding genes. Therefore, more epidemiologic and mechanistic studies were required to assess the roles of pollutant-associated epigenetic changes in human health.

24.3.2 Long-Term Effects

Long-term effects refer to the cumulative effects of continuous exposure to air pollution mixtures that may persist over longer time periods (e.g., ranging 1 year to several decades), which are most frequently determined by using the technique of the cross-sectional and cohort design. Cohort study is one of the main methodologies in testing the causality of the association between air pollution and human health. The Harvard Six Cities study is a landmark study in worldwide that reveals the health effects of long-term exposure [81]. In this well-characterized cohort, 8,111 adults (25–74 years old) living in six US cities underwent 14–16 years of follow-up. Using PM_{10} and $PM_{2.5}$ as exposure metrics, the adjusted rate ratio of total mortality obtained in the most-polluted city relative to the least-polluted city was 1.27 (95% CI: 1.08–1.48) and 1.26 (95% CI: 1.08–1.47), respectively. The effects remained robust after adjusting for a wealth of covariates measured at individuals, including demographics (e.g., age, sex, body mass index, and education levels), behavior risk factors (e.g., smoking status), and cardiometabolic disorders (hypertension and diabetes). Pollutants over the years of exposure were also associated with elevated risk ratios for mortality due to lung cancer and cardiopulmonary diseases. Subsequently, evidence for a wide range of health effects attributed to long-term exposure was derived from a series of high-quality studies, including the American Cancer Society (ACS) study [82], Trucking Industry Particle Study (TrIPS) [83], and Adventist Health Study on Smog (AHSMOG) study [84], as well as European Study of Cohorts for Air Pollution Effects (ESCAPE) [85]. For instance, the ESCAPE study included 17 cohorts from 9 European countries that covered 312,944 participants, and 2095 individuals experienced lung cancer after mean of 12.8 years of follow-up. Concentrations of ambient PM_{10}, $PM_{2.5}$, and NO_x at each participant's baseline residential address were estimated using LUR models. With adjustments for a variety of confounder variables (e.g., age, sex, calendar time, smoking status, socioeconomic status, employment status, education levels, occupation, and fruit intake), Raaschou-Nielsen et al. [85] showed a positive association between lung cancer and ambient PM_{10} concentrations (hazard ratio [HR]: 1.22 [95% CI: 1.03–1.45] per 10 μg/m^3 increase in PM_{10}). In the same project, Beelen et al. [86] found that per 5 μg/m^3 increase in annual average ambient $PM_{2.5}$ was associated with a 7% increased risk of natural-cause mortality (HR: 1.07 [95% CI: 1.02–1.13]). The positive associations (HR: 1.06 [95% CI: 1.00–1.12]) could be still detected at annual average $PM_{2.5}$ concentrations <20 μg/m^3, which is well below the current annual limit value of 25 μg/m^3 in Europe. The data from the US National Institutes of Health-AARP cohort also found that per 10 μg/m^3 increase in annual average ambient $PM_{2.5}$ exposures at residential address increased risks of 3% (HR: 1.03 [95% CI: 1.00–1.05]) for total mortality and 10% (HR: 1.10 [95% CI: 1.05–1.15]) for cardiovascular mortality, despite low levels of $PM_{2.5}$ exposures (ranging from 10 to 13 μg/m^3) [87]. In a meta-analysis of 18 studies, long-term increases in PM concentrations (both PM_{10} and $PM_{2.5}$) were related to increased risks for lung cancer and adenocarcinomas of the lung [88]. In specific, per 10 μg/m^3 increase in exposure to $PM_{2.5}$ was associated with an increased RR of lung cancer by 9% (HR: 1.09 [95% CI: 1.04–1.14]).

Until recently, the impacts and underlying mechanisms of long-term air pollution exposure on health status in China remain poorly unknown. To reduce existing research gaps, a handful of studies has attempted to combine the existing epidemiologic database with state-of-the-art approaches of exposure prediction, such as the hierarchical LUR model and satellite data. Using the same LUR models developed by the ESCAPE study, Su et al. [89] found that significant increases in the maximum left of carotid intima-media thickness were positively associated with 1-year averaged concentrations of PM_{10} and NO_2 exposures, but not associated with $PM_{2.5}$. In a cross-sectional analysis of 8867 patients with suspected coronary heart disease, Wang et al. [90] found that exposure to LUR-derived $PM_{2.5}$ and NO_2 was independently associated with increases in coronary artery calcium (CAC) scores of 27.2% (95% CI: 10.8–46.1) per 30 μg/m^3 increase in concentrations of $PM_{2.5}$ and 24.5% (95% CI: 3.6–49.7) per 20 μg/m^3 increase in concentrations of NO_2, with adjusting for individual-level risk factors and multiple air pollutants. The pro-atherogenic effects of air pollution were stronger among elderly participants (age >60 years) and those with diagnosed diabetes. CAC measure reflects the degree of subclinical atherosclerosis involving plaque calcification and has been consistently associated with the onset of future cardiovascular events [91]. In the Chinese Elderly Health Services Cohort conducted in Hong Kong, Qiu et al. [92] identified 806 incident cases of type 2 diabetes from 53,905 non-diabetic participants at baseline over an approximately 10-year follow up. They found that IQR increases in satellite-based $PM_{2.5}$ at residential address were associated with elevated incident risk of diabetes (HR: 1.15 [95% CI: 1.05–1.25]), after controlling for various risk factors. Selected large cohort studies on associations between long-term air pollution exposure and mortality are summarized in Table 24.2.

A Working Group of scientists who were from 11 countries (including China) were invited by the International Agency for Research on Cancer (IARC) to assess the carcinogenicity of outdoor air pollution in 2013. Based on sufficient evidence from high-quality epidemiologic studies primarily conducted in North America and Europe, the Working Group unanimously agreed that both outdoor air pollution and PM in ambient air can be classified as IARC Group 1 human carcinogens. Given that relevant epidemiologic evidence is limited in China, only one study has been available for evaluation by the IARC Working Group. A national cohort study performed by Cao et al. [97] examined the mortality effects of long-term air pollution exposure in 70,947 middle-aged adults residing in 31 Chinese cities. The average concentrations of ambient total suspended particles (TSP), NO_x, and SO_2 between 1991 and 2000 were estimated from the combination of local air monitoring station and resident zip code. Further, $PM_{2.5}$ concentrations were estimated from TSP data (conversion as $PM_{2.5}/TSP \approx 0.325$). With adjustments for individual characteristics (e.g., demographics and parameters relevant to smoking and socioeconomic status), per 10 μg/m^3 increase in $PM_{2.5}$, NO_x and SO_2 increased the RR of lung cancer

Table 24.2 Summary of selected cohort study results of the risks of long-term ambient air pollution exposure on mortality

Study	Author (published year)	Pollutants	Increases	Hazard ratios for mortality (95% confidence interval)		
				Total	Cardiopulmonary	Lung cancer
Harvard Six-Cities	Lepeule et al. (2012) [93]	$PM_{2.5}$	10 μg/m^3	1.14 (1.07–1.22)	1.26 (1.14–1.40)	1.37 (1.07–1.75)
ACS	Pope et al. (2002) [94]	$PM_{2.5}$	10 μg/m^3	1.06 (1.02–1.11)	1.09 (1.03–1.16)	1.14 (1.04–1.23)
NHIS	Pope et al. (2019) [95]	$PM_{2.5}$	10 μg/m^3	1.12 (1.08–1.15)	1.23 (1.17–1.29)	1.12 (1.00–1.26)
AHSMOG	Beeson et al. (1998) [84]	PM_{10}	24 μg/m^3	–	–	5.21 (1.94–13.99)
		SO_2	3.7 ppb	–	–	2.66 (1.62–4.39)
		NO_2	1.98 ppb	–	–	1.45 (0.67–3.14)
TrIPS	Hart et al. (2011) [96]	PM_{10}	6 μg/m^3	1.10 (1.05–1.15)	–	1.05 (0.94–1.17)
		$PM_{2.5}$	4 μg/m^3	1.04 (1.01–1.07)	–	1.02 (0.95–1.10)
		NO_2	6 ppb	1.15 (1.10–1.20)	–	1.07 (0.96–1.2)
		SO_2	4 ppb	1.11 (1.05–1.17)	–	1.09 (0.95–1.25)
ESCAPE	Raaschou-Nielsen et al. (2013) [85]	PM_{10}	10 μg/m^3	–	–	1.22 (1.03–1.45)
		$PM_{2.5}$	5 μg/m^3	–	–	1.18 (0.96–1.46)

Abbreviations: ACS: American Cancer Society; NHIS, National Health Interview Surveys, TrIPS, Trucking Industry Particle Study; AHSMOG, Adventist Health Study on Smog; ESCAPE, European Study of Cohorts for Air Pollution Effects; PM_{10}, particulate matter (PM) with aerodynamic diameter <10 μm; $PM_{2.5}$, PM with aerodynamic diameter <2.5 μm; SO_2, sulfur dioxide; NO_2, nitrogen dioxide mortality by 0.3% (RR: 1.03 [95% CI: 1.00–1.07]), 0.3% (RR: 1.03 [95% CI: 0.99–1.07]), and 0.4% (RR: 1.04 [95% CI: 1.02–1.06]), respectively. Although this study provided preliminary findings supporting the linkage between $PM_{2.5}/SO_2$ and lung cancer; however, the magnitude of association estimate is low relative to studies conducted in the developed world. The authors speculated that the discrepancy in findings might be partially explained by varied study contexts, including population, local pollutants levels, physical and chemical characteristics of pollutant mixtures, as well as differential shapes of exposure-response curves. It is worth noting that the attenuated risk coefficient may also be caused by possible exposure measurement errors. Indeed, potential measurement errors could have occurred when pollutants concentrations at each participant's residential address were estimated using pollutant data monitored at the fixed monitoring station, along with resident zip code. Selected studies on associations of ambient PM air pollution exposure with lung cancer are summarized in Table 24.3.

Table 24.3 Summary of selected evidence of the risks of ambient $PM_{2.5}$ exposures (per 10 μg/m³ increases) on lung cancer

Author (published year)	Hazard ratios	95% confidence interval
North American		
Hart et al. (2011) [96]	1.18	0.95–1.48
Hystad et al. (2013) [98]	1.29	0.95–1.76
Jerrett et al. (2013) [99]	1.12	0.91–1.37
Krewski, et al. (2009) [100]	1.09	1.05–1.13
Lepeule et al. (2012) [93]	1.37	1.07–1.75
Lipsett, et al. (2011) [101]	0.95	0.70–1.28
McDonnell, et al. (2000) [102]	1.39	0.79–2.46
Europe		
Beelen et al. (2008) [103]	0.81	0.63–1.04
Carey, et al. (2013) [104]	1.11	0.86–1.43
Cesaroni et al. (2013) [105]	1.05	1.01–1.10
Raaschou-Nielsen et al. (2013) [85]	1.39	0.91–2.13
East Asia		
Cao et al. (2011) [97]	1.03	1.00–1.07
Katanoda et al. (2011) [106]	1.24	1.12–1.37

Abbreviations: $PM_{2.5}$, particulate matter (PM) with aerodynamic diameter <2.5 μm

24.4 Summary and Perspectives

In light of the poor air quality disproportionately and continuously affecting hundreds of millions of people worldwide, particularly those residing in developing countries, the WHO has released its first air quality guidelines to policymakers on strengthening air quality management and protecting population health in 2005. In the last decades, emerging findings related to short- and long-term effects of air pollution exposure have resulted in an update of the evidence-based guidance on air quality regulation strategy that has been released by WHO in 2021 [107]. To date, compelling epidemiologic evidence supports approximately linear relationships between ambient pollutants exposures (e.g., $PM_{2.5}$) and adverse health status in North American and European countries [108]. However, little high-quality evidence thus far available for assessing whether the current Chinese NAAQ could sufficiently protect against the public health burden attributable to air pollution.

Different from air pollution sources dominated by traffic emissions in western countries, the source contribution of ambient pollutants in China is largely characterized by a mixed emission type of coal smoke and vehicle emissions. Further, the susceptibility of the Chinese population to air pollution might differ from that of foreign residents due to diversities in genetic characterization and age structure. Consequently, the shapes of the dose-response curves derived from the developed world cannot be simply and directly applied for evaluating the health effects of air pollution exposure in the Chinese population. In this context, further high-quality epidemiologic studies are required to systematically elucidate the casual relationships and dose-response curves between air pollution (particularly long-term exposure) and adverse health status. These actions would generate comprehensive and consolidated evidence for evaluating or revising the current Chinese NAAQS, thereby achieving the blueprint of Healthy China 2030 targeted at improving public health.

References

1. Nemery B, Hoet PH, Nemmar A. The Meuse Valley fog of 1930: an air pollution disaster. Lancet. 2001;357(9257):704–8.
2. Logan WP. Mortality in the London fog incident, 1952. Lancet. 1953;1(6755):336–8.
3. Landrigan PJ, Fuller R, Acosta NJR, et al. The Lancet Commission on pollution and health. Lancet. 2018;391(10119):462–512.
4. Nemmar A, Vanbilloen H, Hoylaerts MF, Hoet PH, Verbruggen A, Nemery B. Passage of intratracheally instilled ultrafine particles from the lung into the systemic circulation in hamster. Am J Respir Crit Care Med. 2001;164(9):1665–8.
5. Nemmar A, Hoet PH, Vanquickenborne B, et al. Passage of inhaled particles into the blood circulation in humans. Circulation. 2002;105(4):411–4.
6. Miller MR, Raftis JB, Langrish JP, et al. Inhaled nanoparticles accumulate at sites of vascular disease. ACS Nano. 2017;11(5):4542–52.
7. Cohen AJ, Brauer M, Burnett R, et al. Estimates and 25-year trends of the global burden of disease attributable to ambient air pollution: an analysis of data from the Global Burden of Diseases Study 2015. Lancet. 2017;389(10082):1907–18.
8. Song Y, Wang X, Maher BA, et al. The spatial-temporal characteristics and health impacts of ambient fine particulate matter in China. J Clean Prod. 2016;112:1312–8.
9. WHO. WHO global air quality guidelines: particulate matter ($PM_{2.5}$ and PM_{10}), ozone, nitrogen dioxide, sulfur dioxide and carbon monoxide. Available at: https://www.who.int/publications/i/item/9789240034228.
10. Sørensen M, Autrup H, Møller P, et al. Linking exposure to environmental pollutants with biological effects. Mutat Res. 2003;544(2–3):255–71.
11. Beelen R, Hoek G, Vienneau D, et al. Development of NO_2 and NOx land use regression models for estimating air pollution exposure in 36 study areas in Europe—The ESCAPE project. Atmos Environ. 2013;72:10–23.
12. Zhang J, Zhu T, Kipen H, et al. Cardiorespiratory biomarker responses in healthy young adults to drastic air quality changes surrounding the 2008 Beijing Olympics. Res Rep. 2013;174:5–174.
13. Rajagopalan S, Brauer M, Bhatnagar A, et al. Personal-level protective actions against particulate matter air pollution exposure: a scientific statement from the American Heart Association. Circulation. 2020;142(23):e411–31.
14. Samet JM, Dominici F, Curriero FC, Coursac I, Zeger SL. Fine particulate air pollution and mortality in 20 U.S. cities, 1987-1994. N Engl J Med. 2000;343(24):1742–9.
15. Katsouyanni K, Touloumi G, Samoli E, et al. Confounding and effect modification in the short-term effects of ambient particles on total mortality: results from 29 European cities within the APHEA2 project. Epidemiology. 2001;12(5):521–31.
16. Wong CM, Vichit-Vadakan N, Kan H, Qian Z. Public Health and Air Pollution in Asia (PAPA): a multicity study of short-term effects of air pollution on mortality. Environ Health Perspect. 2008;116(9):1195–202.
17. Chen R, Kan H, Chen B, et al. Association of particulate air pollution with daily mortality: the China Air Pollution and Health Effects Study. Am J Epidemiol. 2012;175(11):1173–81.
18. Yin P, He G, Fan M, et al. Particulate air pollution and mortality in 38 of China's largest cities: time series analysis. BMJ. 2017;356:j667.
19. Yang G, Wang Y, Zeng Y, et al. Rapid health transition in China, 1990-2010: findings from the Global Burden of Disease Study 2010. Lancet. 2013;381(9882):1987–2015.
20. Shang Y, Sun Z, Cao J, et al. Systematic review of Chinese studies of short-term exposure to air pollution and daily mortality. Environ Int. 2013;54:100–11.
21. Wu R, Song X, Bai Y, et al. Are current Chinese national ambient air quality standards on 24-hour averages for particulate matter sufficient to protect public health? J Environ Sci. 2018;71:67–75.
22. Li M, Wu Y, Tian YH, et al. A Meta-analysis on the relations between short-term exposure to $PM_{2.5}$ and both mortality and related emergency visits in China. Zhonghua liuxingbingxue zazhi. 2018;39(10):1394–401.
23. Wu R, Zhong L, Huang X, et al. Temporal variations in ambient particulate matter reduction associated short-term mortality risks in Guangzhou, China: a time-series analysis (2006-2016). Sci Total Environ. 2018;645:491–8.
24. Zanobetti A, Schwartz J. The effect of fine and coarse particulate air pollution on mortality: a national analysis. Environ Health Perspect. 2009;117(6):898–903.
25. Samoli E, Stafoggia M, Rodopoulou S, et al. Associations between fine and coarse particles and mortality in Mediterranean cities: results from the MED-PARTICLES project. Environ Health Perspect. 2013;121(8):932–8.
26. Lelieveld J, Evans JS, Fnais M, Giannadaki D, Pozzer A. The contribution of outdoor air pollution sources to premature mortality on a global scale. Nature. 2015;525(7569):367–71.
27. Atkinson RW, Mills IC, Walton HA, Anderson HR. Fine particle components and health—a systematic review and meta-analysis of epidemiological time series studies of daily mortality and hospital admissions. J Expo Sci Environ Epidemiol. 2015;25(2):208–14.

28. Chen R, Huang W, Wong CM, et al. Short-term exposure to sulfur dioxide and daily mortality in 17 Chinese cities: the China air pollution and health effects study (CAPES). Environ Res. 2012;118:101–6.
29. Chen R, Samoli E, Wong CM, et al. Associations between short-term exposure to nitrogen dioxide and mortality in 17 Chinese cities: the China air pollution and health effects study (CAPES). Environ Int. 2012;45:32–8.
30. Huang W, Cao J, Tao Y, et al. Seasonal variation of chemical species associated with short-term mortality effects of $PM_{2.5}$ in Xi'an, a central city in China. Am J Epidemiol. 2012;175(6):556–66.
31. Hou B, Dai L, Wang Z, Shang Y, Li J. Time-series analysis of acute mortality effects of air pollution in Xi'an. J Environ Health. 2011;28(12):1039–43. https://doi.org/10.16241/j.cnki.1001-5914.2011.12.003.
32. Wu R, Song X, Chen D, et al. Health benefit of air quality improvement in Guangzhou, China: results from a long time-series analysis (2006–2016). Environ Int. 2019;126:552–59.
33. Gu J, Shi Y, Zhu Y, et al. Ambient air pollution and cause-specific risk of hospital admission in China: a nationwide time-series study. PLoS Med. 2020;17(8):e1003188.
34. Global, regional, and national deaths, prevalence, disability-adjusted life years, and years lived with disability for chronic obstructive pulmonary disease and asthma, 1990-2015: a systematic analysis for the Global Burden of Disease Study 2015. Lancet Respir Med. 2017;5(9):691–706.
35. Zhou M, Wang H, Zhu J, et al. Cause-specific mortality for 240 causes in China during 1990-2013: a systematic subnational analysis for the Global Burden of Disease Study 2013. Lancet. 2016;387(10015):251–72.
36. Samet JM, Zeger SL, Dominici F, et al. The National Morbidity, Mortality, and Air Pollution Study. Part II: Morbidity and mortality from air pollution in the United States. Res Rep. 2000;94(Pt 2):5–70. Discussion 71–9
37. Zhang S, Li G, Tian L, Guo Q, Pan X. Short-term exposure to air pollution and morbidity of COPD and asthma in East Asian area: a systematic review and meta-analysis. Environ Res. 2016;148:15–23.
38. Liang L, Cai Y, Barratt B, et al. Associations between daily air quality and hospitalisations for acute exacerbation of chronic obstructive pulmonary disease in Beijing, 2013-17: an ecological analysis. Lancet Planet Health. 2019;3(6):e270–9.
39. Tian L, Ho KF, Wang T, et al. Ambient carbon monoxide and the risk of hospitalization due to chronic obstructive pulmonary disease. Am J Epidemiol. 2014;180(12):1159–67.
40. Tian L, Qiu H, Pun VC, et al. Ambient carbon monoxide associated with reduced risk of hospital admissions for respiratory tract infections. Am J Respir Crit Care Med. 2013;188(10):1240–5.
41. Tian Y, Liu H, Liang T, et al. Ambient air pollution and daily hospital admissions: a nationwide study in 218 Chinese cities. Environ Pollut. 2018;242(Pt B):1042–9.
42. Tian Y, Liu H, Wu Y, et al. Association between ambient fine particulate pollution and hospital admissions for cause specific cardiovascular disease: time series study in 184 major Chinese cities. BMJ. 2019;367:l6572.
43. Liu C, Chen R, Sera F, et al. Ambient particulate air pollution and daily mortality in 652 cities. N Engl J Med. 2019;381(8):705–15.
44. Guo FH, Comhair SA, Zheng S, et al. Molecular mechanisms of increased nitric oxide (NO) in asthma: evidence for transcriptional and post-translational regulation of NO synthesis. J Immunol. 2000;164(11):5970–80.
45. Rahman I, Biswas SK. Non-invasive biomarkers of oxidative stress: reproducibility and methodological issues. Redox Rep. 2004;9(3):125–43.
46. Bikov A, Horvath I. Methodological issues and possible clinical implications for exhaled breath condensate pH in asthma. Curr Top Med Chem. 2016;16(14):1550–60.
47. Huang W, Wang G, Lu SE, et al. Inflammatory and oxidative stress responses of healthy young adults to changes in air quality during the Beijing Olympics. Am J Respir Crit Care Med. 2012;186(11):1150–9.
48. Lin W, Huang W, Zhu T, et al. Acute respiratory inflammation in children and black carbon in ambient air before and during the 2008 Beijing Olympics. Environ Health Perspect. 2011;119(10):1507–12.
49. Romieu I, Barraza-Villarreal A, Escamilla-Nuñez C, et al. Exhaled breath malondialdehyde as a marker of effect of exposure to air pollution in children with asthma. J Allergy Clin Immunol. 2008;121(4):903–909.e906.
50. Chen J, Zhao Q, Liu BB, et al. Airway oxidative stress and inflammation markers in chronic obstructive pulmonary diseases(COPD) patients are linked with exposure to traffic-related air pollution: a panel study. Chin J Prev Med. 2016;50(5):411–7.
51. Miller MR. The cardiovascular effects of air pollution: prevention and reversal by pharmacological agents. Pharmacol Ther. 2021; https://doi.org/10.1016/j.pharmthera.2021.107996.
52. Peng-Kun LI, Gao ZY, Jiang RF, Gai BB, Qin YQ, Song WM. DNA damage in population exposed to fine particulate. J Environ Occup Med. 2010. https://doi.org/10.13213/j.cnki.jeom.2010.05.014.
53. Zhu CQ, Lam T, Jiang CQ, Wei BX, Chen YH, Xu QR. A study on lymphocyte DNA damage in traffic policemen in Guangzhou. Chin J Ind Hyg Occup Dis. 2003;21(1):41–4.
54. Gong J, Zhu T, Kipen H, et al. Comparisons of ultrafine and fine particles in their associations with biomarkers reflecting physiological pathways. Environ Sci Technol. 2014;48(9):5264–73.

55. Rich DQ, Kipen HM, Huang W, et al. Association between changes in air pollution levels during the Beijing Olympics and biomarkers of inflammation and thrombosis in healthy young adults. JAMA. 2012;307(19):2068–78.
56. Bevan GH, Al-Kindi SG, Brook RD, Münzel T, Rajagopalan S. Ambient air pollution and atherosclerosis: insights into dose, time, and mechanisms. Arterioscler Thromb Vasc Biol. 2021;41(2):628–37.
57. Crea F, Libby P. Acute coronary syndromes: the way forward from mechanisms to precision treatment. Circulation. 2017;136(12):1155–66.
58. Xu H, Wang T, Liu S, et al. Extreme levels of air pollution associated with changes in biomarkers of atherosclerotic plaque vulnerability and thrombogenicity in healthy adults. Circ Res. 2019;124(5):e30–43.
59. Li J, Zhou C, Xu H, et al. Ambient air pollution is associated with HDL (high-density lipoprotein) dysfunction in healthy adults. Arterioscler Thromb Vasc Biol. 2019;39(3):513–22.
60. Mathew AV, Yu J, Guo Y, et al. Effect of ambient fine particulate matter air pollution and colder outdoor temperatures on high-density lipoprotein function. Am J Cardiol. 2018;122(4):565–70.
61. Bell G, Mora S, Greenland P, Tsai M, Gill E, Kaufman JD. Association of air pollution exposures with high-density lipoprotein cholesterol and particle number: the multi-ethnic study of atherosclerosis. Arterioscler Thromb Vasc Biol. 2017;37(5):976–82.
62. Pi X, Xie L, Patterson C. Emerging roles of vascular endothelium in metabolic homeostasis. Circ Res. 2018;123(4):477–94.
63. Zanobetti A, Canner MJ, Stone PH, et al. Ambient pollution and blood pressure in cardiac rehabilitation patients. Circulation. 2004;110(15):2184–9.
64. Huang W, Zhu T, Pan X, et al. Air pollution and autonomic and vascular dysfunction in patients with cardiovascular disease: interactions of systemic inflammation, overweight, and gender. Am J Epidemiol. 2012;176(2):117–26.
65. Langrish JP, Li X, Wang S, et al. Reducing personal exposure to particulate air pollution improves cardiovascular health in patients with coronary heart disease. Environ Health Perspect. 2012;120(3):367–72.
66. Sun Y, Song X, Han Y, et al. Size-fractioned ultrafine particles and black carbon associated with autonomic dysfunction in subjects with diabetes or impaired glucose tolerance in Shanghai, China. Part Fibre Toxicol. 2015;12:8.
67. Baja ES, Schwartz JD, Wellenius GA, et al. Traffic-related air pollution and QT interval: modification by diabetes, obesity, and oxidative stress gene polymorphisms in the normative aging study. Environ Health Perspect. 2010;118(6):840–6.
68. Morita H, Wu J, Zipes DP. The QT syndromes: long and short. Lancet (London, England). 2008;372(9640):750–63.
69. Xu H, Chen J, Zhao Q, et al. Ambient air pollution is associated with cardiac repolarization abnormalities in healthy adults. Environ Res. 2019;171:239–46.
70. Huang W, Wang L, Li J, et al. Short-term blood pressure responses to ambient fine particulate matter exposures at the extremes of global air pollution concentrations. Am J Hypertens. 2018;31(5):590–9.
71. Brook RD, Sun Z, Brook JR, et al. Extreme air pollution conditions adversely affect blood pressure and insulin resistance: the air pollution and cardiometabolic disease study. Hypertension. 2016;67(1):77–85.
72. Liu S, Brook RD, Huang W, et al. Extreme levels of ambient air pollution adversely impact cardiac and central aortic hemodynamics: the AIRCMD-China study. J Am Soc Hypertens. 2017;11(11):754–761.e753.
73. Martens DS, Nawrot TS. Air pollution stress and the aging phenotype: the telomere connection. Curr Environ Health Rep. 2016;3(3):258–69.
74. Rider CF, Carlsten C. Air pollution and DNA methylation: effects of exposure in humans. Clin Epigenetics. 2019;11(1):131.
75. Baccarelli A, Wright RO, Bollati V, et al. Rapid DNA methylation changes after exposure to traffic particles. Am J Respir Crit Care Med. 2009;179(7):572–8.
76. Bind MA, Lepeule J, Zanobetti A, et al. Air pollution and gene-specific methylation in the Normative Aging Study: association, effect modification, and mediation analysis. Epigenetics. 2014;9(3):448–58.
77. Rabinovitch N, Jones MJ, Gladish N, et al. Methylation of cysteinyl leukotriene receptor 1 genes associates with lung function in asthmatics exposed to traffic-related air pollution. Epigenetics. 2021;16(2):177–85.
78. Sasaki F, Yokomizo T. The leukotriene receptors as therapeutic targets of inflammatory diseases. Int Immunol. 2019;31(9):607–15.
79. Bellavia A, Urch B, Speck M, et al. DNA hypomethylation, ambient particulate matter, and increased blood pressure: findings from controlled human exposure experiments. J Am Heart Assoc. 2013;2(3):e000212.
80. Chen R, Meng X, Zhao A, et al. DNA hypomethylation and its mediation in the effects of fine particulate air pollution on cardiovascular biomarkers: a randomized crossover trial. Environ Int. 2016;94:614–9.
81. Dockery DW, Pope CA 3rd, Xu X, et al. An association between air pollution and mortality in six U.S. cities. N Engl J Med. 1993;329(24):1753–9.
82. Pope CA 3rd, Thun MJ, Namboodiri MM, et al. Particulate air pollution as a predictor of mortality in a prospective study of U.S. adults. Am J Respir Crit Care Med. 1995;151(3 Pt 1):669–74.
83. Laden F, Hart JE, Smith TJ, Davis ME, Garshick E. Cause-specific mortality in the unionized U.S. trucking industry. Environ Health Perspect. 2007;115(8):1192–6.

84. Beeson WL, Abbey DE, Knutsen SF. Long-term concentrations of ambient air pollutants and incident lung cancer in California adults: results from the AHSMOG study. Adventist Health Study on Smog. Environ Health Perspect. 1998;106(12):813–22.
85. Raaschou-Nielsen O, Andersen ZJ, Beelen R, et al. Air pollution and lung cancer incidence in 17 European cohorts: prospective analyses from the European Study of Cohorts for Air Pollution Effects (ESCAPE). Lancet Oncol. 2013;14(9):813–22.
86. Beelen R, Raaschou-Nielsen O, Stafoggia M, et al. Effects of long-term exposure to air pollution on natural-cause mortality: an analysis of 22 European cohorts within the multicentre ESCAPE project. Lancet. 2014;383(9919):785–95.
87. Thurston GD, Ahn J, Cromar KR, et al. Ambient particulate matter air pollution exposure and mortality in the NIH-AARP diet and health cohort. Environ Health Perspect. 2016;124(4):484–90.
88. Hamra GB, Guha N, Cohen A, et al. Outdoor particulate matter exposure and lung cancer: a systematic review and meta-analysis. Environ Health Perspect. 2014;122(9):906–11.
89. Su TC, Hwang JJ, Shen YC, Chan CC. Carotid intima-media thickness and long-term exposure to traffic-related air pollution in middle-aged residents of Taiwan: a cross-sectional study. Environ Health Perspect. 2015;123(8):773–8.
90. Wang M, Hou ZH, Xu H, et al. Association of estimated long-term exposure to air pollution and traffic proximity with a marker for coronary atherosclerosis in a nationwide study in China. JAMA Netw Open. 2019;2(6):e196553.
91. Gepner AD, Young R, Delaney JA, et al. Comparison of coronary artery calcium presence, carotid plaque presence, and carotid intima-media thickness for cardiovascular disease prediction in the multi-ethnic study of atherosclerosis. Circ Cardiovasc Imaging. 2015;8(1)
92. Qiu H, Schooling CM, Sun S, et al. Long-term exposure to fine particulate matter air pollution and type 2 diabetes mellitus in elderly: a cohort study in Hong Kong. Environ Int. 2018;113:350–6.
93. Lepeule J, Laden F, Dockery D, Schwartz J. Chronic exposure to fine particles and mortality: an extended follow-up of the Harvard Six Cities study from 1974 to 2009. Environ Health Perspect. 2012;120(7):965–70.
94. Pope CA, 3rd, Burnett RT, Thun MJ, et al. Lung cancer, cardiopulmonary mortality, and long-term exposure to fine particulate air pollution. JAMA. 2002;287(9):1132–41.
95. Pope CA, 3rd, Lefler JS, Ezzati M, et al. Mortality Risk and Fine Particulate Air Pollution in a Large, Representative Cohort of U.S. Adults. Environ Health Perspect. 2019;127(7):77007.
96. Hart JE, Garshick E, Dockery DW, Smith TJ, Ryan L, Laden F. Long-term ambient multipollutant exposures and mortality. Am J Respir Crit Care Med. 2011;183(1):73–78.
97. Cao J, Yang C, Li J, et al. Association between long-term exposure to outdoor air pollution and mortality in China: a cohort study. J Hazard Mater. 2011;186(2–3):1594–600.
98. Hystad P, Demers PA, Johnson KC, Carpiano RM, Brauer M. Long-term residential exposure to air pollution and lung cancer risk. Epidemiology. 2013;24(5):762–72.
99. Jerrett M, Burnett RT, Beckerman BS, et al. Spatial analysis of air pollution and mortality in California. Am J Respir Crit Care Med. 2013;188(5):593–99.
100. Krewski D, Jerrett M, Burnett RT, et al. Extended follow-up and spatial analysis of the american cancer society study linking particulate air pollution and mortality. Research report. 2009(140):5–114; discussion 115–36.
101. Lipsett MJ, Ostro BD, Reynolds P, et al. Long-term exposure to air pollution and cardiorespiratory disease in the California teachers study cohort. Am J Respir Crit Care Med. 2011;184(7):828–35.
102. McDonnell WF, Nishino-Ishikawa N, Petersen FF, Chen LH, Abbey DE. Relationships of mortality with the fine and coarse fractions of long-term ambient PM_{10} concentrations in nonsmokers. J Expo Anal Environ Epidemiol. 2000;10(5):427–36.
103. Beelen R, Hoek G, van den Brandt PA, et al. Long-term exposure to traffic-related air pollution and lung cancer risk. Epidemiology. 2008;19(5):702–10.
104. Carey IM, Atkinson RW, Kent AJ, van Staa T, Cook DG, Anderson HR. Mortality associations with long-term exposure to outdoor air pollution in a national English cohort. Am J Respir Crit Care Med. 2013;187(11):1226–33.
105. Cesaroni G, Badaloni C, Gariazzo C, et al. Long-term exposure to urban air pollution and mortality in a cohort of more than a million adults in Rome. Environ Health Perspect. 2013;121(3):324–31.
106. Katanoda K, Sobue T, Satoh H, et al. An association between long-term exposure to ambient air pollution and mortality from lung cancer and respiratory diseases in Japan. J Epidemiol. 2011;21(2):132–43.
107. Hoffmann B, Boogaard H, de Nazelle A, et al. WHO air quality guidelines 2021—aiming for healthier air for all: a joint statement by medical, public health, scientific societies and patient representative organisations. Int J Public Health. 2021;66(88)
108. Chen J, Hoek G. Long-term exposure to PM and all-cause and cause-specific mortality: a systematic review and meta-analysis. Environ Int. 2020;143:105974.